Approach and Observation in
Clinical Dermatology

Approach and Observation in
Clinical Dermatology

Editors

Jigna Padhiyar MD (DVL)
Associate Professor
Department of Dermatology, Venereology and Leprosy (DVL)
Gujarat Cancer Society Medical College, Hospital and
Research Centre (GCSMCH and RC)
Ahmedabad, Gujarat, India

Nayan Patel MD (DVL)
Professor
Department of Dermatology, Venereology and Leprology (DVL)
Gujarat Cancer Society Medical College, Hospital and
Research Centre (GCSMCH and RC)
Ahmedabad, Gujarat, India

Foreword
Deepika Pandhi

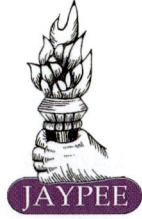

JAYPEE BROTHERS MEDICAL PUBLISHERS
The Health Sciences Publisher
New Delhi | London

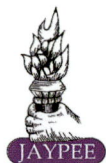 **Jaypee Brothers Medical Publishers (P) Ltd**

Headquarters
EMCA House
23/23-B, Ansari Road, Daryaganj
New Delhi 110 002, India
Landline: +91-11-23272143, +91-11-23272703
+91-11-23282021, +91-11-23245672
E-mail: jaypee@jaypeebrothers.com

Corporate Office
Jaypee Brothers Medical Publishers (P) Ltd.
4838/24, Ansari Road, Daryaganj
New Delhi 110 002, India
Phone: +91-11-43574357
Fax: +91-11-43574314
E-mail: jaypee@jaypeebrothers.com

Overseas Office
JP Medical Ltd.
83, Victoria Street, London
SW1H 0HW (UK)
Phone: +44-20 3170 8910
Fax: +44(0)20 3008 6180
E-mail: info@jpmedpub.com

Website: www.jaypeebrothers.com
Website: www.jaypeedigital.com

© 2023, Jaypee Brothers Medical Publishers

The views and opinions expressed in this book are solely those of the original contributor(s)/author(s) and do not necessarily represent those of editor(s) or publisher of the book.

All rights reserved by the author. No part of this publication may be reproduced, stored or transmitted in any form or by any means, electronic, mechanical, photocopying, recording or otherwise, without the prior permission in writing of the publishers.

All brand names and product names used in this book are trade names, service marks, trademarks or registered trademarks of their respective owners. The publisher is not associated with any product or vendor mentioned in this book.

Medical knowledge and practice change constantly. This book is designed to provide accurate, authoritative information about the subject matter in question. However, readers are advised to check the most current information available on procedures included and check information from the manufacturer of each product to be administered, to verify the recommended dose, formula, method and duration of administration, adverse effects and contraindications. It is the responsibility of the practitioner to take all appropriate safety precautions. Neither the publisher nor the author(s)/editor(s) assume any liability for any injury and/or damage to persons or property arising from or related to use of material in this book.

This book is sold on the understanding that the publisher is not engaged in providing professional medical services. If such advice or services are required, the services of a competent medical professional should be sought.

Every effort has been made where necessary to contact holders of copyright to obtain permission to reproduce copyright material. If any have been inadvertently overlooked, the publisher will be pleased to make the necessary arrangements at the first opportunity.

Inquiries for bulk sales may be solicited at: jaypee@jaypeebrothers.com

Approach and Observation in Clinical Dermatology / Jigna Padhiyar, Nayan Patel

First Edition: **2023**

ISBN: 978-93-5696-083-1

Printed at: Samrat Offset Pvt. Ltd.

Dedication

*To my children and postgraduate students,
for whom I always like to emphasize importance of reading and observations.*
—Jigna Padhiyar

*To my parents for their blessings, my family for love.
Above all to my patients from whom I learn the science of dermatology.*
—Nayan Patel

Contributors

EDITORS

Jigna Padhiyar MD (DVL)
Associate Professor
Department of Dermatology, Venereology and Leprosy (DVL)
Gujarat Cancer Society Medical College, Hospital and Research Centre (GCSMCH and RC)
Ahmedabad, Gujarat, India

Nayan Patel MD (DVL)
Professor
Department of Dermatology, Venereology and Leprology (DVL)
Gujarat Cancer Society Medical College, Hospital and Research Centre (GCSMCH and RC)
Ahmedabad, Gujarat, India

CONTRIBUTING AUTHORS

Akash Kumar Shah MBBS MD (DVL) DNB (DVL)
Senior Resident
Department of Dermatology
Mata Gujri Memorial Medical College
Kishanganj, Bihar, India

Amita Himanshu Sutaria MBBS DVD MD (Dermatology)
Associate Professor
Department of Dermatology, Venereology and Leprosy (DVL)
BJ Medical College
Ahmedabad, Gujarat, India

Amit Mistry MD (DVL)
Professor and Head
Department of Dermatology, Venereology and Leprosy (DVL)
Dharmsinh Desai University
Nadiad, Gujarat, India

Ashish Jagati MD (DVL)
Associate Professor
Department of Dermatology
Smt NHL Medical College and SCL Hospital
Ahmedabad, Gujarat, India

Ashka Shah MD (DVL)
Private Practitioner
Surat, Gujarat, India

Avanitaben Dipakkumar Solanki MBBS MD (DVL)
Professor
Department of Dermatology
Narendra Modi Medical College
Ahmedabad, Gujarat, India

Bhavin Ashokbhai Shah MD (Internal Medicine) DM (Medical Oncology)
Director and Consultant
Hemato-oncologist
Hemato-oncology Clinic
Vedanta and Sterling Hospital
Ahmedabad, Gujarat, India

Bhumesh Kumar Katakam MD (DVL) MD (Pediatrics)
Pediatric Dermatologist
Associate Professor and Head
Department of Dermatology, Venereology and Leprosy (DVL)
GMC/GGH, SRPT
Telangana, India

Bhushan Madke MBBS MD
Professor and Head
Department of Dermatology, Venereology and Leprosy (DVL)
Jawaharlal Nehru Medical College
Datta Meghe Institute of Higher Education and Research
(Deemed to be University)
Nagpur, Maharashtra, India

Chirag Ashwin Desai MBBS DDVL
Fellowship in Diagnostic Dermatology (MUHS)
Fellowship in Dermatopathology (Germany)
Consultant Dermatologist
Divya Sparsh Skin and Hair Clinic
Mumbai, Maharashtra, India

Deblina Bhunia MBBS MD (DVL)
Associate Professor
Department of Dermatology
Mata Gujri Memorial Medical College
Kishanganj, Bihar, India

Feroze Kaliyadan MD DNB MNAMS
Dip EBDV SCE-RCP FRCP (London)
Professor, Department of Dermatology, Venereology and Leprosy (DVL)
Sree Narayana Institute of Medical Sciences
Kerala, Thiruvananthapuram, India

Halak J Vasavada MD (Pediatrics)
Professor (HG)
Department of Pediatrics
NHL Medical College
Ahmedabad, Gujarat, India

Ishan Asutosh Pandya MBBS MD (DVL) MSc (Psychology) PG Diploma in Clinical Hypnosis
Consultant Dermatologist and Psychologist
Lumos Skinic
Ahmedabad, Gujarat, India

Jagadish P MBBS DDVL (Dermatology)
Founder, Director and Chief Dermatologist,
CutiCare (Centre for Skin, Hair and Cosmetology)
Bengaluru, Karnataka, India

Jeta Y Buch MD (DVL)
Consultant Dermatologist and Hair Transplant Surgeon
Ahemadabad, Gujarat, India

Jigna Padhiyar MD (DVL)
Associate Professor
Department of Dermatology, Venereology and Leprosy (DVL)
Gujarat Cancer Society Medical College, Hospital and Research Centre (GCSMCH and RC)
Ahmedabad, Gujarat, India

Kalgi Baxi Majmundar MD DNB (DVL)
Assistant Professor
Department of Dermatology
Smt NHL Medical college and SVP Hospital
Ahmedabad, Gujarat, India

Khushbu R Modi MD
Assistant Professor
Department of Dermatology
LG Hospital
Narendra Modi Medical College
Ahmedabad, Gujarat, India

Kirankumar Madhusudan Solanki MBBS
Junior Resident
Department of Dermatology, Venereology and Leprosy (DVL)
BJ Medical College
Ahmedabad, Gujarat, India

Kiruthika Subburaj MD (DVL)
Senior Resident
Department of Dermatology, Venereology and Leprology (DVL)
Postgraduate Institute of Medical Education and Research
Chandigarh, India

Krina Bharat Patel MD DV&D
Professor and Head
Department of Dermatology
GMERS Medical College Sola
Ahmedabad, Gujarat, India

Krishna Vivek Dave MD (DVL)
Consultant Dermatologist
Ahmedabad, Gujarat, India

Lalit Kumar Gupta MBBS MD (DVL)
Senior Professor and Head
Department of Dermatology, Venereology and Leprosy (DVL)
Ravindra Nath Tagore Medical College
Udaipur, Rajasthan, India

Manisha Balai MBBS MD (DVL)
Assistant Professor
Department of Dermatology, Venereology and Leprosy (DVL)
Ravindra Nath Tagore Medical College
Udaipur, Rajasthan, India

Nainesh P Bhatt MD (Skin, VD)
Consultant Dermatologist
Om Skincare Clinic
Surat, Gujarat, India

Nandita Krishnagopal Patel MBBS MD (DVL)
Consultant
Kira Multispeciality Hospital
Surat, Gujarat, India

Nayan Patel MD (DVL)
Professor
Department of Dermatology, Venereology and Leprology (DVL)
Gujarat Cancer Society Medical College, Hospital and Research Centre (GCSMCH and RC)
Ahmedabad, Gujarat, India

Neela M Patel MD DVD
Professor and Head
Department of Dermatology
LG Hospital
Narendra Modi Medical College
Ahmedabad, Gujarat, India

Neha Sharma MD (DVL)
Consultant Dermatologist
Ahmedabad, Gujarat, India

Nishi Trivedi MBBS MD (DVL)
Consultant Dermatologist
Ahmedabad, Gujarat, India

Nita Radhakrishnan MD (Pediatrics)
Associate Professor and Head
Department of Pediatric Hematology Oncology
Super Speciality Paediatric Hospital and Post Graduate Teaching Institute
Noida, Uttar Pradesh, India

Pooja Agarwal MBBS MD (DVL) Gold Medallist
Associate Professor
Department of Dermatology, Venereology and Leprosy (DVL)
Sardar Vallabhbhai Patel Institute of Medical Science and Research
Smt NHL Municipal Medical College
Ahmedabad, Gujarat, India

Pragya Nair MD (Dermatology and Venereology)
Professor and Head
Department of Dermatology, Venereology and Leprosy (DVL)
Pramukhswami Medical College
Karamsad, Gujarat, India

Pratik R Agarwal MD (Dermatology and Venereology)
Consultant Dermatologist
Dermatologie Klinik, Suit 206-208,
Dev Red Square, Anand Bhalej Road
Anand, Gujarat, India

Puravoor Jayasree MD DNB
Consultant Dermatologist
Medical Trust Hospital
Kochi, Kerala, India

Rahul Mahajan MBBS MD MNAMS
FRCP (Edinburgh)
Associate Professor
Department of Dermatology,
Venereology and Leprology (DVL)
Postgraduate Institute of Medical
Education and Research
Chandigarh, India

Ranjan Raval MBBS MD DVD (Skin)
Professor and Head
Department of Dermatology
Gujarat Cancer Society Medical College,
Hospital and Research Centre
(GCSMCH and RC)
Ahmedabad, Gujarat, India

Ravi Ranjan MBBS MD (DVL)
Assistant Professor
Department of Dermatology,
Venereology and Leprosy (DVL)
Mata Gujri Memorial Medical College
Kishanganj, Bihar, India

Sabha Neazee MBBS MD (DVL)
Senior Resident
Department of Dermatology,
Venereology and Leprosy (DVL)
Shalinitai Meghe Hospital and Research
Hospital, Datta Meghe Medical College
Nagpur, Maharashtra, India

Sejal Hitesh Thakkar MD (DVL) PGDCAH
Professor and Head
Department of Dermatology,
Venereology and Leprosy (DVL)
Medical College Baroda
Vadodara, Gujarat, India

Shravya Rimmalapudi MBBS MD
Assistant Professor
Department of Dermatology,
Venereology and Leprosy (DVL)
Jawaharlal Nehru Medical College
Datta Meghe Institute of Higher
Education and Research
(Deemed to be University)
Nagpur, Maharashtra, India

Smita Nagpal MD (Skin and VD)
Consultant Dermatologist
Anya Skin Clinic
Ahmedabad, Gujarat, India

Sujata Mehta Ambalal MD
Founder and Director
Skin and Hair Research and Education
Initiative (SHREI)
Ahmedabad, Gujarat, India

Vidya Kuntoji MBBS MD (Dermatology)
FRGUHS (Aesthetic Dermatology)
Founder and Consultant Dermatologist
Skinomy Dermatology and Aesthetic
Clinic
Bengaluru, Karnataka, India

Yogesh U Patel MD (Dermatology)
PhD (Dermatology)
Associate Professor
Department of Dermatology
Government Medical College
Surat, Gujarat, India

Foreword

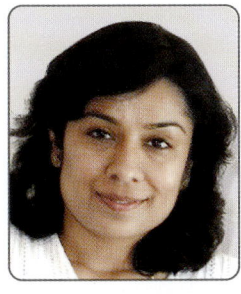

Deepika Pandhi MD FAMS
Director and Professor
Department of Dermatology and STD
University College of Medical Sciences and Guru Teg Bahadur Hospital
New Delhi, India

The specialty of dermatology has evolved tremendously over the years with several new entities being described and a steady rise in the possible management interventions. It has become a challenge to keep abreast with the evolving diagnostic and therapeutic scenario.

Michael Bierut rightly said that "The problem contains the solution" and it is imperative to solve the diagnostic conundrum through a simplified and logical approach. The title *"Approach and Observation in Clinical Dermatology"* is an innovative attempt toward this end, as it presents a succinct, analytic approach to management of common dermatological diseases with an emphasis on clinical presentation and the symptomatology. The editors Dr Jigna Padhiyar and Dr Nayan Patel, are to be commended for envisioning this textbook with its unique approach and have done a stupendous job, including very relevant, 32 chapters covering the—approach to patients with purpura, targetoid lesions, fever with rash, panniculitis, annular lesions, facial melanosis; pediatric patients with primary immunodeficiency, genital lesions, erythroderma; disorders of nail and hair such as trachyonychia, diffuse hair loss, premature canities, cicatricial alopecia, and patients with involvement of specific sites such as oral ulcers, vulval pruritus, vaginal discharge, and indurated lesions on the face. The sections on special considerations in dermatology—a patient with recalcitrant dermatophytosis and systemic steroids in patients with comorbidities would be specifically very useful to the practitioner and postgraduates. The latter would also find the section on Observations in dermatology: Signs, facies, and phenomena in dermatology: cutaneous signs, hair, nail and mucosal in dermatology; facies and phenomenon in dermatology and pattern and named signs in dermoscopy and dermatopathology to be a great help in their preparation for their formative and summative evaluations. The book follows a simplified descriptive approach, embodying the tenets taught to us as medical students that nothing can replace a good history and examination and it includes the clinical presentation, key points for possible differential diagnoses, the diagnostic approach and therapy, and provides practical tips and pointers. It is well illustrated with tables, flow diagrams, and images for greater comprehension, and the inclusion of a summary of the salient points in a table provides the reader with a ready reckoner at a glance, that will be God sent for the practitioner in a busy clinic.

An innovative approach to dermatological disease management can be a huge challenge and has been made possible in this book only due to the inclusion of resource people who are experts in their respective field of contribution. The authors of these chapters must be hugely complemented for their tremendous work. I congratulate the editors and all the authors involved in this project and wish this title serves as a timely aid for the practitioners on how to approach management of common dermatological cases and also as a handy tool for postgraduates to brush up their knowledge with key points provided liberally in this textbook.

As Uri Levine said, "Fall in love with the problem, not the solution," so this book encourages us to analyse the clinical presentation. I sign off with my best wishes for the grand success of this book that breaks the stereotypical fixation on finding the magic solution!

Preface

Dermatology is a science of visual impact on a clinician's mind. In dermatology, we have luxury to see most lesions with our eyes. As the famous saying goes "eyes see what your mind knows", ability of seeing and examining skin lesions with our eyes and a keen mind helps us to diagnose a patient. The art of deductive reasoning to arrive at a conclusive diagnosis has always fascinated us. Clinical dermatology is the subject which has always been nearer to our heart. *"Approach and Observation in Clinical Dermatology"* has been planned with purpose of helping clinician and postgraduate students with the art of differential diagnosis in dermatology. It is always helpful to arrive at a conclusive differential diagnosis before advising a battery of laboratory tests to a patient. This standard protocol has been taught to us since ages as the art of history taking by our teachers.

Postgraduate students are frequently asked a theory question about "How to approach a patient with particular symptoms/lesions?". There are lot of many dermatology books to describe findings of a particular disease. But a patient does not present to us with a readymade diagnosis. They usually present to us with a particular symptom or a lesion. From here we need to ask few history points, observe and examine the patient in relevance to their presentations and need to put relevant differential diagnosis to advise tests to aid our clinical judgment. Hopefully, our plan of symptom or lesion-based approach and art of observatory skills will help clinicians as well as students with the differential diagnosis they should be looking at. We think that this book will aid in clinical judgments regarding diagnostics in dermatology.

This book has been focused on various common symptoms or lesions. Efforts have been made to compile few observations specific to the field of dermatology.

Jigna Padhiyar
Nayan Patel

Acknowledgments and Disclaimer

We thank all the contributors/authors who readily agreed to our requests and work hard to put their vast experience and knowledge in a concise manner as a chapter.

We are thankful to the M/s Jaypee Brothers Medical Publishers (P) Ltd, New Delhi, India, for having faith in our work. Our special thanks to Shri Jitender P Vij (Group Chairman), Mr Ankit Vij (Managing Director), Mr MS Mani (Group President), Ms Chetna Malhotra (Senior Director – Professional Publishing, Marketing & Business Development), Ms Pooja Bhandari (Production Head) and a note of thanks to Ms Himani Pandey (Development Editor) who managed the project well.

Last but not least, we are thankful to all our patients from whom we have learned and progressed so far in field of Dermatology, Venereology and Leprosy.

Disclaimer:
All the authors agree that they have obtained adequate informed consent to publish the images of a patient in this book.

Contents

SECTION 1: Approach in Dermatology

Part 1: General

1. **Fever with Rash in an Adult Patient** — 3
   Amita Himanshu Sutaria, Kirankumar Madhusudan Solanki

2. **A Patient with Purpura** — 11
   Nayan Patel, Bhavin Ashokbhai Shah

   Approach to a Patient with Palpable Purpura 11
   Nayan Patel

   Approach to a Patient with Nonpalpable Purpura 26
   Bhavin Ashokbhai Shah

3. **A Patient with Target or Targetoid Lesions** — 34
   Jigna Padhiyar

4. **A Patient with Suspected Cutaneous Adverse Drug Reaction: Practice Tips** — 46
   Lalit Kumar Gupta, Manisha Balai

5. **A Patient with Generalized Pruritus without Skin Lesions** — 58
   Avanitaben Dipakkumar Solanki, Ishan Asutosh Pandya

6. **A Patient with Annular Skin Lesions** — 74
   Sejal Hitesh Thakkar, Ashka Shah

7. **A Suspected Case of Panniculitis** — 91
   Feroze Kaliyadan, Puravoor Jayasree

8. **A Patient of Facial Melanosis** — 105
   Chirag Ashwin Desai, Nandita Krishnagopal Patel

   Part 1: A Patient of Facial Hypermelanosis 105

   Part 2: A Patient with Facial Hypomelanosis 116

Part 2: Disorders of Nail and Hair

9. **Trachyonychia** — 125
   Shravya Rimmalapudi, Bhushan Madke

10. **A Case of Hirsutism** — 132
    Vidya Kuntoji, Jagadish P

11.	**A Patient with Diffuse Hair Loss** *Smita Nagpal, Neha Sharma*	**141**
12.	**A Patient with Cicatricial Alopecia** *Ranjan Raval, Nishi Trivedi*	**150**
13.	**A Patient with Premature Graying of Hair** *Sujata Mehta Ambalal*	**164**

Part 3: Involvement of Specific Site

14.	**A Patient with Leg Ulcer** *Nainesh P Bhatt, Yogesh U Patel*	**173**
15.	**A Patient with Chronic and Recurrent Oral Ulcers or Erosions** *Jigna Padhiyar*	**181**
16.	**A Patient with Hyperkeratotic Lesions on Palm and/or Sole** *Deblina Bhunia, Ravi Ranjan*	**192**
17.	**A Case of Indurated Facial Plaque** *Kiruthika Subburaj, Rahul Mahajan*	**202**
18.	**A Female with Chronic and Recurrent Vaginal Discharge** *Neela M Patel, Khushbu R Modi*	**222**
19.	**A Female Patient with Vulvar Pruritus** *Neela M Patel, Khushbu R Modi*	**235**

Part 4: Pediatric Dermatology

20.	**A Child with Genital Lesions** *Kalgi Baxi Majmundar, Ashish Jagati*	**247**
21.	**Approach to a Child with Erythroderma** *Jeta Y Buch, Halak J Vasavada*	**278**
22.	**A Child with Fever and Rash** *Sabha Neazee, Pooja Agarwal*	**296**
23.	**A Child with Photosensitivity** *Amit Mistry, Krishna Vivek Dave*	**306**
24.	**A Child with Suspected Primary Immunodeficiency: A Dermatologist's Perspective** *Bhumesh Kumar Katakam, Nita Radhakrishnan*	**315**

Part 5: Special Considerations in Dermatology

25.	**Systemic Steroid in Patient with Comorbidities** *Nayan Patel*	**324**
26.	**A Patient with Recalcitrant Dermatophytosis** *Pratik R Agarwal, Pragya Nair*	**337**

SECTION 2: Observations in Dermatology: Signs, Faces and Phenomena in Dermatology

27. Cutaneous Signs in Dermatology — 367
Vidya Kuntoji

28. Hair, Nail, and Mucosal Signs and Appearance in Dermatology — 392
Akash Kumar Shah

29. Facies in Dermatology — 397
Avanitaben Dipakkumar Solanki, Ishan Asutosh Pandya

30. Phenomenon in Dermatology — 417
Pragya Nair, Pratik R Agarwal

Observable Phenomenon 428

Histopathological Phenomena 435

Laboratory Phenomena 436

Therapeutic Phenomena 438

31. Distinguished Appearance or Pattern and Named Signs in Dermoscopy — 443
Jigna Padhiyar

32. Named Appearance, Cell, or Sign in Dermatopathology — 447
Jigna Padhiyar, Krina Bharat Patel

Index — 455

SECTION 1

Approach in Dermatology

Part 1: General

1

Fever with Rash in an Adult Patient

Amita Himanshu Sutaria, Kirankumar Madhusudan Solanki

INTRODUCTION

An adult patient presenting with fever and cutaneous rash is quite challenging as the differential diagnoses are very extensive. The clinical presentation is different in each of the cases. A doctor needs to decide the probable diagnoses quickly to start the initial treatment. Morphologically, the rash can present differently in each case. It can be categorized into maculopapular, urticarial, vesiculobullous/vesiculopustular rash, diffuse erythema with desquamation, nodular, and petechial rashes.[1] A detailed history and clinical examination have to be done to come the probable differential diagnoses. However, laboratory tests can be done to confirm the diagnosis. A detailed history should be taken including age, gender, residence, personal history, family history, past medical or surgical history, and specific history about cutaneous rash including the site of onset, order of spread, associated other symptoms, and temporal association between rash and fever. The various differential diagnoses according to the morphological types of rash are tabulated in **Table 1**.

Table 2 enumerates causes of fever with maculopapular rash.

DIAGNOSTIC APPROACH

History taking in case of fever with rash should incorporate detail about characteristic of fever and its temporal association with rash **(Table 3)**.

Table 1: Classification of differential diagnoses of fever with rash according to the type of rash.[1-4]	
Maculopapular rash	<ul><li>Drug-induced maculopapular rash</li><li>Dengue fever</li><li>Coronavirus disease 2019 (COVID-19) viral infection</li><li>Chikungunya fever</li><li>Systemic lupus erythematosus</li><li>Erythema multiforme **(Figs. 1A to C)**</li><li>Secondary syphilis</li><li>Drug reaction with eosinophilia and systemic symptoms</li><li>Infectious mononucleosis</li><li>Rubella</li><li>Measles</li><li>Erythema infectiosum (parvovirus B19 infection)</li><li>Typhoid fever</li><li>Adult-onset Still's disease</li><li>Typhus fever</li><li>Rickettsial spotted fever</li><li>Erythema marginatum</li><li>Lyme disease</li></ul>
Urticarial rash	<ul><li>Infection-induced urticaria (e.g., COVID-19 viral infection)</li><li>Urticarial vasculitis</li><li>Drug-induced urticaria</li></ul>

Continued

Continued

Vesiculobullous/ Vesiculopustular rash	• Varicella virus infection (chickenpox) • Disseminated herpes simplex virus infection • Disseminated herpes zoster infection • Kaposi's varicelliform eruption • Id eruption • Acute generalized exanthematous pustulosis
Diffuse erythema with skin desquamation	• Stevens–Johnson syndrome • Toxic epidermal necrolysis • Drug reaction with eosinophilia and systemic symptoms • Staphylococcal toxic shock syndrome • Streptococcal toxic shock syndrome
Nodular rash	• Erythema nodosum • Erythema induratum • Sweet syndrome (a type of panniculitis) • Kaposi sarcoma • Bacillary angiomatosis
Petechial or purpuric rash	• Purpura fulminans • Necrotizing fasciitis • Henoch–Schönlein purpura (a type of cutaneous vasculitis) • Disseminated intravascular coagulation due to septicemia • Infections such as viral hemorrhagic fever and enteroviral infection • Meningococcal infection

Table 2: Enumerates causes of fever with maculopapular rash.

Viral infections	• Dengue fever • Chikungunya fever • Coronavirus disease 2019 (COVID-19) viral infection • Infectious mononucleosis • Rubella* • Measles* • Erythema infectiosum (parvovirus B19 infection)
Bacterial infections	• Scarlet fever • Secondary syphilis • Typhoid fever • Toxic shock syndrome
Rickettsial infections	• Typhus fever • Rickettsial spotted fever • Lyme disease
Drug induced	• Drug reaction with eosinophilia and systemic symptoms (DRESS) • Erythema multiforme • Drug-induced maculopapular (MP) rash • Acute generalized exanthematous pustulosis (AGEP)
Autoimmune etiology	• Systemic lupus erythematosus • Adult-onset Still's disease

*More common in children.

Evaluation of associated complain of patient may give important clue about underlying etiology. It will also help into evaluation of systemic involvement if any **(Table 4)**.

CHARACTERISTICS AND DISTRIBUTION OF RASH

Evaluation of distribution, characteristic color, and pattern of rash is helpful in differentiating underlying etiology. Though characteristic pattern associated with rashes may not be always present on examination, if present some of them have high specificity for particular etiology which may help in prompt diagnosis and avoidance of unnecessary investigations **(Table 5)**.

DRUG-INDUCED MACULOPAPULAR RASH

Drug-induced maculopapular rash is most commonly reported cutaneous adverse drug reaction. Though few classes of drug are very strongly associated with it like antituberculous drugs, antiepileptics, ART, etc., practically any drug can cause the same. Many a time differentiating drug-induced maculopapular rash from infection-induced exanthema is challenging. Few points in history and examination can help differentiate the both from each other though they are not mutually exclusive (see Chapter 4). Drug induced maculopapular eruption when suspected, it is vitally important to rule out more sever cutaneous adverse drug reactions like drug hypersensitivity and drug reaction with eosinophilia and systemic symptoms (DRESS) from simple drug-induced maculopapular exanthema as former required more aggressive investigations for systemic involvement, immediate withdrawal of drug, and prolong corticosteroid therapy while later can be managed symptomatically with continuation of suspected drug under observation ("carry through" or "treat through" approach).

LABORATORY DIAGNOSIS

A detailed history and clinical examination have to be done initially to come to the probable differential diagnoses. Diascopy test should be done differentiate erythema from

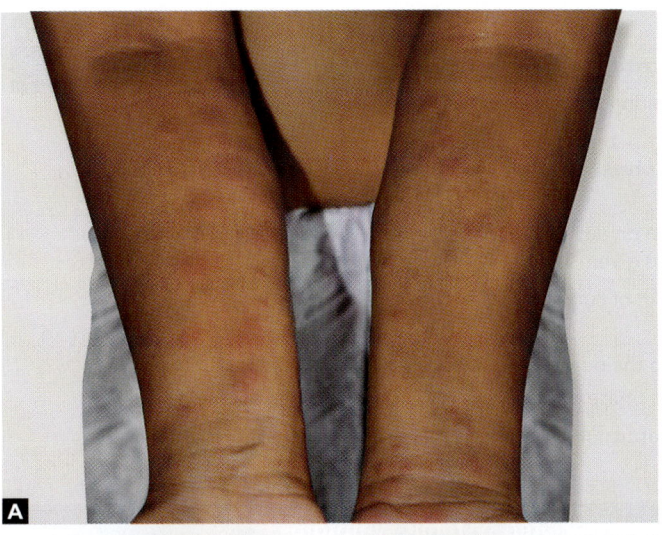
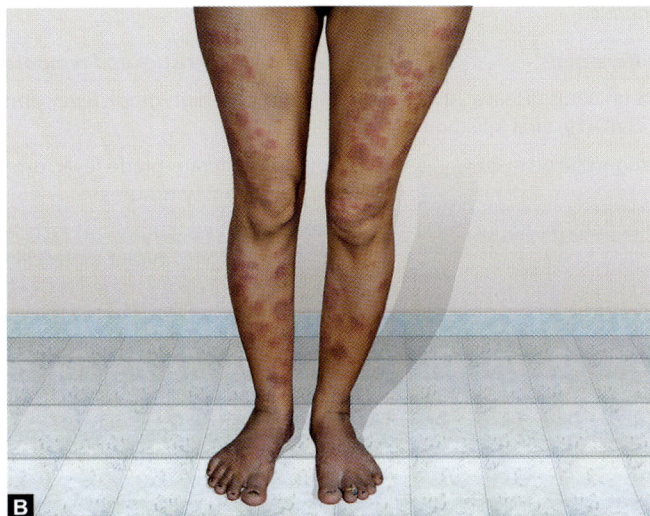
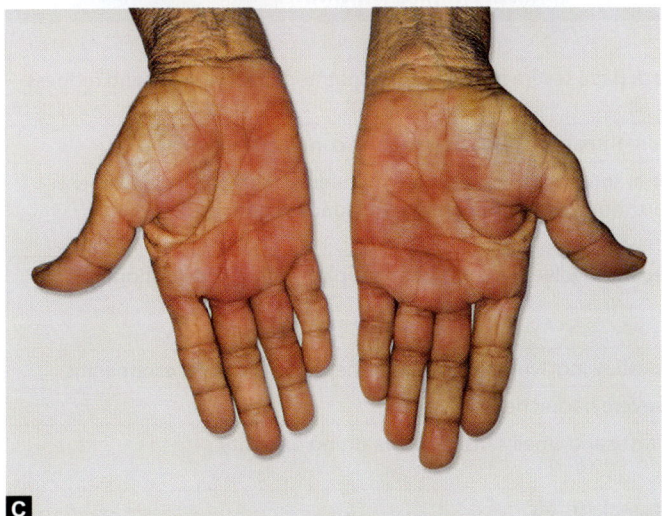

FIGS. 1A TO C: Erythema multiforme minor characteristic targetoid lesions and involvement of palms.

Table 3: Fever characteristics and temporal association between fever and rash.[2,3]	
Differentials	**Fever characteristics and temporal association between fever and rash**
Dengue fever	• Sudden onset high-grade fever, subsides with decrease in viremia usually in 6–7 days • Rash begins on day 3 of fever and persists for 2–3 days
Chikungunya fever	• Sudden onset moderate-to-high-grade fever, occasionally with chills, subsides within 7–10 days, fever may recur after 7–10 days known as "saddle back fever" • Rash begins during the illness or after the fever has subsided
Secondary syphilis	• Low-grade fever, more pronounced at night • Rash can begin earlier or along with the fever
Drug reaction with eosinophilia and systemic symptoms (DRESS)	• Low- to moderate-grade fever, presents along with or after cutaneous rash 2–6 weeks after implicated drug intake • Variable temporal association between fever and rash
Stevens–Johnson syndrome	• Moderate-to-high-grade fever presents along with or after the onset of cutaneous lesions 7–21 days after implicated drug intake • Fever may precede or noticed during the course of cutaneous eruption
Chickenpox	Low-to-moderate-grade fever appearing 2–3 days before the appearance of cutaneous eruption

Continued

Continued

Differentials	Fever characteristics and temporal association between fever and rash
Coronavirus disease 2019 (COVID-19) viral infection	Moderate-to-high-grade fever, appearing few days before the skin rash
Drug-induced rash	Low-to-moderate-grade fever, often presents with or after the skin rash, often associated with constitutional symptoms
Infectious mononucleosis	Low-grade fever, cutaneous rash seen on day 4–6 of the fever in 10% individual which reaches to 95–100% if concomitant amoxicillin is given
Erythema infectiosum (parvovirus B19 infection)	Low-grade fever seen before the onset of cutaneous rash
Measles	• High-grade fever corresponding to the peak of cutaneous rash • Rash starts usually after prodromal phase of 1–7 days
Rubella	Moderate-grade fever with maculopapular rash appears simultaneously with the onset of illness

Table 4: Differentials of fever with maculopapular rash and their associated systemic symptoms.[2,3]

Differentials	Associated systemic features
Dengue fever	Frontal headache, retro-orbital pain, back pain, severe myalgia, adenopathy, palatal vesicles, and redness of eyes
Chikungunya fever	Severe arthralgia, malaise, headache, sore throat, retrobulbar pain, and conjunctival redness
Secondary syphilis	Constitutional symptoms such as malaise, sore throat, headache, lymphadenopathy, eye involvement in the form of uveitis and iridocyclitis, arthritis, bursitis, hepatitis with jaundice, gastritis, and glomerulonephritis
Drug reaction with eosinophilia and systemic symptoms (DRESS)	Yellow discoloration of sclera due to hepatic involvement, lymphadenopathy other constitutional symptoms like malaise, headache, etc.
Stevens–Johnson syndrome	Stinging sensation in eyes, pain while swallowing, lymphadenopathy, hepatitis, diarrhea, esophagitis
Chickenpox	Pruritus, malaise, loss of appetite, and severe backache
Coronavirus disease 2019 (COVID-19) viral infection	Sore throat, myalgia, headache, loss of taste and smell sensation, breathing difficulty
Drug-induced rash	Constitutional symptoms like headache, malaise, etc.
Infectious mononucleosis	• Sore throat, malaise, fatigue, nausea, anorexia without vomiting, palatal petechiae, uvular edema, bilateral transient upper eyelid edema (Hoagland sign) • Triad of fever, pharyngitis and lymphadenopathy
Erythema infectiosum (parvovirus B19 infection)	Severe constitutional symptoms such as sore throat, malaise, joint pain, myalgia, nausea, diarrhea, and erythema may be seen over pharynx
Measles	Running nose, cough, conjunctivitis, malaise, mucosal lesions, Koplik's spot on buccal mucosa against the second molar
Rubella	Sore throat, cough, headache and malaise, cervical and occipital lymphadenopathy, Forchheimer spots (rose pink pinpoint petechiae) on soft palate and uvula, conjunctivitis, and testicular pain

Table 5: Characteristics and distribution of rash.[2,3]

Differentials	Characteristics and distribution of rash
Dengue fever	Generalized erythema, or itchy maculopapular or scarlatiniform rash, starts on the legs and spread to the chest and trunk and spread to the face, arms and legs with areas of sparing known as "White islands in sea of red" **(Fig. 2)**.[2] The rash fades as the fever subsides, but can have a phase with petechiae on the arms and legs due to mild thrombocytopenia
Chikungunya fever	Pruritic maculopapular rash that starts on the trunk, then spread centrifugally to involve palms and soles. Erythema over nose and ears can be seen. Post-illness hyperpigmentation over nose **(Fig. 3)**, cheeks and forehead can be seen

Continued

Continued

Differentials	Characteristics and distribution of rash
Secondary syphilis	Symmetrically distributed, non-itchy, coppery red colored maculopapular **(Figs. 4A and B)** or roseolar rash with scaling known as "papulosquamous syphilide", the cutaneous lesions can be macular or roseolar, papular, papulosquamous, pustular or nodular, predominantly distributed over the flexures and trunk
Drug reaction with eosinophilia and systemic symptoms (DRESS)	Rash begins as a morbilliform eruption **(Figs. 5A and B)**, but may have vesicles, follicular or nonfollicular pustules, erythroderma, and purpuric lesions, initially involves face, upper trunk, with facial edema being a hallmark of DRESS
Stevens–Johnson syndrome	The cutaneous lesions begin as erythematous, dusky red, or purpuric macules, having a tendency to coalesce, followed by vesicles or bullae formation and widespread skin detachment. Skin lesions tend to appear first on the trunk, spreading to the neck, face, proximal upper extremities, and palms and soles sparing distal portions of the arms and legs. Buccal, genital, and ocular mucosal erosions seen in >90% of patients. The skin lesions are tender, and mucosal erosions are painful
Chickenpox	Generalized pruritic rash starting from face and scalp progressing to involve the extremities, begins as macules that become papules followed by vesicles on an erythematous base giving "dew drops on rose petal" appearance. The vesicles turn into pustules and crusts in 2–4 days. Different morphological types of lesions are present at the same time
Coronavirus disease 2019 (COVID-19) viral infection	Urticarial rash, maculopapular rash **(Figs. 6A and B)**, predominantly involving the trunk, purpuric rash, commonly over the extremities, vasculitic lesions and chilblain-like lesions are seen
Drug-induced rash	Maculopapular or diffuse erythematous rash involving, extremities and trunk, face and palms, and soles **(Fig. 7)**
Infectious mononucleosis	Two types of cutaneous rash are seen. First is, a transient maculopapular rash due to direct viral infection seen within 1–2 days of onset of the disease. Second is, after the administration of antibiotics, commonly β-lactam antibiotics **(Fig. 8)**. It is maculopapular eruption, may be pruritic seen over the trunk and the extremities
Erythema infectiosum (parvovirus B19 infection)	• Bright, erythematous macular rash over the cheeks sparing periorbital, perioral, and the nasal bridge area giving "slapped cheek appearance" • The rash on the face gradually fades in 4–5 days and followed by generalized, reticular, occasionally pruritic rash, seen over the trunk and the extensor aspects of the extremities
Measles	Blanchable, erythematous, maculopapular rash that begins behind the ears and anterior hair line, progresses to the neck, trunk and extremities within 2–4 days. The rash fades in the same order and becomes nonblanchable. Fine skin desquamation may be seen
Rubella	The rash begins as light pink-colored macules and papules firstly on the cheeks, followed by retroauricular area and spread caudally to involve trunk and the extremities

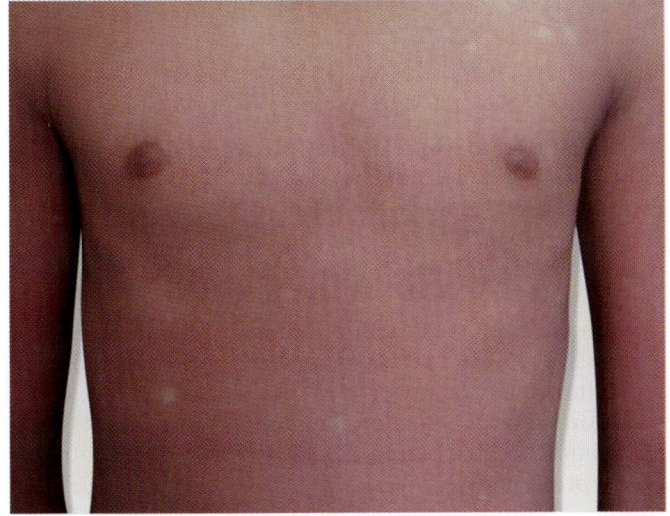

FIG. 2: "White islands in sea of red appearance" in a patient with dengue fever.

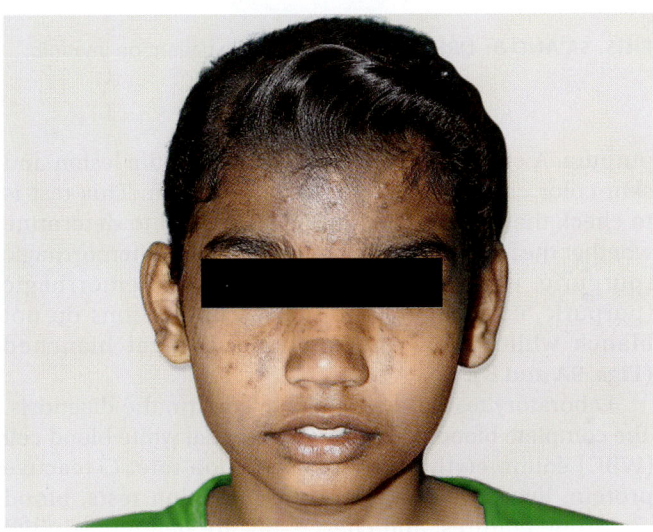

FIG. 3: Post-chikungunya hyperpigmentation over the face.

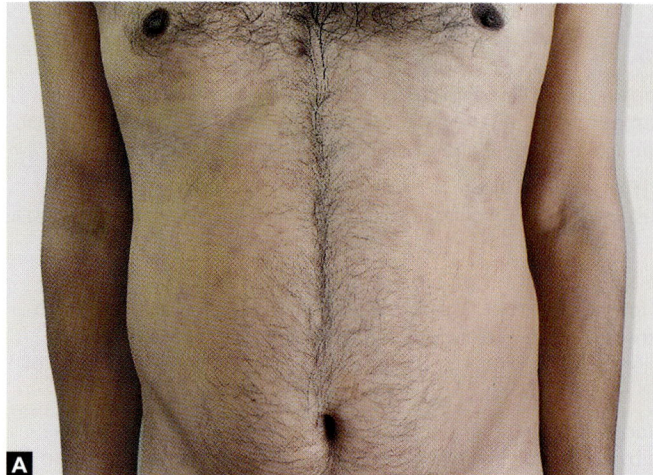
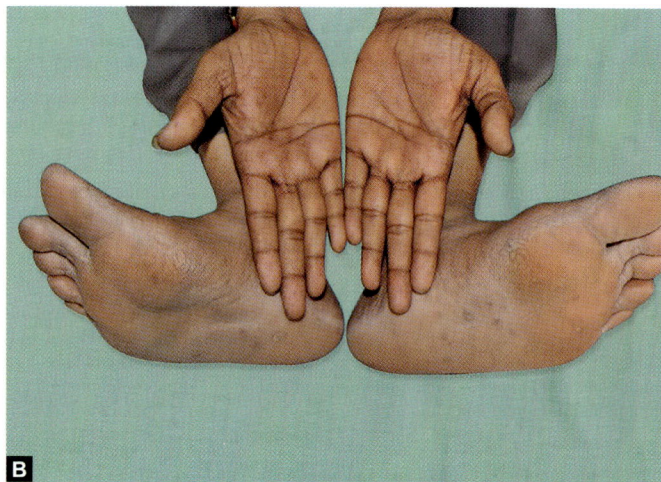

FIGS. 4A AND B: Coppery red colored maculopapular rash in patient of secondary syphilis with involvement of palm and soles.

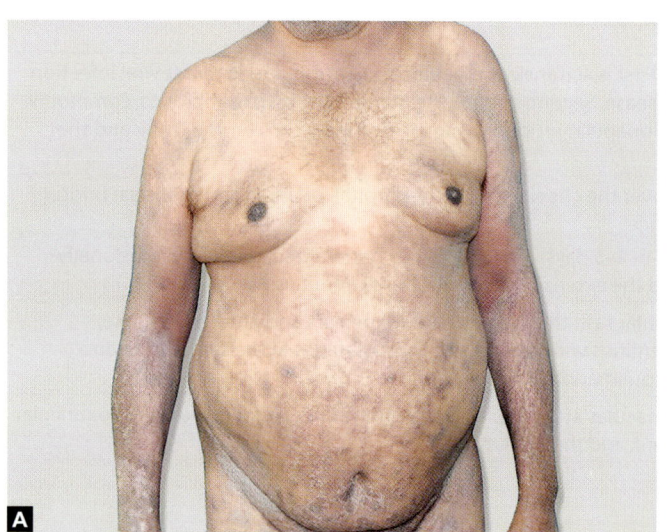
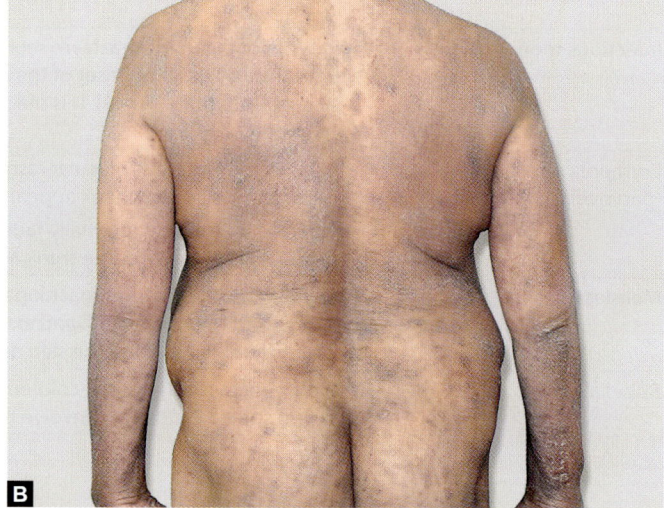

FIGS. 5A AND B: DRESS syndrome in a male patient on imatinib.

purpura. A clear glass slide is pressed upon the lesion and skin color changes over the lesion are seen. This test is to check the blanchability of the lesion and to determine whether the lesion is erythematous (vascular), hemorrhagic (purpuric, ecchymotic), or nonvascular. Hemorrhagic (purpuric, ecchymotic) and nonvascular lesions do not blanch while the erythematous lesions get blanched **(Figs. 9A and B)**.

Laboratory tests are generally to confirm the diagnosis. The complete blood count with differential white blood cell (WBC) count, erythrocyte sedimentation rate, C-reactive protein, liver function tests, renal function tests, blood and urine cultures, and chest X-ray are helpful as initial investigations to come to the probable diagnosis. The common clinical and routine investigation findings **(Table 6)** would guide to the specific tests required.

The serological tests for dengue, chikungunya, syphilis, herpes simplex viral infection, and infectious mononucleosis can be done.

The specific tests include biopsy, slit-skin smear for acid fast bacilli in case of suspected erythema nodosum leprosum, Tzanck smear for herpes virus infection, Gram stain for bacterial infection, antistreptolysin O (ASO) titer for streptococcal infection, C3 levels, antinuclear antibody (ANA) profile for systemic lupus erythematosus, coagulation profile, Mantoux test, and gene expert can be done for

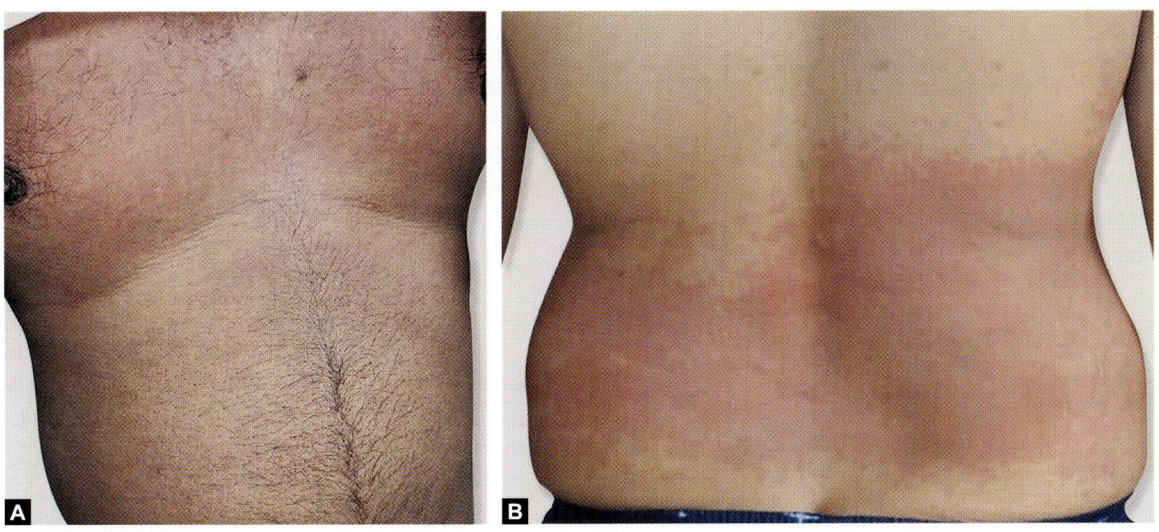
FIGS. 6A AND B: Maculopapular rash in a Coronavirus disease 2019 (COVID-19) patient.

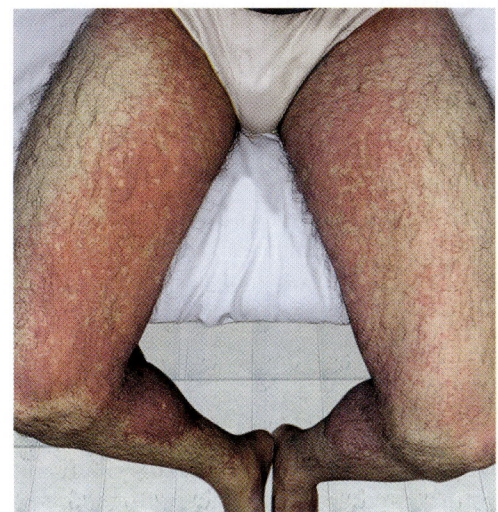
FIG. 7: Drug-induced maculopapular rash.

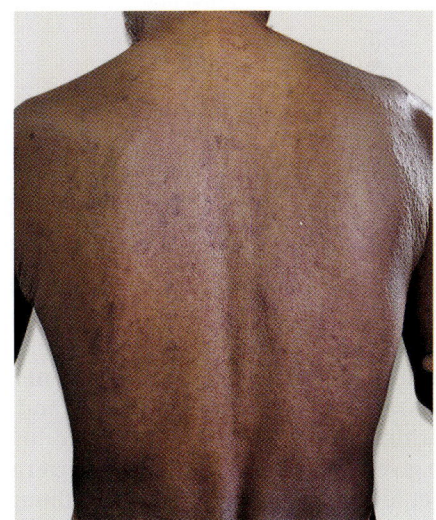
FIG. 8: Ampicillin-induced maculopapular rash.

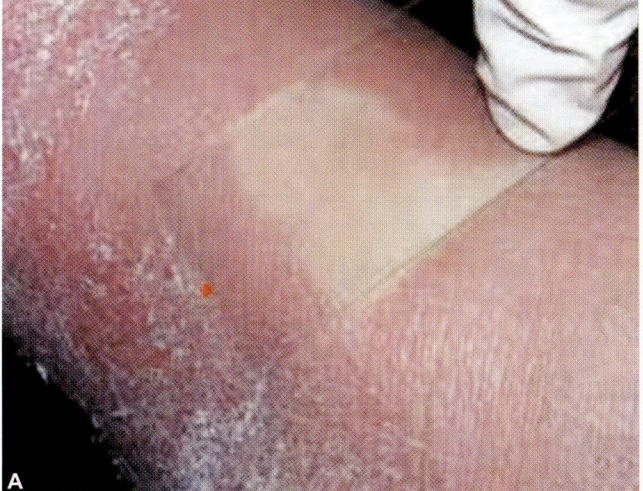
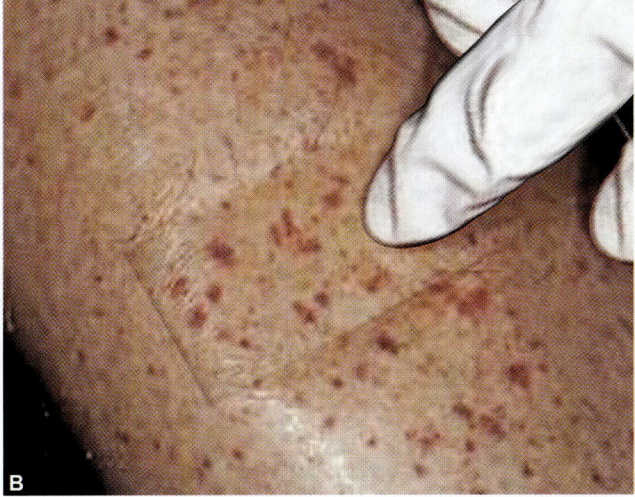
FIGS. 9A AND B: Diascopy test to differentiate erythema (blanchable) from purpura (nonblanchable).

Table 6: Specific clinical and laboratory findings in various differential diagnoses.

Clinical and laboratory finding	Differential diagnosis
Forchheimer's spots on uvula	Rubella
Koplik's spot in oral cavity	Measles
Lymphadenopathy	Secondary syphilis, infectious mononucleosis, rubella, drug reaction with eosinophilia and systemic symptoms (DRESS), Stevens–Johnson syndrome
Leukocytosis with atypical lymphocytes (>10%)	Infectious mononucleosis
Thrombocytopenia	Dengue fever
Eosinophilia	DRESS
Leukopenia	Suggests possibility of viral infections except infectious mononucleosis

Table 7: Specific diagnostic tests for various differential diagnoses.

Disease	Specific tests
Dengue fever	Dengue NS1 antigen test
Chikungunya fever	Chikungunya antibody test
Toxic shock syndrome	Blood culture and sensitivity
Secondary syphilis	• Rapid plasma reagin (RPR) test with titer • Treponema pallidum hemagglutination (TPHA) test
Tuberculosis	Mantoux test and gene expert
Systemic lupus erythematosus (SLE)	Antinuclear antibody (ANA) profile
Bacterial infection	Gram stain
Herpes simplex virus infection	Tzanck smear, herpes simplex virus (HSV), immunoglobulin M (IgM), and IgG antibody test
Erythema nodosum leprosum	Slit-skin smear
Infectious mononucleosis	• Antibody test against Epstein-Barr virus (EBV) antigen • Paul–Bunnell test (screening test)
Coronavirus disease 2019 (COVID-19) infection	COVID RT-PCR test
Parvovirus B19 infection	RTPCR for parvovirus B19, IgM and IgG antibodies against parvovirus B19
Streptococcal infection	Antistreptolysin O (ASO) titer, throat swab for culture

tuberculosis. The specific tests for the suspected diseases are summarized in **Table 7**.

MANAGEMENT APPROACH

Management of maculopapular exanthema will depend on underlying etiology of rash. Most of the time rash per se is self-limiting and only require symptomatic treatment if pruritic. Antihistamine may help to some extent in reducing pruritus so is soothing agent such as calamine and pramoxine hydrochloride in emollient base. Specific antibacterial need to be given for rash if suspected of bacterial in origin (e.g., scarlet fever, toxic shock syndrome) though focus of infection may not be skin. For management of drug-induced maculopapular rash kindly refer to Chapter 4.

In conclusion viral exanthema remains most common cause of fever with rash in adult. Drug-induced maculopapular reaction needs to be always kept in mind while evaluating the case. Most of viral exanthema are self-limiting and unnecessary investigations can be avoided if dermatologist gives enough attention to clues in history, associated complains, and screening investigations.

REFERENCES

1. McKinnon HD Jr, Howard T. Evaluating the febrile patient with a rash. Am Fam Physician. 2000;62(4):804-16.
2. Bolognia JL, Schaffer JV, Cerroni L. Dermatology, 4th editon. London, England: Elsevier Health Sciences; 2017.
3. Griffiths C, Barker J, Bleiker T, Chalmers R, Creamer D (Eds). Rook's Textbook of Dermatology, 9th edition. Hoboken, NJ: Wiley-Blackwell; 2016.
4. Sarkar R, Mishra K, Garg VK. Fever with rash in a child in India. Indian J Dermatol Venereol Leprol. 2012;78(3):251-62.

A Patient with Purpura

Nayan Patel, Bhavin Ashokbhai Shah

For ease of understanding, this chapter is divided in two parts. Section 1 will cover approach to patient with palpable purpura. Section 2 will cover approach to patient with nonpalpable purpura.

APPROACH TO A PATIENT WITH PALPABLE PURPURA

Nayan Patel

INTRODUCTION

Purpura is defined as nonblanchable red or purple spot on the skin resulting from extravasation of red blood cells (RBCs) due to underlying platelet, vascular or coagulation disorders. In clinical practice, very first thing required is to differentiate purpura from nonpurpuric lesions. Traditionally to differentiate purpura from other red- or purple-looking lesion is diascopy done where pressure is applied on lesion using glass slide to differentiate blanchable from nonblanchable lesion. One has to be little cautious here as many lesions of nonvascular origin too can be nonblanchable for papules and plaques of sweet syndrome, cutaneous lymphoma and lymphocytoma cutis, and early lesion of vascular origin that could be blanchable as at the time of examination, sufficient RBCs extravasation may not have occurred. Next step is to differentiate palpable purpura from macular purpura. Palpable purpura is hallmark of vasculitis process whereas macular purpura could be secondary to varied etiology causing red cell extravasation **(Table 1)**.

Table 1 shows possible differential diagnosis according to morphology of purpura.[1]

APPROACH TO A PATIENT WITH PALPABLE PURPURA

Palpable purpura most commonly represents inflammation of small vessels. All intraparenchymal vessels including arteries, arterioles, capillaries, and venules are considered small vessels for classification purpose. Branches of named vessels before entering the parenchyma are considered medium vessels. Small biopsies only contain small vessels for examination so involvement of even largest intraparenchymal arteries in skin biopsies is considered small vessels disease. Medium-size vessels may be involved along with small vessels in some instances such as granulomatosis with polyangiitis (Wegner's granulomatosis) (GPA), microscopic polyangiitis (MPA), eosinophilic granulomatosis with polyangiitis (Churg–Strauss syndrome) (EGPA), and polyarteritis nodosa (PAN).[2] Approach to patient with palpable purpura should be centered around establishing diagnosis, finding possible etiology, establishing possible systemic involvement, and selecting best possible treatment. **Flowchart 1** shows possible causes of small- and medium-vessels vasculitis based on Chapel Hill Consensus Conference on the Nomenclature of Systemic Vasculitides (CHCC, 2012).

Table 1: Differential diagnosis according to morphology of purpura.

Petechia (≤4 mm in size)	Purpuric macules (>1 cm in size)
Due to thrombocytopenia: 1. *Infections*: Dengue, malaria, rickettsia, meningococci, and leptospirosis 2. *Immune mediated*: 　○ Idiopathic thrombocytopenic purpura (ITP) 　○ Thrombotic thrombocytopenic purpura (TTP) 　○ Gestational thrombocytopenia 3. *Neonatal alloimmune thrombocytopenia*: 　○ Drug-induced thrombocytopenia 4. Hemolytic uremic syndrome (HUS) 5. *Due to platelet function defect*: 　• Von Willebrand disease 　• Bernard–Soulier syndrome 　• Glanzmann thrombasthenia 6. *With normal platelets*: 　• Trauma 　• Scurvy (perifollicular pattern) 　• Pigmented purpuric dermatoses (PPDs) 　• Hypergammaglobulinemic purpura (Waldenstrom)	1. *Infections*: 　• DIC due to any cause (purpura fulminans) 　• Sepsis 2. *Coagulation defect*: 　• Anticoagulant therapy 　• Liver failure 　• Vitamin K deficiency 3. *Defect in connective tissue*: 　• Ehlers–Danlos syndrome 　• Actinic purpura 　• Senile purpura 　• Corticosteroid purpura 　• Scurvy 　• Amyloidosis 4. *Other causes*: Gardner–Diamond syndrome
Purpuric macules (5–9 mm): • Early lesions of vasculitis • Hypergammaglobulinemic purpura (Waldenstrom)	*Palpable purpura*: Possible causes include various types of vasculitis **(Flowchart 1)**

(DIC: disseminated intravascular coagulation)

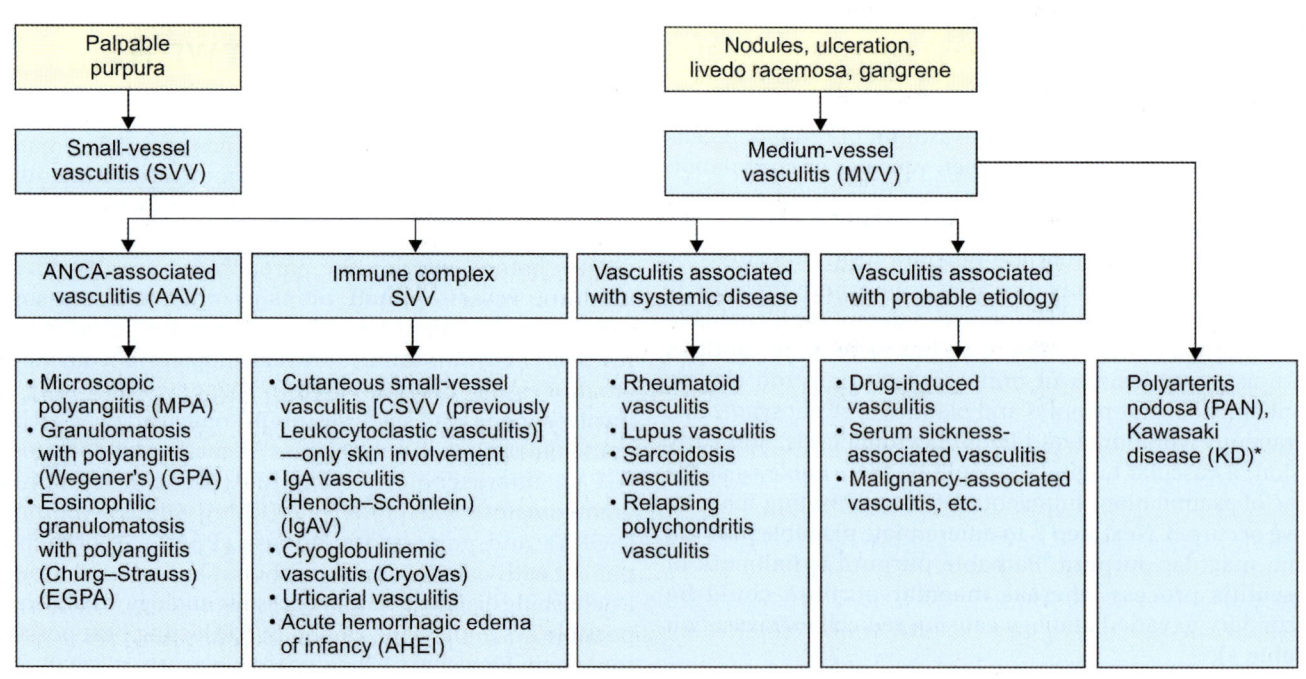

*No vasculitis in skin lesions of Kawasaki disease. Most common involvement is of medium size coronary arteries.[3]

FLOWCHART 1: Possible causes of small- and medium-vessels vasculitis based on Chapel Hill Consensus Conference on the Nomenclature of Systemic Vasculitides (CHCC, 2012).

(ANCA: antineutrophil cytoplasmic antibody)

Table 2: Age and sex predilection.								
Disease	CSVV[4]	IgAV[5]	UV[6]	Vasculitis associated with rheumatic disorders	MPA[7]	GPA[8]	EGPA[9]	PAN[10]
Age distribution	All ages	Predominantly children, adult cases 1/10th of pediatric. Majority 5–10 years	Middle aged adults. Median age 43 years	Follow the pattern of primary connective tissue disorder	Average age of presentation 50–60 years	Wide age distribution peak at 64–75 years (8–15% cases in children)[11]	Average age of onset 55 years	Mean age of onset 47 years
Sex predilection	Equal	M>F (1.3–2:1)	M<F (1:2)	Overall female predominant	Slight male preponderance (1.8:1)	No sex predilection	M<F (1:2)	M>F (1:1.8)

[CSVV: cutaneous small-vessel vasculitis; EGPA: eosinophilic granulomatosis with polyangiitis; F: female; GPA: granulomatosis with polyangiitis; IgAV: IgA vasculitis (Henoch–Schönlein); M: male; MPA: microscopic polyangiitis; PAN: polyarteritis nodosa; UV: urticarial vasculitis]

AGE AND SEX PREDILECTION

Table 2 shows age and sex predilection for common vasculitis.

Drug and malignancy-induced vasculitis is well-recognized entity now. Temporal relationship with introduction of drug or associated symptoms suggestive of malignancy should prompt search for these etiologies of vasculitis irrespective of age or sex of patient.[12,13] Cryoglobulinemic vasculitis is commonly associated with B-cell lymphoproliferative malignancy, hepatitis C virus infection, HIV, and autoimmune disorder. Acute hemorrhagic edema of infancy (AHEI) is more common in male child in first 2 years of life.[14]

PRESENTING SYMPTOMS

Palpable purpura is uniformly a presenting symptoms of small-vessels vasculitis. Small-vessel involvement is seen exclusively in cutaneous small-vessel vasculitis (CSVV), IgAV, and AHEI. Vesiculation or necrosis in center of lesion is not uncommon if inflammation is severe. Hemorrhagic or necrotic purpura is seen in one-third of adults with IgA vasculitis.[15] Associated livedoid reticularis, dermal nodules, large ulcerations, and digital gangrene suggest some degree of medium-vessel vasculitis either exclusively or with small-vessel involvement which is feature of MPA, GPA, EGPA, CryoVas, and PAN. Differential diagnosis of medium-vessel vasculitis also includes disorders showing coagulopathy such as antiphospholipid antibody (APLA), livedoid vasculopathy, Sneddon syndrome, etc. (not discussed in this Chapter).

Urticarial wheals with or without angioedema, not disappearing in 24 hours, leaving behind bruising or hyperpigmentation, showing prominent central clearing, not limited to dependant areas and one which burn more than itch should raise suspicion for UV.[16]

ORIGIN AND PROGRESS

Acute onset of corps of purpura with or without systemic complain is feature of CSVV, IgAV, UV, and AHEI. Recurrent corps is seen in more commonly in IgAV, UV, vasculitis associated with rheumatic disorders, CryoVas, and antineutrophil cytoplasmic antibody (ANCA)-associated vasculitis (AAV). Recurrent corps of purpura set up of pre-existing systemic disease should guide the further work up for diagnosis. Symptoms of AAV and PAN are more chronic in nature (see associated symptoms in **Table 3**). Palpable purpura associated with mix CryoVas is not typically cold induced whereas vascular occlusive lesion of monoclonal CryoVas (Raynaud's phenomena, livedo reticularis, acrocyanosis, and gangrene) is more cold induced.

Lesions of CSVV and IgAV prefer dependent area to start with and in due course can become generalized. Lesion of UV can be generalized from onset. Face and scrotum are involved in AHEI.

SIGNIFICANT PAST/PRECEDING HISTORY

Preceding history of sore throat, abdominal pain, diarrhea, and vomiting can be present in CSVV, IgAV, and AHEI. Acute hemorrhagic edema of infancy can follow vaccination in children.[17] Past history of asthma and allergic rhinitis suggests possibility of EGPA. Preceding history of drug or substance abuse should alert dermatologist for drug-induced vasculitis **(Table 4)**. Systemic involvement in any type of vasculitis is dynamic process. Other system involvement can be preceding, concomitant, or following cutaneous involvement. History taking should also focus around evaluating symptoms of any malignancy, as malignancy is important etiology for cutaneous vasculitis. Detail history taking in this regard can help to establish not only extent of

Table 3: Evaluation of associated symptoms in patient of palpable purpura.	
Symptom	**Diagnostic/Prognostic clue**
Fever	Fever is a nonspecific symptom. Almost all form of vasculitis can present with fever. In fact, persistent or prolong fever in patient with purpura should prompt investigation for systemic involvement[18]
Arthralgia	Mild arthralgia in absence of joint swelling or effusion is common with CSVV, UV.[19] Severe arthritis with joint swelling in patient of UV indicates possibility of HCUV syndrome. IgAV may present with joint swelling and pain of elbow, knee, and ankle joint.[20] Frank arthritis with joint swelling of long duration is feature of vasculitis associated with primary rheumatic disorder and CryoVas[21]
Weight loss	Significant weight loss can be associated with CryoVas, GPA, and vasculitis associated with primary rheumatic disorders. Patient of PAN can present with weight loss. Significant weight loss should initiate search for malignancy also
Upper respiratory symptoms:	
Nasal blockage/discharge	Suggest possibility of GPA particularly recurrent and long-standing symptoms. More than 90% patients of GPA have upper respiratory symptoms.[22] Long-standing allergic rhinitis and nasal polyp precede development of EGPA[23]
Epistaxis	
Nasal deformity	
Lower respiratory symptoms:	
Cough	Asthma precedes for years before development of EGPA. Alveolar hemorrhage, pulmonary infiltrate, pulmonary edema, and interstitial fibrosis are reported in 25–55% patients with MPA.[24] Large number of patients with GPA develop pulmonary symptoms which include dyspnea due to pulmonary infiltrate and pleural effusion and hemoptysis secondary to pulmonary hemorrhage.[25] Chronic obstructive pulmonary disease and other lower respiratory symptoms in patient of UV are strongly associated with HUVS[26]
Dyspnea	
Hemoptysis	
Chest pain	
Gastrointestinal:	
Abdominal pain	• GI manifestations are common with IgAV. Occult GI bleeding manifesting as melena, intussusception, and perforation presenting as acute abdomen are associated with IgAV[27,28] • Acute abdomen secondary to involvement of intestinal arteries and infract could be presentation of PAN[29] • Abdominal pain can be presenting symptom of MPA. Abdominal bleeding and perforation too reported with MPA though less common than PAN[30] • Anorexia and jaundice could be indication of chronic active hepatitis. Association of PAN with hepatitis B and CryoVas (mix) with hepatitis C virus is well documented
Anorexia and jaundice	
Melena and hematochezia	
Peripheral nervous system:	
Paresthesia	Symptom suggestive of peripheral nerve involvement should initiate search for systemic involvement in case of CSVV.[17] Mononeuritis multiplex is reported more commonly with PAN, MPA, CryoVas, and EGPA and rarely with IgAV.[23,31] Symmetrical or asymmetrical polyneuropathy is also reported with above-mentioned vasculitis disorders
Neuritic pain	
Motor weakness	
Cranial nerve palsies	Cranial nerve palsies could be due to extension of granuloma in GPA[32]
Central nervous system	Headache, mood change, vision change, ataxia, chorea, convulsion, and disturbance of consciousness in case of IgAV suggest cerebral vasculitis. CNS vasculitis can be associated with cutaneous vasculitis in patient of lupus erythematosus
Ophthalmic:	
Conjunctival injection	• Almost 30–50% patients of GPA have associated eye involvement.[33] Symptoms range from red eye, loss of vision, photophobia, proptosis, and diplopia depending on the structure involved within ocular system. Dry eye can be presentation of Sjogren syndrome and associated mix CryoVas • Uveitis and episcleritis are one of the minor diagnostic criteria for HUVS[34]
Dry eye	
Blurring of vision	
Diplopia	
Proptosis	
Auditory:	
Hearing loss and ear discharge	Sudden onset sensorineural hearing loss can be presentation of PAN.[35] Recurrent serous otitis media could be secondary to involvement of nose and nasopharynx in GPA and EGPA

Continued

Continued

Symptom	Diagnostic/Prognostic clue
Renal:	
Hematuria	Hematuria and proteinuria are indicators of renal involvement in vasculitis. CSVV is diagnosis of exclusion renal involvement should raise suspicion for other form of systemic vasculitis. Renal involvement in patients of UV may be manifestation of HCUV or HUVS and possible association with SLE.[36] PAN does not cause glomerulonephritis but infract and hematoma due to rupture of microaneurysms can occur which can manifest as haematuria.[23,29] Approximately 30–50% patients of IgAV develop renal involvement proportion of which progress to glomerulonephritis and around 1–7% develop end-stage renal disease.[37] Lower urinary track involvement in form of urethritis and stricture is also known to occur with IgAV.[38] Acute or chronic renal involvement is common with type 2 CryoVas. Renal involvement can be feature of all three AAV in decreasing order of prevalence in MPA > GPA > EGPA
Frothy urine (s/o proteinuria)	
Edema	
Reproductive:	
Testicular pain	Although rare, unilateral orchitis due to testicular artery ischemia is highly specific for PAN.[39] Epididymitis, orchitis, and hematoma around the testis and testicular torsion are reported with IgAV[40]
Vascular system:	
Raynaud's phenomenon	Presence of Raynaud's phenomenon and acrocyanosis are seen in CryoVas associated with type I cryoglobulinemia which is almost always associated with malignant or benign lymphoproliferative disorder.[41] Medium-vessel involvement in GPA, EGPA, MPA, and PAN can give rise to similar vascular symptoms. Peripheral vascular symptoms are also feature of systemic sclerosis and antiphospholipid antibody mediated lupus vasculopathy
Acrocyanosis	
Digital ulceration	

[AAV: ANCA-associated vasculitis; CryoVas: cryoglobulinemic vasculitis; CSVV: cutaneous small-vessel vasculitis; EGPA: eosinophilic granulomatosis with polyangiitis; GPA: granulomatosis with polyangiitis; HCUV: hypocomplementemic urticarial vasculitis; HUVS: hypocomplementemic urticarial vasculitis syndrome; IgAV: IgA vasculitis (Henoch–Schönlein); PAN: polyarteritis nodosa; S/O: suggestive of; SLE: systemic lupus erythematosus; UV: urticarial vasculitis]

Table 4: Drug-induced vasculitis—salient features.

Drug-induced vasculitis is present in following three distinct clinical, pathological, and serological patterns.[13]

Type of drug-induced vasculitis	Reported culprit drugs	Features
Drug-induced cutaneous leukocytoclastic vasculitis[44]	• Antibiotics • Analgesics • Allopurinol • Antiepileptics • Antihypertensive • Anecdotal reports of metformin, clopidogrel, isoniazid, rifampicin, adalimumab, ceritinib	Internal organ involvement is more common compared to primary CSVV. Joint involvement in almost half of the patients, kidney, and GI involvement in third of patients[13]
Drug-induced IgA vasculitis and other small-vessel vasculitis	• Adalimumab • Infliximab[45] • Etanercept[46] • Palbociclib[47]	Cutaneous purpura associated with renal or GI involvement
Drug-induced antineutrophil cytoplasmic antibodies-associated vasculitis	Antithyroid drugs propylthiouracil, methimazole, and carbimazole	Asymptomatic circulating ANCA is more common. Clinical manifestations range from only cutaneous involvement to systemic vasculitis affecting lungs and kidney. Vasculitis may manifest years after starting therapy.[48,49] Both C- and P-ANCA can be detected
	Hydralazine	Cutaneous involvement is not common, predominantly affects kidneys. Median duration from onset of drug is 22 months. Clinical presentation overlaps with drug-induced lupus erythematosus as almost all patients have concomitant ANA and ANCA (majority P-ANCA) reactivity and hypocomplementemia[50]

Continued

Continued

Type of drug-induced vasculitis	Reported culprit drugs	Features
	• Cocaine/levamisole • Cocaine is commonly snorted via nose by addicts • Levamisole is used as bulking agent in illicit cocaine to increase weight. It is also found to potentiate neurostimulatory effect of cocaine by inhibition of monoamine oxidase and catecholamine-O-methyltransferase. Therapeutic use of levamisole can also induce similar vasculitis syndrome[51]	• Cocaine due to its effect on nasal mucosa produces midline destructive lesion involving nose clinically indistinguishable from GPA. Both C-ANCA and P-ANCA may be positive in patient[52] • Levamisole-induced vasculitis presents with skin manifestations such as palpable purpura, cutaneous ulceration, and digital gangrene. Leukopenia, pulmonary, and renal involvements are also common. Almost all patients show P-ANCA positivity, half of which can also have C-ANCA[53]

(ANCA: antineutrophil cytoplasmic antibodies; CSVV: cutaneous small-vessel vasculitis; GI: gastrointestinal; GPA: granulomatosis with polyangiitis)

systemic involvement but also possible etiology of vasculitis also (see associated symptoms in **Table 3**).

ASSOCIATED SYMPTOMS

It is important to remember CSVV, NCUV, and AHEI are majority time skin limited disease though mild constitutional symptom such as fever and arthralgia can be associated with purpura but otherwise patient is fine. Any prolong or significant systemic symptoms should prompt search for more serious systemic vasculitis syndrome.

Careful evaluation of associated symptoms helps closing on possible diagnosis, severity of disease, and ultimately selection of treatment **(Table 3)**.

GENERAL EXAMINATION

General examination in patient of palpable purpura is of vital importance as it may give possible clue about etiology as well as identify the systemic involvement **(Table 5)**.

CUTANEOUS EXAMINATION

Remember palpable purpura is hallmark of small-vessel vasculitis. **Flowchart 2** shows important points on cutaneous examination of palpable purpura.

Lesions of UV appear in corps involving extremity and trunk with or without angioedema. Any urticarial lesion lasting >24 hours should be investigated for UV.

Lesions of AHEI are large erythematous or urticarial plaques, which evolve into annular or targetoid lesion favoring head and extremities. Tender nonpitting edema of face ears, extremities, and scrotum are characteristic of this condition.

DERMOSCOPY FINDINGS

Dermoscopy in suspected case of palpable purpura helps into diagnosis of vasculitis with findings correlating with histological features but as of now, histopathological examination remains gold standard for diagnosis of vasculitis. **Figure 8** shows dermoscopic findings in patient of palpable purpura with histological correlation.[43] Dermoscopic examination also helps in differentiating UV from CIU **(Fig. 9)** and vasculopathy from vasculitis **(Fig. 10)**.

INVESTIGATIONS

Purpose of laboratory and radiological investigations in patients of palpable purpura should be two prongs: (1) to establish definitive type of vasculitis, and (2) to know the extent of systemic involvement. As ordering all the investigations in all patients of vasculitis does not make sense in term of scientific utility, additionally it can put immense stress on patient's expense. Other than screening investigations, associated suspected systemic involvement should guide selection for further specialized investigations. Following basic investigations should be ordered as screening:
- Complete blood count with differential leukocyte count
- Routine urine analysis
- Stool routine analysis
- Erythrocyte sedimentation rate
- C-reactive protein levels
- Liver function study
- Renal function study
- Skin biopsy for histopathological and direct immunofluorescence (DIF) study

If primary cutaneous examination (nodule, livedo reticularis, acrocyanosis, gangrene, or large cutaneous

Table 5: Important findings on general examination in patient of palpable purpura.

Area of examination	Examination findings	Possible interpretation and associations
Scalp	Diffuse hair loss, telogen effluvium	Look for systemic disorder such as SLE, RA, SS, and chronic telogen effluvium secondary to systemic disorder or nutritional deficiencies including anemia associated with renal involvement
	Lupus hair	Lupus-associated vasculitis
	Cicatricial alopecia of DLE	Lupus-associated vasculitis
Eye	Conjunctival pallor	Anemia secondary to systemic involvement
	Dry eye	Vasculitis associated with Sjogren syndrome
	Proptosis	Orbital involvement in GPA
	Red eye, scleritis, and episcleritis	HUVS
Facial features	Malar rashes	SLE-associated vasculitis
	Nasal mass, nasal septum deviation, saddle nose deformity	GPA
Oral cavity	Chronic recurrent ulcers	Rheumatic disorders, SLE, Sjögren's syndrome-associated vasculitis
	Ulcer, induration, perforation of hard palate and gingival hyperplasia (strawberry gingiva)[42]	GPA
Nail	Clubbing	COPD associate with HUVS. Chronic lung insufficiency in GPA, EGPA, and MPA
	Splinter hemorrhages	Feature of SLE and RA
	Periungual telangiectasias	SLE-associated vasculitis
	Tortures capillaries with prominent subpapillary plexus on nail fold capillaroscopy	
Hypertension	Diastolic BP > 90 mm Hg or systolic BP > 140 mm Hg	Renal artery involvement in PAN produces renovascular hypertension
Lymph node	Enlarged cervical/axillary/inguinal lymph nodes	Enlarge lymph node can be marker of infection, e.g., streptococcal, EBV, and CMV. Lymphoreticular malignancy should be suspected if morphology of lymph node enlargement suggests the same (CryoVas, malignancy-associated CSVV)

(BP: blood pressure; CMV: cytomegalovirus; COPD: chronic obstructive pulmonary disease; DLE: discoid lupus erythematosus; EBV: Epstein–Barr virus; EGPA: eosinophilic granulomatosis with polyangiitis; GPA: granulomatosis with polyangiitis; HUVS: hypocomplementemic urticarial vasculitis syndrome; MPA: microscopic polyangiitis; PAN: polyarteritis nodosa; RA: rheumatoid arthritis; SLE: systemic lupus erythematosus; SS: systemic sclerosis)

In patient of CSVV, lesions usually begin from area with high venous pressure such as around ankle, other dependant sites, as well as areas under tight fitting clothing. Lesions spare intertriginous regions. In general, lesions are asymptomatic or they may be painful or associated with burning and stinging. Size of lesions ranges from one millimeter to several centimeter. Secondary changes of vesiculation, ulceration, necrosis, and postinflammatory hyperpigmentation may be present. Associated edema in lower limb is not unusual finding **(Figs. 1 and 2)**

↓

Symmetrical distribution involving extensor of elbow, knee, and buttocks. Severe vesiculation, bullae formation, hemorrhage, necrosis, and retiform pattern within lesion are more common with adult IgAV **(Fig. 3)**

↓

Lesions above waist line with fever and elevated ESR in adult patient of IgAV have more chances of developing severe renal involvement **(Fig. 4)**

↓

Purpura over background of, or in association with livedo reticularis, cutaneous nodules, acrocyanosis, and digital gangrene suggests involvement of medium-vessel vasculitis **(Figs. 5 to 7)**

FLOWCHART 2: Important points in cutaneous examination of palpable purpura.
(CSVV: cutaneous small-vessel vasculitis; ESR: erythrocyte sedimentation rate)

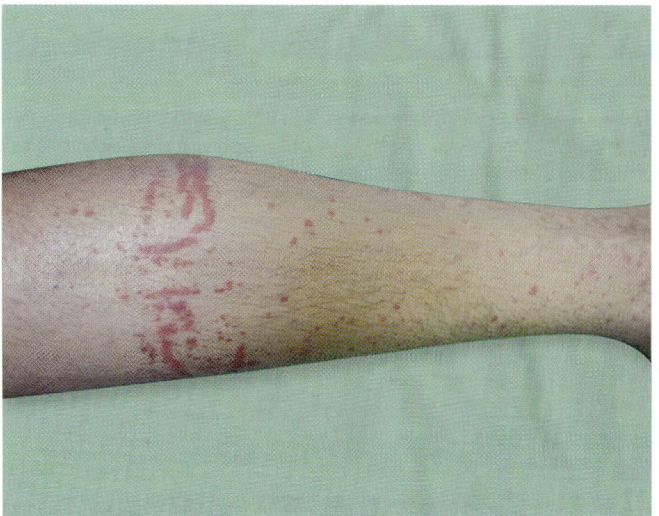

FIG. 1: Case of cutaneous small-vessel vasculitis showing palpable purpura of varying size in lower limb marks the congregation of purpura around area of contact with tight fitting shocks.

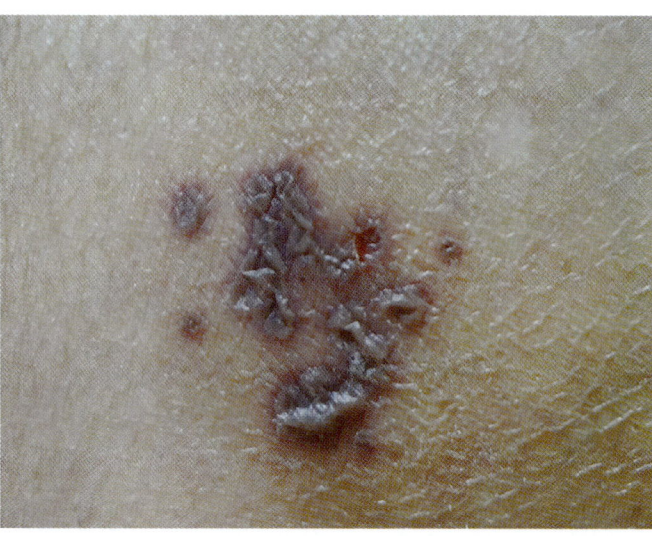

FIG. 2: Vesiculation and ulceration within purpura due to intense inflammation.

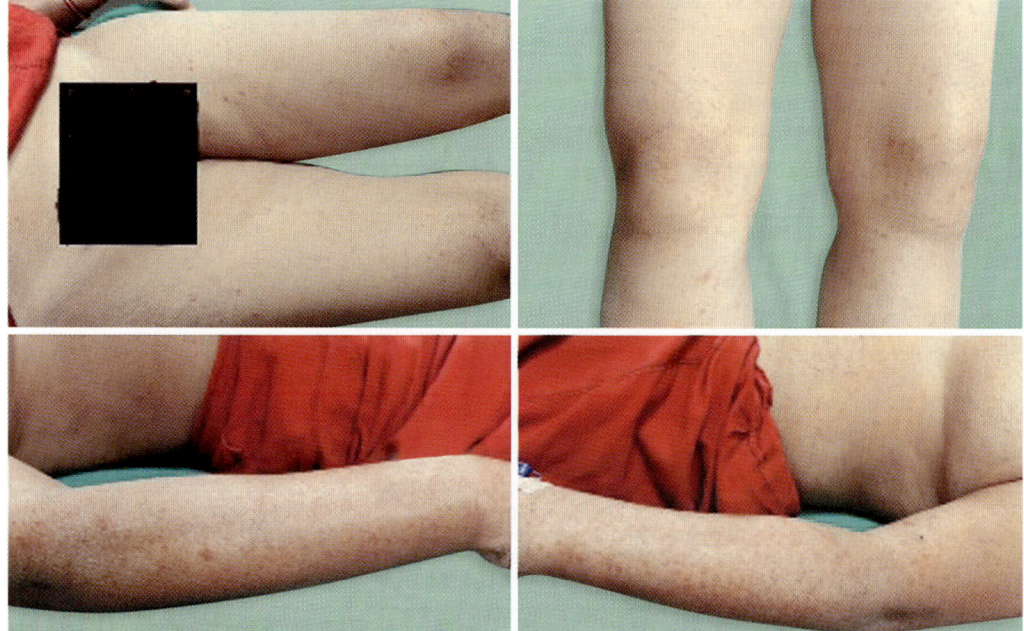

FIG. 3: Case of IgA vasculitis with associated IgA nephropathy showing corps of palpable purpura distributed bilateral and symmetrically in lower and upper limb.
(IgA: immunoglobulin A)

ulceration) or associated systemic symptoms **(Table 3)** suggest additional medium-vessel involvement, add ANCA, chest X-ray, ANA, and APLA testing as initial screening. Detail of positive findings in history and examination on presentation should clearly be mentioned in case paper of patient to justify your rationale behind ordered investigations. Inclusion of ANA and ANCA in all patient of cutaneous vasculitis adds additional financial burden to patient.

Biopsy Technique

For best possible specimen for pathologist to comment about, it is very important to select correct lesion and correct technique for biopsy. Only biopsy extending to subcutis can incorporate medium-sized vessels situated in subcutis. So preferably biopsy from most tender and purpuric lesion which is <48 hours old extending up to subcutis is preferable.[54] Lymphocytes start to replace

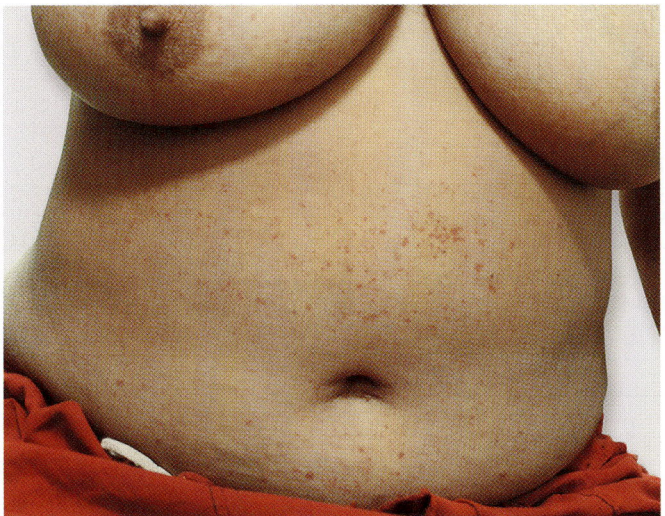

FIG. 4: Purpura above the waistline in patient of IgAV is associated with severe renal disease.
(IgAV: IgA vasculitis)

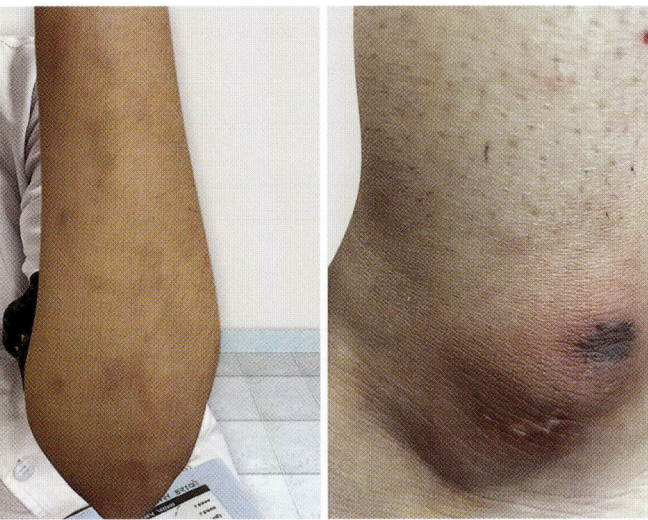

FIG. 5: Patient of polyarteritis nodosa showing livedo changes in upper limb and erythematous indurated nodules with overlying necrosis in lower limb.

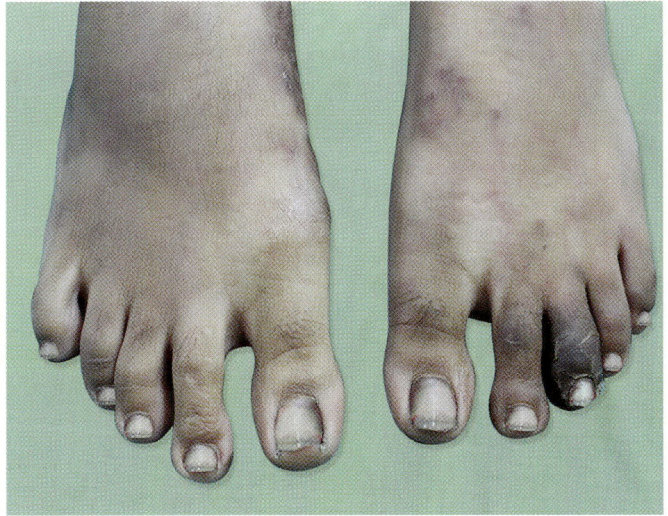

FIG. 6: Patient with livedo-like erythema in association with acrocyanosis involving toe.

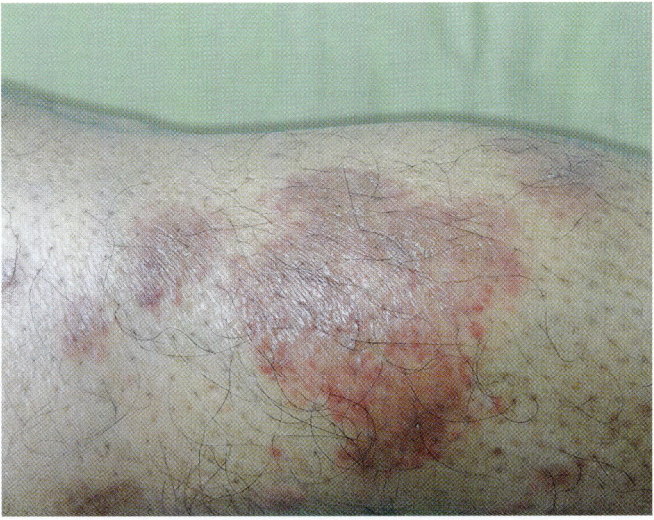

FIG. 7: Purpura with indurated plaque in patient of GPA.
(GPA: granulomatosis with polyangiitis)

neutrophil after 24 hours of onset of lesion so any biopsy from lesion >48 hours old will demonstrate lymphocyte-rich infiltrate irrespective of actual type of vasculitis.[55] In case of livedo racemosa type lesion, biopsy should be taken from central white area and not from erythematous periphery. If superficial ulcer is present, biopsy should be taken from edge of lesion. In case of deep punched out lesion biopsy incorporated central base of lesion will incorporate arteries for examination.[56] For immune complex mediated vasculitis yield of immunoglobulin is 100% in lesion less than 24 hours old, 70% between 24 and 48 hours. Biopsy from lesion >72 hours will not show immunoglobulin deposition though compliment can be visible.[18]

Based on results of preliminary investigations and clinical presentation advanced investigation should be performed **(Table 6)**.

MANAGEMENT

Management of vasculitis largely depends on etiology, extent of systemic involvement, and possible precipitating factors. **Table 7** shows broad approach in management of various types of vasculitis in concise. Readers are advised to refer other resources for details.

Dermoscopic features of vasculitis and its correlation with histological findings.	
Dermoscopic features	Histopathological features
Purpuric blotches (Red arrow)	Associated with perivascular extravasation and degradation of red blood cells
Purpuric dots and globules (Yellow arrow)	Dermal erythrocyte extravasation secondary to fibrinoid degeneration of small blood vessels, with a mixed neutrophilic infiltrate
Puruple and yellow background (Green arrow)	Intact extravasated erythrocytes and extravasated siderophages respectively
Whitish blue patches (Blue)	Epidermal necrosis
Homogenous purpuric pattern	Extravasated erythrocytes in the dermis with capillaries devoid of inflammatory cells
Mottled purpuric pattern	Extravasated erythrocytes in the dermis with capillaries showing variable inflammatory changes
• Irregular/tortuous vessels and arborizing vessels • Round vessels	• Deeper dilated horizontal subpapillary capillaries • Papillary capillaries

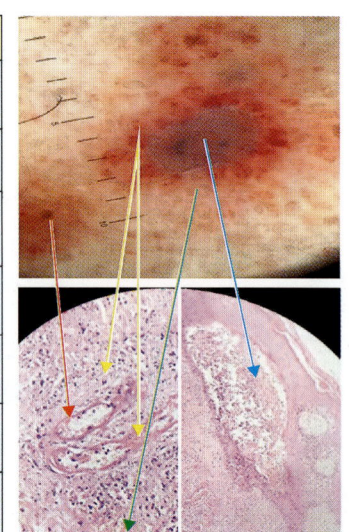

FIG. 8: Dermoscopic findings in patient of palpable purpura with histological correlation.

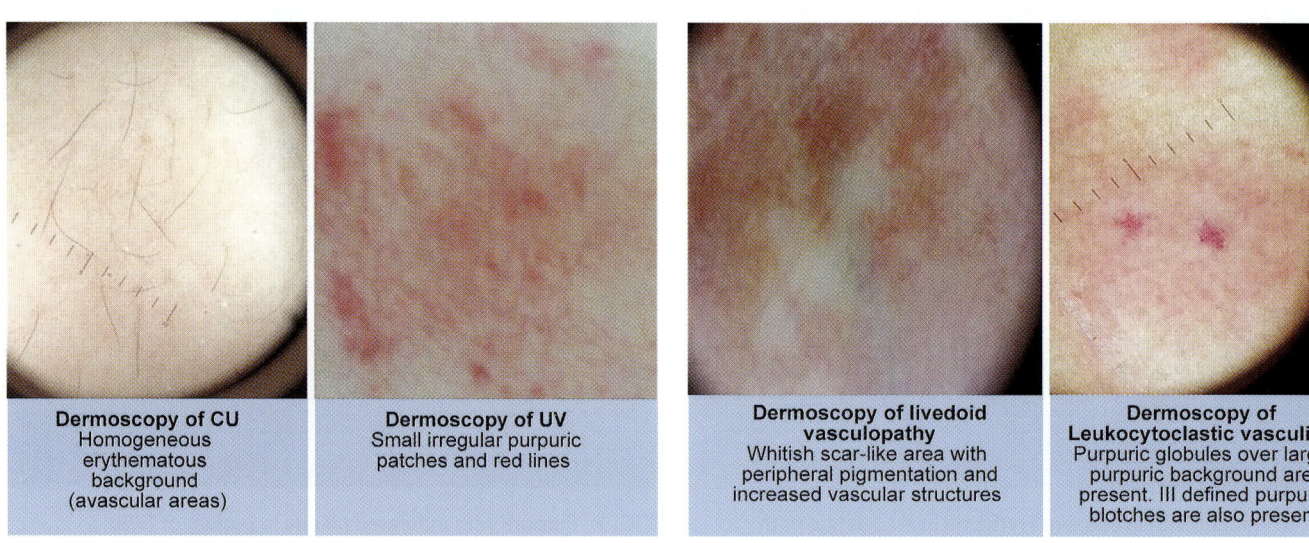

Dermoscopy of CU
Homogeneous erythematous background (avascular areas)

Dermoscopy of UV
Small irregular purpuric patches and red lines

Dermoscopy of livedoid vasculopathy
Whitish scar-like area with peripheral pigmentation and increased vascular structures

Dermoscopy of Leukocytoclastic vasculitis
Purpuric globules over large purpuric background are present. Ill defined purpuric blotches are also present

FIG. 9: Dermoscopic examination helps in differentiating UV from CIU.

FIG. 10: Dermoscopic examination helps in differentiating vasculopathy from vasculitis.

Table 6: Interpretation of preliminary investigation and suggested advance investigations.		
Clinical findings	*Results of preliminary investigations*	*Advance investigations and interpretation*
Palpable purpura with minimal systemic complaints	CBC—mild leukocytosis, elevated CRP. Normal urine and stool analysis, Biopsy s/o leukocytoclastic vasculitis involving only small vessels in superficial dermis **(Fig. 11)** ± perivascular IgG or IgM ± complement deposition	Most likely skin-limited CSVV. No further investigations required. Search for infective foci as precipitating cause. Keep patient under close follow-up for any systemic involvement

Continued

Continued

Clinical findings	Results of preliminary investigations	Advance investigations and interpretation
Palpable purpura with joint pain, fever, malar rash, oral ulceration, and photosensitivity	Cytopenia ± low Hb, elevated ESR, proteinuria ± hematuria. Biopsy s/o leukocytoclastic vasculitis of small ± medium-size vessels with lymphocyte-rich infiltrate around vessels ± other changes of CTD (**Fig. 12**) ± perivascular immunoglobulin IgM or IgG on DIF. Presence of immunoreactant at DEJ strongly suggests associated SLE	• Vasculitis associated with CTD (commonly SLE, RA, and Sjögren's syndrome; uncommonly DM and SS) • ANA by IF, ANA profile for extractable nuclear antigen. Serum C3 and C4
Palpable purpura, with any one of following:* • Acute abdominal pain • Leukocytoclastic vasculitis on biopsy (proliferative glomerulonephritis with IgA deposition in kidney biopsy if already done) • Acute arthralgia or arthritis • Hematuria or proteinuria	±Leukocytosis ±Thrombocytosis ±Elevated ESR ±Occult blood in stool ±Elevated BUN and creatinine Bx s/o leukocytoclastic vasculitis involving small vessels in superficial dermis, occasionally whole dermis;[57] on biopsy ± predominant IgA deposition around vessels (IgA deposit not necessary for diagnosis of IgAV)	p/o IgA vasculitis • ASO titer may be elevated and suggests streptococcal infection as precipitating cause • D-dimer is elevated in sizable patients. Serum IgA may be elevated. Factor XIII and serum C3 and C4 decreased in some patients
Urticarial lesions lasting >24 hours ± angioedema ± joint pain	± Mild leukocytosis ±Leukocytoclastic vasculitis Not all features may be present on histology[34]	p/o NUV
Urticarial lesions with joint pain ± other features of SLE	±Proteinuria ± hematuria ± perivascular immunoreactant ± BMZ immunoreactant (lupus band)[58]	p/o HCUV • Serum C3, C4, and C50, if low, suggest HCUV. Most common association with SLE advises ANA study
Symptoms of HCUV ± eye involvement, COPD, and abdominal pain	Same as above	p/o HUVS • Same as above plus low Serum C1q with anti-C1q antibody[52]
• Palpable purpura ± h/o viral hepatitis ± joint pain ± s/o peripheral neuropathy ± s/o cranial nerve involvement ± s/o CNS involvement ± fever, fatigue and fibromyalgia*[59] • S/o hyperviscosity state such as livedo, Raynaud's phenomenon, and digital infract	Elevated ESR ± elevated liver enzymes ± proteinuria ± hematuria ± Bx s/o LCV affecting both small- and medium-size vessels on biopsy with eosinophilic deposits in vessel wall and lumen.[60] Immunoreactant on DIF	p/o CryoVas • Test for cryoglobulin (on two separate occasions at least 12 weeks apart* • Serum C4 can be low. • Serum protein electrophoresis for monoclonal or polyclonal globulin band • RA factor test is positive in mixed CryoVas. ANA profile for anti-SSA/SSB as mixed CryoVas is associated with SS and SLE. Malignancy screen if symptom suggests as type I CryoVas is almost always associated with lymphoproliferative disorder
Palpable purpura ± cutaneous nodules, ulcerated nodules, s/o upper airway involvement*[61] ± s/o lung involvement ± s/o renal involvement ± s/o GI involvement	Elevated ESR and CRP. Hematuria ± proteinuria* Bx s/o necrotizing vasculitis involving small- and medium-size vessels (if Bx from purpura). Granulomatous inflammation* (if Bx from nodule). DIF study may show immune reactant deposition from skin biopsy (remember pauci-immune is term coined for renal biopsy)[62,63]	p/o GPA • ANCA study of majority of patients of GPA shows C-ANCA positivity[64] • Sinus and lung X-ray and CT scan to evaluate upper respiratory and lung involvement. Look for sinus thickening, fixed pulmonary infiltrate, cavitating, and noncavitating nodules present ≥ 1 month, alveolar hemorrhage*

Continued

Continued

Clinical findings	Results of preliminary investigations	Advance investigations and interpretation
Palpable purpura ± s/o renal involvement ± s/o pulmonary involvement (According to EMA diagnostic algorithm, MPA is diagnosis of exclusion of GPA and EGPA in setting of renal and lung involvement with ANCA positivity)[65]	• Elevated ESR and CRP ± anemia ± leukocytosis ± thrombocytosis • Proteinuria ± hematuria • Skin Bx s/o leukocytoclastic vasculitis ± absence of immune reactant on DIF	p/o MPA • ANCA study: 50–75% positive for P-ANCA. Further lung and renal work-up according to presentation
Palpable purpura ± s/o obstructive airway disease* ± nasal polyp* ± s/o mononeuritis multiplex*[66]	• Eosinophilia ≥ 10% of differential leukocyte count* • Hematuria in urine analysis* • Bx suggestive of necrotizing vasculitis upper dermis ± mid dermis and subcutis showing eosinophil-rich infiltrate*	p/o EGPA • ANCA study shows P-ANCA (74%) and C-ANCA (38%). Lung and paranasal sinus imaging shows sinus thickening, polyp, and pulmonary infiltrates which may be transient
Palpable purpura (not very common) ± livedo reticularis* ± Raynaud's phenomenon ± cutaneous ulceration ± nodules ± gangrene associated with weight loss*, myalgia, weakness*, testicular pain*, diastolic hypertension >90 mm Hg*	• ± Elevated ESR • ± Lymphocytosis • ± Elevated liver enzymes • Pan mural necrotizing vasculitis [involvement of medium-size arteries is a must in subcutis (Fig. 13)][67,68]	p/o PAN • Angiographic evaluation of involved organ (mesenteric, renal, and hepatic arteries) showing saccular and fusiform microaneurysm with stenosis[58] • Viral hepatitis screening to check for association with hepatitis B[69]

*Component of diagnostic criteria.
(±: with or without; ANA: antinuclear antibodies; ANCA: antineutrophil cytoplasmic antibodies; BMZ: basement membrane zone; BUN: blood urea nitrogen; Bx: biopsy; CBC: complete blood count; COPD: chronic obstructive pulmonary disease; CRP: C-reactive protein; CSVV: cutaneous small vessel vasculitis; CTD: connective tissue diseases; DEJ: dermoepidermal junction; DIF: direct immunofluorescence; DM: dermatomyositis; EGPA: eosinophilic granulomatosis with polyangiitis; EMA: European Medicines Agency; ESR: erythrocyte sedimentation rate; GI: gastrointestinal; GPA: granulomatosis with polyangiitis; Hb: hemoglobin; HCUV: hypocomplementemic urticarial vasculitis; HUVS: hypocomplementemic urticarial vasculitis syndrome; IF: immunofluorescence; MPA: microscopic polyangiitis; P/O: possibility of; PAN: polyarteritis nodosa; RA: rheumatoid arthritis; S/O: suggestive of; SLE: systemic lupus erythematosus; SS: systemic sclerosis)

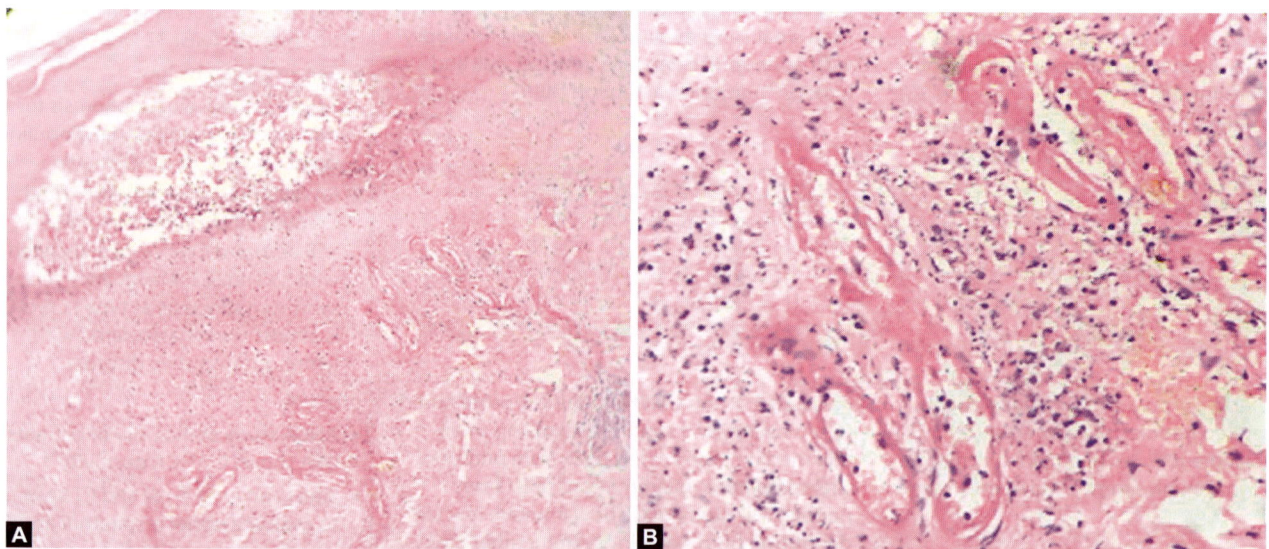

FIGS. 11A AND B: (A) Leukocytoclastic vasculitis showing epidermal necrosis H&E, 100×. (B) Dermal perivascular neutrophils and few lymphocyte infiltration. Vessel wall damage and fibrinoid changes are observed along with extravasated RBCs, karyorrhexis, and endothelial cell swelling H&E, 400×.

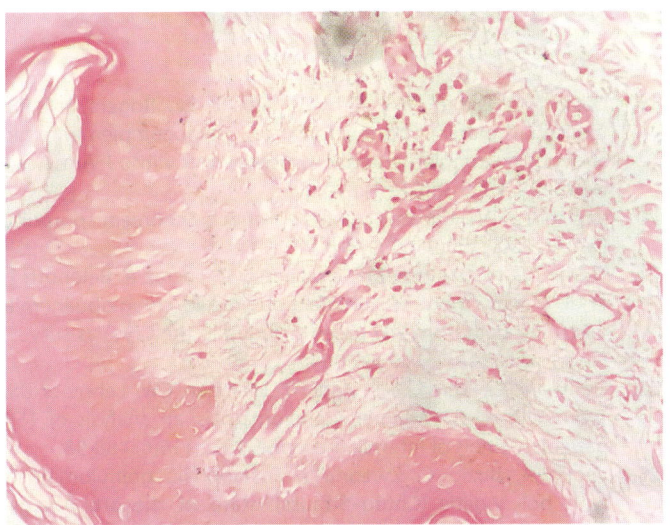

FIG. 12: Lymphocyte-rich perivascular infiltrate with endothelial cell swelling and red cell extravasation H&E, 400×.

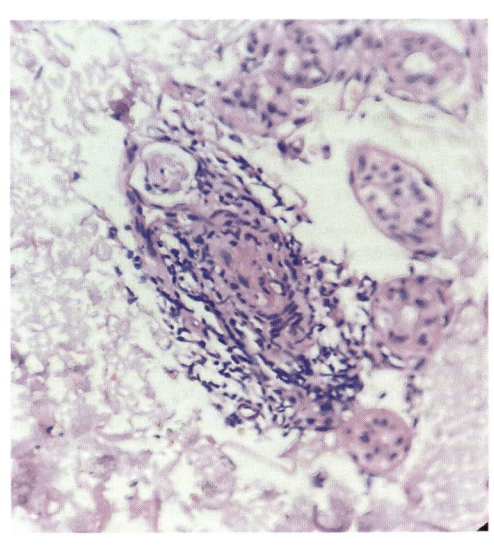

FIG. 13: Pan-mural neutrophilic infiltrates with fibrinoid necrosis of vessel wall involving medium-size muscular arteries of deep dermis in case of cutaneous polyarteritis nodosa.

Table 7: Broad approach in management of vasculitis.

Type of vasculitis	CSVV	IgAV	UV	CryoVas	GPA	EGPA	MPA	PAN
First-line treatment	Address underlying cause (infection, drug, malignancy), NSAIDs, antihistamines	Supportive	Antihistamines, indomethacin, dapsone ± pentoxifylline, CS	IFN + Ribavirin (for HCV associated) CS	CS + MTX, CS + CYC ± RTX for severe renal disease CS + CYC + PEX	CS ± CYC	CS ± RTX ± CYC	• For cutaneous PAN • Address underlying cause (infection, drug), NSAIDs, CS • For classic PAN (± HBV) • CS + PEX ± IFN/lamivudine
Second-line treatment	Colchicine, dapsone, CS, HCQS	Dapsone, colchicine, CS ± AZA/CSA/CYC	Colchicine, HCQS, AZA, and MTX	CS + CYC	TMP–SMX ± CS		MTX	• For cutaneous MTX, dapsone, IVIg • For classic CS + CYC
Third-line treatment	AZA, MTX, IVIg, CSA, CYC, PEX	IVIg, RTX, MMF, PEX	MMF, IVIg, RTX, CSA, PEX	IVIG, RTX, PEX	MMF, IVIg, PEX, infliximab, and alemtuzumab	IVIg ± PEX, RTX, AZA, MMF, MTX, IFN-α	AZA, MMF, IVIg, RTX, infliximab	• For cutaneous pentoxifylline, colchicine, AZA, MMF, and TNF-α inhibitors • For classic IVIg

[AZA: azathioprine; CryoVas: cryoglobulinemic vasculitis; CS: corticosteroids; CSA: cyclosporine; CSVV: cutaneous small-vessel vasculitis; Cyc: cyclophosphamide: RTX: rituximab; EGPA: eosinophilic granulomatosis with polyangiitis; GPA: granulomatosis with polyangiitis; HBV: hepatitis B virus; HCQS: hydroxychloroquine; HCV: hepatitis C virus; IFN: interferon; IgAV: IgA vasculitis (Henoch–Schönlein); IVIg: intravenous immunoglobulin; MMF: mycophenolate mofetil; MPA: microscopic polyangiitis; MTX: methotrexate; NSAIDs: nonsteroidal anti-inflammatory drugs; PAN: polyarteritis nodosa; PEX: plasmapheresis; TMP–SMX: trimethoprim–sulfamethoxazole; UV: urticarial vasculitis]

REFERENCES

1. Pipette WW. Purpura: Mechanisms and Differential Diagnosis. In: Bolognia JL, Jorizzo JL, Schaffer JL (Eds). Dermatology, 3rd edition. India: Elsevier; 2013. p. 359.
2. Jennette JC, Falk RJ, Bacon PA, Basu N, Cid MC, Ferrario F, et al. 2012 revised international chapel hill consensus conference nomenclature of vasculitides. Arthritis Rheum. 2013;65(1):1-11.
3. Sato N, Sagawa K, Sasaguri Y, Inoue O, Kato H. Immunopathology and cytokine detection in the skin lesions of patients with Kawasaki disease. J Pediatr. 1993;122(2):198-203.
4. Lotti T, Ghersetich I, Comacchi C, Jorizzo JL. Cutaneous small-vessel vasculitis. J Am Acad Dermatol. 1998;39(5):667-90.
5. Du L, Wang P, Liu C, Li S, Yue S, Yang Y. Multisystemic manifestations of IgA vasculitis. Clin Rheumatol. 2020;40(1):43-52.
6. Mehregan DR, Hall MJ, Gibson LE. Urticarial vasculitis: a histopathologic and clinical review of 72 cases. J Am Acad Dermatol. 1992;26(3):441-8.
7. Chung SA, Seo P. Microscopic polyangiitis. Rheum Dis Clin North Am. 2010;36(3):545-58.
8. Kubaisi B, Samra KA, Foster CS. Granulomatosis with polyangiitis (Wegener's disease): An updated review of ocular disease manifestations. Intractable Rare Dis Res. 2016;5(2):61-9.
9. Sada KE, Amano K, Uehara R, Yamamura M, Arimura Y, Nakamura Y, et al. A nationwide survey on the epidemiology and clinical features of eosinophilic granulomatosis with polyangiitis (Churg-Strauss) in Japan. Mod Rheumatol. 2014;24(4):640-4.
10. Mahr A, Guillevin L, Poissonnet M, Aymé S. Prevalences of polyarteritis nodosa, microscopic polyangiitis, Wegener's granulomatosis, and Churg-Strauss syndrome in a French urban multiethnic population in 2000: a capture–recapture estimate. Arthritis Care Res. 2004;51(1):92-9.
11. Gajic-Veljic M, Nikolic M, Peco-Antic A, Bogdanovic R, Andrejevic S, Bonaci-Nikolic B. Granulomatosis with polyangiitis (Wegener's granulomatosis) in children: report of three cases with cutaneous manifestations and literature review. Pediatr Dermatol. 2013;30(4):e37-42.
12. Fain O, Hamidou M, Cacoub P, Godeau B, Wechsler B, Parlès J, et al. Vasculitides associated with malignancies: analysis of sixty patients. Arthritis Care Res. 2007;57(8):1473-80.
13. Misra DP, Patro P, Sharma A. Drug-induced vasculitis. Indian J Rheumatol. 2019;14(5):3-9.
14. Savino F, Lupica MM, Tarasco V, Locatelli E, Viola S, di Montezemolo LC, et al. Acute hemorrhagic edema of infancy: a troubling cutaneous presentation with a self-limiting course. Pediatr Dermatol. 2013;30(6):e149-52.
15. Audemard-Verger A, Pillebout E, Guillevin L, Thervet E, Terrier B. IgA vasculitis (Henoch–Shönlein purpura) in adults: Diagnostic and therapeutic aspects. Autoimmun Rev. 2015;14(7):579-85.
16. Venzor J, Lee WL, Huston DP. Urticarial vasculitis. Clin Rev Allerg Immunol. 2002;23(2):201-16.
17. Fiore E, Rizzi M, Ragazzi M, Vanoni F, Bernasconi M, Bianchetti MG, et al. Acute hemorrhagic edema of young children (cockade purpura and edema): a case series and systematic review. J Am Acad Dermatol. 2008;59(4):684-95.
18. Sais G, Vidaller A, Jucgla A, Servitje O, Condom E, Peyrí J. Prognostic factors in leukocytoclastic vasculitis: a clinico-pathologic study of 160 patients. Arch Dermatol. 1998;134(3):309-15.
19. Davis MD, Daoud MS, Kirby B, Gibson LE, Rogers 3rd RS. Clinicopathologic correlation of hypocomplementemic and normocomplementemic urticarial vasculitis. J Am Acad Dermatol. 1998;38(6 Pt 1):899-905.
20. Saulsbury FT. Clinical update: Henoch-Schönlein purpura. Lancet. 2007;369(9566):976-8.
21. Terrier B, Krastinova E, Marie I, Launay D, Lacraz A, Belenotti P, et al. Management of noninfectious mixed cryoglobulinemia vasculitis: data from 242 cases included in the CryoVas survey. Blood. 2012;119(25):5996-6004.
22. Hoffman GS, Kerr GS, Leavitt RY, Hallahan CW, Lebovics RS, Travis WD, et al. Wegener granulomatosis: an analysis of 158 patients. Annals of internal medicine. 1992;116(6):488-98.
23. Vaglio A, Buzio C, Zwerina J. Eosinophilic granulomatosis with polyangiitis (Churg–Strauss): state of the art. Allergy. 2013;68(3):261-73.
24. Lhote F, Cohen P, Guillevin L. Polyarteritis nodosa, microscopic polyangiitis and Churg–Strauss syndrome. Lupus. 1998;7(4):238-58.
25. Li J, Li C, Li J. Thoracic manifestation of Wegener's granulomatosis: Computed tomography findings and analysis of misdiagnosis. Exp Ther Med. 2018;16(1):413-9.
26. David C, Jachiet M, de Chambrun MP, Gamez AS, Mehdaoui A, Zenone T, et al. Chronic obstructive pulmonary disease associated with hypocomplementemic urticarial vasculitis. J Allergy Clin Immunol. 2020;8(9):3222-4.
27. Lai HC. Henoch-Schönlein purpura with intussusception: a case report. Pediatr Neonatol. 2010;51(1):65-7.
28. Ebert EC. Gastrointestinal manifestations of Henoch-Schonlein purpura. Digest Dis Sci. 2008;53(8):2011-9.
29. Stone JH. Polyarteritis nodosa. JAMA. 2002;288(13):1632-9.
30. Pagnoux C, Mahr A, Cohen P, Guillevin L. Presentation and outcome of gastrointestinal involvement in systemic necrotizing vasculitides: analysis of 62 patients with polyarteritis nodosa, microscopic polyangiitis, Wegener granulomatosis, Churg-Strauss syndrome, or rheumatoid arthritis-associated vasculitis. Medicine (Baltimore). 2005;84(2):115-28.
31. Cattaneo L, Chierici E, Pavone L, Grasselli C, Manganelli P, Buzio C, et al. Peripheral neuropathy in Wegener's granulomatosis, Churg–Strauss syndrome and microscopic polyangiitis. J Neurol Neurosurg Psychiatr. 2007;78(10):1119-23.
32. Nishino H, Rubino FA, DeRemee RA, Swanson JW, Parisi JE. Neurological involvement in Wegener's granulomatosis: an analysis of 324 consecutive patients at the Mayo Clinic. Ann Neurol. 1993;33(1):4-9.
33. Abdou NI, Kullman GJ, Hoffman GS, Sharp GC, Specks U, McDonald T, et al. Wegener's granulomatosis: survey of 701 patients in North America. Changes in outcome in the 1990s. J Rheumatol. 2002;29(2):309-16.
34. Davis MD, Brewer JD. Urticarial vasculitis and hypocomplementemic urticarial vasculitis syndrome. Immunol Allergy Clin North Am. 2004;24(2):183-213,
35. Tsunoda K, Akaogi J, Ohya N, Murofushi T. Sensorineural hearing loss as the initial manifestation of polyarteritis nodosa. J Laryngol Otol. 2001;115(4):311-2.
36. Aydogan K, Karadogan SK, Adim SB, Tunali S. Hypocomplementemic urticarial vasculitis: a rare presentation of systemic lupus erythematosus. Int J Dermatol. 2006;45(9):1057-61.

37. Chen JY, Mao JH. Henoch-Schönlein purpura nephritis in children: incidence, pathogenesis and management. World J Pediatr. 2015;11(1):29-34.
38. Siomou E, Serbis A, Salakos C, Papadopoulou F, Stefanidis CJ, Siamopoulou A. Masked severe stenosing ureteritis: a rare complication of Henoch-Schönlein purpura. Pediatr Nephrol. 2008;23(5):821-5.
39. Hughes LB, Bridges SL Jr. Polyarteritis nodosa and microscopic polyangiitis: etiologic and diagnostic considerations. Curr Rheumatol Rep. 2002;4(1):75-82.
40. Clark WR, Kramer SA. Henoch-Schönlein purpura and the acute scrotum. J Pediatr Surg. 1986;21(11):991-2.
41. Terrier B, Karras A, Kahn JE, Le Guenno G, Marie I, Benarous L, et al. The spectrum of type I cryoglobulinemia vasculitis: new insights based on 64 cases. Medicine (Baltimore). 2013;92(2):61-8.
42. Handlers JP, Waterman J, Abrams AM, Melrose RJ. Oral Features of Wegener's Granulomatosis. Arch Otolaryngol. 1985;111(4):267-70.
43. Ashfaq AM, Alon S, Vazquez-Lopez F, García-García B, Sanchez-Martin J, Argenziano G. Dermoscopic patterns of purpuric lesions. Arch Dermatol. 2010;146(8):938.
44. Ortiz-Sanjuán F, Blanco R, Hernández JL, Pina T, González-Vela MC, Fernández-Llaca H, et al. Drug-associated cutaneous vasculitis: study of 239 patients from a single referral center. J Rheumatol. 2014;41(11):2201-7.
45. Nishikawa J, Hosokawa A, Akashi M, Mihara H, Nanjo S, Yoshita H, et al. IgA vasculitis associated with anti-TNF-α inhibitors in a patient with Crohn's disease. Nihon Shokakibyo Gakkai Zasshi. 2015;112(10):1852-7.
46. Rolle AS, Zimmermann B, Poon SH. Etanercept-induced Henoch-Schönlein purpura in a patient with ankylosing spondylitis. J Clin Rheumatol. 2013;19(2):90-3.
47. Guillemois S, Patsouris A, Peyraga G, Chassain K, Le Corre Y, Campone M, et al. Cutaneous and gastrointestinal leukocytoclastic vasculitis induced by palbociclib in a metastatic breast cancer patient: A case report. Clin Breast Cancer. 2018;18:e755-8.
48. Lee JY, Chung JH, Lee YJ, Park SS, Kim SY, Koo HK, et al. Propylthiouracil-induced nonspecific interstitial pneumonia. Chest. 2011;139(3):687-90.
49. Koike KJ, Blice JP, Kylstra JA, Ralston JS, Self SE, Ruth NM, et al. Frosted branch angiitis in methimazole-induced antineutrophil cytoplasmic antibody-positive vasculitis. Retin Cases Brief Rep. 2018;12(2):136-9.
50. Kumar B, Strouse J, Swee M, Lenert P, Suneja M. Hydralazine-associated vasculitis: Overlapping features of drug-induced lupus and vasculitis. Semin Arthritis Rheum. 2018;48(2):283-7.
51. Chang A, Osterloh J, Thomas J. Levamisole: a dangerous new cocaine adulterant. Clin Pharmacol Ther. 2010;88(3):408-11.
52. Trimarchi M, Gregorini G, Facchetti F, Morassi ML, Manfredini C, Maroldi R, et al. Cocaine-induced midline destructive lesions: clinical, radiographic, histopathologic, and serologic features and their differentiation from Wegener granulomatosis. Medicine (Baltimore). 2001;80(6):391-404.
53. McGrath MM, Isakova T, Rennke HG, Mottola AM, Laliberte KA, Niles JL. Contaminated cocaine and antineutrophil cytoplasmic antibody-associated disease. Clin J Am Soc Nephrol. 2011;6(12):2799-805.
54. Chen KR, Carlson JA. Clinical approach to cutaneous vasculitis. Am J Clin Dermatol. 2008;9(2):71-92.
55. Carlson JA. The histological assessment of cutaneous vasculitis. Histopathology. 2010;56(1):3-23.
56. Ricotti C, Kowalczyk JP, Ghersi M, Nousari CH. The diagnostic yield of histopathologic sampling techniques in PAN-associated cutaneous ulcers. Arch Dermatol. 2007;143(10):1331-44.
57. Magro CM, Crowson AN. A clinical and histologic study of 37 cases of immunoglobulin A-associated vasculitis. Am J Dermatopathol. 1999;21(3):234-40.
58. Buck A, Christensen J, McCarty M. Hypocomplementemic urticarial vasculitis syndrome: a case report and literature review. J Clin Aesthetic Dermatol. 2012;5(1):36.
59. De Vita S, Soldano F, Isola M, Monti G, Gabrielli A, Tzioufas A, et al. Preliminary classification criteria for the cryoglobulinaemic vasculitis. Ann Rheum Dis. 2011;70(7):1183-90.
60. Kazandjieva J, Antonov D, Kamarashev J, Tsankov N. Acrally distributed dermatoses: Vascular dermatoses (purpura and vasculitis). Clin Dermatol. 2017;35(1):68-80.
61. Leavitt RY, Fauci AS, Bloch DA, Michel BA, Hunder GG, Arend WP, et al. The American College of Rheumatology 1990 criteria for the classification of Wegener's granulomatosis. Arthritis Rheum. 1990;33:1101-7.
62. Brons RH, de Jong MC, de Boer NK, Stegeman CA, Kallenberg CG, Tervaert JW. Detection of immune deposits in skin lesions of patients with Wegener's granulomatosis. Ann Rheum Dis. 2001;60(12):1097-102.
63. Chhabra S, Minz RW, Rani L, Sharma N, Sakhuja V, Sharma A. Immune deposits in cutaneous lesions of Wegener's granulomatosis: Predictor of an active disease. Indian J Dermatol. 2011;56(6):758.
64. Finkielman JD, Lee AS, Hummel AM, Viss MA, Jacob GL, Homburger HA, et al. ANCA are detectable in nearly all patients with active severe Wegener's granulomatosis. Am J Med. 2007;120(7):643-e9.
65. Watts R, Lane S, Hanslik T, Hauser T, Hellmich B, Koldingsnes W, et al. Development and validation of a consensus methodology for the classification of the ANCA-associated vasculitides and polyarteritis nodosa for epidemiological studies. Ann Rheum Dis. 2007;66(2):222-7.
66. Robson J, Grayson P, Ponte C, Suppiah R, Craven A, Khalid S, et al. 110. Classification criteria for the ANCA-associated vasculitides. Rheumatology. 2019;58(Suppl 2): kez058-050.
67. Guillevin L, Lhote F. Polyarteritis nodosa and microscopic polyangiitis. Clin Exp Immunol. 1995;101(Suppl 1):22.
68. Jennette JC. Implications for pathogenesis of patterns of injury in small- and medium-sized vessel vasculitis. Clevel Clin J Med. 2002;69:SII33-8.
69. Guillevin L, Mahr A, Callard P, Godmer P, Pagnoux C, Leray E, et al. Hepatitis B virus-associated polyarteritis nodosa: clinical characteristics, outcome, and impact of treatment in 115 patients. Medicine (Baltimore). 2005;84(5):313-22.

APPROACH TO A PATIENT WITH NONPALPABLE PURPURA

Bhavin Ashokbhai Shah

INTRODUCTION

Bleeding, either gross or extravasation occurs chiefly via the following possible mechanisms: trauma and physical disruption or hemostatic failure; neither is necessarily exclusive.

Sudden hemorrhage due to macrovascular disruption often presents with shock and pain. While, in microvascular disruption, extravasated blood presents characteristically as petechiae and purpura. The presence of both shock and purpura is a strong pointer of an infectious etiology.

According to a study, up to 65% and 25% of healthy women and men respectively report that they bruise easily,[1] which actually is mild day-to-day traumatic purpura. Characteristically, (1) they are never true (i.e., palpable) hematomas, (2) <4–6 in number, and (3) <3 centimeters in size.

Petechiae are pinpoint lesions usually <3 mm in diameter with sharply demarcated margins. They soon fade to a salmon color in a few days, becoming less demarcated, and then finally become brownish spots caused by retention of hemosiderin from extravasated blood.

Ecchymosis refers to large extravasations that result from coalescence of separate petechial lesions or, more commonly, a bleed from a slightly larger vessel. **Table 8** shows pathophysiologic categories of purpura.

Table 8: Pathophysiologic categories of purpura.	
Benign causes	**Pathological causes**
Mechanical purpura	*Platelet abnormalities*: Immune thrombocytopenia, platelet functional abnormalities
Factitious/psychogenic purpura	*Microbial endothelial damage*: Viral hemorrhagic fever
Senile purpura	*Microthrombus related*: Disseminated intravascular coagulopathy, thrombotic thrombocytopenic purpura, heparin-induced thrombocytopenia, Warfarin-induced skin necrosis, fat embolism syndrome, and leukostasis
Purpura simplex	Amyloidosis
Bruises and hematoma: Post-traumatic	Vasculitis

NONHEMATOLOGICAL CAUSES OF PURPURA

Mechanical Purpura

Any pressure that exceeds the finite mechanical strength of vessels/capillaries (e.g., vacuum of 200 mm Hg)[2,3] could well lead to extravasation of red cells. Petechiae on the face and neck may result from increased venous pressure after vomiting,[4] seizures, or even from prolonged hanging upside down by.[5] Purpura on the palms and soles could be due to leisure activities such as weight-lifting, from traumatic blows.[6] Petechiae could be a result of choking,[7] asphyxiation,[8] seizure,[9] barotrauma,[10] and electrocution[11] and may be seen on normal infants.[12] So, history remains of gold standard in such scenarios.

Factitious/Psychogenic Purpura[13,14]

History that is vague or not credible, when the patient has been seen repeatedly by multiple physicians but no hemostatic or underlying medical conditions can be found on investigating are soft pointers toward factitious purpura.

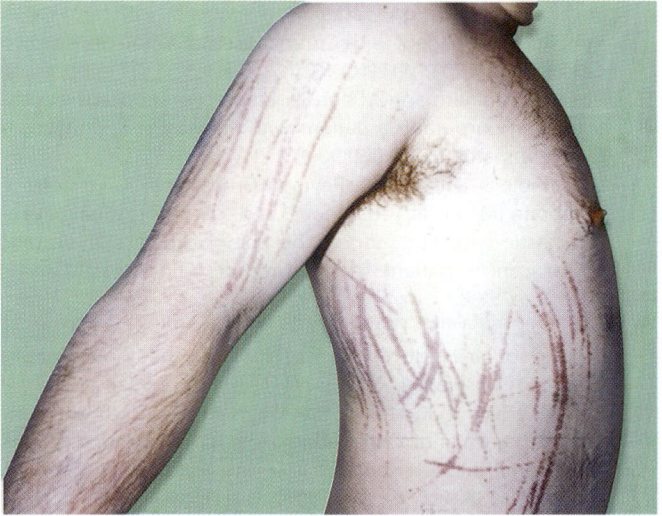

FIG. 14: Factitious purpura: These long linear lesions with very sharply demarcated borders appear only in places that the patient can reach.

Usually, the lesions are well circumscribed and are found chiefly on accessible areas **(Fig. 14)**. Characteristically, factitious purpuric lesions may come and go without an easy explanation; long "remissions" may occur.

"Senile," "Atrophic," or "Actinic" Purpura

Senile purpura is most encountered purpuric condition in dermatology outpatient department (OPD). Apart from older and debilitated patients, any extremely ill patient who

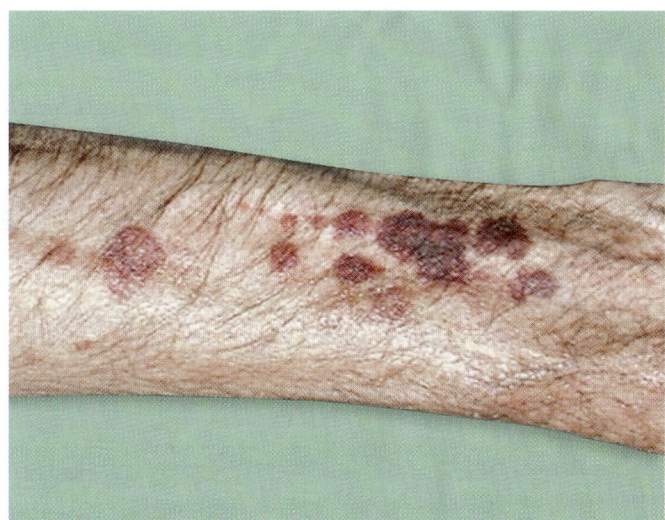

FIG. 15: Senile purpura: Older patient with extremely thin skin with purpura on extensor surface of forearm.

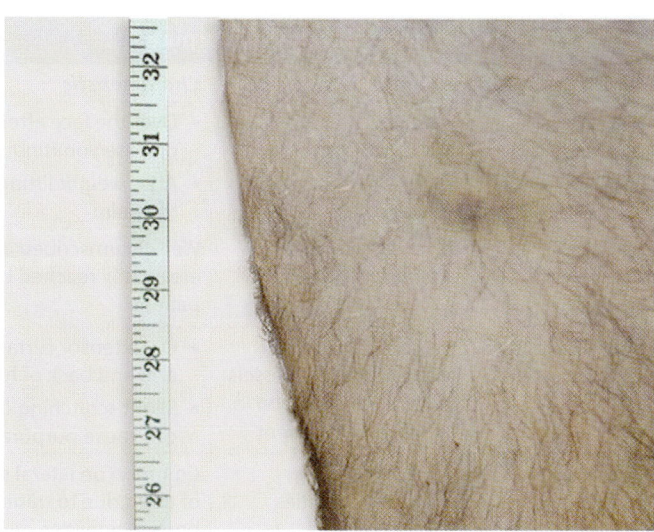

FIG. 16: Purpura simplex: Simple bruise due to day-to-day trauma. Such bruises are caused by encounters with objects on a daily basis. As shown, these lesions occur on the external surface of the thigh and are typically 30 inches above the ground.

exhibits weight loss and negative nitrogen balance, and even healthy patients who have excessive solar exposure, are also likely to get these lesions. Extensor surfaces of the forearms are characteristic sites of this purpura, particularly in those who work outdoors with short or no sleeves. Usually, the skin appears extremely thin **(Fig. 15)** and atrophic epidermis and dermis on histopathology. So, even the slightest trauma or stretching causes this entity, no specific treatment is available.

Purpura Simplex

This refers to small bruises that are associated with trauma of daily living occurring in healthy individuals. Women report bruising more frequently than men.[1] **Figure 16** shows an ecchymotic area on the lateral surface of the thigh. It is striking that these bruises appear on body parts that are approximately 30 inches above the floor—the height of most furniture, cabinets, and tables. Purpura simplex may result from being pinched; and is known as "devil's pinches" if one has no recall of being pinched. Such patients may safely undergo surgery or invasive procedures.

Bruises and Hematomas

Bruises (including purpura simplex) are not palpable. Bruises result from trauma but of course can be exacerbated by platelet or coagulation defects to become larger bruises or even true hematomas. Simple bruises are usually <3 cm in diameter and not palpable, and no more than four to six over the body. "Normal bruising" has been quantified in healthy infants up to four bruises up to 10-mm maximum diameter. Such bruises tend to occur over bony prominences and increase in frequency as the child's mobility increases.[15] Bruises not confined to bony prominences or in unusual places (soles or palms) may raise questions of abuse. If

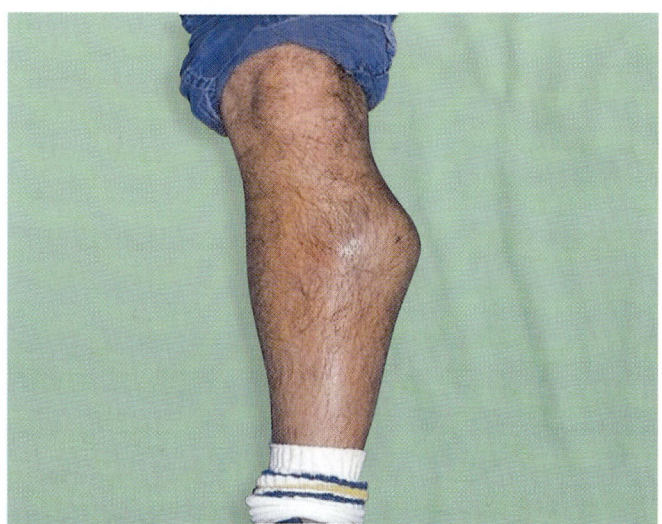

FIG. 17: Hematoma in patient with hemophilia.

bruises are larger and more numerous, consideration may be given to a hemostatic defect, especially if the masses are palpable **(Fig. 17)** (i.e., true hematomas).

Table 9 shows major differentiating points among purpura due to nonhematological causes.

PURPURA ASSOCIATED WITH HEMATOLOGICAL DISORDERS

Amyloidosis

Purpuric bleeding was detected in 15% of all cases and it could be a very initial finding leading to a diagnosis.[16]

Table 9: Nonhematological causes of purpura.				
Types of purpura	Etiology	Characteristic	Diagnosis	Treatment
Mechanical purpura	Increased pressure leads to extravasation of red blood cells	• Over the face after profuse vomiting • After weight lifting on the palm	History of activities prior to purpura	No specific treatment required. Purpura subsides after 7–10 days
Factitious/Psychogenic purpura	Psychological issue or attention sickness	Well circumscribed and on area easily reached by the patient	• No underlying hemostatic issue • Psychological issues	Psychiatric treatment
Senile purpura	Loss of subcutaneous tissue makes the vessels very fragile, common in elderly and ill patient	• On extensor surface of arm and back of hand • Slight scratching on skin can cause purpura	• Clinical diagnosis • No hemostatic abnormality	No specific treatment required
Purpura simplex	• Trauma during routine activities • Nonpathological purpura	Common on lateral surface of thigh due to trauma in normal activities	• Clinical diagnosis • No hemostatic abnormality	No specific treatment required
Bruises/Hematoma	Post-traumatic, usually exacerbated with platelet or coagulation disorders	• Nonpalpable and flat • Simple bruise <3 cm and less than 4–6 in numbers • In hemostatic defect or platelet disorder, hematoma can be elevated, >3 cm	• Simple bruise—normal coagulation parameters • Hematoma—coagulation parameters can be altered (platelet counts low/functional defect, PT, aPTT, or fibrinogen deranged)	• Simple bruise: No treatment • Hematoma: Supplement abnormal parameter, like platelet-rich concentrate, or specific factors such as VIII and IX. Antifibrinolytic agent such as tranexamic acid

(aPTT: activated partial thromboplastin time; PT: prothrombin time)

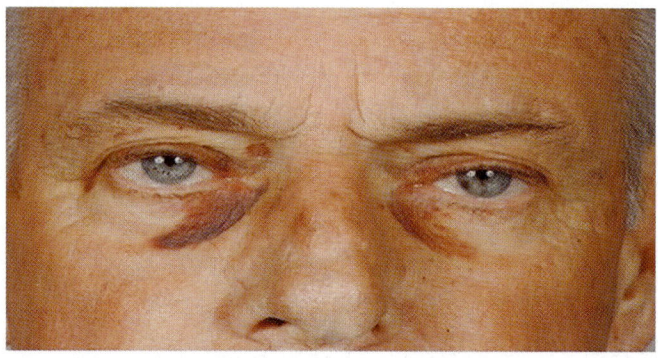

FIG. 18: Periorbital purpura in case of amyloidosis.

Amyloid material gets deposited between the endothelium and the basement membrane, and, therefore, can be found in any organ. Amyloid leads to probable increased capillary fragility and impedes the ability to constrict, thereby failing to limit regional flow and bleeding from injured vessels. Coagulation abnormalities are frequent, multiple, and of varying patterns in amyloidosis,[17] which may confuse the clinician about the true cause of the purpura, which is the deposition of amyloid. Characteristically the distribution of purpura is somewhat unusual and more likely to occur along pressure points, with a peculiar periorbital predilection **(Fig. 18)**.

PURPURA ASSOCIATED WITH ABNORMALITIES OF PLATELETS

Thrombocytopenic purpura results most commonly from mild trauma but may also be found in patients with qualitative platelet defects.

Thrombocytopenic Purpura

Sudden, spontaneous petechial hemorrhage is the clinical hallmark of acute idiopathic thrombocytopenic purpura. Epistaxis is also a common finding in thrombocytopenia (<10,000/dL). Ecchymosis can occur even in absence of trauma. Platelets repair the defect/leak through adhesion to disrupted endothelium and subendothelial tissues with subsequent aggregation.[18]

PURPURA ASSOCIATED WITH ABNORMAL PLATELET FUNCTION

When platelets function are impaired even with sufficient in number, patient may present with bleeding, which usually manifest as purpura or epistaxis. Theoretically, this can be seen with antiplatelet agents, which are being increasingly used in the treatment of patients with ischemic heart disease or stroke.[19] Congenital defects of platelet function that cause purpura are such as Bernard–Soulier syndrome or Glanzmann thrombasthenia.

PURPURA ASSOCIATED WITH MICROBIAL ENDOTHELIAL DAMAGE

Viral Hemorrhagic Fevers

Certain viruses have been implicated in destroying endothelial cells, which result in various hemorrhagic fevers. Although bleeding could be due to thrombocytopenia or even disseminated intravascular coagulation, petechial manifestations of these hemorrhagic fevers are believed to represent endothelial damage caused by direct invasion and destruction by virus. The common hemorrhagic fevers include dengue and yellow fever. The mortality rate of these diseases varies from rather low to extremely high.[20] A periodically discovered and rediscovered hemorrhagic fever with a mortality rate as high as 90% is Ebola hemorrhagic fever, which directly causes endothelial cell damage.[21] Hemorrhage in all these disorders not only is cutaneous in the way of purpura but also involves multiple organs, the dysfunction of which results from hemorrhage and ultimately causes death. Unfortunately, treatment is currently nonexistent. If any of these viral hemorrhagic diseases is seriously considered in the differential diagnosis, especially in persons who have recently been abroad, rapid consultation with infectious disease experts is mandatory.[22]

PURPURA ASSOCIATED WITH MICROTHROMBI

Microthrombi obstructing microcirculation in dermis may result in microinfarction and disruption of endothelial membrane resulting in extravasation of red blood cells (RBCs). In its most expressive form, the process is called *purpura fulminans*. When microthrombi involve multiple organs, end-organ damage may occur, leading to multiorgan dysfunction syndrome (MODS).

DISSEMINATED INTRAVASCULAR COAGULATION

Occlusive deposition of fibrin, particularly in the microcirculation, leads to this life-threatening condition due to various etiological factors. Clinically, it manifests as purpuric skin lesions and frank purpura fulminans. One of the foremost causes of the latter is meningococcemia, which results in characteristic rapidly progressive necrotizing purpura fulminans **(Fig. 19)**. Morbidity and mortality in

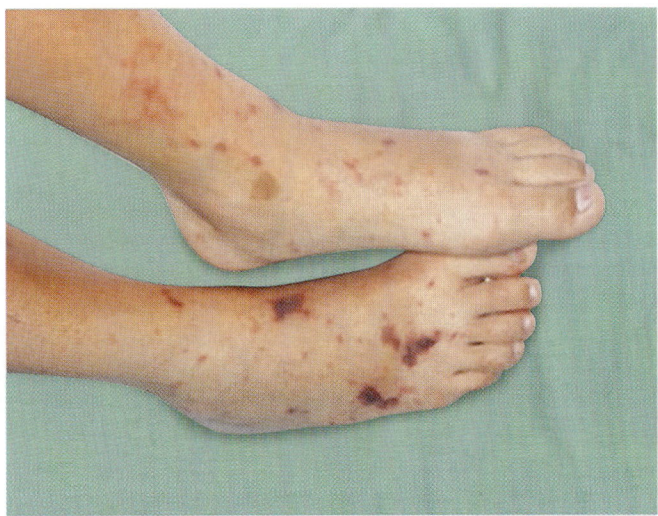

FIG. 19: Disseminated intravascular coagulopathy.

purpura fulminans are high (~50%) because of multiorgan involvement.[23,24] Purpura fulminans of postinfectious etiology is greatly accelerated by any asplenic state.[25]

WARFARIN SKIN NECROSIS

This is a special cause of fibrin deposition that appears limited to the dermal microcirculation.[26] It is now believed to be due to drop in levels of protein C because of warfarin. The half-life of protein C is only 4–5 hours; which is why it results in early hypercoagulable state. In case of genetic deficiency of protein C or consumption in thrombotic stage, warfarin could further decrease its level resulting in localized hypercoagulable stage resulting in necrosis. Because protein S is the cofactor of protein C, congenital or acquired protein S deficiency is also a risk factor for warfarin skin necrosis.

Due to some unknown reasons, women are more frequently affected (9:1 ratio) and it usually occurs in areas with generous adipose tissue, such as the thighs, buttocks, or breasts **(Fig. 20)**. Stinging or burning sensation approximately 2–4 days after the initiation of warfarin therapy is the first symptom. The site becomes hemorrhagic a day or 2 later. If it is not recognized and treated at this stage, the site becomes necrotic and requires subsequent skin grafting. On biopsy, fibrin deposition is prominent in the microcirculation. As loading dose (1 mg/kg) is not used frequently and patients are first treated by other rapidly acting anticoagulants, now it is rarely seen. One can start with a dose that approximates the estimated maintenance dose to prevent or decrease its occurrence. If the diagnosis of warfarin skin necrosis is entertained, prompt initiation of heparin therapy and cessation of warfarin and intravenous vitamin K are considered the best treatment.

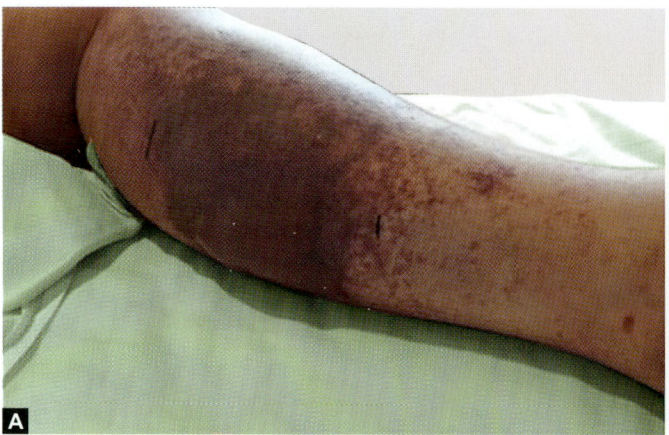
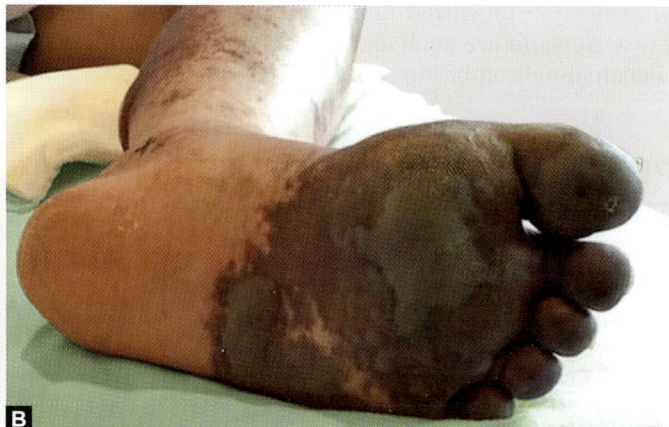

FIGS. 20A AND B: Warfarin-induced skin necrosis.

FAT EMBOLISM SYNDROME

Characteristically, the petechiae in this entity are distributed around the neck, shoulders, and especially the axillary folds in the upper chest area. They can be observed occasionally on the conjunctivae. It is believed that this distribution may be because these are counter-dependent areas of the body. So, circulating fat particles may rise and embolize in this pattern. These petechiae rarely represent a problem, but their presence may serve for diagnosing fat embolism syndrome.[27]

Fat embolization can be encountered as a result of bone marrow necrosis in patients with hemoglobinopathies.[28] Fat embolism may also be seen after liposuction or after fracture of major bones and blunt trauma.[29]

Along with characteristic distribution of petechiae, shortness of breath and hypoxia are seen in 50% of patients; the shortness of breath is ironically worse on sitting up and improves in recumbency and hypoxia is worse on standing up, a situation referred to as platypnea–orthodeoxia.[30] 30% of patients experience confusion or coma. Retinal changes may occur, and platelet count may drop lightly in 50% of cases. Fever is characteristic, and diagnosis hinges on recognition of the probability of this syndrome. Symptoms may occur as late as 24–72 hours after the traumatic event.[31]

LEUKOSTASIS

Leukostasis is seen with a large number of circulating myeloblasts and promyelocytes, for example, in acute myeloid leukemia, acute promyelocytic leukemia, or blast crisis of chronic myeloid leukemia. These large malignant myeloid cells may embolize within the dermal microcirculation and cause infarctive lesions that are far in excess of the degree of thrombocytopenia that may accompany leukemia and its treatment. When it involves cerebral and pulmonary capillary beds, patient presents with central nervous system dysfunction and hypoxia.[32] The therapy is cytoreduction of malignant cells.

THROMBOTIC THROMBOCYTOPENIC PURPURA

It is a type of microangiopathic hemolytic anemia characterized by pentad–microangiopathic hemolytic anemia (Coombs' negative), thrombocytopenia, fever, renal dysfunction, and neurologic dysfunction. Although very less in number, petechial, purpuric, and infarctive lesions are occasionally present, and are overshadowed by other manifestations of this disorder.

HEPARIN-INDUCED THROMBOCYTOPENIA WITH THROMBOSIS

Ischemia of the extremities in patients who have received or are receiving heparin and in those who have become thrombocytopenic should alert the clinician to this possibility.

Table 10 shows salient differentiating points among hematological causes of purpura.

CONSULTATION POINTS TO PONDER

In hospitalized patients with purpura, high probabilities exist for cutaneous vasculitis, DIC, thrombocytopenia due to viral infection, and heparin-induced thrombocytopenia (HIT). In healthy ambulatory patients, the most commonly encountered processes are senile purpura, purpura simplex, immune thrombocytopenic purpura, cutaneous vasculitis, and factitious purpura.

Table 10: Hematological disorders associated with purpura.				
Disorder	**Etiology**	**Characteristic**	**Diagnosis**	**Treatment**
Amyloidosis	Due to amyloid deposit in blood vessels, there is a increase capillary fragility which impair the vasoconstriction	Purpura along pressure points with peculiar periorbital predilection	Histopathological diagnosis, monoclonal band on protein electrophoresis, altered serum-free light chain ratio	• *AL amyloidosis*: Treat with chemotherapy • *AA amyloidosis*: No specific treatment available
Immune thrombocytopenic purpura	Low platelet counts due to immune destruction	Spontaneous petechial hemorrhage more on dependent part	Low platelet count usually < 10,000/mm^3 with normal white blood cells and differential counts	Prednisolone, immunoglobulin, rituximab, thrombopoietin-stimulating agents, and splenectomy
Platelet function disorder (Glanzmann thrombocythemia, Bernard–Soulier syndrome)	Qualitative platelet dysfunction	Purpura, menorrhagia since menarche, epistaxis	Platelet functional studies abnormalities	Platelet-rich concentrate, antifibrinolytic agent
Viral hemorrhagic fever (dengue hemorrhagic fever)	Vascular endothelial damage, immune destruction	Petechiae due to low-platelet count, occasional mucosal bleed	Viral antigen and antibody study, PCR for specific viral infection	Supportive treatment, hydration, antipyretic, blood component if bleeding
Disseminated intravascular coagulopathy (DIC)	Occlusion of fibrin in microcirculation leads to consumptive coagulopathy and organ dysfunction	Sick patient with purpuric skin lesions, occasionally purpura fulminans	Low-platelet count and fibrinogen with altered PT, aPTT and raised FDP (fibrinogen degradation product)	• Treat the cause. • Antibiotics, blood component therapy • Role of heparin is controversial
Warfarin skin necrosis	Due to protein C or S deficiency, sudden onset of hypercoagulable state	Usually after 2–4 days of starting Warfarin, more common in female Skin necrosis is more common with high adipose tissue such as thigh, buttocks, or breast	Low protein S or C level	• Stop warfarin • Start heparin • Vitamin K supplement can be given
Fat embolism syndrome	Fat particles in circulation and embolize in microcirculation	• Purpura around neck, shoulder, and axilla • Conjunctiva is common site	Post-trauma or fracture, liposuction, hemoglobinopathies are precipitating factors. Platypnea–orthodeoxia is commonly found	• Supportive treatment • Hydration, oxygenation, and DVT prophylaxis
Leukostasis	Hyperviscosity due to very high WBC count or high number of blast cells	• Dermal microcirculation blockage leads to infarct • Associated hypoxia/neurological symptoms	High WBC count. Common with acute myeloid leukemia, CML with blast crisis or acute promyelocytic leukemia	Hydration, leukapheresis, treatment of underlying leukemia
Thrombotic thrombocytopenic purpura	Von Willebrand factor-rich microthrombi affecting vessels	Bleeding is uncommon. Thrombus is more common	• Schistocytes in peripheral smear, low-platelet count, anemia • ADAMTS-13 deficiency	Plasma exchange, steroids, rituximab
Heparin-induced thrombocytopenia (HIT)	Formation of antibodies after heparin usage that activates the platelet and forms thrombus	Petechiae are very rare, thrombosis is more common at extremities	• PF4 antibodies present • Thrombocytopenia • Previous history of heparin usage	Direct thrombin inhibitors such as lepirudin and fondaparinux

(aPTT: activated partial thromboplastin time; PCR: polymerase chain reaction; PT: prothrombin time)

Table 11: Clues in distribution.

Areas involved	Disease to be suspected
Head and face	Postictal petechiae, petechiae secondary to fat embolization, and the purpura associated with amyloidosis
Gum bleeding	Scurvy
Body and trunk ecchymoses and purpura	Hemophilia, factor VIII inhibitors, concomitant anticoagulant use, amyloidosis, and even purpura simplex, especially when the patient's activities involve leaning over and bearing weight on the lower ribcage
Dependent purpura	Acute and chronic ITP and cutaneous vasculitis
Painful acral purpuric lesions	Indicative of ischemia from emboli such as those seen in subacute bacterial endocarditis, cholesterol embolization, or cardioembolization from atrial myxoma or nonbacterial thrombotic emboli (marantic endocarditis)[33]
Nearly mirror image, symmetrical involvement of the legs and trunk in the palpable purpura	HSP
High degree of asymmetry	Factitious process

(HSP: Henoch–Schönlein purpura; ITP: immune thrombocytopenic purpura)

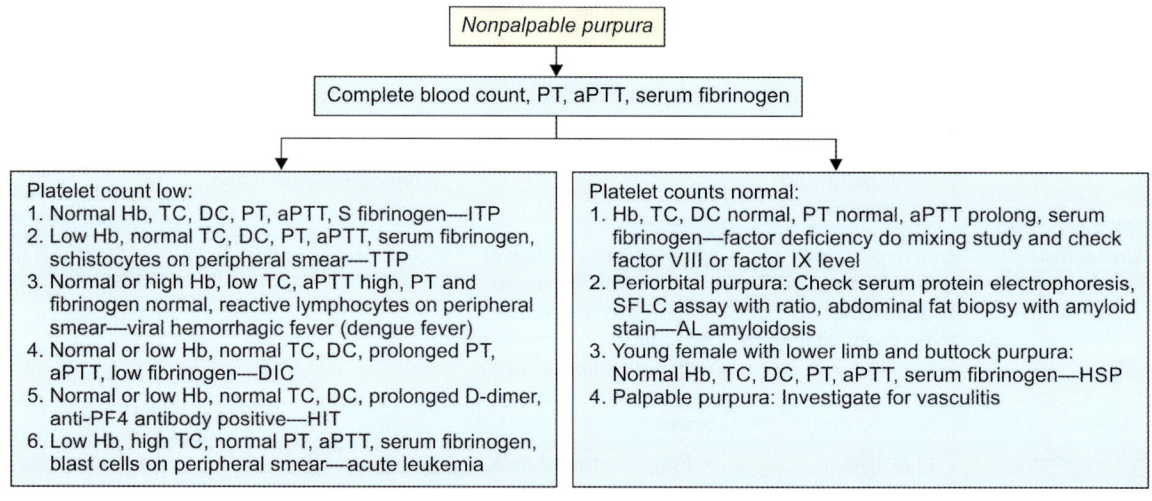

FLOWCHART 3: Approach and interpretation to laboratory investigations in cases of nonpalpable purpura.

(aPTT: activated partial thromboplastin time; DC: differential WBC count; Hb: hemoglobin; HIT: heparin-induced thrombocytopenia; HSP: Henoch–Schönlein purpura; ITP: immune thrombocytopenic purpura; PT: prothrombin time; SFLC assay: serum free light chain assay; TC: total WBC count; TTP: thrombotic thrombocytopenic purpura)

Clues exist in the distribution of purpura **(Table 11)**. Acute-onset purpura generally has a worse prognosis than chronic purpura, and hence rapid evaluate should be done to rule out infectious causes, DIC, cholesterol embolism, and other catastrophic processes such as TTP and DIC in the microthrombotic category.

LABORATORY EVALUATION

In patient with purpura, complete blood count (CBC) with a platelet count and differential white cell count, as well as a prothrombin time and a partial thromboplastin time should be used for screening purposes.

The bleeding time or platelet function assay (PFA) is normal, except in qualitative and quantitative platelet disorders. Normal bleeding time is consistent with the fact that other purpuric disorders do not primarily interfere with platelet-endothelial interaction, as is tested by bleeding time.

Skin biopsy is frequently helpful and is usually ordered in collaboration with a dermatologist.

After a complete history and physical examination, the following laboratory investigations should be considered:
- *Always*:
  - Complete blood count and review of blood smear
  - Activated partial thromboplastin time (aPTT) and prothrombin time (PT)

Additional tests to be considered if diagnosis not apparent:
- Thrombin time
- Fibrinogen level
- Analyses for fibrin degradation products and D-dimers

Additional tests to be considered in cases of cutaneous vasculitis:
Refer to part: Approach to a Patient with Palpable Purpura of this chapter.

Additional tests to be considered in obscure cases:
- Blood cultures
- Viral studies
- Bone marrow aspirate/biopsy

Flowchart 3 shows approach and interpretation to laboratory investigations in cases of nonpalpable purpura.

REFERENCES

1. Lackner H, Karpatkin S. On the "easy bruising" syndrome with normal platelet count. Ann Intern Med. 1975;83:190-6.
2. Elliott RHE. The suction test for capillary resistance in thrombocytopenic purpura. JAMA. 1938;110:1177-9.
3. Urkin J, Katz M. Suction purpura. Isr Med Assoc J. 2000;2:711.
4. Kaliyadan F, Kuruvilla JP. Post-vomiting purpura. Indian Dermatol Online J. 2016;7:456-7.
5. Friberg TR, Weinreb RN. Ocular manifestations of gravity inversion. JAMA. 1985;253:1755-7.
6. Rashkovsky I, Safadi R, Zlotogorski A. Black palmar macules: Palmar petechiae ("black palm"). Arch Dermatol. 1998;134:1020, 1023-4.
7. Ely SF, Hirsch CS. Asphyxial deaths and petechiae: A review. J Forensic Sci. 2000;45:1274-7.
8. Maxeiner H. Congestion bleedings of the face and cardiopulmonary resuscitation: An attempt to evaluate their relationship. Forensic Sci Int. 2001;117:191-8.
9. Grunfeld J, Klein C. Seizure-induced purpura: A rare but useful clue. Isr Med Assoc J. 2001;3:779.
10. Mader C. Barotrauma in diving. Wien Med Wochenschr. 1999;151:126-30.
11. Karger B, Suggeler O, Brinkmann B. Electrocution: Autopsy study with emphasis on "electrical petechiae." Forensic Sci Int. 2002;23:210-3,126.
12. Downes AJ, Crossland DS, Mellon AF. Prevalence and distribution of petechiae in well babies. Arch Dis Child. 2002;86:291-2.
13. Yucel B, Kiziltan E, Aktan M. Dissociative identity disorder presenting with psychogenic purpura. Psychosomatics. 2000;41:279-81.
14. Sarkar S, Ghosh SK, Bandyopadhyay D, Nath S. Psychogenic purpura. Indian J Psychiatry. 2013;55:192-4.
15. Carpenter RF. The prevalence and distribution of bruising in babies. Arch Dis Child. 1999;80:363-6.
16. Gertz MA, Lacy MQ, Dispenzieri A. Amyloidosis. Hematol Oncol Clin North Am. 1999;13:1211-33.
17. Mumford AD, O'Donell J, Gillmore JD, Manning RA, Hawkins PN, Laffan M. Bleeding symptoms and coagulation abnormalities in 337 patients with AL-amyloidosis. Br J Haematol. 2000;110:454-60.
18. Nachman RL, Rafii S. Platelets, petechiae, and preservation of the vascular wall. N Engl J Med. 2008;359:1261-70.
19. Tsuda T, Okamoto Y, Sakaguchi R, Katayama N, Hara I, Hayashi H, et al. Purpura due to aspirin-induced platelet dysfunction aggravated by drinking alcohol. J Int Med Res. 2001;29:374-80.
20. Schnittler HJ, Feldmann H. Viral hemorrhagic fever: A vascular disease? Thromb Haemost. 2003;89:967-72.
21. Connolly BM, Steele KE, Davis KJ, Geisbert TW, Kell WM, Jaax NK, et al. Pathogenesis of experimental Ebola virus infection in guinea pigs. J Infect Dis. 1999;179(suppl1):S203-17.
22. Borio L, Inglesby T, Peters W, Schmaljohn AL, Hughes JM, Jahrling PB, et al. Hemorrhagic fever viruses as biological weapons: Medical and public health management. JAMA. 2002;287: 2391-405.
23. Faust SN, Heyderman RS, Levin M. Disseminated intravascular coagulation and purpura fulminans secondary to infection. Bailliere's Clin Haematol. 2000;13:179-97.
24. Gamper G, Oschatz E, Herkner H, Paul G, Burgmann H, Janata K, et al. Sepsis-associated purpura fulminans in adults. Wien Klin Wochenschr. 2001;113:107-12.
25. Okabayashi T, Hanazaki K. Overwhelming postsplenectomy infection syndrome in adults – a clinically preventable disease. World J Gastroenterol. 2009;14:176-9.
26. Nazarian RM, Van Cott EM, Zembowicz A, Duncan LM. Warfarin-induced skin necrosis. J Am Acad Dermatol. 2009;61:325-32.
27. Fabian TC. Unraveling the fat embolism syndrome. N Engl J Med. 1993;329:961-3.
28. Gangaraju R, Reddy VV, Marques MB. Fat embolism syndrome secondary to bone marrow necrosis in patients with hemoglobinopathies. South Med J. 2016;109:549-53.
29. Eriksson EA, Pellegrini DC, Vanderkolk WE, Minshall CT, Fakhry SM, Cohle SD. Incidence of pulmonary fat embolism at autopsy: an undiagnosed epidemic. J Trauma. 2011;71:312-5.
30. Gourgiotis S, Aloizos S, Gakis C, Salemis NS. Platypnea-orthodeoxia due to fat embolism. Int J Surg Case Rep. 2011;2:147-9.
31. Jarner J, Ampanozi G, Thali MJ, Bolliger SA. Role of survival time and injury severity in fatal pulmonary fat embolism. Am J Forensic Med Path. 2017;38:74-7.
32. McKee LC Jr, Collins RD. Intravascular leukocyte thrombi and aggregates as a cause of morbidity and mortality in leukemia. Medicine (Baltimore). 1974;53:463-78.
33. McAllister SM, Bornstein AM, Callen JP. Painful acral purpura. Arch Dermatol. 1998;134:789-91.

A Patient with Target or Targetoid Lesions

Jigna Padhiyar

DEFINITION

Target lesion: An erythema multiforme (EM) lesion with three distinct zones—a darker central area with blister/crust, a pallor edematous rim surrounding central area and an outer erythematous rim. Individual lesion is usually round and regular in shape with well-defined border and <3 cm in size **(Fig. 1)**.

Targetoid lesion: A lesion that looks like target lesion, but it is not EM.

TYPES

Classical/Typical target lesion: It is as described in definition of target lesion. The prototype of this category is EM.

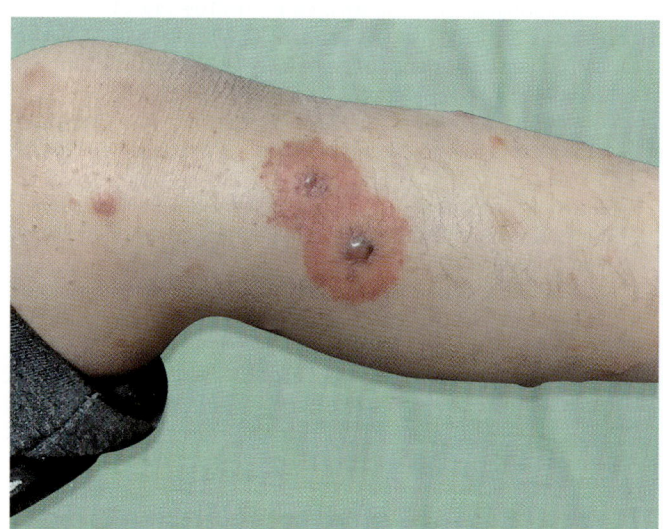

FIG. 1: Classical target lesions with three zones.

Atypical target lesion: A lesion with only two zones and/or indistinct border.

Raised/Flat: Raised lesions are defined as edematous and palpable lesions. Flat lesions might have central potential blister, but they are nonpalpable due to absence of edema. Both typical and atypical target lesions can be raised or flat as per revised classification.[1] Raised lesions suggest infective etiology while flat lesions point toward drug as culprit for the lesions.[1]

Macules with or without blister: Erythematous or purpuric macules of ill-defined size and shapes which can be confluent at places. This presentation usually suggests diagnosis toward drug reaction with few exceptions mentioned in **Table 1**.

Iris lesion: An early target lesion with central dusky and outer red zone.

Herpes iris of Bateman: A distinctive lesion sometimes noted in EM major characterized by central bulla over erythematous background surrounded by a ring of vesicles at the margin.[2]

CLASSIFICATION OF EM/SJS/TEN

According to body surface area (BSA) and mucosal involvement:

Erythema multiforme: <10% detachment of total BSA, localized symmetrical typical target or raised atypical target lesions mainly on extremities. EM minor involves only one mucous membrane in contrast to EM major which involves two or more mucous membrane along with more variability in target lesions.[3]

Stevens–Johnson syndrome (SJS): <10% detachment of total BSA, widespread erythematous or purpuric macules or

Table 1: Differential diagnosis.			
Flat (macular)	Raised (papular/plaque)		TEN (toxic epidermal necrolysis)/ TEN like (acute syndrome of apoptotic pan-epidermolysis)
	Infective	Noninfective	
Generalized bullous fixed drug eruption (GBFDE)	*Herpes viruses* (70–80%), *adenovirus*, *Cytomegalovirus, Epstein–Barr virus*, associated EM	Drug-induced EM (10%) (Antibiotics, NSAIDs, anticonvulsants, allopurinol, antifungal, etc.)	Drug-induced SJS/TEN (Antibiotics, NSAIDs, anticonvulsants, allopurinol, antifungal, etc.)
Linear IgA bullous dermatosis	*Enteroviruses, Coxsackie* viruses (hand foot mouth disease)	Serum sickness like reaction	Lupus erythematosus
Paraneoplastic pemphigus	*Mycoplasma, Borrelia*, associated EM	Urticaria multiforme	Acute graft-versus-host disease
	Human immunodeficiency virus (HIV)	Polymorphic eruptions of pregnancy	Generalized bullous fixed drug eruption
	Toxic shock syndrome	Leukocytoclastic vasculitis	Pseudoporphyria
	Legionella	Rowell's syndrome	
	Corynebacterium diphtheriae	Acute hemorrhagic edema of infancy	
	Salmonella	Sweet's syndrome	
	Chlamydia	Bullous pemphigoid and pemphigoid gestationist	
	Pneumococci	Cockade nevus	
	Congenital and secondary syphilis	Hobnail hemangioma	

(EM: erythema multiforme; IgA: immunoglobulin A; NSAIDs: nonsteroidal anti-inflammatory drugs; SJS: Stevens–Johnson syndrome)

flat atypical targets along with two or more mucosal site involvements.

Toxic epidermal necrolysis (SJS/TEN) overlap: 10–30% detachment of total BSA, widespread purpuric macules or flat atypical targets along with two or more mucosal site involvements.

TEN with spots: >30% detachment of total BSA, widespread purpuric macules or flat atypical targets along with two or more mucosal site involvements.

TEN without spots: >10% detachment of total BSA, large epidermal sheets and no purpuric macules along with two or more mucosal site involvements.

Table 1 summarizes various disorders presenting as target or targetoid lesions.

FOCUSED HISTORY POINTS

- *Age*: It can help us to narrow down the possibilities in differential diagnosis. In general, apart from drug-induced EM, urticaria multiforme (UM), mycoplasma-induced rash and mucositis (MIRM), and serum sickness-like reactions (SSLRs) are more common in children.
- *Duration and onset of lesions*: Acute versus chronicity of lesions is important in differential diagnosis, drug-induced, and infection-induced lesions are acute while other autoimmune disease associated targetoid lesions are chronic.
- *Progression of lesion*: This is summarized in **Tables 2 and 3**.
- *History of associated symptoms*: This is summarized in **Tables 2 and 3**. History of triggering factors, relieving factors, and systemic symptoms can be obtained accordingly.

EXAMINATION POINTS

- *Distribution points*: Drug-induced targetoid lesions are more on trunk compared to extremities while infection-induced are more common on extremities. Autoimmune disease associated targetoid lesions can involve any part of the body. It may be distributed on photoexposed parts in cases of polymorphous light eruption (PMLE) and connective tissue diseases.
- *Typical versus atypical lesions*: As described earlier.
- *Mucosal involvement*: Absence of involvement and number of mucosae involved is important and highlighted in **Tables 2 and 3**.
- *Involvement of total body surface area*: This important diagnostically as well as therapeutic purpose.

INVESTIGATIONS AND MANAGEMENT

These are summarized in **Tables 2 and 3** briefly.

Apart from the specific treatment mentioned in tables, fluid management is also important when larger BSA is

Table 2: Distinguished features of EM and alike conditions.

	EM	UM	AHOI	SSLR	UV	Rowell's syndrome
Age	All ages Average age range: 20–40 years	0–4 years	<24 months	All age but more in children	Adults Median age is 45 years	All age Median age is 32 years
Sex	F > M	Not known	Not known	Not known	F > M	F > M (8:1)
Prevalence	0.01–1%	Rare	Not known	Not known	0.5/100,000-person years	Not known
Etiology/Triggers	Infections (90%) Drugs and food colors (10%) Trauma, sun exposure	Infections, drugs (mainly antibiotics), vaccines	Infections, drugs, vaccines	Drugs mainly β-lactams, vaccines, infections	Idiopathic, infections, autoimmune disease, drugs, malignancy	Sunlight exposure
Pathophysiology	T-cell-mediated cytotoxic response (HSV), TNF-α-mediated tissue damage (drugs)	Histamine-mediated hypersensitivity reaction	Immune complex-mediated disease	Haptens-induced immunological response, direct toxic effect of drug metabolite	Type 3 hypersensitivity reaction	Antibody-mediated autoimmune disease
Prodromal symptoms/Associated symptoms	+/- Mild fever dysarthria, dysphonia, dysphagia	Mild fever + pruritus, facial and acral edema	Fever, facial and acral edema	High-grade fever, myalgia, soreness, burning, lymphadenopathy, arthralgia	Variable fever, facial and acral edema, arthralgia, pain, or burning	Mild fever, photosensitivity
Onset	2–3 days	1–3 days	1–3 days	7–10 days	Weeks to months	Weeks to months
Duration of individual lesion	Days to weeks	<24 hours	Few days	Days to weeks	Days to weeks	Days to weeks
Total duration of disease	2–3 weeks	2–12 days	Days to weeks	1 to 6 week	1 to 6 weeks	Weeks
Progress	Maculopapular → color change in center with vesicle formation → target lesions → confluence of lesions	Small blanchable urticarial lesions → large arciform plaques with violaceous center	Purpuric lesions → spread outward	Varied morphology of lesions which includes urticarial, maculopapular rash and EM form fixed lesions	Urticarial lesions with center color change (violaceous or gray)	Fixed targetoid lesions along with other lesions suggestive of LE/SCLE/CCLE
Sites	Acral and face EM minor: Symmetric EM major: Asymmetric	Trunk, extremities, and face	Symmetric Face and extremities, spares trunk	Face, trunk, extremities, lateral aspect of hands and feet	Face, trunk, extremities	Mainly on photoexposed part
Clinically distinguished features	Rarely lesions persists for more than a month	Dermographism and evanescent lesions	–	No blister formation Disabling joint pain may last for weeks	Pain and burning in lesions	–
Mucosal involvement	EM minor: One mucosa EM major: Two mucosae	Absent	Rarely involved	Absent	Absent	+/–

Continued

Continued

	EM	UM	AHOI	SSLR	UV	Rowell's syndrome
Dermoscopy	Center shows clod of different colors like red, blue, purple, or black areas surrounded by featureless plain area and outer most ring of homogenous erythema	Not described	Not described	Not described	Purpuric patches and globules	Not described
Investigation	Elevated ESR, CRP, or liver enzymes	Elevated ESR, CRP, or liver enzymes and IgE	Elevated ESR, eosinophils, WBCs, platelets Hematuria and proteinuria	Elevated ESR, CRP, lymphocytes and eosinophils neutopenia	Elevated ESR, C3↓, hematuria, and proteinuria	ANA, anti-SjT, anti-Ro, anti-La, RA positivity
Histopathology	Spongiosis with exocytosis, colloid bodies throughout epidermal layers, dermal edema and dilated capillaries, lymphocytic infiltrate	Perivascular lymphocytic and eosinophilic infiltrate	Leukocytoclastic vasculitis with or without fibrinoid necrosis. Perivascular C1q and IgA positivity (30%)	Perivascular lymphocytic infiltrate with few eosinophils	Leukocytoclastic vasculitis with fibrinoid necrosis, erythrocyte extravasation DIF: Complement and immunoglobulin +/−	Necrotic keratinocytes with perivascular lymphocytic infiltrate, dermal edema, endothelial cell swelling
Management	Symptomatic Tetracycline or antivirals as per etiology. Steroids and immunomodulators for lesions persisting beyond few weeks	Symptomatic Antihistamines Steroids for persisting lesions	Symptomatic Role of steroids is controversial	Antihistamines, NSAIDs, steroids	Antihistamines, steroids, immunosuppressives, biologics	Steroids, immunosuppressives, HCQ, photoprotection and symptomatic treatment
Complication	Dyspigmentation	–	PIH	PIH	PIH, depends on renal involvement	Depends on organ involvement
Prognosis	Self-limiting	Good	Self-limiting No relapse	Self-limiting, good	Depends on renal involvement	Depends on organ involvement

(AHOI: acute hemorrhagic edema of infancy; ANA: antinuclear antibody; CCLE: chronic cutaneous lupus erythematosus; CRP: C-reactive protein; DIF: direct immunofluorescence; EM: erythema multiforme; ESR: erythrocyte sedimentation rate; HCQ: hydroxychloroquine; HSV: herpes simplex virus; IgE: immunoglobulin E; LE: lupus erythematosus; NSAIDs: nonsteroidal anti-inflammatory drugs; PIH: postinflammatory hyperpigmentation; RA: rheumatoid arthritis; SCLE: subacute cutaneous lupus erythematosus; SSLR: serum sickness-like reaction; TNF-α: tumor necrosis factor α; UM: urticaria multiforme; UV: urticarial vasculitis; WBCs: white blood cells)

Table 3: Distinguished features of TEN and TEN-alike disorders.

	SJS/SJS–TEN overlap/TEN	GBFDE	TEN like LE	Acute GVHD	Pseudoporphyria
Age	Any age	Mainly older age Median age of 78 years	Mean age 43 years But can also affect children	All age	–
Sex	F > M	M > F	F > M (6.5:1)	–	–
Incidence	0.93–1.89/million	Extremely rare	Rare	Stage 3 and 4: 22–27%	Only one case reported
Genetic association	HLA-B 5,802/1,502	Not evaluated	Not evaluated	Not evaluated	–
Etiology/triggering factors	Drugs (90%) Infections (10%)	Drugs	UV light, rarely Infections or drugs	Stopping of immunosuppressives, sex disparity	Drugs, hemodialysis
Pathophysiology	Fas, FasL, perforin and granzyme B activation by cytotoxic T cells	CD8+ memory T cells	IL6, Fas, FasL, upregulations and cytotoxic T cell-mediated injury	Donor lymphocytes	Accumulations of porphyrins because of renal dysfunction
Origin/onset	Abrupt and acute (<14 days)	Few hours (3–24 hours), interval ↓ with recurrent episodes	Subacute over a period of 14 or more days	Acute (<100 days of stem cell transplant) Late acute onset (>100 days of stem cell transplant)	Abrupt
Total duration of disease with treatment	3–4 weeks	1–2 weeks	1–2 weeks	Weeks/Months Few patients shift to chronic GVHD	–
Progression	Atypical targets/purpuric macules → increase in size and coalesce → blisters → sheet like peeling	Diffuse to well-defined purpuric/livid patches → postinflammatory hyperpigmentation. Intervening areas of normal skin: +	Initial photodistributed vesiculobullous lesions → generalized sheet like	Lesions begins around follicle → coalesce and become generalized	Large areas of bullae → rapid extension and generalized involvement
Associated symptoms	Flu like prodromal symptoms like malaise, fever and RTI × 2–3 days	Absent	Low-grade fever, joint pain, photosensitivity. ~60% are already diagnosed as LE before	Involvement of GI mucosa is associated with GI symptoms	Absent
Sites involved	Face, trunk, limbs	Recurrence at same site, three out of six anatomical sites (head and neck, anterior trunk, posterior trunk, upper limbs, lower limbs, and genitalia)	Photoexposed sites → generalized	Cheeks, neck, back, palms, and soles → generalized	Thigh, trunk, genitalia
Nikolsky's sign	Positive	Negative	Positive/Negative	–	Negative
Mucosal involvement	Severe Internal and external both are involved	No to minimal involvement (oral and genital) Never involves conjunctiva	No to less severe usually asymptomatic	GI mucosal involvement	Involves mucous membranes

Continued

Continued

	SJS/SJS–TEN overlap/TEN	GBFDE	TEN like LE	Acute GVHD	Pseudoporphyria
Dermoscopic findings	Erythema, purpuric dots, black dots ++, epidermal detachment, necrotic borders, erosions	Erythema, purpuric dots, occasional black dots ++, epidermal–dermal separation	Not described	Not described	Not described
Vitals	Stable/Unstable	Stable	Stable	Stable/Unstable	Stable
Investigations	CBC, RFT, LFT, serum glucose, serum bicarbonate, swabs	Hepatic enzymes and serum electrolytes	ANA and ANA profile (dsDNA, Ro/La +/−)	CBC, RFT, LFT, and as required after clinical examination Chimerism may suggest GVHD	Porphyrin levels <10 μg/dL compared to porphyria
Histopathology	Full thickness epidermal necrosis: + Eosinophils: + Melanophages: −/+ CD4: + CD56: ++/+++	Full thickness epidermal necrosis: +/− Civatte bodies: + Eosinophils: ++ Melanophages: +++ CD4: ++ CD56: +	Full thickness epidermal necrosis extending to adnexal epithelium: + Superficial perivascular lymphocytic and neutrophilic infiltrate Mucin: +	Subepidermal necrotic bulla, lichenoid inflammation of adnexa, extensive satellite cell necrosis	Festooning of dermal papillae, PAS positive material in vessel walls
DIF	Negative	Negative	Positive (IgG, IgM, IgA, C3)	–	Positive/Negative
Serum granulysin levels	++/+++	+	+	–	–
Management	Cutaneous and mucosal care, IV fluids steroids, cyclosporine, IVIg, infliximab, etanercept, thalidomide, G-CSF	Antihistamines, analgesics, steroids, cyclosporine, IVIg	Corticosteroids, HCQ, MMF, azathioprine, cyclophosphamide, IVIg, plasmapheresis, rituximab, and dapsone	Steroids, cyclosporine, methotrexate, infliximab, anti-thymocyte globulin, MMF, CD5-specific immunotoxin, Anti-IL2 receptor, phototherapy	Local wound care
Mortality	30–40%	Not reported	~10%	87%	Not evaluated
Prognosis	Depends on SCORETEN	Good	Relatively good, depends on organ involvement	Stage 4 acute GVHD has extremely poor prognosis	Not evaluated
Complications	Infections, airway compromise, scarring, pigmentary changes	Pigmentary changes	Organ specific involvement has varied complications	PIH, pulmonary GVHD, infections, pneumonia, GI bleed, multisystem failure	Hepatorenal syndrome

(ANA: antinuclear antibody; CBC: complete blood count; DIF: direct immunofluorescence; dsDNA: double-stranded deoxyribonucleic acid; GBFDE: generalized bullous fixed drug eruption; G-CSF: granulocyte colony-stimulating factor; GI: gastrointestinal; GVHD: graft-versus-host disease; HCQ: hydroxychloroquine; HLA-B: human leukocyte antigen B; IgG: immunoglobulin G; IL6: interleukin 6; IV: intravenous; IVIg: intravenous immune globulin; LE: lupus erythematosus; LFT: liver function test; MMF: mycophenolate mofetil; PAS: periodic acid–Schiff; PIH: postinflammatory hyperpigmentation; RFT: renal function test; RTI: respiratory tract infection; SJS: Stevens–Johnson syndrome; TEN: toxic epidermal necrolysis; UV: ultraviolet)

affected. Local part care in terms of dressings is important part of management in TEN and TEN alike conditions.

Erythema Multiforme

Erythema multiforme usually affects young adults with age ranging between 20 and 40 years though cases in children have been reported.[3] Females are more commonly affected. Genetic predisposition has been reported in Asian ethnic group. Increased susceptibility has been reported with HLA-B15 (B62), HLA-B35, HLA-A33, HLA-Dr53, HLA DQ3 (herpes-associated EM), and HLA-DQB1*0301. Extensive oral involvement has been reported in association with HLA-DQB1*0402.[4] As documented in **Table 1** most common etiology for EM is infections in approximately 90% of cases and rest 10% can be due to drugs and other causes.[4] Among infectious etiology, 70–80% of cases are due to *herpes* virus. Very rarely EM can be caused by malignancy, food additives, or chemicals.

Oral involvement has been reported in 35–65% of patients.[5] Oral lesions can precede the lesions on skin. Anterior part of oral cavity being mostly involved, lip is the most common site. Hemorrhagic crust and pseudomembrane formation is characteristic. Other mucosae can be involved in EM major. Cutaneous lesions are classical target lesions **(Figs. 1 and 2)**. Dermoscopic features[6] of EM is elaborated in **Table 2**.

Mycoplasma-induced Rash and Mucositis[1]

Recently, it has been classified as a distinct entity from EM and SJS. It usually affects children with age ranging from 5 to 15 years. Prodromal symptoms such as fever, malaise, and cough precede skin lesions approximately by 1 week. Cutaneous lesions vary from vesiculobullous lesions, targetoid lesions, maculopapular rash to macular, or popular lesions. Lesions are predominantly distributed over extremities involving <10% of BSA. Hallmark of MIRM is severe mucosal involvement involving two or more mucosae. Overall MIRM has milder disease course compared to SJS though systematically atypical pneumonia is a characteristic finding.

Urticaria Multiforme[7,8]

This is relatively a benign condition but clinically it might look alarming **(Fig. 3)**. Diagnosis of UM is mainly based on clinical history taking and examinations. Laboratory examinations and skin biopsy are rarely needed. Diagnostic criteria proposed by Sempau L et al. are as follows:
- Large annular plaques with a transient ecchymotic center
- Individual lesions with a duration of <24 hours
- Associated episode of fever
- Total duration of disease of <10 days
- Edema of the limbs

Acute Hemorrhagic Edema of Infancy

It is also known as Finkelstein disease, Seidlmayer syndrome, medallion-like purpura, and infantile postinfectious iris-like purpura and edema.[9] In comparison to UM lesions of acute hemorrhagic edema of infancy (AHOI) lasts for several days and leaves residual pigmentations.[8] Visceral involvement is rare and uncommon in AHOI unlike Henoch–Schönlein purpura.[10]

Serum Sickness-like Reaction[11]

Unlike classical serum sickness which is usually precipitated by heterologous serum, SSLR is usually precipitated by drugs, vaccines, and infections and it is not associated with antigen-antibody complex formation. Morphology of cutaneous

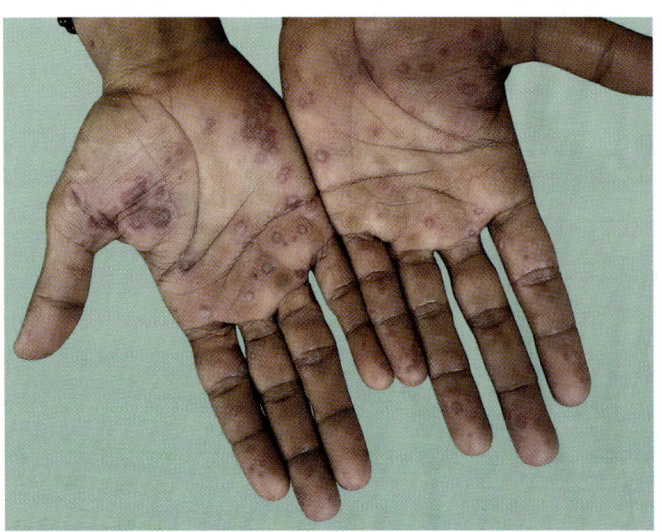

FIG. 2: Erythema multiforme on palms in a patient with herpes labialis.

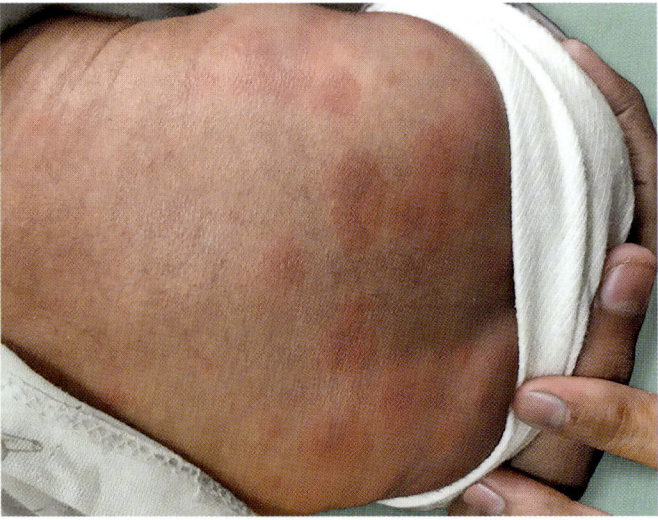

FIG. 3: Urticaria multiforme in an infant.

lesions varies widely. It can present as morbilliform rash, urticarial lesions, annular urticarial plaques, and EM-like lesions. The lesions of SSLR usually starts after 7-10 days of triggering factors and remains fixed until resolution. Patients might experience swelling of lip and periorbital area, but it never involves tongue and laryngeal mucosa. Itching is usually absent. SSLR lesions do not have typical three zones like EM and they never show blister formation. Along with skin lesions, arthralgia affecting mainly joints of hands and feet presenting as joint swelling, pain, and purple discoloration of overlying skin may be present. In adult associated lymphadenopathy may be found unlike pediatric patients.

Urticarial Vasculitis[12,13]

About 9-21% of leukocytoclastic vasculitis are urticarial vasculitis (UV). 2-27% of patients initially presenting as urticaria were reported to have UV. Pediatric cases are rare. Of all vasculitis patients in pediatric age group, only 1% has UV.

Approximately 10-20% cases of UV have hypocomplementemic UV or HUVS (hypocomplementemic urticarial vasculitis syndrome/McDuffie syndrome). Diagnostic criteria for HUVS are as follow:
- *Major criteria*: Urticarial lesions of >6 months, low C1q, C3 and C4.
- *Minor criteria*: Anti-C1q dermal vasculitis, arthralgia/arthritis, uveitis/episcleritis, glomerulonephritis, and/or recurrent abdominal pain.

Normocomplementemic UV is limited to skin involvement. It is sometimes difficult to differentiate it from chronic spontaneous urticaria and a definitive diagnosis requires biopsy. However, dermoscopy might help to differentiate it from urticaria along with classical clinical features.

Unlike EM, the lesion of UV never shows blister formation and site predilection. Mucosal involvement is also absent.

Rowell's Syndrome

This entity is being debated recently for being overlap syndrome, a real association or coincidence, a subentity, or a different variant of lupus erythematosus (LE).[14] It is a rare disease and <100 cases have been described till date. Usually, diagnosis of LE precedes EM form lesions **(Fig. 4)**.[15] Latest diagnostic criteria proposed by Torchia et al.[16] are as follows:
- *Major criteria*:
  o Presence of chronic cutaneous lupus erythematosus (CCLE)-discoid lupus erythematosus (DLE)/chilblain
  o Presence of EM-like typical or atypical targetoid lesions
  o Antinuclear antibody (ANA) speckled pattern/anti-Ro (SSA)/anti-La (SSB) antibody positivity
  o Negative direct immunofluorescence (DIF) on lesional EM-like lesions

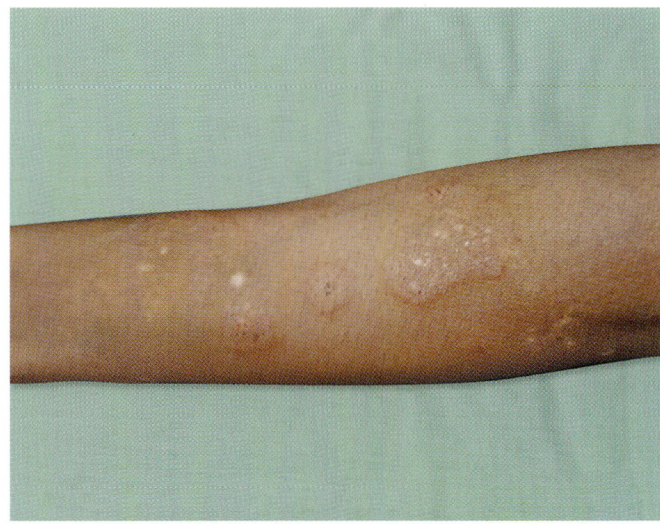

FIG. 4: Erythema multiforme in a patient with subacute cutaneous lupus erythematosus who was positive for anti-Ro antibodies.

- *Minor criteria*:
  o Absence of infectious or pharmacological triggers
  o Absence of typical EM location (acral/mucosal)
  o Presence of at least one additional American Rheumatism Association (ARA) criterion for diagnosis of systemic lupus erythematosus (SLE) besides DLE, ANA, photosensitivity, malar rash, and oral ulcers.

All major and one minor criteria are required for diagnosis.

The targetoid EM-like lesions in Rowell's syndrome are usually characterized by two zones—raised erythematous lesions with vesicular border.[1]

Linear IgA Bullous Disease

Linear IgA bullous disease (LABD) is an autoimmune disease occurring spontaneously or triggered/induced by drugs. In adults, it can present as widely varied morphology. It usually presents as flat target lesions with tense bulla in center which further coalesce though in children, polycyclic plaques, and papules with vesicles at periphery (string of pearls appearance) is common **(Fig. 5)**. It commonly involves trunk and extremities with variable mucosal involvement. Biopsy and DIF findings are very characteristic revealing subepidermal blister with linear IgA deposition at basement membrane zone (BMZ).

Other Diseases Presenting as EM-like Conditions

Bullous pemphigoid **(Fig. 6)**, Kawasaki disease, toxic shock syndrome, Sweets syndrome, syphilis **(Fig. 7)**,

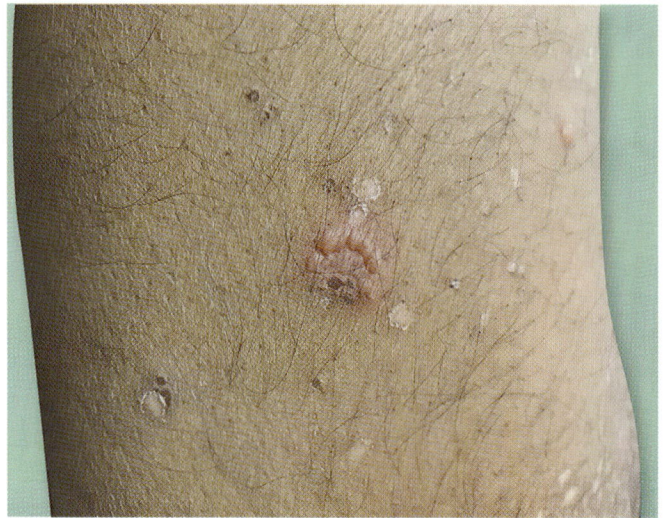

FIG. 5: Targetoid lesions in linear immunoglobulin A (IgA) bullous dermatosis.

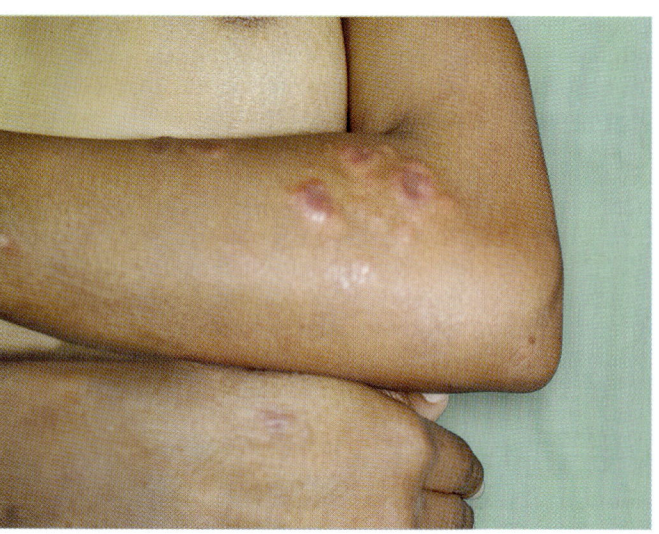

FIG. 7: Targetoid annular lesions of secondary syphilis.

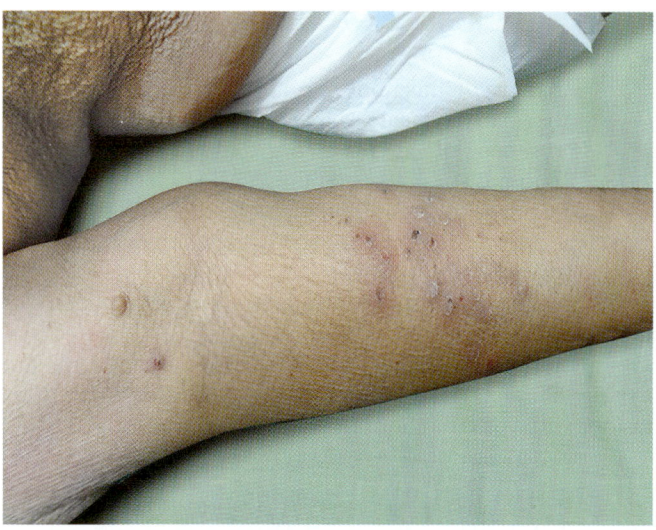

FIG. 6: Targetoid lesions in bullous pemphigoid.

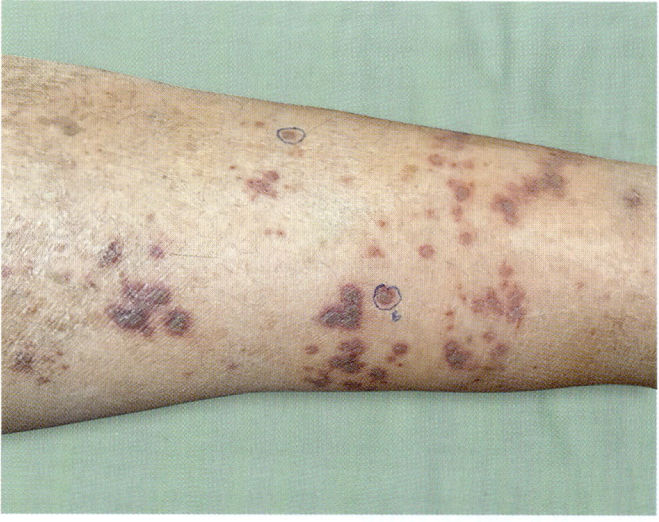

FIG. 8: Atypical target lesions in lekocytoclastic vasculitis.

leukocytoclastic vasculitis **(Fig. 8)** and polymorphic eruptions of pregnancy has been reported to present as EM-like lesions very rarely with only few case reports published.

Table 2 summarizes the features of EM and majority of EM-alike common conditions.

Toxic Epidermal Necrolysis/Lyell's Syndrome[17,18]

It is characterized by full thickness epidermal necrosis caused mainly by drugs and drug metabolites. It has also been reported following measles-mumps, rubella vaccine and mycoplasma infections. Incidence of TEN is considerably higher in patients with HIV infections.

Clinically three phases can be distinguished in TEN:
1. *Prodromal period*: Fever, cough, conjunctivitis, anorexia, malaise, runny nose, etc., lasting from 2 days to few weeks.
2. *Necrolysis period*: Painful and burning macular erythema involving body areas symmetrically and generally does not involve scalp. This over the time become diffuse erythema usually avoiding pressure area progressing rapidly in 3–4 days. Epidermal detachment takes 5–7 days.
3. *Re-epithelialization period*: This stretches from 1 to 3 weeks.

Mucosal involvement is seen in 95% of patients, and both internal and external mucosae can be involved.

Consequences of mucosal involvement can be severe and requires a team approach.

Paraneoplastic Pemphigus

Severe and chronic mucosal involvement is characteristic. Oral mucosa is most common site of involvement. Cutaneous lesions of paraneoplastic pemphigus (PNP) have varied morphology compared to SJS/TEN. But clinical similarity is striking and it is difficult to differentiate the two. It can be differentiated from later by characteristic findings on histopathology (suprabasal acantholysis along with necrotic keratinocyte and vacuolar interphase dermatitis) and DIF (intercellular as well as linear granular deposits at BMZ).[19] IIF and immunoprecipitations can also help it to be differentiate from SJS/TEN.

Generalized Bullous Fixed Drug Eruption

Though exact mechanisms are not known, when offending drug binds to intercellular adhesion molecule-1, CD4+, and CD8+ cells are recruited causing tissue damage by interferon-γ, granulysin, perforin via Fas receptor—Fas ligand system. After this CD8+ cell remains quiescent at DEJ until next trigger.[20] So, in subsequent attacks durations of appearing lesions after triggers get shorter and number of lesions increases.[21]

Abrupt onset and absence of prodromal phase help in differentiation from SJS/TEN. Target lesions in generalized bullous fixed drug eruption (GBFDE) have two zones: darker, dusky center, and peripheral erythematous rim **(Figs. 9 and 10)**. Lesions are usually flat. Though oral and genital mucosae can be involved, conjunctival mucosa is never involved.[1] Interweaving areas of skin appears normal and are not tender. At least three out of six anatomical sites should be involved as summarized in **Table 3**.[20] Serum granulysin levels does not correlate with disease severity unlike SJS/TEN.[22] As the detachment of skin is quite comparative to SJS/TEN it should be treated as vigilantly as the later because prognosis can be guarded.[23] Cyclosporine has claimed to be associated with less PIH.[20]

Acute Graft-versus-host Disease[24,25]

Acute acute graft-versus-host disease (GVHD) usually presents within 100 days of transplant. But delayed presentations have been reported. The lesions begin around a hair follicle. GVHD also affects gastrointestinal (GI) mucosa as a result of T cell mediated injury and bone marrow suppression.

Four stages have been described for acute GVHD as follow:
- *Stage 1*: Macular/purpuric lesions affecting <25% BSA.
- *Stage 2*: Macular/purpuric lesions affecting 25–50% BSA **(Fig. 11)**.
- *Stage 3*: Generalized erythroderma.
- *Stage 4*: TEN like.

Stage four represents 2% of acute GVHD patients. Overall survival is better in late onset acute GVHD.

Toxic Epidermal Necrolysis-like Acute Cutaneous Lupus Erythematosus

Acute syndrome of apoptotic panepidermolysis (ASAP) includes entity like TEN-like LE, acute GVHD, and TEN-like pseudoporphyria. Proposed mechanism in TEN-like LE is ultraviolet light which induces apoptosis and necrosis resulting in increased levels of chemokines CCL27.[26] Extreme

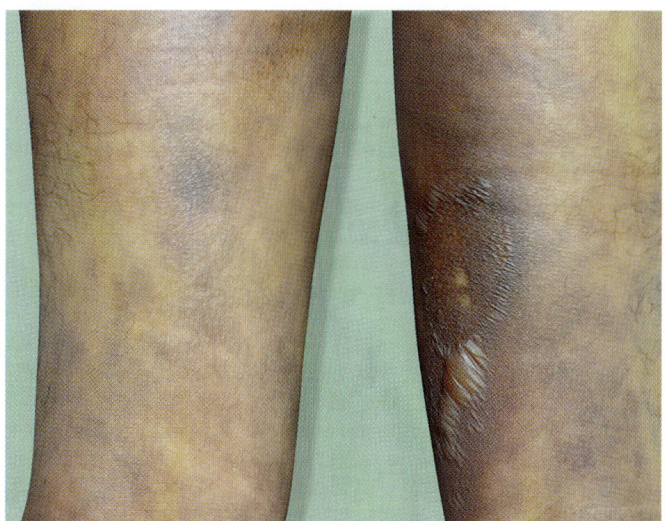

FIG. 9: Generalized bullous fixed drug eruption in an elderly male. Note the characteristic spared areas of normal skin in between the lesions.

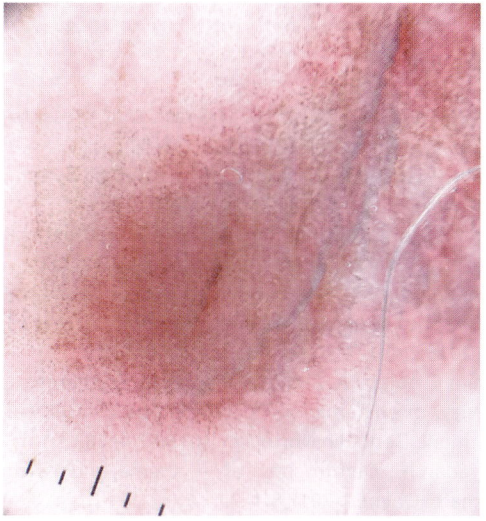

FIG. 10: Dermoscopic features of generalized bullous fixed drug eruption (GBFDE) showing epidermal-dermal separation.

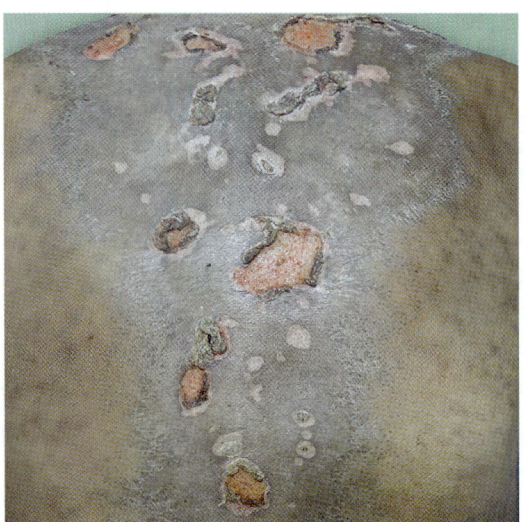

FIG. 11: Stage-2 acute graft-versus-host disease (GVHD) presented after 100 days of transplant.

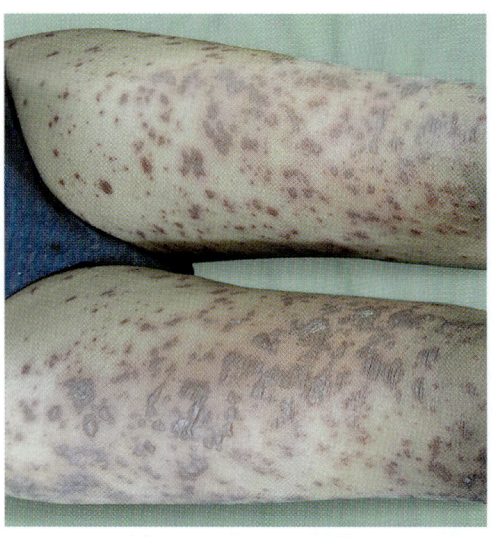

FIG. 12: Toxic epidermal necrolysis (TEN)-like lupus erythematosus (LE) in an already diagnosed patient of lupus erythematosus.

interphase dermatitis is also considered to be responsible for it.

Classification of vesiculobullous diseases in patients of LE includes following entities:[27]

- *LE-specific vesiculobullous skin diseases*:
  - TEN-like acute cutaneous lupus erythematosus (ACLE) **(Fig. 12)**
  - TEN-like subacute cutaneous lupus erythematosus (SCLE)
  - TEN occurring in patients with LE without conventional LE-specific skin lesions
  - Vesiculobullous annular SCLE
  - Vesiculobullous CCLE
- *LE nonspecific vesiculobullous disease—autoimmune conditions*:
  - Dermatitis herpetiformis like LE
  - Epidermolysis bullosa acquisita like LE
  - Bullous pemphigoid like LE

Lesions in bullous LE are situated mainly on photo distributed area and histopathologically it shows neutrophil rich infiltrate. Bullous LE responds very well to dapsone.[28]

TEN-like pseudoporphyria[29] is extremely rare and only a case report has been published till date.

Table 3 summarizes features of TEN and TEN-alike conditions including dermoscopic features of TEN and GBFDE.[30]

REFERENCES

1. Wolf R, Parish JL, Parish LC. The rash that presents as target lesions. Clin Dermatol. 2019;37(2):148-58.
2. Kumar P, Anand V, Hassan S. Herpes iris of Bateman. Indian Dermatol Online J. 2014;5 (Suppl S2):138-9.
3. Hasan S, Jangra J, Choudhary P, Mishra S. Erythema Multiforme: A Recent Update. Biomed Pharmacol J. 2018;11(1).
4. Krishnankutty K, Chaudhuri K, Ashok L. Erythema multiforme: a case series and review of literature. Open Access J Trans Med Res. 2018;2(4):124-30.
5. Samim F, Auluck A, Zed C, Williams PM. Erythema multiforme: a review of epidemiology, pathogenesis, clinical features, and treatment. Dent Clin North Am. 2013;57(4):583-96.
6. Kaliyadan F. Dermoscopy of erythema multiforme. Indian Dermatol Online J. 2017;8(1):75.
7. Emer JJ, Bernardo SG, Kovalerchik O, Ahmad M. Urticaria multiforme. J Clin Aesthet Dermatol. 2013;6(3):34-9.
8. Sempau L, Martín-Sáez E, Gutiérrez-Rodríguez C, Gutiérrez-Ortega MC. Urticaria multiforme: A report of 5 cases and a review of the literature. Actas Dermosifiliogr. 2016;107(1):e1-5.
9. Thakur P, Negi B, Chandrashekhar, Attri P, Basit R, Bhardwaj V, et al. Acute haemorrhagic oedema of infancy. JMSCR. 2019; 7(8):549-51.
10. Jindal SR, Kura MM. Acute hemorrhagic edema of infancy-a rare entity. Indian Dermatol Online J. 2013;4:106-8.
11. Del Pozzo-Magaña BR, Lazo-Langner A. Serum sickness like-reaction in children: review of the literature. EMJ Dermatol. 2019;7(1):106-11.
12. Kolkhir P, Grakhova M, Bonnekoh H, Krause K, Maurer M. Treatment of urticarial vasculitis: A systematic review. J Allergy Clin Immunol. 2019;143(2):458-66.
13. García-García B, Aubán-Pariente J, Munguía-Calzada P, Vivanco B, Argenziano G, Vázquez-López1 F. Development of a clinical-dermoscopic model for the diagnosis of urticarial vasculitis. Sci Rep. 2020;10:6092.
14. Bhat RY, Varma C, Bhatt S, Balachandran C. Rowell syndrome. Indian Dermatol Online J. 2014;5(Suppl 1):S33-5.
15. Gallo L, Megna M, Festa B, Stellato P, di Pinto R, Fabbrocini G, et al. Rowell Syndrome: A Diagnostic Challenge. J Clin Aesthet Dermatol. 2020;13(4):40-2.

16. Torchia D, Romanelli P, Kerdel FA. Erythema multiforme and Stevens-Johnson syndrome/toxic epidermal necrolysis associated with lupus erythematosus. J Am Acad Dermatol. 2012;67(3):417-21.
17. Estrella-Alonso A, Aramburu JA, González-Ruiz MY, Cachafeiro L, Sánchez MS, Lorente JA. Toxic epidermal necrolysis: a paradigm of critical illness. Rev Bras Ter Intensiva. 2017;29(4):499-508.
18. Harris V, Jackson C, Cooper A. Review of Toxic Epidermal Necrolysis. Int J Mol Sci. 2016;17(12):2135.
19. Padhiyar JK, Patel NH, Ninama K, Bilimoria FE, Mahajan R, Gajjar T, et al. Paraneoplastic pemphigus presenting as toxic epidermal necrolysis: A case report. Nepal J Dermatol Venereol Leprol. 2018;16(1):59-62.
20. Barootes HC, Peebles ER, Matsui D, Rieder M, Abuzgaia A, Mohammed JA. Severe Generalized Bullous Fixed Drug Eruption Treated with Cyclosporine: A Case Report and Literature Review. Case Rep Dermatol. 2021;13(1):154-63.
21. Girisha BS, Noronha TM, Alva AC, Menon A. Generalized bullous fixed drug eruption mimicking toxic epidermal necrolysis caused by paracetamol. Clin Dermatol Rev. 2018;2:34-7.
22. Cho YT, Lin JW, Chen YC, Chang CY, Hsiao CH, Chung WH, et al. Generalized bullous fixed drug eruption is distinct from Stevens-Johnson syndrome/toxic epidermal necrolysis by immunohistopathological features. J Am Acad Dermatol. 2014;70(3):539-48.
23. Lipowicz S, Sekula P, Ingen-Housz-Oro S, Liss Y, Sassolas B, Dunant A, et al. Prognosis of generalized bullous fixed drug eruption: comparison with Stevens-Johnson syndrome and toxic epidermal necrolysis. Br J Dermatol. 2013;168(4):726-32.
24. Goyal PKK, Xu S, Choi J. Delayed presentation of toxic epidermal necrolysis-like cutaneous acute graft-versus-host disease in the setting of recent immunosuppressant discontinuation. Dermatol Online J. 2017;23(10):13030/qt7j12q9rk.
25. Macedo FI, Faris J, Lum LG, Gabali A, Uberti JP, Ratanatharathorn V, et al. Extensive toxic epidermal necrolysis versus acute graft versus host disease after allogenic hematopoietic stem-cell transplantation: challenges in diagnosis and management. J Burn Care Res. 2014;35(6):e431-5.
26. Romero LS, Bari O, Forbess Smith CJ, Schneider JA, Cohen PR. Toxic epidermal necrolysis-like acute cutaneous lupus erythematosus: report of a case and review of the literature. Dermatol Online J. 2018;24(5):13030/qt5r79d67k.
27. Singthong S, Kwangsukstid O, Sudtikoonaseth P. Toxic epidermal necrolysis-like lupus erythematosus: A case report. Thai J Dermatol. 2019;35(1):25-33.
28. Yu J, Brandling-Bennett H, Co DO, Nocton JJ, Stevens AM, Chiu YE. Toxic Epidermal Necrolysis-Like Cutaneous Lupus in Pediatric Patients: A Case Series and Review. Pediatrics. 2016;137(6):e20154497.
29. Papadopoulos AJ, Schwartz RA, Fekete Z, Kihiczak G, Samady JA, Atkin SH, et al. Pseudoporphyria: an atypical variant resembling toxic epidermal necrolysis. J Cutan Med Surg. 2001;5(6):479-85.
30. Rossi G, da Silva Cartell A, Marchiori Bakos R. Dermoscopic Aspects of Cutaneous Adverse Drug Reactions. Dermatol Pract Concept. 2021;11(1):e2021136.

4
A Patient with Suspected Cutaneous Adverse Drug Reaction: Practice Tips

Lalit Kumar Gupta, Manisha Balai

"Primum non nocere"
(First, do no harm to patient)

—*Hippocrates*

INTRODUCTION

With the advent of newer drugs almost on a daily basis and the adverse effects caused by them, clinicians need to keep themselves abreast with the adverse events related to them. Skin is one of the most frequent and visible site of drug reactions. Cutaneous adverse drug reactions (CADRs) are great imitators and can virtually mimic almost any inflammatory dermatoses. They have got a very wide clinical spectrum ranging from innocuous or benign rash on one hand to serious life-threatening rash also called serious cutaneous adverse drug reactions (SCARs). In the absence of reliable and validated laboratory investigative tools, the diagnosis of CADR is essentially based on clinical judgment and expertise. A clinician should have a thorough knowledge of the various reaction patterns induced by drugs and be able to differentiate from mimics that produce identical reaction pattern.[1] This chapter is intended to guide clinicians on the practical aspects of dealing with a case who presents with a rash suspected to be drug related.

When to suspect a rash to be drug induced?[1]
Not all rash in skin are drug induced. A possibility of rash caused by drug is suspected in the following setting:
- The rash that has developed after consumption of a drug by the patient.
- There is a temporal correlation between drug intake and appearance of rash.
- The rash is itchy and generalized [exception being fixed drug eruption (FDE) which is localized].
- There has been similar episode(s) in the past.
- The rash that improves following dose reduction/withdrawal of the drug (dechallenge)
- There is aggravation/reappearance of rash upon reintroduction (rechallenge).

It is important to enquire in details about the prescriptional as well as nonprescriptional/over-the-counter (OTC), herbal, and alternative medications. Very often patients do not consider home remedies and OTC medications to be responsible for reaction and do not reveal it unless they are specifically and repeatedly probed. The reactions to drugs generally appear immediately within hours or days, if the patient is already sensitized to that particular drug. However, a latent period of few weeks and even months may elapse if the drug is consumed for the first time. This is usually seen in drug hypersensitivity syndrome (DHS), Stevens–Johnson syndrome-toxic epidermal necrolysis (SJS-TEN) and lichenoid eruption. Physicians often ignore this fact and fail to pinpoint the drug as the cause that the patient is taking for such a long-time. This is very commonly noticed in case of anticonvulsant-induced DHS or SJS-TEN and in such cases the antibiotics and nonsteroidal anti-inflammatory drugs (NSAIDs) that the patient takes for the prodromal phase of drug reaction with eosinophilia and systemic symptom (DRESS) or TEN is erroneously implicated. The reaction to drugs generally subsides almost immediately after its withdrawal or reduction in the dose (dechallenge). But this may not happen if the reaction is caused by drugs that have longer half-life, e.g., anticonvulsants where despite the stoppage of the offending drug the rash may progress. The reaction in such instances is caused by the metabolites of the drug and not the parent drug itself.[2,3]

Are there any "at risk" groups prone for drug reactions?
Not all individuals are at equal risk of developing reaction to a drug. Some factors (**Box 1**) predispose a person to have higher propensity of reactions to drugs. Likewise there some drug/drug groups which are more likely to cause reactions such as anticonvulsants, anticancer drugs, antiretroviral drugs, sulfonamides, NSAIDs, and allopurinol. Clinicians should execute extreme caution while prescribing these medications in high-risk group of subjects.[1]

Box 1: High-risk subjects for CADR.

- Polypharmacy/patients on multiple drugs
- History of drug reaction/allergy
- Patients with autoimmune connective tissue diseases such as SLE and rheumatoid arthritis
- Immunocompromised patients, e.g., AIDS
- *Viral infections*: Cytomegalovirus and Epstein–Barr virus, HHV6, 7, CMV, and HIV greatly enhance the risk and severity of drug reactions. (HIV/AIDS patients have up to 100-fold risk to develop reactions to cotrimoxazole, anticonvulsants, and antiretrovirals, particularly nevirapine; patients with infectious mononucleosis on ampicillin have 60–100% risk of maculopapular rash (In contrast to 3–7% normal subjects)
- Renal/hepatic impairment
- *Genetic predisposition*: Human leukocyte antigen (HLA) association, e.g., HLA-B*5801 in allopurinol induced SJS/TEN and DRESS, HLA-B*1502 with carbamazepine induced SJS/TEN, HLA-B*22 and fixed drug eruption
- Atopic patients

(AIDS: acquired immunodeficiency syndrome; CADR: cutaneous adverse drug reaction; CMV: cytomegalovirus; HIV: human immunodeficiency virus; SJS/TEN: Stevens–Johnson syndrome/toxic epidermal necrolysis; SLE: systemic lupus erythematosus)

Table 1: Differentiating features between exanthematous drug rash and infective exanthema.

Feature	Exanthematous drug rash	Infective exanthem
History of drug intake	Always elicited	Usually absent
Itching	Generally present, moderate to intense	Usually absent or mild
Distribution and spread	Usually begins from trunk and proximal arms, spreads centrifugally	Begins from face and cephalocaudal spread
Lymphadenopathy	Generally absent	Usually present
Conjunctival erythema	Usually not seen	Common
Enanthem	Generally absent	May be present
Seasonal and family clustering	Generally not seen	May be commonly seen

How to approach a patient with suspected drug reaction?
Suspect a possibility of drug reaction in any patient who is on any medication and develops a rash that is usually itchy, generalized, and symmetrically distributed. Generally, a recently added drug is thought to be the culprit but any drug consumed by the patient during last 2 months should be evaluated as a possible suspect.[3,4]

The three basic steps in approaching a drug reaction are:
1. Recognizing the morphology/pattern of drug reaction
2. Assessing the severity of reaction (benign or simple vs. serious or complex)
3. Recognition of causal drug—ascertaining drug causality

"Medicine is a science of uncertainty and an art of probability"
—**William Osler**

Except for the FDE there is no reaction pattern that can be attributed specific to the drugs. The reaction to a drug is neither predictable nor reproducible always. A particular drug may elicit multiple reaction patterns and on the contrary multiple drugs may result in a common reaction pattern. The rash may involve only skin when it is termed as *benign* or *simple rash*. But when it involves internal organs in addition to skin it is called complex or serious reaction. Fortunately benign reactions are much more common than complex reactions and do not pose any threat to the patient. It is also important to differentiate between a simple or complex/serious rash as in a case of serious reaction, immediate stoppage of the culprit drug(s) is mandatory along with prompt institution of supportive and specific therapeutic measures, while in simple rash the drug may be continued with a close observation on the progression of reaction ("*carry through*" or "*treat through*" approach). It is important to note that sometimes a rash may begin as a simple rash (maculopapular rash) but in due course of time progresses into a serious rash (DRESS/DHS or TEN)

Maculopapular drug rash is the most common reaction pattern reported in most studies, followed by urticaria and FDEs. It is sometimes practically difficult to differentiate between exanthematous/maculopapular rash from an infective exanthem. **Table 1** shows some important points that may help to differentiate between them.

RECOGNIZING THE PATTERN OF DRUG REACTION

Some of the common morphology of simple or benign reaction pattern and the drugs that commonly cause them are highlighted in **Table 2**.[1]

ASSESSING THE SEVERITY OF THE RASH

This is the most important step in the evaluation of any case with suspected drug reaction and guides the further therapy and predicts the prognosis. A rash is termed as serious if it shows extensive involvement of skin, is associated with internal organ involvement, leads to hospitalization/prolongs hospital stay, has significant morbidity/sequelae or results in death. The serious reactions often show some prodromal and warning signs. It is very important to identify some of the *warning signs* or *red flag signs* that indicate serious nature of a drug reaction early so as to diagnose the

Table 2: Morphological pattern of drug reaction with causative drugs.	
Morphological pattern	**Causative drugs**
Maculopapular rash (**Fig. 1**)	Penicillins, sulfonamides, antiepileptics, antiretrovirals, NSAIDs, and antimalarials
Urticaria/angioedema (**Fig. 2**)	Aspirin/NSAIDs, penicillins, ACE-I, radiocontrast media, morphine, dextran, and polymyxin
Fixed drug eruption (**Fig. 3**)	Sulfonamides, NSAIDs, fluoroquinolones, metronidazole, ornidazole, tetracyclines, and pseudoephedrine
Photosensitivity	Quinolones, tetracyclines, sulfonamides, antimalarials, thiazides, griseofulvin, amiodarone, and psoralens
Acneiform (**Fig. 4**)	Corticosteroids, phenytoin, isoniazid, oral contraceptives, androgens, iodides, vitamin B6 and B12, lithium, and EGFRI
Lichenoid (**Fig. 5**)	Chloroquine, gold salts, phenothiazines, β-blockers, ACE-I, methyldopa, penicillamine, quinidine, and NSAIDs
Pigmentation	Minocycline, antimalarials, phenothiazines, alkylating agents, zidovudine, gold and silver salts, arsenic, clofazimine, and amiodarone
Pityriasis rosea like eruption (**Fig. 6**)	Gold, captopril, isotretinoin, omeprazole, allopurinol, barbiturates, terbinafine, vaccines, and metronidazole
Psoriasiform	Antimalarials, β-blockers, lithium, ACE-I, and NSAIDs
Erythema multiforme	Sulfonamides, penicillins, quinolones, tetracycline, rifampicin, anticonvulsants, NSAIDs, nevirapine, phenothiazines, and thiazides
Vasculitis	Antibiotics, antithyroid drugs, levamisole, and phenytoin
Hypertrichosis	Corticosteroids, phenytoin, cyclosporine, and minoxidil
Alopecia	Chemotherapeutic agents, anticonvulsants, isoniazid, indinavir, warfarin, antithyroid drugs, and retinoids
Scleroderma like	d-penicillamine, bleomycin, L-tryptophan, carbidopa, taxanes, pentazocine, and vitamin K
(ACE-I: angiotensin-converting enzyme inhibitor; EGFRI: epidermal growth factor receptor inhibitor; NSAIDs: nonsteroidal anti-inflammatory drugs)	

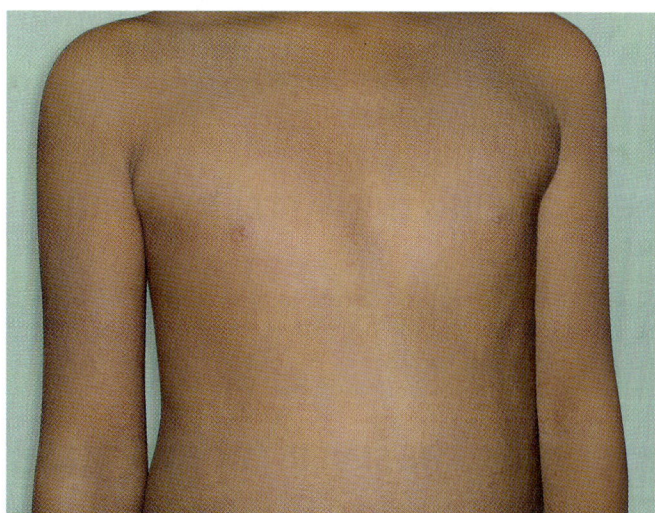

FIG. 1: Maculopapular rash to amoxicillin.

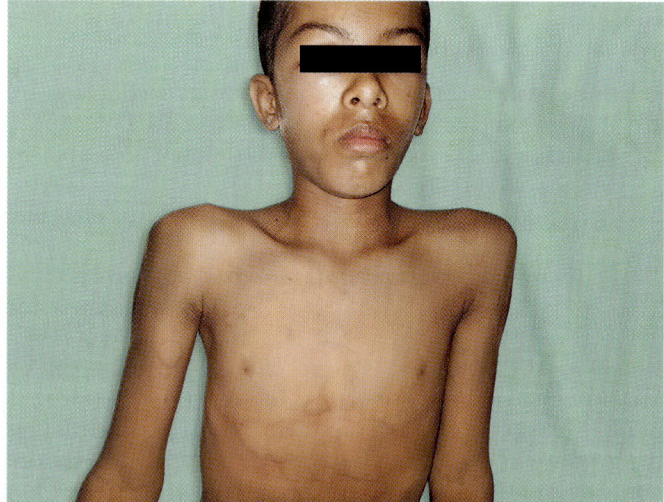

FIG. 2: Urticaria and angioedema in a child with paracetamol.

reaction promptly, stop the offending drug immediately, start supportive and specific treatment and save life.[3] The warning signs that indicate seriousness of rash include:
- Facial edema (DRESS > AGEP)
- Mucosal involvement—two or more (SJS/TEN)
- Skin tenderness, atypical target lesions, bullous skin lesions, purpura, skin necrosis, and necrolysis (SJS/TEN)
- Presence of signs and symptoms such as fever, malaise, pharyngitis, lymphadenopathy, and arthritis (DRESS, TEN)
- Reduced urine output (SJS-TEN)

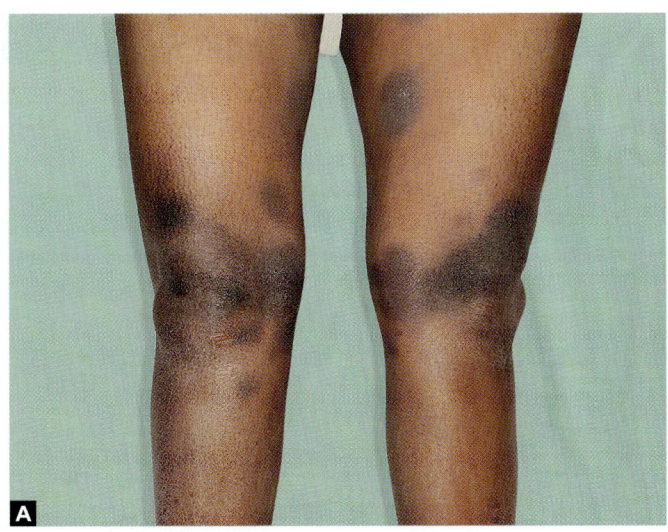
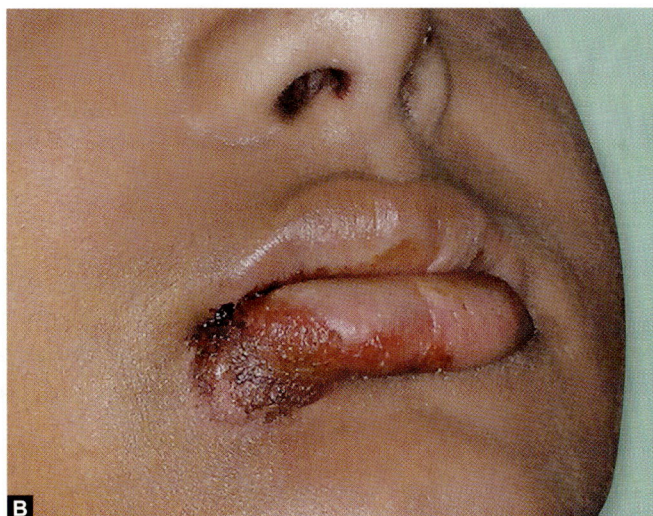

FIGS. 3A AND B: (A) Widespread fixed drug eruption (FDE) to cotrimoxazole; and (B) Mucosal FDE in a patient on cotrimoxazole.

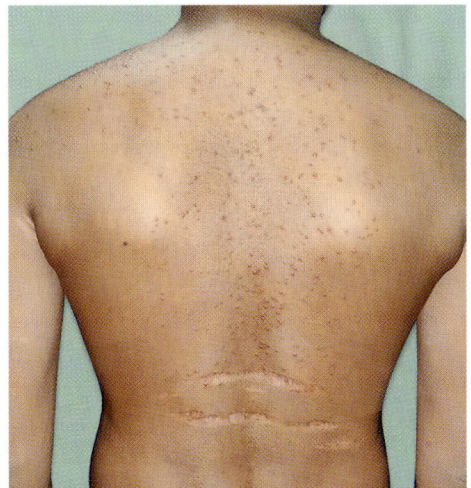

FIG. 4: Steroid-induced acneiform eruptions.

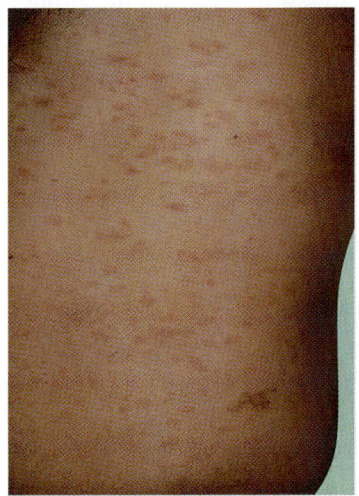

FIG. 6: Pityriasis rosea-like rash to metronidazole.

- Systemic involvement, e.g., hepatitis, pneumonitis (DRESS/SJS-TEN)
- Breathlessness, eye, and tongue swelling (anaphylaxis)
- Laboratory abnormalities: Anemia, thrombocytopenia, neutropenia, eosinophilia, atypical lymphocytes in blood film, deranged hepatic, and renal functions

Whenever a patient with suspected drug reaction arrives, it is important to observe how anxious, toxic or sick the patient feels and whether the patient has fever or is afebrile. Presence of fever is an important pointer toward SCAR. **Table 3** shows that similar morphology of rash in the presence of fever will qualify for SCAR while those without fever will be benign drug reactions. Likewise joint pains and lymphadenopathy in a patient with urticaria may indicate a possibility of serum sickness like reaction (vasculitis) rather than simple urticaria.[1]

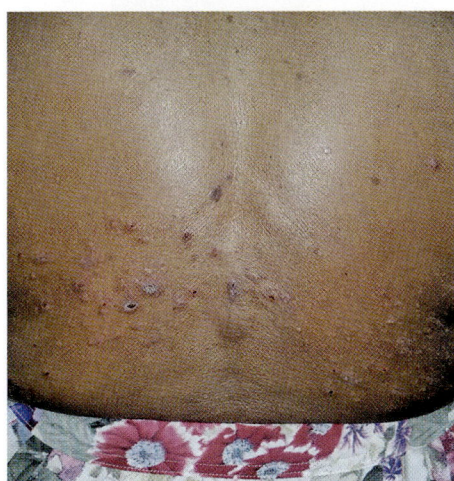

FIG. 5: Lichenoid drug reaction to amlodipine.

Stevens–Johnson syndrome-toxic epidermal necrolysis spectrum represents the prototype example of SCARs, with widespread skin necrosis and multiorgan involvement that requires urgent and appropriate intervention. Some of the other SCARs with drugs commonly causing them are shown in **Table 4**.

ASSESSING DRUG CAUSALITY

This is perhaps the most important albeit most difficult step in the evaluation of a patient, particularly so in patient consuming multiple drugs and not carrying a formal prescription which is often a case in the Indian scenario.

Table 3: Diagnosis based on constitutional signs/symptoms.				
Constitutional signs/symptoms/morphology of rash	*Exanthematous*	*Urticaria*	*Blisters*	*Pustular*
No fever	MP drug rash	Urticaria	FDE	Acneiform eruptions
Fever	DRESS/DHS	Serum sickness-like skin reaction (SSLR)	SJS/TEN	Acute generalized exanthematous pustulosis (AGEP)
(DHS: drug hypersensitivity syndrome; DRESS: drug reaction with eosinophilia and systemic symptom; FDE: fixed drug eruption; SJS/TEN: Stevens–Johnson syndrome/toxic epidermal necrolysis)				

Table 4: Various SCARs and causative drugs.	
Morphological pattern	*Causative drugs*
Stevens–Johnson syndrome/toxic epidermal necrolysis **(Fig. 7)**	Phenytoin, phenobarbitone, carbamazepine, lamotrigine, aminopenicillins, cephalosporins, cotrimoxazole, and nevirapine
Drug reaction with eosinophilia and systemic symptoms **(Fig. 8)**	Phenytoin, phenobarbitone, carbamazepine, lamotrigine, dapsone, minocycline, allopurinol, nevirapine, abacavir, and NSAIDs
Acute generalized exanthematous pustulosis (AGEP) **(Fig. 9)**	Aminopenicillins, sulfonamides, quinolones, hydroxychloroquine, terbinafine, and diltiazem
Anaphylaxis	Penicillins, cephalosporins, vaccines, radiocontrast media, animal sera, aspirin, ibuprofen, anesthetics, and dextrans
Serum sickness	Cefaclor, minocycline, penicillins, and propranolol
Erythroderma **(Fig. 10)**	Anticonvulsants, chloroquine, antitubercular drugs, chlorpromazine, lithium, sulfonamides, and nevirapine
(NSAIDs: nonsteroidal anti-inflammatory drugs; SCARs: serious cutaneous adverse drug reactions)	

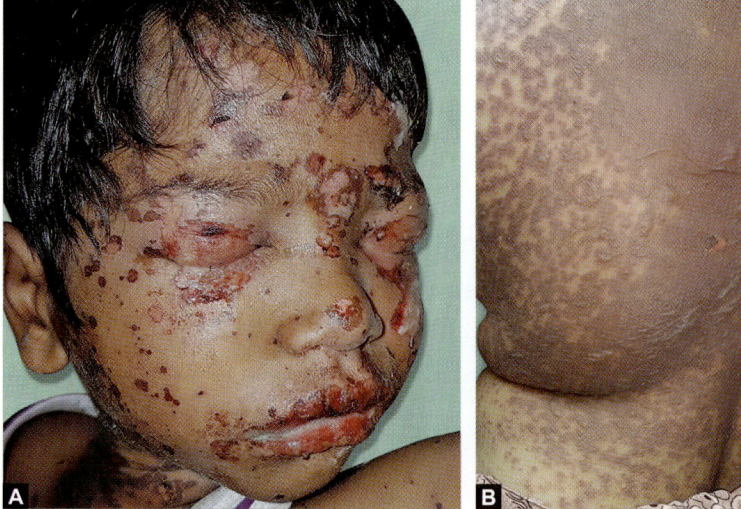

FIGS. 7A AND B: (A) Stevens–Johnson syndrome (SJS) in a child to carbamazepine and (B) Sheet like peeling of skin in TEN due to carbamazepine.

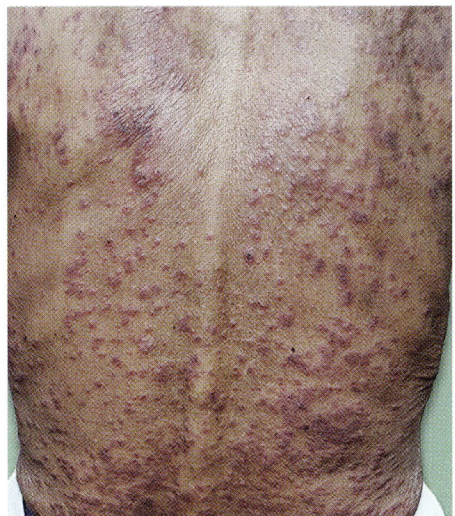

FIG. 8: Drug hypersensitivity syndrome/drug reaction with eosinophilia and systemic symptom (DHS/DRESS) to allopurinol.

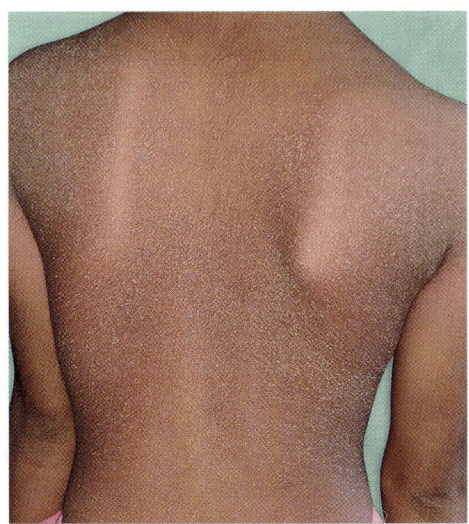

FIG. 10: Erythroderma to nevirapine.

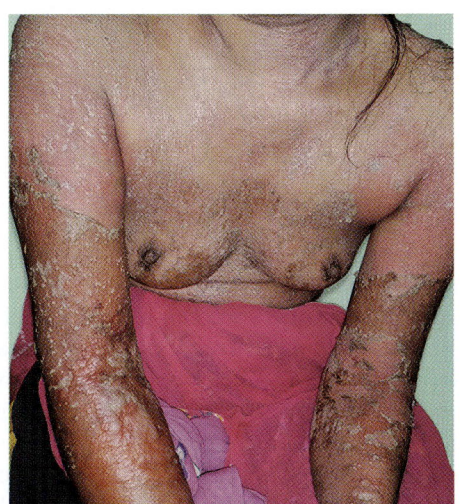

FIG. 9: Acute generalized exanthematous pustulosis (AGEP) to griseofulvin.

It is also a further guide whether suspected drug(s) needs to be continued, substituted or discontinued immediately. Certain scales and scoring systems are available to assess the drug causality; however, none of them is universally accepted and practically applicable in the individual patient care. The two most commonly causality assessment tools that can be used are: (1) Naranjo adverse drug reaction probability scale **(Table 5)** and (2) World Health Organization (WHO)—Uppsala Monitoring Center (UMC) causality assessment criteria **(Table 6)**. A thorough search of literature (DERM index, PUBMED, Litt's DERM, MEDLINE) regarding the frequency with which the specific morphologic pattern is caused by a particular drug is also a useful resource to refer to.[1,3]

Table 5: Naranjo adverse drug reaction probability scale—items and score.

Questions	Yes	No	Do not know
1. Are there previous conclusion reports on this reaction?	+1	0	0
2. Did the adverse event appear after the suspected drug was administered?	+2	−1	0
3. Did the adverse reaction improve when the drug was discontinued or a specific antagonist was administered?	+1	0	0
4. Did the adverse event reappear when the drug was readministered?	+2	−1	0
5. Are there alternative causes (other than the drug) that could on their own have caused the reaction?	−1	+2	0
6. Did the reaction reappear when a placebo was given?	−1	+1	0
7. Was the drug detected in blood (or other fluids) in concentrations known to be toxic?	+1	0	0
8. Was the reaction more severe when the dose was increased or less severe when the dose was decreased?	+1	0	0
9. Did the patient have a similar reaction to the same or similar drugs in any previous exposure?	+1	0	0
10. Was the adverse event confirmed by any objective evidence?	+1	0	0

Scoring for Naranjo algorithm: >9 = definite ADR; 5–8 = probable ADR; 1–4 = possible ADR; 0 = doubtful ADR.

Table 6: WHO-UMC causality categories.

Causality terms	Assessment criteria
Certain	• Rash with plausible time relationship to drug intake • Cannot be explained by disease or other drugs • Response to withdrawal plausible (pharmacologically, pathologically) • Event definitive pharmacologically or phenomenologically (i.e., an objective and specific medical disorder or a recognized pharmacologic phenomenon) • Positive rechallenge test
Probable/likely	• Rash that has reasonable time relationship to drug intake • Unlikely to be attributed to disease or other drugs • Response to withdrawal clinically reasonable • Rechallenge not required
Possible	• Rash with reasonable time relationship to drug intake • Could also be explained by disease or other drugs • Information on drug withdrawal may be lacking or unclear
Unlikely	• Rash with a time to drug intake that makes a relationship improbable (but not impossible) • Disease or other drugs provide plausible explanation
Conditional/unclassified	• Event or laboratory test abnormality • More data for proper assessment needed • Additional data under examination
Unassessable/unclassifiable	• Report suggesting an adverse reaction • Cannot be judged because information is insufficient or contradictory • Data cannot be supplemented or verified

(WHO-UMC: World Health Organization-Uppsala Monitoring Center)

Do laboratory and other diagnostic tests help?
Several laboratory tests are available to evaluate and confirm the diagnosis of CADR, assess reaction severity, detect other organ(s) involvement, identify offending drug, and to exclude other close mimics. However, none of the available in vivo and in vitro tests are specific, reproducible and validated and hence the diagnosis of drug reactions still is mainly clinical. Some of the investigations that can support/aid in making diagnosis are listed here.[1,4]

- *Blood investigations*: It may be useful in some cases as an adjunct. These include complete blood count (atypical lymphocytosis in DRESS, neutropenia in TEN, eosinophilia in DRESS, etc.) and liver and renal function tests. Other blood tests [enzymes, electrolytes, biochemistry, erythrocyte sedimentation rate (ESR), antinuclear antibody (ANA), bacterial and viral serology, etc.] can be requested depending upon the suspected diagnosis. Culture (skin, blood, tissue, etc.) and medical imaging can also be in appropriate clinical settings to confirm or rule out potential differential diagnoses. The following blood specialized tests may sometimes be undertaken if the facility exists and patient can afford.
  - *Elevated serum tryptase levels*: Anaphylactic reaction
  - *Low C4 levels*: Angioedema alone (not in urticaria)
  - *Antibodies to single-stranded DNA/histone*: Drug-induced lupus
  - *Antibodies to double-stranded DNA*: SLE
- *Histopathological examination*: Histopathology and direct immunofluorescence can sometimes distinguish between lesions that are drug induced and due to other diseases. For example, TEN can mimic a staphylococcal scalded skin syndrome, but a biopsy would differentiate between the two, particularly the frozen sections. Infiltration of eosinophilic polymorphonuclear leukocytes may suggest a drug-induced lesion. In DRESS the most common finding on histologic examination is a dense, superficial perivascular lymphocytic infiltrate, spongiotic or lichenoid dermatitis, and variable degree of edema. However, biopsies do not allow for identification of the causative drug.
- *In vitro tests:* These tests are apparently safer than in vivo tests. However, they are not freely available and are practically research tools currently. Their results should be interpreted in conjunction with patient history and clinical findings only. These include:
  - Histamine release test
  - Basophil degranulation test
  - Passive hemagglutination
  - Leukocyte and macrophage migration inhibition tests
  - Lymphocyte transformation test
- *In vivo tests:* In vivo tests include skin testing, dechallenge, and provocation or rechallenge test.

- *Prick and intradermal testing:* They have been found to be useful for confirmation of immunoglobulin E (IgE)-mediated immediate hypersensitivity reactions. Skin testing has only been validated for a few drugs, such as penicillin.
- *Patch testing:* It may be useful in FDE, AGEP, DHS, and maculopapular drug rash. In patients with DHS due to carbamazepine or phenytoin (CBZ/PHT), a concentration of 1% and 10% carbamazepine/phenytoin (CBZ/PHT) in petrolatum has been recommended. Patch test should generally be undertaken 6–8 weeks after the eruption has subsided in order to rule out false positive reactions due to heightened activity or false negative reactions due to a refractory state.
- *Dechallenge and rechallenge:* Dechallenge is improvement after a decrease in dosage or stopping of a suspected drug and is a strong pointer to the rash due to drug. Rechallenge is recurrence or exacerbation of eruption after re-exposure to a drug and strongly suggests a drug-induced lesion. Oral rechallenge is time consuming and generally avoided in cases of serious drug reactions. Oral rechallenge protocol with antitubercular drugs is shown in **Flowchart 1**.

MANAGEMENT

Management of a drug reaction is essentially based on accurate clinical diagnosis keeping a strong clinical suspicion in a patient who is on drug(s), establishing a temporal correlation, identifying the morphological pattern of rash, looking for the warning signs that indicate a serious nature of the rash and promptly withdrawing the offending agent and instituting supportive and specific treatment. Prevention of reaction in future is also important part of the management. As highlighted earlier the diagnosis of drug reaction is still primarily clinical in the absence of any validated, specific, accurate, and reproducible laboratory investigations therefore a need for a meticulous history and thorough clinical examination is very important. Management depends whether the rash is benign or represents a serious drug reaction or SCAR. Some of the practical management essentials for both benign and serious reactions are discussed here.

Managing Benign/Simple Drug Reaction

Maculopapular rash is a prototype example of benign rash. These patients may be managed in the outpatient settings as these reactions do not pose threat to life. Immediate

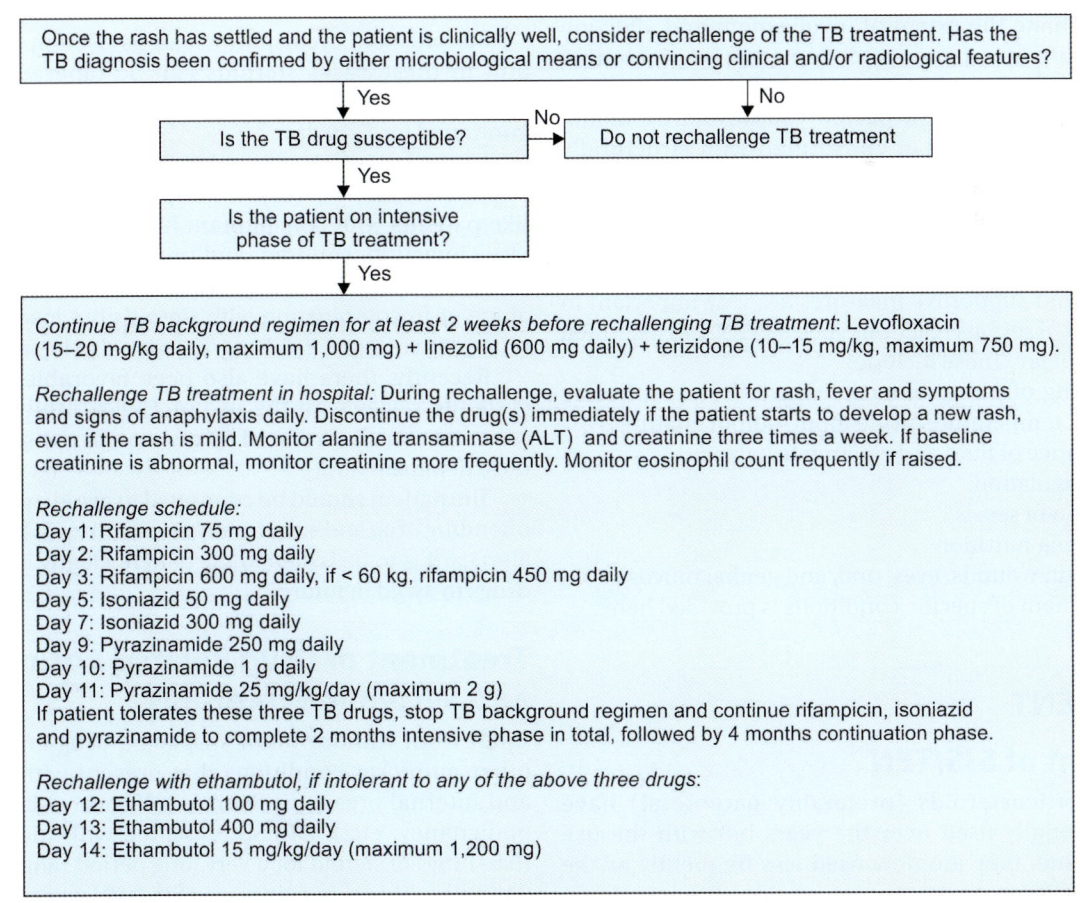

FLOWCHART 1: TB drug rechallenge after skin reaction.

stoppage of drug may not be necessary in all the cases and a wait and watch approach or "treat through approach" may be adopted as in many instances the rash may subside spontaneously even with the continuation of drug. However, a close watch should be kept on the possible progression of maculopapular rash to serious rash like DRESS. If a drug causing reaction is essential in the management of patient's primary medical condition, it should be substituted by a safer and chemically unrelated drug. Example of this includes carbamazepine or phenytoin replaced with relatively safer antiepileptic valproate sodium, clobazam or levetiracetam and sulfonamides replaced with nonsulfa drugs.[1,2]

Symptomatic antipruritic agents such as oral antihistamines, emollients, calamine lotion, and topical steroids may be used. In refractory or generalized cases, a short course of systemic steroids and immunosuppressants may be justified.

Managing Serious Drug Reactions

Severe reactions, such as SJS, TEN, and hypersensitivity reactions, warrant immediate hospital admission ideally in ICU or burn care unit or high dependency unit. However where facility is not available they can also be managed in isolation ward or general dermatology ward with proper sepsis care. Initial assessment of patient is made to evaluate the extent of involvement and affection of internal organs. A proper documentation, including photodocumentation of the condition should be made in the bed head ticket. The suspected/causative drug should be stopped immediately or substituted with structurally unrelated drugs if the medical condition warrants the use of medication, e.g., in epilepsy or septicemia. Treatment of underlying comorbidities is undertaken in consultation with multidisciplinary team.[1,3]

General and supportive measures are very important in management of serious reactions such as TEN and instituted without any delay. These include:
- Monitoring of pulse, blood pressure (BP), respiratory rate (RR), temperature, urine input/output charting
- Maintenance of fluid and electrolyte balance
- Thermoregulation
- Prevention of sepsis
- Maintaining nutrition
- Care of skin wounds, eyes, oral, and genital mucosa

The management of specific conditions is provided here.

TREATMENT

Treatment of SJS/TEN

Systemic corticosteroids (preferably parenteral) have been traditionally used over the years but with the use of cyclosporine, they are now used less frequently as the disease-modifying treatment of choice. Prednisolone, dexamethasone or methylprednisolone should be given early (preferably within 72 hours) in high dosage (1–2 mg/kg/day prednisolone or 8–16 mg/day of dexamethasone intravenous or intramuscular) and tapered quickly such that the total duration of steroid therapy is around 7–10 days.[5,6]

Cyclosporine is used in the dose of 3–5 mg/kg/day for 10–14 days, and is especially useful in patients with relative contraindications to corticosteroid use, (e.g., patients with tuberculosis and severe hyperglycemia). Despite a lack of randomized control trials, cyclosporine at a dose of 3–5 mg/kg/day orally or via nasogastric administration has been shown to have a mortality benefit in the treatment of SJS/TEN in most studies.[7-9] In a meta-analysis on the efficacy of various immunomodulators in the treatment of epidermal necrolysis, Zimmermann et al.[10] reported beneficial effects of cyclosporine [odds ratio (OR) 0.1; 95% confidence interval (CI) 0.0–0.4] and a distinct benefit of corticosteroid treatment (OR 0.7; 95% CI 0.5–0.97). In another meta-analysis of nine studies involving a total of 256 SJS/TEN patients, cyclosporine was associated with improved mortality, with a pooled standardized mortality ratio (SMR) of 0.320 (95% CI 0.119–0.522; $p = 0.002$). Most other case series, retrospective studies, and open, phase II trial have documented the efficacy, safety, and beneficial effects of cyclosporine in SJS/TEN patients which is now regarded as the first-line treatment of SJS/TEN. Our personal experience also supports the view that cyclosporine should be used as a first-line agent in SJS/TEN.[5]

Steroids and cyclosporine can be used in combination and in these cases steroids can be tapered even more quickly (2–3 days) and cyclosporine (3–5 mg/kg/day) can be continued for 7–10 days.[5]

Intravenous immunoglobulins (IVIgs), once very popular are rarely used now except in some special situation like patients with concomitant human immunodeficiency virus infection, children, and pregnant women in the first trimester. Variable dosing schedules have been used either alone or in combination with steroids but low-dose of IVIg (cumulative dose 0.2–0.5 mg/kg) may also be useful.[5]

Recently, there have also been favorable reports and systemic reviews on the use of TNF-α inhibitors (single subcutaneous injection of 50 mg etanercept single 300 mg dose of infliximab).[11,12]

The patient should be counseled to avoid exposure to the offending drug and structurally similar drug in future. A drug alert card is to be issued to the patient clearly indicating the drugs to avoid in future.

Treatment of Drug Related Eosinophilia and Systemic Symptoms

Apart from withdrawal of suspected drug and ruling out other mimicker conditions that present with fever, rash, and internal organs (infective, collagen vascular disease, malignancy, etc.), DRESS is treated with moderate dose (0.5–1 mg) of steroid for a very long period ranging from 3 to 6 months. This is in contrast to SJS-TEN where a high-dose (1–2 mg/kg) steroid is used for a short period (7–10 days).

The role of cyclosporine and other immunosuppressants is not well established in DRESS.[1]

Treatment of AGEP

Acute generalized exanthematous pustulosis (AGEP) is a relatively milder SCAR and withdrawal of drug, supportive treatment, topical steroids mixed with emollients is usually sufficient. In some unresponsive cases, systemic steroids (0.3–0.5 mg/kg/day) over 5–7 days may be used.[1,2]

Treatment of Anaphylaxis

Anaphylaxis is a multisystem acute, life-threatening emergency, and requires a team management. Apart from stoppage of drug, checking the airway, intravenous cannulation, BP, and pulse monitoring, O_2/assisted respiration, immediate administration of injection adrenaline, 0.3–0.5 mg, 1:1,000 IM in lateral thigh is administered and is life-saving. It can be repeated after 5–20 minutes if needed, until tachycardia/hypertension appears. For bronchospasm injection aminophylline 250 mg IV, given over 5 minutes and 250 mg by slow infusion over 6 hours in 500 mL normal saline or terbutaline/salbutamol nebulizer is used. For cutaneous symptoms injectable chlorpheniramine maleate (CPM), 10–20 mg IV or hydroxyzine (25–50 mg intramauscular is administered. Role of steroids is doubtful in treatment of anaphylaxis but are often used to decrease/prevent the occurrence of delayed (biphasic) anaphylaxis. Injection hydrocortisone 250 mg stat IV followed by 100 mg IV every 6 hourly for 24 hours is given. Oral prednisolone (40 mg/day × 3 days) is then used to prevent biphasic reaction.[1,3]

Desensitization

When a drug is essential for patient's well-being and no alternative is available, it is possible to induce a state of antigen-specific mast cell unresponsiveness with type I IgE-mediated reactions. Penicillin is the most common example; desensitization must be carried out in an intensive care unit (ICU) setting. Classical protocol for oral and intravenous desensitization is to start at 1/10,000–1/100 of the target dose; doubled doses are administered every 15–20 minutes till the therapeutic dose is reached **(Table 7)**. Same technique has been used for sulfonamide desensitization in HIV patients **(Table 8)** and severe reactions with multidrug anti-TB treatment.[13]

MANAGEMENT OF ADVERSE DRUG REACTIONS IN SPECIAL SITUATIONS

Contrast Media-induced Reactions

Adverse side effects from the administration of contrast media vary from minor physiological disturbances to rare severe life-threatening situations. Patients who have had a prior allergic-like reaction or unknown-type reaction, (i.e., a reaction of unknown manifestation) to contrast medium have an approximately 5-fold increased risk of developing a future allergic-like reaction if exposed to the same class of contrast medium again. In general, patients with unrelated allergies are at a 2- to 3-fold increased risk of an allergic-like contrast reaction. There is no cross-reactivity between different classes of contrast medium. Intradermal skin testing with contrast media to predict the likelihood of adverse reactions has not been shown to be useful in minimizing reaction risk.[14]

Premedication strategies: Oral premedication is preferable to IV premedication in most settings due to lower cost, more convenience, and greater evidentiary support in the literature.

Table 7: Oral penicillin desensitization protocol.

Step*	Penicillin (mg/mL)	Amount (mL)	Dose (mg)	Cumulative dose (mg)
1	0.5	0.1	0.05	0.05
2	0.5	0.2	0.1	0.15
3	0.5	0.4	0.2	0.35
4	0.5	0.8	0.4	0.75
5	0.5	1.6	0.8	1.55
6	0.5	3.2	1.6	3.15
7	0.5	6.4	3.2	6.35
8	5.0	1.2	6.0	12.35
9	5.0	2.4	12.0	24.35
10	5.0	5.0	25.0	49.35
11	50.0	1.0	50.0	100.0
12	50.0	2.0	100.0	200.0
13	50.0	4.0	200.0	400.0
14	50.0	8.0	400.0	800.0

*The interval between doses is 15 minutes.

Table 8: Oral desensitization protocol of sulfamethoxazole/trimethoprim.

		Sulfamethoxazole (mg)	Trimethoprim (mg)
Day 1	9 AM	4	0.8
	11 AM	8	1.6
	1 PM	20	4
	5 PM	40	8
Day 2	9 AM	80	16
	3 PM	160	32
	9 PM	200	40
Day 3	9 AM	400	80

1. *Prednisone-based*: 50 mg prednisone by mouth at 13 hours, 7 hours, and 1 hour before contrast medium administration, plus 50 mg diphenhydramine intravenously, intramuscularly, or by mouth 1 hour before contrast medium administration.
2. *Methylprednisolone-based*: 32 mg methylprednisolone by mouth 12 hours and 2 hours before contrast medium administration. 50 mg diphenhydramine may be added as in option 1.

If a patient is unable to take oral medication, option 1 may be used substituting 200 mg hydrocortisone IV for each dose of oral prednisone. If a patient is allergic to diphenhydramine in a situation where diphenhydramine would otherwise be considered, an alternate antihistamine without cross-reactivity may be considered, or the antihistamine portion of the regimen may be dropped.[14]

Anesthetic Induction Drugs

It has been suggested to avoid other barbiturates in patients with allergy to thiopental since immunologic cross-reactivity may occur. Cross-reactivity does not occur between the different pharmaceutical classes. Therefore, propofol can be helpful in patients with sensitivity to barbiturates. Desmethyldiazepam seems to be responsible for the cross-reactivity of diazepam with other benzodiazepines. Patients with a history of allergy to products such as medications, vaccines, cosmetics, and foods containing propylene glycol solvent should avoid diazepam that also contains this solvent.[14]

Reaction to Dyes

Blue dyes are used particularly in lymphangiography and lymphatic mapping in sentinel lymph node biopsy. There is an immunologic cross-reactivity between patent blue V and isosulfan blue, which share the same formula. Methylene blue is structurally unrelated with patent blue V and can be used after negative skin testing results.[14]

Opioid Reaction

Morphine may commonly induce a cutaneous rash, urticaria, and rarely hypotension or bronchospasm through a non-IgE-mediated mechanism. When analgesia is required in patients who experienced an adverse reaction, a nonopioid alternative drug should be given.

Reactions to Antihistamines

Paradoxical reactions to antihistamines though not common in clinical practice have been reported and should be kept in mind. FDE and urticaria have been reported to hydroxyzine, cetirizine, and levocetirizine. This scenario requires a high degree of suspicion and in such a case it is advised to switch over to other class of antihistaminics. For instance in a patient reacting to piperazines (hydroxyzine, cetirizine, and levocetirizine), the use of alternative structurally unrelated group of antihistamines as ethanolamines (diphenhydramine), alkylamines (CPM), phenothiazines (promethazine), piperidines (cyproheptadine hydrochloride), or second-generation piperidines (loratadine or fexofenadine) may be done.

DEALING WITH REFERRALS FROM OTHER SPECIALTIES, PROVIDING SAFE DRUG LIST AND MEDICOLEGAL ASPECT: CASE SCENARIOS

Quite often dermatologist receives referrals from other specialties to guide them on the use of safer drugs when a patient under their care has developed reaction to a particular drug. Although drug reactions are an unpredictable event and any drug can theoretically produce reaction in any subject, but a certain general guidelines can be suggested to them to ensure drug safety.

- *Patient with reaction to anticonvulsant drugs:* A very common situation is when a patient develops reaction to aromatic anticonvulsants (phenytoin, phenobarbitone, carbamazepine, and lamotrigine). In such case avoidance of all the drugs belonging to this group may be substituted with other drugs such as sodium valproate, clobazam, gabapentin, etc. Although lamotrigine and sodium valproate belong to different groups but they should not be combined as the latter increases the half-life of lamotrigine making it more prone to serious reactions. The family members of these patients are also advised against the use of aromatic anticonvulsants.
- *Patient with local anesthetic agent reaction:* In case of reaction to lidocaine (amide group of local anesthetic), this can be substituted with drugs from ester group (procaine and benzocaine). However, the skin prick test and intradermal test sometimes may help to ascertain the possibility of reaction to local anesthetic drug and can be advised in suspected settings.
- *Patient with penicillin allergy*: Approximately 10% of all patients report history of penicillin allergy, although in around 90% of such cases, penicillin can finally be tolerated over the years. There is a cross-reactivity among penicillins themselves as well as with the other β-lactams including cephalosporins (1–5%) and carbapenems. However, aztreonam and monobactams are relatively safe to use in penicillin-sensitive patients.
- *Patient with sulfa allergy:* The antibiotics and nonantibiotics containing sulfa moiety should be avoided in case of suspected sulfa reactions. These include carbonic anhydrase inhibitor (acetazolamide), loop diuretics (furosemide), thiazide, and related diuretics, sulfonylureas (glimepiride, gliclazide, and tolbutamide), rheumatologic agents (sulfasalazine, probenecid, celecoxib, valdecoxib), dapsone, and topiramate.

- *Patient with analgesic sensitivity:* In case of sensitivity to NSAIDs, opioid analgesics like tramadol can be used.

In author's view dermatologist should stick to diagnosing the CADR, providing management and providing list of drugs "commonly" causing particular type of CADR. In our view even such list should clearly mention that it is based on most commonly reported drugs for such CADR and need not be complete. Drugs within or outside that list can still cause similar or other CADR. Dermatologist can advise for alternative safer drugs whenever such guidelines are available. Onus of deciding the efficacy of such alternative drug in managing patient's underlying condition should be left to treating physician. Dermatologist can also help in desensitizing or rechallenge of particular drug if situation demand. For most of CADR possibility of developing future reactions is always higher in patient with documented episode of CADR than on without it. Drug reactions are highly unpredictably and depend of multitude of factors as discussed earlier in chapter in view of which dermatologist should refrain from making close-ended statement about safety of future drugs, which can be requested by specialist from other disciplines as it provide them with sense of security. Rather than documenting that "particular drug will be safe to use in future", "particular class of drug is less likely to cause this type of CADR" is legally more balanced statement. For serious CADR like anaphylaxis note about "use of any future drug or contrast media in facility where immediate CPR can be performed" should be added in documentation.

REFERENCES

1. Gupta LK, Martin AM, D'Souza P, Pande S (Editors). IADVL's Textbook on Cutaneous Adverse Drug Reactions: A comprehensive guide, 1st edition. New Delhi: Bhalani Publishing House; 2018.
2. Griffiths C, Barker J, Bleiker T, Chalmers R, Creamer D (Editors). Rook's Textbook of Dermatology, 9th edition. UK: Wiley-Blackwell Publication; 2016.
3. Pujara SB, Shah BJ. Drug reactions. In: Sacchidanand S (Editors). IADVL Textbook of Dermatology, 4th edition. Mumbai: Bhalani Publishing House; 2015. pp. 2344-95.
4. Shear NH, Dodiuk-Gad RP (Editors). Advances in Diagnosis and Management of Cutaneous Adverse Drug Reactions: Current and Future Trends. Singapore: Springer Nature Singapore Pte Ltd.; 2019.
5. Gupta LK, Martin AM, Agarwal N, D'Souza P, Das S, Kumar R, et al. Guidelines for the management of Stevens–Johnson syndrome/toxic epidermal necrolysis: An Indian perspective. Indian J Dermatol Venereol Leprol. 2016;82:603-25.
6. McPherson T, Exton LS, Biswas S, Creamer D, Dziewulski P, Newell L, et al. British Association of Dermatologists' guidelines for the management of Stevens–Johnson syndrome/toxic epidermal necrolysis in children and young people, 2018. Br J Dermatol. 2019;81:37-54.
7. Shelley WB, Shelley ED (Editors). Advanced Dermatologic Therapy II. Philadelphia: WB Saunders Company; 2001. p. 330-7.
8. González-Herrada C, Rodríguez-Martín S, Cachafeiro L, Lerma V, González O, Lorente JA, et al. Cyclosporine use in epidermal necrolysis is associated with an important mortality reduction:Evidence from three different approaches. J Invest Dermatol. 2017;1347:2092-100.
9. Morgado-Carrasco D, Fustà-NovellX, Iranzo P. FR-Ciclosporin as a First-Line Treatment in Epidermal Necrolysis. Actas Dermosifiliogr. 2019;110:601-3.
10. Zimmermann S, Sekula P, Venhoff M, Motschall E, Knaus J, Schumacher M, et al. Systemic immunomodulating therapies for Stevens-Johnson syndrome and toxic epidermal necrolysis: A systematic review and meta-analysis. JAMA Dermatol. 2017;153:514-22.
11. Frantz R, Huang S, Are A, Motaparthi K. Stevens-Johnson Syndrome and Toxic Epidermal Necrolysis: A Review of Diagnosis and Management. Medicina (Kaunas). 2021;57:895.
12. Zhang S, Tang S, Li S, Pan Y, Ding Y. Biologic TNF-alpha inhibitors in the treatment of Stevens-Johnson syndrome and toxic epidermal necrolysis: a systemic review. J Dermatol Treat. 2020;31(1):66-73.
13. National HIV & TB HCW Hotline. Management of suspected drug-induced rash, kidney injury and liver injury in adult patients on TB treatment and/or antiretroviral treatment, 2nd edition. South Africa: Medicines Information Centre Division of Clinical Pharmacology, University of Cape Town; 2020.
14. American College of Radiology (ACR). ACR Committee on Drugs and Contrast Media. ACR manual on contrast media, 2021. [online]. Available from https://www.acr.org/-/media/ACR/files/clinical-resources/contrast_media.pdf [Last accessed December, 2022].

A Patient with Generalized Pruritus without Skin Lesions

Avanitaben Dipakkumar Solanki, Ishan Asutosh Pandya

INTRODUCTION

Definition of Pruritus[1]

- Pruritus (syn.: itch) is an unpleasant sensory perception which causes an intense desire to scratch and which has a high impact on quality of life. Pruritus is the most frequently encountered symptom in dermatology and can occur in acute or chronic forms.
- Generalized pruritus without skin lesions has a significant impact on quality of life that causes various problems related to sleep, anxiety, attention, and sexual function. It also poses significant burden on society in terms of healthcare cost and treatment challenges. Recent studies have suggested a point prevalence of chronic pruritus to be approximately 13.5% in general adult population and 16.8% in those undergoing cancer screening.[2]

CLASSIFICATION OF PRURITUS ACCORDING TO MECHANISM (TWYCROSS CLASSIFICATION)[3]

- *Acute itch*: Itch lasting <6 weeks
- *Chronic itch*: Itch lasting >6 weeks

A two-tier classification system for pruritus has been proposed by International Forum for the Study of Itch.[4]

- *First-tier*: Pruritus with unknown diagnosis and it consists of three groups:
  - *Group 1*: Pruritus on diseased (inflamed) skin
  - *Group 2*: Pruritus on nondiseased skin, such as pruritus related to kidney disease, cholestatic pruritus, or neuropathic pruritus
  - *Group 3*: Pruritus presenting with severe, chronic secondary skin lesions like prurigo nodularis or excoriations
- *Second-tier*: Pruritus with known origin and it involves the following categories:
  - *Skin-derived itch (pruritoceptive itch)*: Skin-derived itching is originated from the skin, which is caused by inflammation, dryness, or damage of the skin. It is produced and irritated by conduction of C nerve fiber. *Example*: urticaria, scabies, and insect bite dermatitis.
  - *Neurogenic itch*: Neurogenic itch is derived from the central nervous system, in which itch is produced by the induction and transmission of mediators and receptors without nerve damage. *Example*: itching due to bile stasis, which is caused by opioid peptides acting on mu opioid receptor.
  - *Neuropathic itch*: Neuropathic pruritus is associated with pathological alteration in afferent pathway of sensory nerve fibers. *Example*: postherpetic neuralgia.
  - *Psychogenic itch*: Psychogenic itch is caused by psychological factors or psychiatric comorbidities. *Example*: delusional parasitosis.
  - *Mixed*: Pruritus due to more than one cause.

CAUSES OF GENERALIZED PRURITUS WITHOUT UNDERLYING DERMATOSES[5]

Generalized pruritus without skin lesions can be a manifestation of a dermatological disorder or underlying systemic diseases. The causes of generalized pruritus without skin lesions are discussed here.

- *Pruritic skin disease before rash*:
  - Bullous pemphigoid
  - Dermatitis herpetiformis
  - *Autoimmune connective tissue disorders*: Systemic sclerosis and dermatomyositis

- *Disorders of iron metabolism*:
  - Iron deficiency anemia (IDA)
  - Hemochromatosis
- *Infections and infestations*:
  - *Viral*: Human immunodeficiency virus (HIV), viral hepatitis, chikungunya, and varicella zoster infection
  - *Parasitic*: Strongyloidosis, onchocerciasis, schistosomiasis, and malaria
- *Uremia*: End-stage kidney disease
- Hepatic disease
- *Malignancies*:
  - Solid tumors
  - Hematological malignancies
- Neurological disorders
- Psychological itch (functional itch)
- Drugs
- *Endocrine disorders*:
  - Thyroid disorders
  - Diabetes mellitus
- Generalized pruritus with unknown origin (GPUO)
- *Pruritus in special populations*:
  - Pruritus in elderly
  - Pruritus in pregnancy

Approach to a patient of generalized pruritus without primary skin lesions **(Fig. 1)**:

- Before proceeding to a diagnosis of generalized pruritus without rash (GPWOR), a detailed history should be taken **(Table 1)** and a thorough clinical examination should be carried out **(Table 2)** to rule out the dermatological diseases that can mimic GPWOR but may have transient or minimal skin lesions such as urticaria, atopic dermatitis, scabies, viral exanthem, drug-induced maculopapular rash, etc.
- Once a diagnosis of GPWOR is made, a battery of screening tests should be advised to identify the underlying cause **(Table 3)**.

Regardless of whatever the cause might be in a particular patient, some general measure as mentioned in **Table 4** can be effective along with the specific treatment.

UNDERSTANDING THE CAUSES OF GENERALIZED PRURITUS WITHOUT SKIN LESIONS

Dermatological Diseases without Primary Skin Lesions

- *Bullous pemphigoid*:[34]
  - In preclinical stage of bullous pemphigoid, pruritus without skin lesions can be the only clinical manifestation. Patients complain of pruritus all day long without specific reference to time and aggravation after emotional stress.
  - Diagnosis of bullous pemphigoid can be confirmed by taking a skin biopsy for direct immunofluorescence (DIF) which demonstrates deposits of immunoglobulin G (IgG) and complement C3 in a linear band at the dermoepidermal junction (DEJ).
  - A salt split skin technique is performed in which the skin specimen is incubated in 1 mol/L solution of salt prior to performing the DIF. This technique helps to differentiate between bullous pemphigoid and other subepidermal blistering disorders. In bullous pemphigoid, deposition of IgG is seen on the roof (epidermal side of DEJ).
- *Autoimmune connective tissue disorders*:[34]
  - Although rare, a few autoimmune connective tissue disorders may present with generalized pruritus.
  - *Systemic sclerosis*: Pruritus is a common symptom of systemic sclerosis (SSc) which affects not only

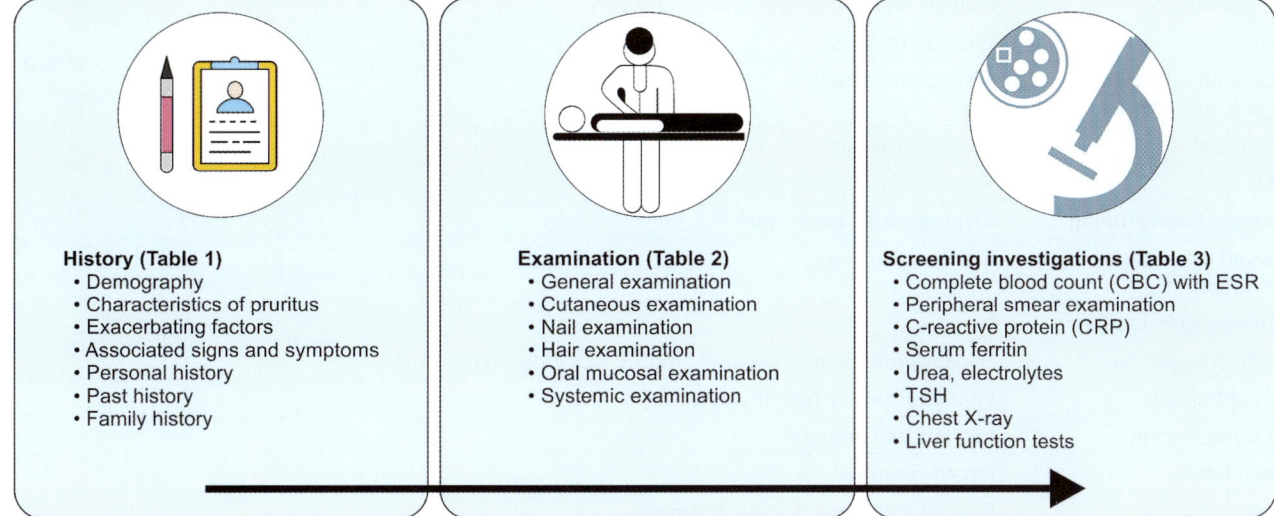

FIG. 1: Approaching a patient of generalized pruritus without skin lesions.

(ESR: erythrocyte sedimentation rate; TSH: thyroid-stimulating hormone)

Table 1: Points to consider while taking the history of a patient with generalized pruritus without skin lesions.	
History	
Demography	
Age	• Generalized pruritus without skin lesions is relatively rare in pediatric population • Prevalence of pruritus increases with age which is partially attributed to the decline in the physiological status of the skin[6] • *Geriatric population*: Common causes of generalized pruritus without skin lesions include bullous pemphigoid, malignancies, GPUO and drugs. Due to loss of free fatty acids in stratum corneum leads to xerosis and superficial cracking of skin resulting in a steatotic eczema which can cause intense pruritus in the elderly patients[5]
Gender	• Females in reproductive age group with generalized pruritus without rash should be evaluated for iron deficiency anemia, hepatic pruritus (exacerbation in premenstrual period, advanced pregnancy, hormone replacement therapy), intrahepatic cholestasis of pregnancy (if pregnancy is detected) as causes[5] • Neuropathic and psychosomatic causes of pruritus are more commonly associated with female gender[6] • Pruritus due to malignancies is more common in males
Occupation	• *Drivers, CSW, health professionals*: HIV, hepatitis B, and C • *Occupations associated with frequent travelling*: Parasitic infections such as schistosomiasis, onchocerciasis, malaria, strongyloidosis; chikungunya, hepatitis A and E
Socioeconomic status	• *Lower socioeconomic status*: Infections and infestations • *Higher socioeconomic status*: Endocrine disorders, malignancies
Residence	Parasitic and vector-borne infections should be ruled out in patients residing in endemic regions
Characteristics of pruritus	
Acute	Infections, drug-induced pruritus
Chronic	Hepatic, uremic, malignancies, psychological pruritus, GPUO
Continuous	Uremic pruritus, malignancies
Nocturnal	Hepatic pruritus, psychological pruritus, lymphoma, pruritus in pregnancy[5]
During rest/inaction	Psychological pruritus[5]
Hands and feet	Hepatic pruritus[5]
Volar aspects of hands and feet	Pruritus in pregnancy[7]
Back and face	Uremic pruritus[5]
Scapular region	Multiple endocrine neoplasm syndromes[2]
Trunk	Diabetes mellitus[2]
Associated with burning, tingling, paresthesias	Neuropathic pruritus[5]
Paroxysmal	Multiple sclerosis[8]
Nasal	Associated with brain tumors[2]
Associated with flushing	Atypical gastric carcinoids[4]
Relieved by ice pack application	Brachioradial pruritus[4]
Exacerbating factors	
Psychological stress	Hepatic pruritus, psychological pruritus, HES-induced pruritus[8]
Dry, cold climate	Pruritus in elderly, hypothyroidism[5,9]
Hot water, friction	HES-induced pruritus[8]
Irritant fabrics	Hepatic pruritus[5]
Water	Polycythemia vera, multiple sclerosis[8]
Sudden movements	Multiple sclerosis[8]

Continued

Continued

History	
Associated signs and symptoms	
Iron deficiency anemia	Headache, irritability, exercise intolerance, hair loss, soreness or burning of tongue, pica, disturbances of gastrointestinal function, dysphagia, chronic fatigue, and muscular weakness
Strongyloidosis	Recurrent urticaria, larva currens (a pathognomonic serpiginous, pruritic, erythematous eruption along the course of larval migration that may advance up to 10 cm/hour), abdominal pain, nausea, diarrhea, bleeding, and weight loss[9]
Onchocerciasis	Transient rash associated with ocular symptoms[9]
Schistosomiasis	Fever, myalgia, general malaise, fatigue, headache, cough, abdominal tenderness, dysuria, hematuria, urinary retention, dribbling and incontinence, seizures[9]
Malaria	Headache, fatigue, myalgias, febrile paroxysms[9]
Chikungunya	Fever, severe arthralgias, migratory polyarthritis mainly affecting small joints[9]
Viral hepatitis	Malaise, nausea, vomiting, diarrhea, dark urine, low-grade fever[9]
HIV infection	Fever persisting for >1 month, involuntary weight loss of >10% of baseline, diarrhea for >1 month[9]
Varicella-zoster infection	High-grade fever associated with fluid-filled skin lesions, malaise, dermatomal pain[9]
Uremic pruritus	Anorexia, weight loss, dyspnea, fatigue, sleep and taste disturbance, and confusion[8]
Hepatic pruritus	Fatigue, deranged sleep patterns, cognitive symptoms, mood changes, anxiety, depression, suicidal ideations[8]
Malignancies	Fever, loss of appetite, lethargy, weight loss (tumor-specific signs and symptoms are discussed in **Table 8**)[5]
Psychogenic pruritus	Presence of psychiatric morbidities such as depression, anxiety, obsessive compulsive disorders, psychoses[5]
Hypothyroidism	Lethargy, dry hair and skin, cold intolerance, hair loss, difficulty in concentrating, poor memory, constipation, mild weight gain with poor appetite, dyspnea, hoarse voice, muscle cramping, menorrhagia[9]
Hyperthyroidism	Warm and moist skin, nervousness, irritability, heat intolerance, excessive sweating, palpitations, fatigue and weakness, weight loss with increased appetite, frequent bowel movements, oligomenorrhea[9]
Diabetes mellitus	Polyuria, polydipsia, polyphagia, fatigue, weakness, weight loss, blurred vision, frequent superficial infections, poor wound healing, paresthesias[9]
Pruritus of pregnancy	Second trimester of pregnancy, abdominal pain, nausea vomiting, insomnia, irritability, depression[7]
Personal history	
Diet	• *Vegetarian/vegan*: Iron deficiency anemia, helminthic infections • *Nonvegetarian/mixed*: Helminthic infections, Creutzfeldt–Jakob disease[8] • *Exacerbation after gluten containing diet*: Dermatitis herpetiformis
Appetite	• *Decreased*: Iron deficiency anemia, HIV infection, malignancies, hypothyroidism, hepatic pruritus • *Increased*: Hyperthyroidism, diabetes mellitus
Sleep	• *Decreased*: Uremic pruritus, hepatic pruritus, lymphoma, psychogenic pruritus, pruritus of pregnancy, neuropathic pruritus • *Increased*: Iron deficiency anemia • *Excessive day time sleepiness, sleep disorders (sleep apnea, restless leg syndrome, periodic limb movement disorder)*: Uremic pruritus[10]
Bowel	• *Diarrhea*: Parasitic infections, viral hepatitis, HIV infection, hyperthyroidism, malignancies, drugs, psychogenic pruritus • *Constipation*: Iron deficiency anemia, hypothyroidism, drugs, psychogenic pruritus, malignancies, pruritus of pregnancy • *Blood in stool*: Iron deficiency anemia, parasitic infections, malignancies, drugs
Bladder	• *Oliguria*: Uremic pruritus • *Polyuria*: Diabetes mellitus • *Discoloration of urine*: Viral hepatitis, hepatic pruritus, drugs • *Hematuria*: Schistosomiasis, malignancies

Continued

Continued

History	
Addictions (tobacco, alcohol, drugs, etc.)	Viral hepatitis, HIV infection, hepatic pruritus, malignancies, neuropathic pruritus, psychogenic pruritus
Recent travel history, contact with pets	Infections
Tattooing, body piercing	HIV infection, viral hepatitis
Sexual history	Infections
Drug history	Drug-induced pruritus (see **Table 13**)
History of pica	Iron deficiency anemia, infections
Past history	
Recent major surgery	Iron deficiency anemia
Blood transfusion	HIV infection, viral hepatitis
Jaundice	Hepatic pruritus
Malignancies	Treated/Untreated
Other illnesses	Diabetes mellitus, thyroid disorders, hypertension, dyslipidemia
Family history	
	• Similar complaints in family • Major medical illnesses • Infections and infestations • Psychiatric disorders • Neurological disorders[11] • Malignancies • Presence of pets in family
(CSW: clinical social worker; GPUO: generalized pruritus with unknown origin; HES: hydroxyethyl starch; HIV: human immunodeficiency virus)	

Table 2: Points to consider while examining a patient with generalized pruritus without skin lesions.

Examination	
General[12]	
Vitals	• *Hyperthermia*: Infections, malignancies, hyperthyroidism • *Hypothermia*: Hypothyroidism, infections • *Tachycardia*: Infections, hyperthyroidism, drugs, iron deficiency anemia[9] • *Bradycardia*: Hypothyroidism, drugs • *Tachypnea*: Infections, hyperthyroidism • *Bradypnea*: Malignancies • *Hypertension*: Uremic pruritus, drugs, hyperthyroidism (systolic), hypothyroidism (diastolic) • *Hypotension*: Drugs, infections
Weight	• *Weight loss*: Iron deficiency anemia, infections, malignancies, hyperthyroidism, psychogenic pruritus, drugs • *Weight gain*: Hypothyroidism, drugs
Orientation	*Disoriented and confused*: Hepatic pruritus, uremic pruritus, neurological pruritus, psychogenic pruritus, infections
Pallor	Iron deficiency anemia, malignancies, HIV infections, drugs, connective tissue disorders
Icterus	Hepatic pruritus, viral hepatitis, drugs, pruritus of pregnancy
Cyanosis	Connective tissue disorders, iron deficiency anemia, drugs, malignancies, neurological pruritus, HIV infection

Continued

Continued

Examination	
Clubbing	Malignancies, iron deficiency anemia, hepatic pruritus
Lymphadenopathy	Malignancies, HIV infection, drugs
Edema	Iron deficiency anemia, hepatic pruritus, uremic pruritus, hypothyroidism,[12] drugs
Cutaneous examination	
	Secondary skin changes such as xerosis, dyspigmentation, excoriations, lichenification, erosions, prurigo, and eczematization are commonly seen in patients with generalized pruritus without primary skin lesions
Dermatitis herpetiformis	Excoriated skin lesions—predominantly on extensor surfaces of limbs and buttocks
Systemic sclerosis	Generalized hyperpigmentation, "salt and pepper" appearance of the skin
HIV infection, viral hepatitis	Cutaneous puncture marks of IV drug abuse, spider nevi, palmar erythema[12]
Onchocerciasis	A history of transient erythematous rash may be given by the patient[9]
Parasitic infections	Lichenification, loss of elasticity, atrophy and/or depigmentation[9]
Uremic pruritus	• Uremic frost is specifically seen in uremic pruritus. Uremic frost is a whitish friable and crystalline powdery frost seen all over body, especially on face and limbs[13] • Secondary skin changes are predominantly seen on back, face, and at the sites of AV fistula
Hepatic pruritus	Secondary skin changes such as excoriations and hyperpigmentation are present predominantly on hands and feet along with spider nevi, palmar erythema[12]
Hodgkin's lymphoma	Ichthyotic skin lesions[14]
Neurogenic and psychogenic pruritus	Lichen simplex chronicus and amyloidosis are predominantly seen in neurogenic and psychogenic pruritus. Even when unconscious, patients having neuropathic pruritus tend to rub or scratch their nostrils[8]
Thyroid disorders	Spider nevi, palmar erythema[12]
Diabetes mellitus	Lichenification and amyloidosis
Drug-induced pruritus	Xerosis[4]
Hair examination	
Hair thinning	Iron deficiency anemia, connective tissue disorders
Diffuse hair loss	Malignancies, drugs, hypothyroidism, infections
Patchy hair loss	Psychogenic pruritus, thyroid disorders
Madarosis	Thyroid disorders
Hypertrichosis	Drugs
Nails[15]	
Koilonychia	Reverse curvature in the transverse and longitudinal axes giving a concave dorsal aspect to the nail—spoon-shaped nails: iron deficiency anemia, hemochromatosis, malignancies, hypothyroidism
Pallor	Iron deficiency anemia, malignancies, HIV infection, drugs, connective tissue disorders
Splinter hemorrhages	*Linear brown black or red streaks on the basal nail plate*: Malignancies, connective tissue disorders, pruritus of pregnancy
Beau's lines	Infections, uremic pruritus
Onycholysis	Malignancies, iron deficiency anemia, pruritus of pregnancy, connective tissue disorders, diabetes mellitus
Plummer's nail	*Undulated and curved upward nails, commonly seen on fourth and fifth finger nail*: Hyperthyroidism
Pitting	*Punctate depression in the nail plate*: Connective tissue disorders
Mees' lines	*Single transverse narrow whitish line runs the width of the nail plate, present in multiple nails that do not disappear on blanching*: Hodgkin's lymphoma
Muehrcke's lines	*Double white transverse line of the nail vascular bed that temporarily disappear on squeezing the distal digit, seen on second, third, and fourth finger nail*: Hepatic pruritus, uremic pruritus, drugs, iron deficiency anemia
Half and half nails	*Normal proximal half and distinctly abnormal distal brownish portion*: Uremic pruritus

Continued

Continued

Examination	
Terry's nails	*White proximally and normal distally*: Hepatic pruritus, diabetes, uremic pruritus, HIV infection
Fragile and brittle nails	Viral hepatitis, hemochromatosis, leukemia, diabetes mellitus
Longitudinal striations	Viral hepatitis, HIV infection, hemochromatosis
Blue lunula	Hemochromatosis
Gray lunula	Malaria
Red lunula, periungual erythema, telangiectasia	Diabetes mellitus
Longitudinal melanonychia	HIV infection
Striated leukonychia, onychotillomania	Psychogenic pruritus
Increased transverse curvature	Systemic sclerosis
Oral mucosa	
Bullous pemphigoid	Oral ulcerations
Autoimmune connective tissue disorders	Periodontitis, dental caries, xerostomia, oral ulcers, microstomia (systemic sclerosis), oral/dental infection, dysphagia[16]
Iron deficiency anemia	Glossitis, glossodynia, angular cheilitis, recurrent oral ulcer, oral candidiasis, erythematous mucositis, and pallor of oral mucosa[17]
HIV infection	Oral ulcers (HSV, aphthous, nonspecific), hairy tongue, coated tongue, fissured tongue, purpuric lesions, hyperpigmentation, cheilitis, tooth decay[18]
Viral hepatitis	Bleeding gums, cheilitis, smooth tongue, xerostomia, bruxism, sialadenitis, and oral lichen planus[19]
Malaria	Gingival bleeding, glossitis, oral ulcer, pigmentation, bitter taste, sore throat[20]
Chikungunya	Ulcers and oral thrush, gingival bleeding, pain and burning of the oral mucous membranes, temporomandibular joint (TMJ) arthralgia, opportunistic infections, and changes in taste[21]
Uremic pruritus	Uremic stomatitis, xerostomia, gingival bleeding, ulcers, gingival hyperplasia, uremic fetor, premature loss of teeth[22]
Hepatic pruritus	Oral lichen planus, oral submucus fibrosis, yellowish discoloration, glossitis, angular cheilitis, taste alterations, petechiae[23]
Hematological malignancies	Pallor of the mucosa, gingival enlargement, bleeding, trismus, and bone changes[24]
Neurogenic pruritus	Mucosal neurofibromas, alteration in taste sensations, enlarged papillae[25]
Psychogenic pruritus	Lichen planus, xerostomia, bruxism, aphthous ulcers[26]
Diabetes mellitus	Candidial infections, fissured tongue, irritation fibroma, dysgeusia, burning mouth syndrome, traumatic ulcers, gingival erythema and edema, periodontal disease, xerostomia, diabetic sialadenosis[25]
Thyroid disorders	Swollen, thickened lips[25]
Drugs	Xerostomia, ulcers, salivary gland enlargement and pain, discoloration of salivary secretions, mucus membrane pigmentation, gingival enlargement, dental caries, taste disorders, halitosis[27]
Systemic examination[12]	
Cardiovascular	Abnormal heart sounds can be heard in iron deficiency anemia
Abdomen	• *Tenderness*: Hepatitis • *Hepatomegaly*: Hepatitis, schistosomiasis, malaria, malignancies • *Splenomegaly*: Connective tissue disorders, hepatitis, malaria, schistosomiasis, hematologic malignancies • *Hepatosplenomegaly*: Malaria, hepatitis, hematologic malignancies • *Ascites*: Iron deficiency anemia, uremic pruritus, parasitic infections, connective tissue disorders, hypothyroidism
Respiratory	*Rhonchi*: Localized malignancies *Rales*: Systemic sclerosis, dermatomyositis, neurofibromatosis (neurogenic pruritus)
(AV: arteriovenous; HIV: human immunodeficiency virus; HSV: herpes simplex virus)	

Table 3: Investigations and their interpretations in context of a patient with generalized pruritus without skin lesions.	
Screening investigations	
Hemoglobin[12]	• *Decreased*: Iron deficiency anemia, connective tissue disorders, human immunodeficiency virus (HIV) infection, uremic pruritus, hepatic pruritus, malignancies, drugs, hypothyroidism • *Increased*: Polycythemia vera
Total leukocyte count[12]	• *Decreased*: Connective tissue disorders, HIV infection, malaria, viral hepatitis, hematologic malignancies, drugs • *Increased*: Uremic pruritus, hepatic pruritus, pruritus of pregnancy, polycythemia vera, malignancies, psychological pruritus
Differential leukocyte count[12]	• *Neutrophilia*: Uremic pruritus, hepatic pruritus, pruritus of pregnancy, polycythemia vera, malignancies, psychological pruritus • *Neutropenia*: Connective tissue disorders, HIV infection, malaria, viral hepatitis, hematologic malignancies, drugs • *Lymphocytosis*: Lymphomas • *Lymphopenia*: Hodgkin's disease, HIV infection, viral hepatitis • *Monocytosis*: Malaria, viral hepatitis, connective tissue disorders, malignancies • *Basophilia*: Polycythemia vera, hypothyroidism • *Eosinophilia*: Drugs, parasitic infections, dermatitis herpetiformis, bullous pemphigoid, malignancies
Platelet count[12]	• *Increased*: Iron deficiency anemia, polycythemia vera • *Decreased*: Connective tissue disorders, viral infections, drugs, malignancies
Peripheral smear examination[12]	• *Hypochromic microcytic anemia*: Iron deficiency anemia, malignancies • *Normochromic normocytic anemia*: Uremic pruritus, connective tissue disorders • *Macrocytic anemia*: Hepatic pruritus, drugs, hypothyroidism • *Acanthocytes, echinocytes*: Uremic pruritus, hepatic pruritus • *Target cells*: Iron deficiency anemia • *Erythrocyte dimorphism*: Iron deficiency anemia, HIV infection • *Schistocytes*: Iron deficiency anemia, uremic pruritus, malignancies • *Basophilic stippling*: Hepatic pruritus
Erythrocyte sedimentation rate (ESR)	• *Increased*: Connective tissue disorders, iron deficiency anemia, HIV infection, malignancies, pruritus of pregnancy • *Decreased*: Polycythemia vera
C-reactive protein (CRP)	• *Increased*: Connective tissue disorders, infections, malignancies, pruritus of pregnancy • *Decreased*: Drugs
Serum ferritin	• *Increased*: Hemochromatosis, infections, malignancies, connective tissue disorders, hepatic pruritus, hyperthyroidism[28] • *Decreased*: Iron deficiency anemia
Urea[29]	• *Increased*: Uremic pruritus, dehydration, drugs, pruritus of elderly, psychological pruritus • *Decreased*: Hepatic pruritus, pruritus of pregnancy[30]
Electrolytes[31]	• *Hyponatremia*: Hepatic pruritus, diabetes • *Hypernatremia*: Pruritus of elderly • *Hyperkalemia*: Diabetes mellitus, uremic pruritus, drugs • *Hypercalcemia*: Malignancies • *Hypomagnesemia*: Hepatic pruritus, drugs • *Hypochloremia*: Uremic pruritus • *Hyperphosphatemia*: Uremic pruritus

Liver function tests	• *Elevated transaminases*: Connective tissue disorders, viral hepatitis, drugs, endocrine diseases, hepatic pruritus, malignancies
	• *Hyperbilirubinemia*:[32]
	  ○ *Conjugated hyperbilirubinemia*: Viral hepatitis, hepatic pruritus, drugs, pruritus of pregnancy, malignancies, parasitic infections
	  ○ *Unconjugated hyperbilirubinemia*: Hyperthyroidism
	• *Elevated alkaline phosphatase (ALP)*: Malignancies, drugs, pruritus of pregnancy, hepatic pruritus, HIV infection, viral hepatitis
	Low ALP levels: Hypothyroidism[33]

Thyroid-stimulating hormone (TSH)[9]	• *Elevated*: Primary hypothyroidism: drugs, hemochromatosis, connective tissue disorders, malignancies • *Low*: Hyperthyroidism
Chest X-ray	Useful in detection of HIV infection and malignancies

Table 4: General measures to manage generalized pruritus without rash.[2]			
Avoid	Use	Relaxation therapy	Educate
Dry climate, heat, alcoholic compresses, ice packs, frequent bathing and washing, very hot and spicy food, alcohol, contact with irritant substances such as chamomile, tea tree oil, etc., excitement, strain and stress, allergens (house dust)	Mild nonalkaline soaps, moisturizers, bathing oils, lukewarm water while bathing, bathe for not >20 minutes, soft cotton clothing, night creams/lotions, after contact with water the skin should be dabbed dry without rubbing it	Relaxation therapy, autogenic training	Psychosocial education, educating patients to cope with itching and scratching, educational training programs

the affected areas, but it is also generalized and on extremities.
  ○ *Sjogren's syndrome*: The pruritus is mainly due to the xerosis with shins being the most common site of the pruritus.

Disorders of Iron Metabolism
- *Iron deficiency anemia*:[5]
  ○ The most common cause of generalized pruritus in patients with underlying systemic disease was found to be IDA.
  ○ *Specific investigations*:
    – Serum ferritin
    – Serum iron
    – Serum total iron binding capacity (TIBC)
    – Tissue transglutaminase (TTG) antibodies
    – Endoscopy
    – Small bowel biopsy
  ○ Management of IDA **(Flowchart 1)**
- *Iron overload*:[5]
  ○ It is associated with hemochromatosis or hyperferritinemia
  ○ Liver infiltration and diabetes mellitus are confounding variables
  ○ *Investigations*: Complete blood count (CBC), liver function tests, serum ferritin levels, serum transferrin saturation
  ○ *Treatment*: Venesection (vascular surgeons)

Infections and Infestations[5,9]
- *Specific investigations*:
  ○ Absolute eosinophil counts (eosinophilia suggests parasitic infection)
  ○ Serological viral markers
  ○ Stool routine and microscopic examination for ova and cysts (for parasitic infections)
  ○ Stool culture
  ○ Peripheral smear
  ○ Skin-snip biopsy sample (onchocerciasis)
  ○ CD4 cell counts (HIV infection)
  ○ Antigen detection tests for specific organisms
  ○ Sputum examination
  ○ Blood culture (recurrent signs of infection)
  ○ Lactate dehydrogenase (LDH)

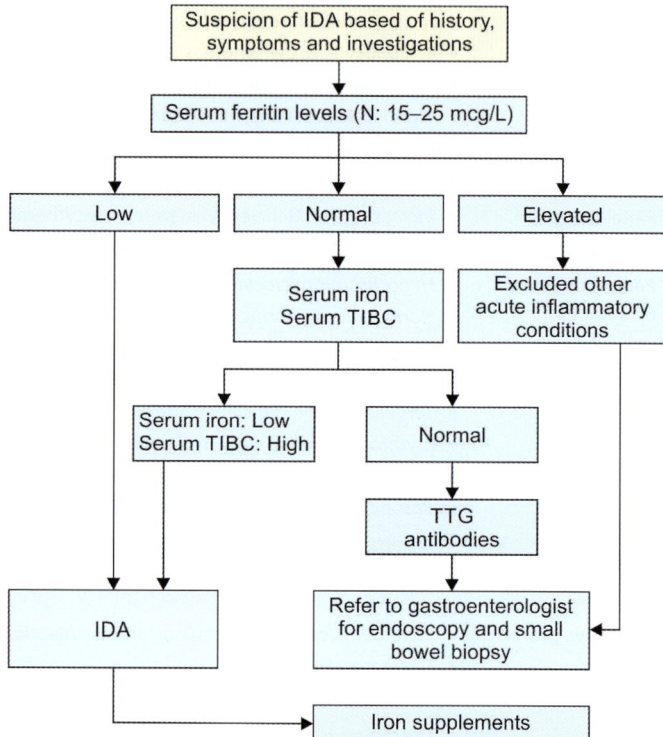

FLOWCHART 1: Management of pruritus associated with iron deficiency anemia.
(IDA: iron deficiency anemia; TIBC: total iron binding capacity)

  ○ Reticulocyte count
  ○ Haptoglobin
  ○ Glucose-6-phosphate dehydrogenase (G6PD) deficiency (malaria)
  ○ Abdominal ultrasonography
  ○ Abdominal computed tomography (CT)
  ○ Thorax CT
- *Specific treatment*: Detailed discussion of the treatment of aspect is beyond the scope of this chapter. Treatment plan for infections is mentioned in **Table 5**.

Uremic Pruritus[5]
Uremic pruritus can be treated by various pharmacological and nonpharmacological measures; however, treating the

CHAPTER 5 A Patient with Generalized Pruritus without Skin Lesions

Table 5: Treatment plan for selected infections responsible for generalized pruritus without skin lesions.

Infection	Treatment
Strongyloidosis	• *Drug of choice*: Ivermectin 200 µg/kg for 1–2 days • Albendazole 400 mg BD for 7 days • *Hyperinfection*: Ivermectin 200 µg/kg daily until stool and sputum becomes negative for 2 weeks, corticosteroids are given concomitantly to prevent hypersensitivity reactions
Onchocerciasis	• Ivermectin 200 µg/kg repeated every 3–6 months for 10–12 years • Doxycycline 100–200 mg/day for 6 weeks • Combination is more effective than monotherapy • Moxidectin 8 mg orally once
Schistosomiasis	Praziquantel 40 mg/kg/day in two divided doses in one day

Malaria	• Treat according to the guidelines from NVBDCP (National Vector-borne Disease Control Program)
	• *Four major drug classes*:
	  i. Quinoline-related compounds
	  ii. Antifolates
	  iii. Artemisinin derivatives
	  iv. Antimicrobials

Chikungunya	Treat according to the guidelines from NVBDCP

Table 6: Pharmacological and nonpharmacological treatments for uremic pruritus.

Treatment (nonpharmacological)	Treatment (pharmacological)

• Ensure adequate dialysis
• Simple emollients for xerosis
• Phototherapy
• Acupuncture
	• Normalize calcium-phosphate balance
	• Control parathyroid hormone (PTH) to accepted levels
	• Correct anemia with erythropoietin
	• Capsaicin (0.025–0.03% cream) four times a day
	• Topical calcipotriol once a day
	• Oral gabapentin 100–300 mg three times a week after dialysis
	
	Experimental therapies:
	• *Topical*:
	  ○ Tacrolimus
	  ○ Cromolyn sodium (4%)
	  ○ Gamma-linoleic acid with evening primrose oil
	• *Systemic*:
	  ○ Ketotifen 1 mg daily
	  ○ Doxepin 10 mg twice daily
	  ○ Pregabalin 75 mg twice daily
	  ○ Granisetron 1 mg daily, tropisetron 5 mg daily
	  ○ Naltrexone 50 mg daily
	  ○ Thalidomide 100 mg daily
	  ○ Mirtazapine 15–30 mg daily
	  ○ Sertraline 25–200 mg daily
	  ○ Oral activated charcoal

underlying cause for uremia remains the mainstay of the treatment **(Table 6)**.

Hepatic Pruritus[5]

- *Specific investigations*:
  ○ Liver function tests
  ○ Bile acids
  ○ Antimitochondrial antibodies
- *General measures to manage hepatic pruritus*:
  ○ Use of emollients and soothing agents (e.g., menthol)
  ○ Showering with cold water
  ○ Wearing light clothes made with natural fibers like cotton
  ○ Avoid clothing that is woollen or tight and the use of scented detergents
  ○ Psychological interventions in cases of addictive scratching
- Pharmacological treatment **(Table 7)**[35]

Malignancies

- *Solid tumors*:[5]
  ○ Generalized pruritus associated with solid tumors can be multifactorial. It can be (a) a true paraneoplastic symptom, (b) a feature of paraneoplastic dermatoses, (c) secondary to paraneoplastic neuropathy, (d) a consequence of secondary skin involvement by cutaneous or noncutaneous primary tumors, or (e) side effect of cancer treatment.
  ○ Various tumors can present with different signs and symptoms and one should be aware of identifying them **(Table 8)**.
  ○ 50% patients with brain tumors have associated nasal pruritus.[2]
  ○ Unilateral pruritus over scapular region has been associated with multiple endocrine neoplasm syndromes.[2]
  ○ *Cancer treatments that can cause pruritus*:[5]
    – Radiotherapy
    – Biological therapies
    – Epidermal growth factor inhibitors (very common)
  ○ *Investigations*:
    – Pruritus with systemic symptoms of malignancy needs tailored investigations to rule out specific cancers. Common investigations include CT of neck, chest, abdomen, and pelvis.

Table 7: Pharmacological treatment modalities for hepatic pruritus.

First line	Cholestyramine 4–16 mg daily (always maintain a 4-hour interval between other drugs)
Second line	*Rifampicin*: Start from 150 mg twice daily, can be given up to 600 mg twice daily. Monitor for hepatotoxicity
Third line	Bezafibrate 200–400 mg daily
Fourth line	Naltrexone 50 mg daily (start with 12.5 mg/day; increase every third day up to 50 mg/day) OR nalmefene 0.25 µg/kg/day IV
Fifth line	Sertraline 75–100 mg daily
Sixth line	• Systemic dronabinol • Phenobarbitone • Propofol • Topical tacrolimus ointment • Phototherapy • Extracorporeal dialysis technique • Nasobiliary drainage • Liver transplantation
Newer treatments	*Ileal bile acid transporter (IBAT) inhibitors*: • Linerixibat 90 mg/day for 3 days, followed by 180 mg/day for 4–14 days • Maralixibat • Odevixibat

Table 8: Tumor-specific signs and symptoms.

Cancer	Symptoms	Signs
Breast cancer	Breast/axillary lump, change in breast shape, blood-stained nipple discharge	
Colorectal cancer	Persistent change in bowel habits, diarrhea, abdominal pain, discomfort/bloating brought on by eating	Blood in stool, in the absence of hemorrhoids
Lung cancer	Persistent cough and breathlessness, persistent chest or shoulder pain	Persistent chest infections, wheeze, facial swelling, hoarse voice, clubbing
Gastric cancer	Persistent nausea, reflux symptoms, dysphagia/vomiting	Melaena, jaundice
Cholangio-carcinoma	Nonspecific upper abdominal discomfort	Jaundice, pale stools, dark urine
Testicular cancer	Intermittent dull ache or sharp pain in testicles or scrotum	Clinical difference between one testicle and the other in texture or firmness
Thymoma	Persistent cough, shortness of breath, pain or pressure in the chest, diplopia, dysphagia	Anemia, frequent infections, muscle weakness, ptosis, arm or facial swelling
Insulinoma	Intermittent double vision or blurred vision, confusion, anxiety and irritability, dizziness, mood swings, weakness, sweating, and hunger	Symptoms correlate with episodic hypoglycemia
Gastric carcinoid tumor	Abdominal pain, diarrhea, intermittent facial swelling, facial flushing	Very rarely, cardiac valve murmurs, cutaneous stigmata of neurofibromatosis type 1 or tuberous sclerosis

- *Treatment*:[5]
    - Antihistamines are not effective in treatment of paraneoplastic pruritus.
    - Paroxetine 20 mg daily
    - Mirtazapine 15–30 mg daily
    - Granisetron—continuous infusion of 3 mg per 24 hours—in advanced malignancies
    - Refer to hematooncologist/oncosurgeon
- *Hematological malignancies*:[5]
    - Amounts for 2% of total cases presenting with GPWOR
    - Investigations and management of pruritus due to hematological malignancies are presented in **Table 9**.

Neuropathic Pruritus[2,5]

Neuropathic pruritus can arise from localized or systemic causes addressed in **Table 10**:
- Itching is frequently associated with burning, tingling, stinging, and paresthesia.
- *Investigations*:
    - *Multiple sclerosis and brain tumors*: Cerebrospinal fluid (CSF) analysis, electroencephalogram (EEG), magnetic resonance imaging (MRI), and CT of brain, and functional tests
    - *Notalgia paresthetica*: MRI of thoracic spine
    - *Brachioradial pruritus*: MRI of thoracic and cervical spine
    - Refer to relevant specialist for further management

Psychological Pruritus (Functional Itch Disorders)[5]

Diagnostic criteria and management of psychogenic pruritus are given in **Tables 11 and 12** respectively

Drug-induced Pruritus[36]

- *History*: A detailed history regarding all the ingested medications including over the counter pharmaceuticals and herbal remedies.

Table 9: Investigations and management of pruritus due to hematological malignancies.

Investigations	Management of pruritus
• CBC, ESR, peripheral blood smear, LDH, immunoglobulins, urinary paraproteins • Skin biopsy • Excision or ultrasound-assisted core biopsy of enlarged lymph nodes or masses • In suspected cases of polycythemia vera (PV), analysis of JAK2 V617F mutation (present in 97% cases of PV) If it turns out to be negative, serum erythropoietin levels, measurement of oxygen saturation, chest X-ray, abdominal ultrasound should be done to rule out secondary causes of PV	*Lymphoma*: • Cimetidine • Gabapentin • Carbamazepine • Mirtazapine • Phototherapy *Incurable lymphoma*: • Oral corticosteroids *Polycythemia vera*: • Cytoreductive therapy • Aspirin • Interferon-α • SSRIs • Phototherapy • Cimetidine • Atenolol

(CBC: complete blood count; ESR: erythrocyte sedimentation rate; LDH: lactate dehydrogenase; SSRIs: selective serotonin reuptake inhibitors)

Table 10: Causes of neuropathic pruritus.

Localized causes	Systemic causes
• Postherpetic neuropathy • Brachioradial pruritus • Notalgia paresthetica	• Neurofibromatosis type 1 • Diabetes mellitus • Guillain–Barré syndrome • Sarcoidosis • HIV • Transverse myelitis • CVA (poststroke pruritus) • Multiple sclerosis • Creutzfeldt–Jakob disease

(CVA: cerebrovascular accident; HIV: human immunodeficiency virus)

Table 11: Diagnostic criteria for psychogenic pruritus.

Compulsory criteria (3 out of 3)	Optional criteria (3 out of 7)
1. Generalized pruritus without primary skin disease 2. Chronic pruritus (>6 weeks) 3. No somatic cause (cutaneous/systemic)	1. Chronological relationship of the occurrence of pruritus with one or several life events that could have psychological repercussions 2. Variations in intensity associated with stress 3. Pruritus that is worse at night 4. Predominance during rest or inaction 5. Associated psychological disorder 6. Pruritus that could be improved by psychotropic drugs 7. Pruritus that could be improved by psychological therapy

Table 12: Management of psychogenic pruritus.

Nonpharmacological measures	Pharmacological treatment
• Psychiatric and psychosomatic exploration • Psychiatric short questionnaires for depression and anxiety • *Psychosocial and behavioral interventions*: Education on how to avoid trigger factors, how to apply treatment, lifestyle interventions, relaxation techniques, cognitive restructuring, behavior modification including habit reversal training • Patient support groups can be beneficial • Referral to social workers, psychologist and psychiatrist can be helpful in individual cases	• Gabapentin • Antidepressants • Low-dose neuroleptics • Mirtazapine

- *Proposed mechanisms*:
  - Cholestasis
  - Direct drug/metabolite deposition
  - Alteration of neural signaling
  - Idiopathic (most common)
- Common medications that can cause GPWOR are mentioned in **Table 13**.

Drug-induced pruritus can be treated with a variety of modalities as mentioned in **Table 14**.

Pruritus Associated with Endocrine Disorders

- Thyroid disorders[9]
- **Table 15** reflects the investigations that can be done to identify the thyroid disorders.
- *Diabetes mellitus*:[9]
  - Pruritus is due to diabetic neuropathy, and predominantly involves trunk.[2]
  - A complete medical history should be obtained with special emphasis on weight, exercise, smoking, ethanol use, family history of DM, and risk factors for cardiovascular diseases.
  - *Symptoms*:
    - Polyuria, polydipsia, weight loss, fatigue, weakness, blurred vision, frequent superficial infections, poor wound healing, and paresthesias.
  - *Investigations*:
    - *Blood sugar levels*: Fasting and postprandial
    - HbA1c
- *Treatment*:
  - Vitamin D supplementation may help in some cases.
  - Refer to endocrinologist for management of underlying disorder

Table 13: Medications that can cause pruritus without skin lesions.

Class of medications	
ACE inhibitors	Captopril, enalapril, lisinopril
Alkaloids	Atropine, papaverine
Antiarrhythmic drugs	Amiodarone, disopyramide, flecainide
Antianxiety drugs	Diazepam, nitrazepam, oxazepam
Antibiotics	Amoxicillin, ampicillin, cefotaxime, erythromycin, josamycin, minocycline, ofloxacin, penicillin, tetracycline
Anticoagulant	Ticlopidine
Antiepileptics	Carbamazepine, clonazepam, gabapentin, lamotrigine
Antigout drugs	Allopurinol, colchicine, probenecid
Antimalarials	Amodiaquine, chloroquine, halofantrine, hydroxychloroquine
Antirheumatic drugs	Gold salts
Antitubercular drugs	Isoniazid, rifampicin
Beta-adrenergic blockers	Acebutolol, atenolol
Calcium antagonists	Amlodipine, diltiazem, nifedipine, verapamil
Catecholamines	Dobutamine
Cytokines	Interleukin-2
Cytostatic drugs	Bleomycin, peplomycin
Hormones	Estrogens, insulin, oral contraceptives, tamoxifen
Neuroleptics	Chlorpromazine, haloperidol, risperidone
Opioids	Codeine, fentanyl, morphine
Plasma volume expanders	HES
Targeted anticancer drugs	Cetuximab, erlotinib, panitumumab, vemurafenib

(HES: hydroxy ethyl starch)

Table 14: Treatment of drug-induced pruritus.

Type	First-line treatment	Second-line treatment	Third-line treatment
Opioid induced	MOR antagonists, κ-opioid receptor agonist	Dopamine receptor antagonist	Serotonin 5HT3 antagonists, sedating antihistaminics
Chloroquine induced	Antihistamines	MOR antagonists	Prednisolone
HES induced	MOR antagonists	Phototherapy	Topical capsaicin
Drug-induced cholestasis	Ursodeoxycholic acid, rifampicin	Cholestyramine	MOR antagonists
EGFRi induced	Antihistamines, topical corticosteroids, menthol	Gabapentin, pregabalin, systemic corticosteroids	Aprepitant
Other type of drug-induced itch	High doses of antihistamines	MOR antagonists	Gabapentin, paroxetine, amitriptyline

(EGFRi: epidermal growth factor receptor inhibitor; HES: hydroxy ethyl starch; MOR: mu-opioid receptor)

Generalized Pruritus with Unknown Origin[5]

- Once both underlying pruritic skin disease and other secondary causes have been excluded, an individual can be considered to have idiopathic GPUO.
- GPUO can be managed by various topical and systemic medications mentioned in **Table 16**.

Pruritus in Elderly (Willan's Itch)[5]

- It is defined as chronic itching occurring in those aged over 65 years.
- Loss of free fatty acids in the stratum corneum leads to superficial cracks and fissures in the epidermis that causes pruritus by producing asteatotic eczema.

Table 15: Investigations and interpretation of thyroid disorders.	
Investigations	
Hypothyroidism	**Hyperthyroidism**
Thyroid function tests: • *Serum TSH*: Elevated • *Free T4*: Decreased • *Anti-TPO antibodies*: Elevated *Other tests*: • Elevated cholesterol • Elevated CPK • Anemia *ECG changes*: Bradycardia, low amplitude QRS complex, flattened or inverted T wave	*Thyroid function tests*: • *Serum TSH*: Low • *Unbound T3*: Elevated • Microsomal thyroid antibodies *Other tests*: • Elevated ESR • Elevated bilirubin • Elevated liver enzymes • Elevated ferritin • Thyroid radioiodine uptake • Color Doppler USG

(anti-TPO: anti-thyroid peroxidase; CPK: creatine phosphokinase; ESR: erythrocyte sedimentation rate; TSH: thyroid-stimulating hormone; USG: ultrasound)

Table 16: Treatment of GPUO.	
Topical	**Systemic**
• *Doxepin*: Limited to 8 days, 10% of BSA, 12 g daily • Clobetasone butyrate • Menthol	• *Nonsedative antihistamines*: Fexofenadine, loratadine, cetirizine • Paroxetine, fluvoxamine, mirtazapine, naltrexone, butorphanol, gabapentin, pregabalin, ondansetron, aprepitant • H1 and H2 antagonists in combination, i.e., fexofenadine and cimetidine • Sedative antihistamines in short term or palliative care setting, i.e., hydroxyzine

(BSA: body surface area; GPUO: generalized pruritus with unknown origin)

- Other factors responsible for the pruritus in the elderly may include GPUO, malignancy, ageing in the nerve fiber bundles and drugs.
- Pruritus alone may be a presenting feature of bullous pemphigoid in elderly.
- *Treatment*:
  - Emollients and topical steroids for a minimum of 2 weeks for the treatment of asteatotic eczema
  - Nonresponding patients should be reassessed.
  - Moisturizers with high lipid content should be preferred.
  - Gabapentin 300 mg daily can be useful in refractory cases.
  - Nonsedative antihistamines should be avoided due to their potential to cause dementia.

Table 17: Management of pruritus in pregnancy without skin lesions.	
Investigations	**Treatment**
• *Total bile acids*: Increased (>40 µmol/L) • Levels of cholic acid (CA) and chenodeoxycholic acid (CDCA), and their ratio (CA/CDCA) • Liver enzymes • Alkaline phosphatase • Lipid profile • Blood coagulation profile • Abdominal ultrasound (USG) • Fetal assessment	• Light and low-fat diet • Ursodeoxycholic acid 300 mg 2–3 times/day (10–16 mg/kg/day) • Vitamin K 10 mg (to prevent postpartum bleeding) • Refer to gynecologist

Pruritus in Pregnancy[2,7]

- Intrahepatic cholestasis of pregnancy (ICP) is characterized by severe pruritus without any primary skin lesions.
- *Risk factors*: Advanced maternal age, multiple gestations, history of cholestasis on oral contraceptives, winter months, second/third trimester of pregnancy, genetic predisposition.
- It is necessary to diagnose ICP as it is associated with increased fetal mortality as pruritus is the only recognizable sign.
- Management of pruritus in pregnancy mentioned in **Table 17**.

SUMMARY

Generalized pruritus without skin rash can be caused by a variety of causes and it becomes important for a dermatologist to be aware of them. A stepwise approach can help the dermatologist to identify and manage the GPWOR effectively. **Flowchart 2** represents how to approach a patient of GPWOR in a summarized way.[37]

CONCLUSION

"Diagnosis by recognition is easy, diagnosis by cognition is hard."

—**Shelley and Shelley**

Pruritus is the first and the most common ailment a dermatologist faces in day-to-day life. It is challenging for the dermatologist and agitating for the patient. Generalized pruritus without skin lesions poses a test for the dermatologist in terms of his/her knowledge, history taking, patience, experience and at times, intuition. We have to tried to provide a scientific approach for a patient with generalized pruritus without skin lesions in the most understandable way.

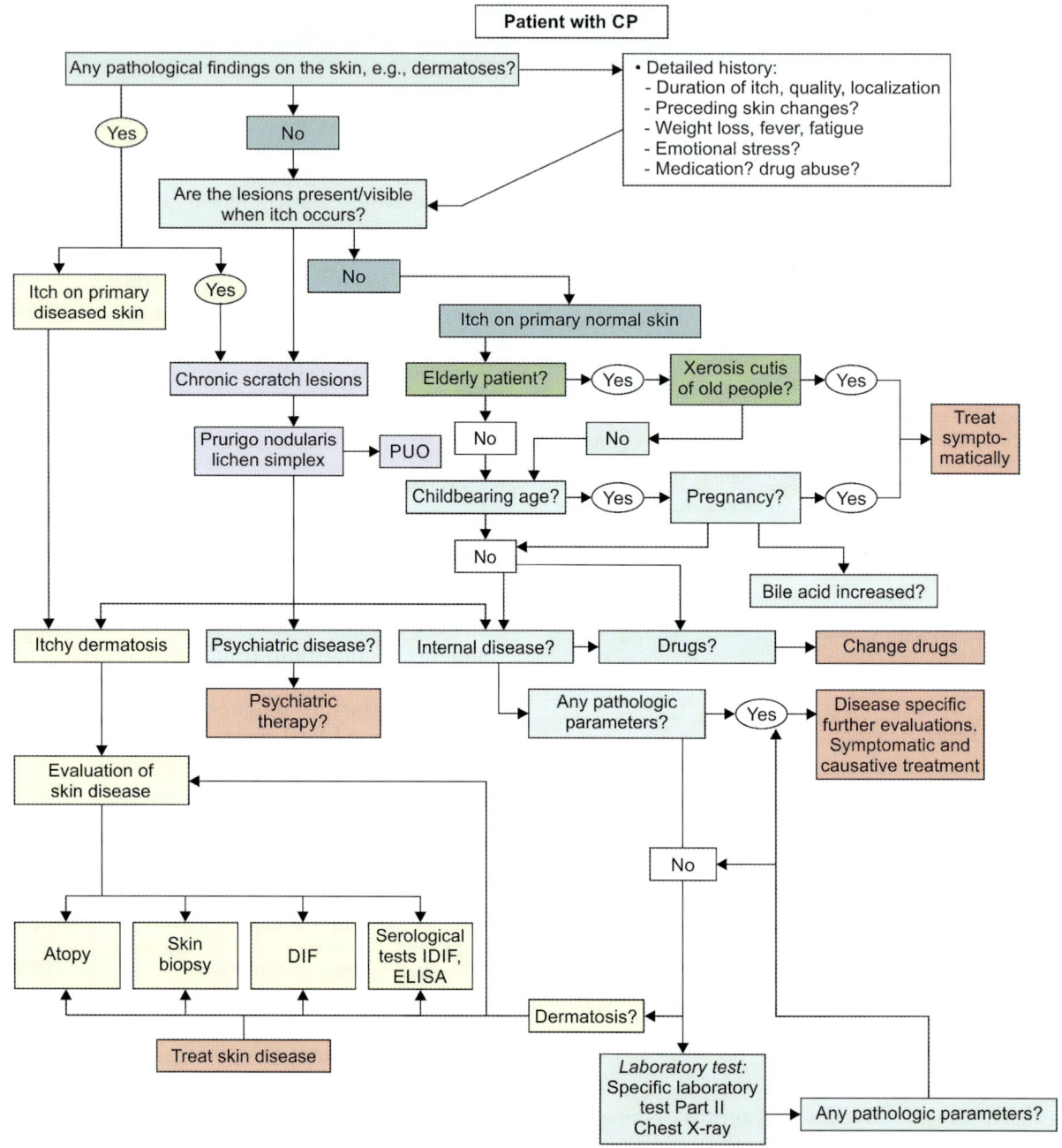

FLOWCHART 2: Approach to a patient of generalized pruritus without skin lesions.[37]
(DIF: direct immunofluorescence; ELISA: enzyme-linked immunosorbent assay; IDIF: indirect immunofluorescence; PUO: pruritus with unknown origin)

REFERENCES

1. Grundmann S, Ständer S. Chronic pruritus: clinics and treatment. Ann Dermatol. 2011;23(1):1-11.
2. Rajagopalan M, Saraswat A, Godse K, Shankar D, Kandhari S, Shenoi S, et al. Diagnosis and management of chronic pruritus: An expert consensus review. Indian J Dermatol. 2017;62(1):7-17.
3. Song J, Xian D, Yang L, Xiong X, Lai R, Zhong J. Pruritus: Progress toward Pathogenesis and Treatment. Biomed Res Int. 2018;2018:9625936.
4. Fazio SB, Yosipovitch G. (2022). Pruritus: Etiology and patient evaluation. [online]. Available from https://www.uptodate.com/contents/pruritus-etiology-and-patient-evaluation#! [Last accessed December, 2022].
5. Millington G, Collins A, Lovell C, Leslie T, Yong A, Morgan J, et al. British Association of Dermatologists' guidelines for the investigation and management of generalized pruritus in adults without an underlying dermatosis, 2018. Br J Dermatol. 2018;178(1):34-60.

6. Renganathan A, Selvaraj N. Chronic pruritus without skin rash—evaluation of systemic causes. J Evid Based Med Healthcare. 2017;4(19):1076-81.
7. Piechota J, Jelski W. Intrahepatic Cholestasis in Pregnancy: Review of the Literature. J Clin Med. 2020;9(5):1361.
8. Szepietowski J, Weisshaar E. Itch—management in clinical practice. Curr Probl Dermatol. 2016;50.
9. Jameson J, Fauci A, Kasper D, Hauser S, Longo D, Loscalzo J. Harrison's Manual of Medicine, 20th edition. New York: McGraw-Hill; 2020.
10. Mahowald MW, Bornemann MA. Sleep and ESRD: a wake-up call. Am J Kidney Dis. 2006;48(2):332-4.
11. Cohen O, Chapman J, Lee H, Nitsan Z, Appel S, Hoffman C, et al. Pruritus in familial Creutzfeldt–Jakob disease: a common symptom associated with central nervous system pathology. J Neurol. 2010;258(1):89-95.
12. Mehta J, Mehta S, Joshi S, Mehta N. PJ Mehta's Practical Medicine for Student and Practitioners. Hari Bhavan, Mumbai: National Book Depot; 2016.
13. Mathur M, D'Souza A, Malhotra V, Agarwal D, Beniwal P. Uremic frost. Clin Kidney J. 2014;7(4):418-9.
14. Zirwas M, Seraly M. Pruritus of unknown origin: A retrospective study. J Am Acad Dermatol. 2001;45(6):892-6.
15. Singh G. Nails in systemic disease. Indian J Dermatol Venereol Leprol. 2011;77(6):646-51.
16. Pandey A, Pandey M, Pandey V, Ravindran V. Oral manifestations of autoimmune connective tissue diseases. Indian J Rheumatol. 2018;13(4):264-72.
17. Nilofer H, Kalkur C, Padmashree S, Anusha LR. Diagnosis of Iron-deficiency Anemia through Oral Manifestation: A Case Report. JOJ Case Stud. 2018;7(4):555724.
18. Pakfetrat A, Falaki F, Delavarian Z, Dalirsani Z, Sanatkhani M, Marani MZ. Oral manifestations of human immunodeficiency virus-infected patients. Iran J Otorhinolaryngol. 2015;27(78):43-54.
19. Bagewadi SB, Arora MP, Mody BM, Krishnamoorthy B, Baduni A, Oral manifestations of Hepatitis B and C: A case series with review of literature. J Dent Spec. 2015;3(1):96-101.
20. Shuai Y, Liu B, Zhou G, Rong L, Niu C, Jin L. Oral manifestations related to malaria: A systematic review. Oral Diseases. 2020; 27(7):1616-20.
21. Brostolin da Costa D, De-Carli A, Probst L, Grande AJ, Guerrero AT. Oral manifestations in chikungunya patients: A systematic review. PLoS Negl Trop Dis. 2021;15(6):e0009401.
22. Dioguardi M, Caloro G, Troiano G, Giannatempo G, Laino L, Petruzzi M, et al. Oral manifestations in chronic uremia patients. Renal Failure. 2015;38(1):1-6.
23. Natarajan K, Manne RK, Anumula A, Bhargavi N, Pulimi S, Nasreen A, et al. Oral manifestations in patients with liver diseases a prospective observational study at a tertiary health care center in India. Int J Development Res. 2018;8(5).
24. Rohani B, Gholizadeh N, poorfar HK, Pourshahidi S, Ebrahimi H. (2015). Oral Manifestations of Hematologic Malignancies. Jundishapur Sci Med J. 2015;14(4):478-85.
25. Sacchidanand S, Oberoi C, Inamdar A. IADVL Textbook of Dermatology, 4th edition. New Delhi: Bhalani Publishing House; 2015.
26. Kaur D, Behl A, Isher P. Oral manifestations of stress-related disorders in the general population of Ludhiana. J Indian Acad Oral Med Radiol. 2016;28(3):262-9.
27. Bakhtiari S, Sehatpour M, Mortazavi H, Bakhshi M. Orofacial Manifestation of Adverse Drug Reactions: A Review Study. Med Pharm Rep. 2018;91(1):27-36.
28. Koperdanova M, Cullis J. Interpreting raised serum ferritin levels. BMJ. 2015;h3692.
29. Higgins C. (2016). Urea and the clinical value of measuring blood urea concentration. [online]. Available from https://acutecaretesting.org/en/articles/urea-and-the-clinical-value-of-measuring-blood-urea-concentration [Last accessed December, 2022].
30. Cheung K, Lafayette R. Renal Physiology of Pregnancy. Adv Chronic Kidney Dis. 2013;20(3):209-14.
31. Shrimanker I, Bhattarai S. Electrolytes. In: StatPearls [Internet]. Treasure Island (FL): StatPearls Publishing; 2021.
32. Joseph A, Samant H. Jaundice. In: StatPearls [Internet]. Treasure Island (FL): StatPearls Publishing; 2021.
33. Lowe D, Sanvictores T, John S. Alkaline Phosphatase. In: StatPearls [Internet]. Treasure Island (FL): StatPearls Publishing; 2021.
34. Zeidler C, Pereira M, Huet F, Misery L, Steinbrink K, Ständer S. Pruritus in Autoimmune and Inflammatory Dermatoses. Front Immunol. 2019;10:1303.
35. Düll M, Kremer A. Newer Approaches to the Management of Pruritus in Cholestatic Liver Disease. Curr Hepatol Rep. 2020;19(2):86-95.
36. Ebata T. Drug-induced Itch Management. Curr Probl Dermatol. 2016;50:155-63.
37. Weisshaar E, Szepietowski J, Darsow U, Misery L, Wallengren J, Mettang T, et al. European Guideline on Chronic Pruritus. Acta Derm Venereol. 2012;92(5):563-81.

6
A Patient with Annular Skin Lesions

Sejal Hitesh Thakkar, Ashka Shah

INTRODUCTION

Visibility, a unique characteristic of dermatological disorders, contributes a great extent to the diagnosis of a clinical condition. Description in terms of morphology (primary and secondary skin lesions), distribution, color, configuration, nature of the borders, and shape of lesions provides an important clue to establish the diagnosis. The annular shape of a lesion is striking in appearance, offering probable diagnosis at a glance. Distinguishing various clinical conditions with such lesions needs thorough evaluation with a methodological, algorithmic approach to reach a precise diagnosis and rule out the differentials.

The term "annular" is derived from the Latin word "annulus," meaning ring shaped. These lesions have a characteristic appearance, described as round to oval-shaped lesions with central clearing. Annular lesions can occur either as a confluence of many circular lesions or as an extension of lesions toward periphery with central clearing. The same dermatological disorder may present with an annular, arciform, or polycyclic configuration. In some instances, nummular circular or coin-shaped lesions, may turn into annular lesions by central clearing on progression of the disease.

Various mechanisms have been proposed to explain the annular configuration of lesions. There may be a centrifugal spread of the lesion by mass extension (e.g., sarcoidosis) or along the plane of skin (e.g., tinea infection). It could also be based on irrigation, so that each round macule represents the territory irrigated by a single arteriole (e.g., figurate erythema). When inflammation extends from superficial/deep dermis to the epidermis, scales may appear over the lesions which help narrowing down the differential diagnoses.[1,2]

DIFFERENTIAL DIAGNOSES OF ANNULAR OR ARCIFORM OR POLYCYCLIC SKIN LESIONS

Annular lesions can present in various conditions, from something as common as dermatophytosis to an infrequent condition such as sarcoidosis. Certain common skin diseases may present with diversified lesions which may happen to include annular configurations, while a few uncommon disorders present with characteristic annular lesions.[3] While dealing with patients having annular skin lesions, common conditions should be ruled out first before considering the not-so-common or rare conditions **(Flowchart 1)**.

APPROACH TO A PATIENT WITH ANNULAR LESIONS

Proper history and thorough examination are the key to reaching the diagnosis. Along with the characteristic annular lesions, features such as age of the patient, associated symptoms, morphology, distribution of the lesions and any other relevant features must be explored.

HISTORY

Age of the Patient

Age of the patient may give us the clue towards the diagnosis. Neonatal lupus may be commonly seen in pediatric patients while syphilis is seen in patients of reproductive age-group.

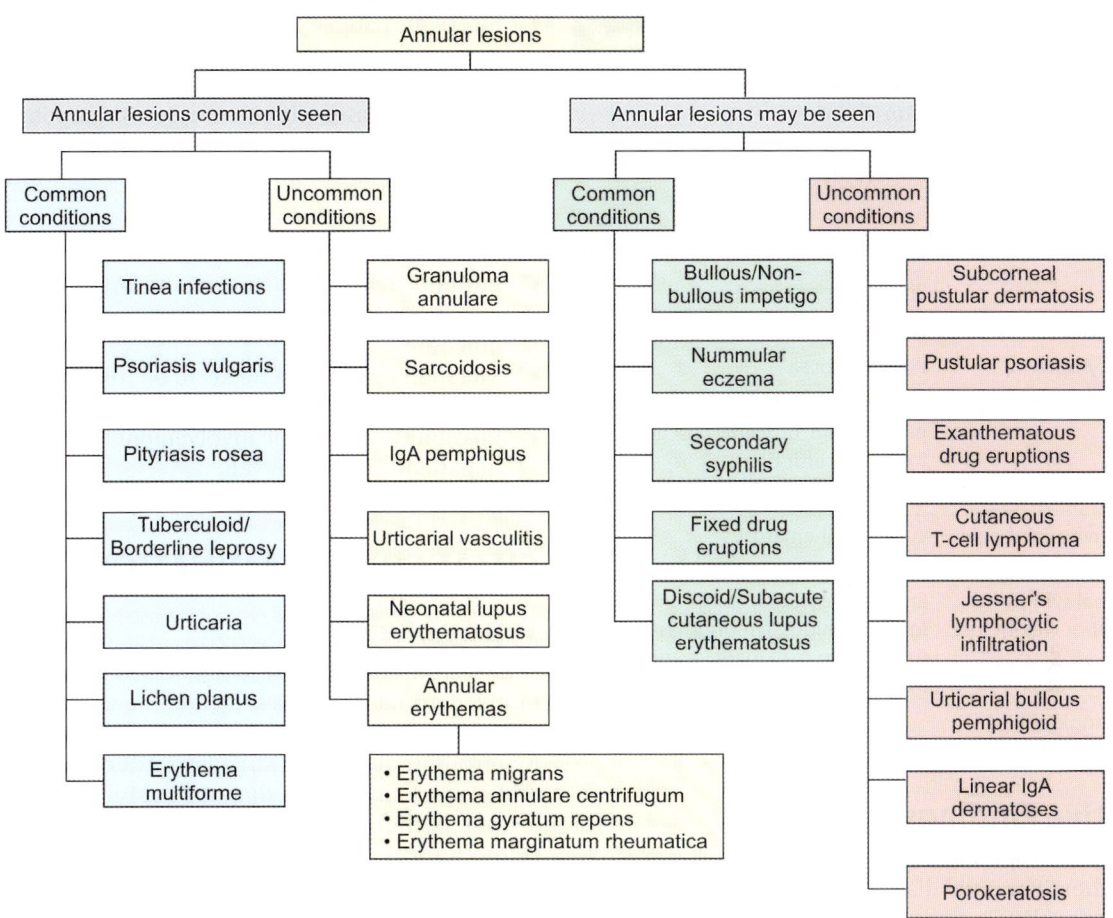

FLOWCHART 1: Skin diseases presenting with annular lesions categorized on basis of frequency of annular lesions seen. (IgA: immunoglobulin A)

Tinea infections, psoriasis and leprosy can be seen in all age-groups, although they are more prevalent in middle-aged patients **(Table 1)**.

PRESENTING SYMPTOMS

Itching may be a presenting symptom in many of the conditions. Apart from itching, patients may present with certain other symptoms which may hint to the diagnosis of the dermatosis **(Table 2)**.

Duration of the Disease

Disorders with acute onset and shorter duration may include urticaria or drug reactions while tinea infections or psoriasis-like conditions may be of variable duration with a remitting and relapsing course. Leprosy and granuloma annulare present with lesions of a longer duration.

Pustular psoriasis or erythema annulare centrifugum are rapidly progressive in nature while tinea and psoriasis progress at a moderate pace.

Leprosy and granuloma annulare evolve very slowly over a period of few months to years.

Table 1: Age predilection for skin disorders with annular lesions.	
Age-group	**Skin disorder**
Infants	Neonatal erythema, neonatal lupus, and erythema marginatum rheumatica
Preschool age-group	Impetigo and pityriasis alba
Up to 12 years	Urticaria and chronic bullous dermatosis of childhood
20–50 years	Tinea infections, psoriasis, leprosy, urticaria, erythema multiforme, fixed drug eruptions, urticarial vasculitis, secondary syphilis, and annular lichen planus
>50 years	Granuloma annulare, sarcoidosis, urticarial bullous pemphigoid, cutaneous T-cell lymphoma, and basal cell carcinoma

Table 2: Symptoms to explore in a patient with annular lesions.	
Symptoms	Skin disorder
Asymptomatic	Granuloma annulare and sarcoidosis
Itching	
Significant	Tinea infections and psoriasis
Mild	Pityriasis rosea
Loss of sensation	Leprosy
Prodromal symptoms	Pityriasis rosea
Burning over the lesions	Erythema multiforme, bullous pemphigoid, urticarial vasculitis, or fixed drug eruptions
Joint pain	Psoriasis
Photosensitivity, joint pain, and fever	Lupus erythematosus
Constitutional symptoms such as fever or weight loss	Erythema gyratus repens, IgA pemphigus, lymphomas (underlying malignancy), and pustular psoriasis
(IgA: immunoglobulin A)	

Supportive Findings

Leading questions pertaining to other symptoms can aid in ruling out the differential diagnosis, to confirm the existing diagnosis as well to assess the systemic involvement or severity of the disease.
- Treatment history (self-medication or prescribed ones) prior to onset of the disorder will help to identify drug reaction if any.
- History of preexisting chronic plaque psoriasis along with history of triggering factor such as sudden withdrawal of corticosteroids can lead to the diagnosis of pustular psoriasis patients.
- Past history of treatment will help to identify the lesions of tinea incognito.
- Family and/or contact history will substantially contribute to diagnose the conditions such as tinea infections, psoriasis, and leprosy.
- History suggestive of motor/sensory deficit such as slippage of footwear while walking, loss of fine grip, or presence of a trophic ulcer can give a clue to diagnose leprosy.
- History suggestive of systemic lupus erythematosus (LE) in mother may lead to the diagnosis of neonatal lupus in a newborn with annular lesions.

Aggravating and Relieving Factors

- Seasonal aggravation is commonly seen with tinea infections and psoriasis showing summer and winter exacerbation, respectively.
- Stress and alcohol may trigger psoriasis.
- Stress and sun-exposure contribute to exacerbate LE. Raynaud's phenomenon with lupus is aggravated during winter.
- Partial response with incomplete treatment followed by relapse is commonly seen in tinea infections.
- Pityriasis alba is commonly seen during winter season.

Associated Comorbidities

- Patients with tinea infections may have associated obesity and/or diabetes which may impact the treatment outcome.
- Metabolic syndrome needs to be ruled out in patients of psoriasis.
- Possibility of systemic involvement needs to be explored in patients of systemic LE.

CUTANEOUS EXAMINATION

Type of Lesion

Skin lesions need to be categorized morphologically in terms of primary lesions seen and the associated secondary lesions, if any. Color of the lesions, e.g., erythematous or hyperpigmented, can suggest underlying pathogenesis and gives a clue to the diagnosis. Morphology of the skin lesions is the key component in reaching the diagnosis **(Flowchart 2)**.

Site Distribution

Patient should be thoroughly examined to determine the sites involved, with special focus on the sites of predilection. Tinea infections are more commonly seen in flexures along with other body sites, while psoriatic lesions are more prevalent on extensors. Annular lesions of leprosy can be found anywhere on the body, more on trunk and extremities. Annular lesions on genitals should raise the suspicion of lichen planus, secondary syphilis, and fixed drug eruptions **(Fig. 1)**. Annular lesions of syphilis most commonly involve facial region.

Characteristics of the Lesions

Annular, centrifugal lesions with fine scaling in intertriginous area may be seen in tinea infections. Annular lesions with micaceous scaling along with nail changes are seen in psoriasis. Erythematous infiltrated lesions are characteristics of leprosy and granuloma annulare. Loss of sensation over these lesions aid in the diagnosis of leprosy. Figurate erythemas may reflect underlying conditions such as infection or malignancy.

Hair, Nail, and Mucosal Examination

Hair, nail, and mucosae are an integral part of dermatology and can give a clue to diagnose many of the dermatological disorders.

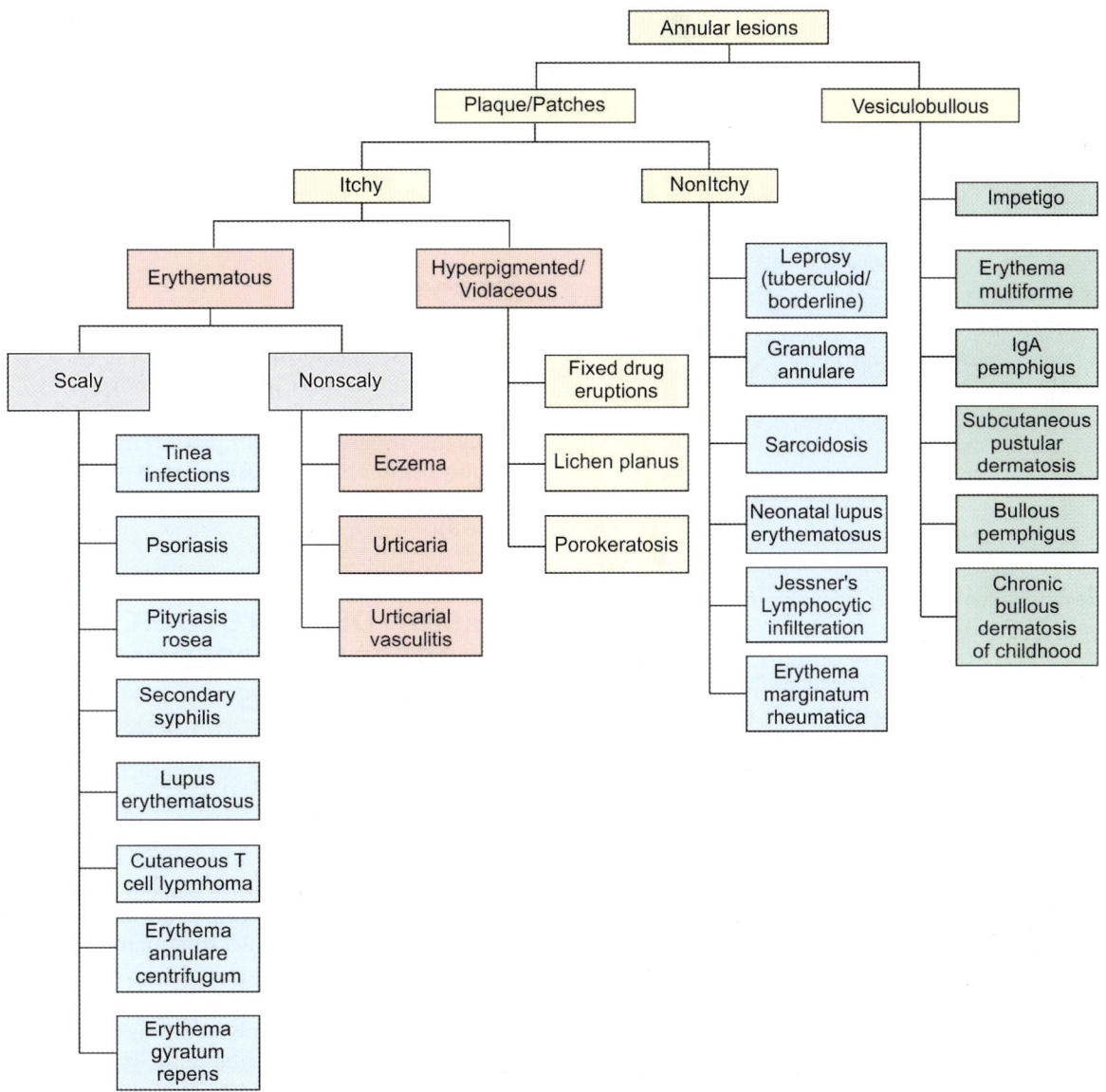

FLOWCHART 2: Morphological characteristics of annular skin lesions in various dermatoses.
(IgA: immunoglobulin A)

- Mucosal involvement may be seen in patients with annular lesions of drug reactions such as erythema multiforme (EM), fixed drug eruptions as well as lichen planus.
- Scalp, nail, and mucosae may show findings of lichen planus along with annular lesions on genitalia.
- Discoloration of nail along with/without dystrophy can be seen in patients with tinea infections.
- Pitting, oil drop sign, and onychodystrophy may be present in patients with psoriasis.

Diagnostic Tests for Differential

Majority of the conditions with annular lesions can be diagnosed at a glance, among which, few can be confirmed after a thorough examination. Some of the patients might need confirmatory diagnostic tests.

- Skin/nail scrapping subjected to potassium hydroxide wet mount test to identify hyphae helps in confirmation of tinea infection.
- Scrapping of scale and identification of bleeding points (Auspitz's sign) might be positive in some of the psoriatic patients.
- Slit skin smear examination may identify acid-fast bacilli in patients of leprosy.
- Rapid antigen reagent test or treponemal tests help to identify the case of secondary syphilis.
- Antinuclear antibody profile may help to diagnose a case of systemic LE.

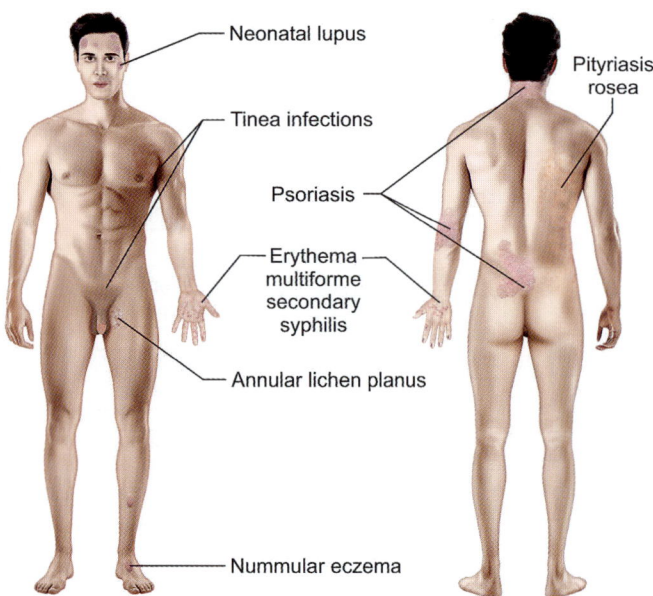

FIG. 1: Site distribution of annular lesions in various cutaneous disorders.

- Routine blood and urine investigations along with liver and renal profile may help to rule out any systemic involvement, especially in conditions such as systemic LE or internal malignancy.
- Resolution of the annular lesion with injection of intralesional normal saline may provide clue to the diagnosis of granuloma annulare.

Dermoscopy Findings

Dermoscope may precisely diagnose certain conditions by identifying characteristic pattern of pigmentary and vascular changes in many of the conditions.
- Psoriasis is identified by a reddish pink background on dermoscopy, with red dots and glomerular vessels, and white or yellow thick scales.
- Dermoscopy might help in diagnosing lichen planus by identifying Wickham's striae or polymorphic pearly white structures, blue black globules, and radiating vessels.
- Pityriasis rosea shows collarette scaling.
- There is minimal literature on dermoscopic findings of EM. A typical target lesion shows central dusky zone with clods of different colors—red, blue, purple, and black. Plain featureless areas corresponding to the pale edematous zone and and homogenous erythema corresponding to the outer red ring can be seen.
- Granulomatous lesions show yellowish-orange structureless areas.

Skin Biopsy

Histopathological examination may not be needed in all patients when clinical diagnosis is apparent and supported by certain noninvasive tests or dermoscopic findings. It may be needed in cases with diagnostic dilemma.
- Histopathology may be confirmatory in a suspected smear negative patient of leprosy.
- Biopsy with genotyping is the diagnostic for cutaneous T-cell lymphoma (CTCL).
- Histopathological examination is the key to diagnose sarcoidosis, Jessner's lymphocytic infiltration, and porokeratosis.

Management

Once diagnosed, patients presenting with annular lesions require disease-specific management.

Various features such as history, morphology, and site of lesion, and its key features as described below help us identify the disease and appropriately manage them.

Many common dermatoses seen in practice present with predominant or occasional occurrence of annular lesions **(Table 3)**.

COMMON DERMATOLOGICAL DISORDERS WITH PREDOMINANTLY ANNULAR LESIONS

Tinea Infections

- Easy to diagnose but challenging to treat this condition **(Figs. 2A to D)**
- History of recurrence and family history are the key components responsible for recalcitrant tinea infection.
- Contributory factors playing a role in recurrence:
  ○ Inadequate or irregular treatment
  ○ Inconsistent follow-up
  ○ Self-medication (re-use of old prescription/prescription of friends or family members/over-the-counter products containing combination therapy including steroids)
  ○ Inadvertent treatment by quacks and steroid abuse by patients or practitioners
- Positive family history needs education and counseling to avoid sharing of towels/clothes.
- Rational and consistent treatment with consistent follow-up may help avoid recurrence. Along with this, taking care of underlying comorbid conditions such as diabetes or obesity is also necessary.[4,5]

Psoriasis

- Psoriasis can be spot-diagnosed **(Figs. 3A and B)**.
- Nail changes and Auspitz's sign may support the diagnosis.
- Dermoscopy and/or biopsy may be confirmatory.
- Along with medical management with topicals or systemic therapy, general measures play a substantial role in management. Education and counseling regarding course of the disease as well as precipitating/

Table 3: Salient features with diagnostic clue and preferred management for common dermatoses with annular skin lesions.

Condition	History	Description of lesions	Key features	Diagnosis and management
Tinea infections	• Itchy skin lesions for few days to few weeks • H/o partial treatment/self-medication • H/o recurrence • Family history • Comorbidity such as obesity or diabetes	Scaly, erythematous annular plaques with raised borders that spread centrifugally	• Groin folds/axillae may be involved • Nails and scalp to be examined	• Clinical diagnosis is evident. KOH mount may show hyphae • Consistent and complete course of oral and/or topical antifungals leads to complete recovery
Psoriasis	• Itchy skin lesions over few weeks • Scaling • Recurrent with winter exacerbation, stress, or alcohol	Well-demarcated, erythematous, annular plaques with silvery white scales	• Koebnerization may be present. • Nail and scalp involvement may be present	• Diagnosis is clinically evident. Auspitz's sign may be positive • Localized lesions respond well to topical keratolytic/corticosteroids/vitamin-D analogs • Extensive lesions need systemic drugs such as methotrexate/phototherapy/biologics
Pityriasis rosea	• Absent or mild itching and skin lesions for few days to 2 weeks, may be with prodromal symptoms • Oldest lesion is the largest one known as Herald patch	Annular, scaly, usually asymptomatic, ovoid patches with collarette scales	• Christmas tree pattern distribution of lesions over trunk • Self-limiting condition over 6–12 weeks	• Diagnosis is clinically evident • Treatment options include calamine lotion, topical corticosteroids, oral antihistamines, and/or phototherapy with ultraviolet rays • Systemic corticosteroids may be used for severe symptoms
Tuberculoid/borderline leprosy	• Asymptomatic skin lesion for few months to years • History suggestive of peripheral nerve involvement (muscle weakness/sensory impairment/deformity)	Erythematous/coppery red/hypopigmented annular plaques vary in number from one to many	• Associated sensory loss and nerve thickening • Granulomatous reaction and periadnexal infiltration on histopathological examination	• Thorough clinical evaluation is needed to diagnose it along with history of belonging to high endemic zone. • Slit skin smear and skin/nerve biopsy helps in diagnostic confirmation • Patients are treated with multidrug therapy containing antileprosy drugs
Urticaria	Itchy red skin lesions of acute onset (few hours duration), transient wheal formation	Itchy, erythematous, annular, or polycyclic plaques	• Lesions usually last for 2–24 hours. Pruritus may be intense. Drug, food, viral infection, or stress may be the underlying causes	• Acute urticaria responds well by eliminating the cause and prescribing antihistamines and/or corticosteroids • Chronic urticaria may require long-term treatment with antihistamines, corticosteroids, cyclosporine, or omalizumab • If individual lesion lasts for >24 hours, biopsy may be needed to rule out urticarial vasculitis
Lichen planus	• Itchy hyperpigmented or violaceous skin lesions of few weeks to months' duration • Scalp, nail, and mucosae may be involved	Flat-topped violaceous, papular lesions may present occasionally with annular configuration	• Annular LP lesions are usually localized, more commonly seen on genitals • Scalp, nail, and mucosae may be involved	Diagnosis is clinically evident. Dermoscopy shows prominent Wickham striae. Biopsy confirms the diagnosis by presence of basal cell vacuolar degeneration, lymphocytic infiltration, and colloid bodies

Continued

Continued

Condition	History	Description of lesions	Key features	Diagnosis and management
Erythema multiforme	• Itchy skin lesions with vesicles of acute onset • H/o fever and/or drugs may be there	• Erythematous, itchy, target lesions with central vesicle. Site predilection may be extremities, and palms-soles • It may present with arciform or annular pattern	Acute onset of lesions in reaction to drug, infections (especially herpes simplex) or any other trigger	• Diagnosis is usually clinically evident • Biopsy may help in diagnosis when clinical picture is not clear • Identification and avoiding trigger factor help in clearance of the lesions as well as preventing recurrence • Symptomatic and supportive treatment helps in resolving the condition • Steroids may be needed in severe cases
Bullous/nonbullous impetigo	• Crusted skin lesions with minimal or no itching and/or pain of acute onset • Contact history may be positive	Superficial crusted and erosive lesion, commonly on face and upper extremities. Common in pediatric age-group	May spread peripherally with central clearing-impetigo circinata	• Clinical diagnosis is evident • Staphylococci can be identified on Gram's stain • It responds well to topical antibiotics. Systemic antibiotics may be needed for severe cases
Nummular eczema	• Itchy skin lesions, more on easily accessible sites, of varied duration • H/o off and on lesions. • H/o off and on treatment—may be a self-medication	Coin-shaped, erythematous, scaly, annular lesions; commonly seen on extensors of extremities	• Precipitated/exacerbated during winter; more commonly present with dry skin • Patient may have associated history of asthma and/or atopic dermatitis	• Clinically may mimic tinea infection, which can be excluded by absence of fungal hyphae on KOH mount • Proper care of skin with vigilant application of moisturizers is the key for management • Topical steroid resolves milder/localized lesions • Systemic steroids can be used for extensive/severe cases
Secondary syphilis	• Red skin lesion with or without itching on face, genitalia, or extremities • History of risky sexual behavior is usually present in such patients • Patient may or may not present with past history of primary syphilis	Diffuse, generalized, bilaterally symmetrical, erythematous papular/annular lesions including palms and soles are present in secondary syphilis	Mucosal lesions and lymphadenopathy are present	Diagnosis is supported by rapid antigen reagent test which may be confirmed by treponemal tests Patient should be treated with injectable benzathine penicillin or tetracycline/macrolide group of antibiotics Counseling and partner treatment must be an integral part of management
Fixed drug eruptions	• Hyperpigmented or erythematous skin lesions of acute onset. It may be associated with mild itching or burning or may be asymptomatic • History of offending drug may be within 1–72 hours before the onset of lesions	Ovoid or annular, erythematous or hyperpigmented patches more commonly on extremities, mucosa, or genitalia	History of recurrence at the same site may be there with similar drug ingestions	• Precipitating drugs must be identified and withdrawn • Sulfonamides and nonsteroidal anti-inflammatory drugs are the most common culprit • Topical corticosteroids and oral antihistaminic help in symptomatic relief • Post-inflammatory hyperpigmentation may persist
Subacute cutaneous lupus erythematosus	Erythematous, scaly, slightly itchy skin lesions on photo exposed area, more common in female	Discoid or annular plaque on a face or neck of a young female patient	• Photosensitivity may be present • Associated symptoms such as joint pain and fever may be there • History of precipitating drugs may be there	• Antinuclear and anti-Sjögren-A antibodies may be positive while anti-double-stranded DNA antibodies are negative • Sun protection is the key for management • Lesions respond to topical corticosteroids. Systemic corticosteroids or other immunomodulators may be required for severe disease

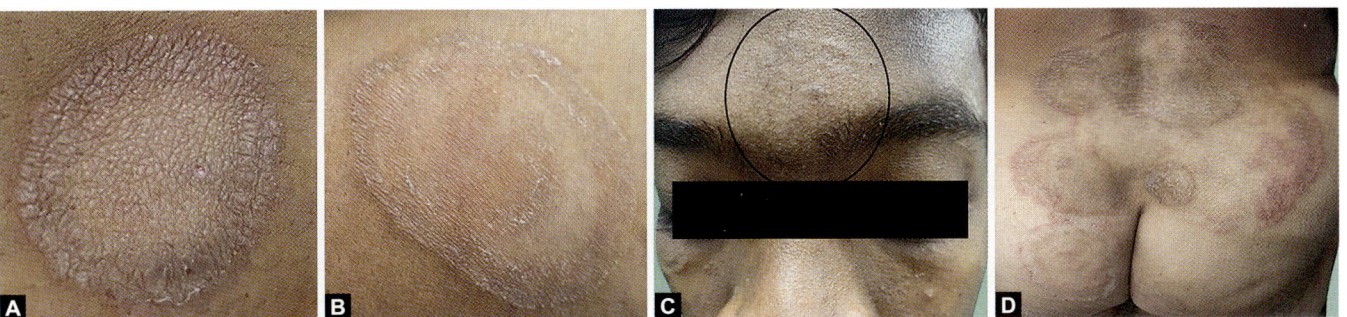

FIGS. 2A TO D: Annular and concentric lesions in tinea infections (members of the same family).

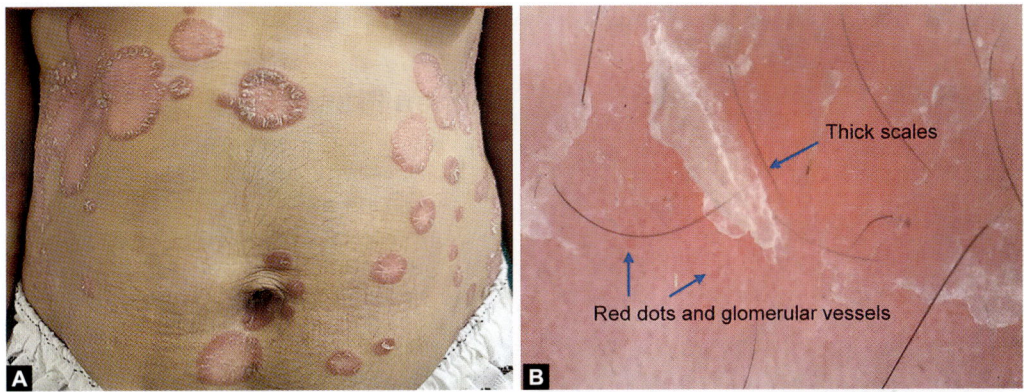

FIGS. 3A AND B: Annular, erythematous, scaly plaques of psoriasis showing supportive dermoscopic findings.

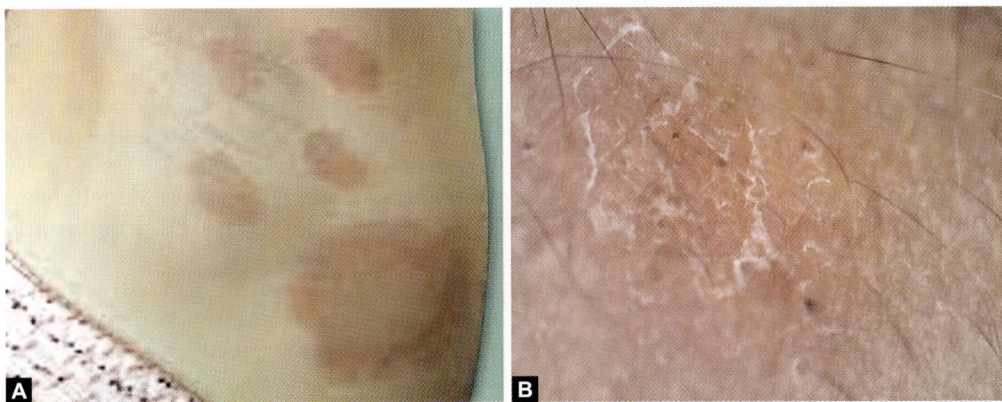

FIGS. 4A AND B: Multiple annular lesions showing collarette scaling clinically and dermoscopic findings in a case of pityriasis rosea.

exacerbating factors along with vigilant application of moisturizer and emollients will help in improving quality of life and better patient compliance.[6]

Pityriasis Rosea

- Annular scaly plaques with collarette scale distributed along the cleavage lines.
- Largest lesion (Herald patch) gives a clue to the diagnosis.
- Dermoscopy highlighting collarette scales **(Figs. 4A and B)**
- It is important to explore for drugs causing pityriasis rosea-like lesions, if any. Common culprits are gold, bismuth, arsenic, barbiturates, or captopril.[7]
- Patients need to be explained about the course of the disease being self-limiting in nature and having transient pigmentary changes.

Tuberculoid/Borderline Leprosy

- Annular, infiltrated, anesthetic, hypopigmented/erythematous plaque

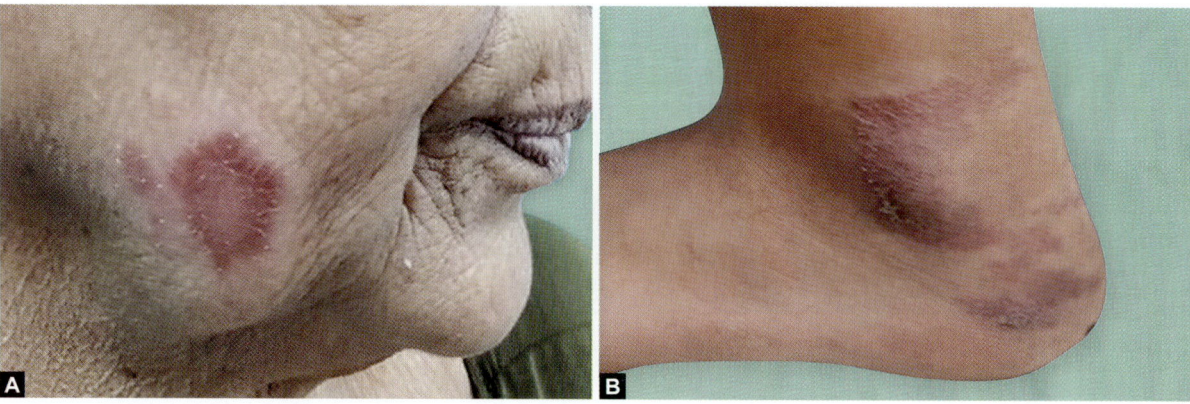

FIGS. 5A AND B: Annular plaques of borderline tuberculoid leprosy with satellite lesions.

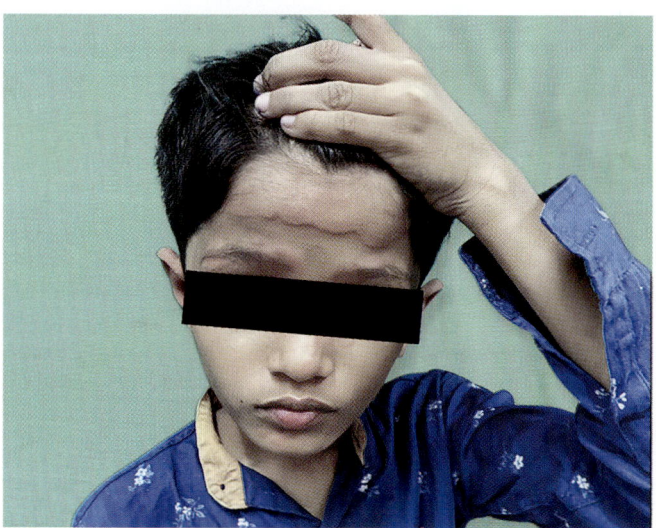

FIG. 6: Annular, polycyclic wheal formation in a case of urticaria.

- Satellite lesions may be seen in the periphery of the lesions **(Figs. 5A and B)**.
- Motor/sensory neurological manifestations with nerve thickening
- Slit-skin smear may be negative for acid–fast bacilli but biopsy confirms the diagnosis in most of the cases by identifying granuloma.
- Patient should be counseled regarding prevention of deformities/prevention of the worsening of the deformities.
- Patient should be kept under surveillance to ensure that they complete course of the treatment.

Urticaria

- Wheal formation or annular lesions with itching **(Fig. 6)**
- Many times, patient presents with history suggestive of urticarial lesions.
- Diagnosis is easy but to identify the etiology and management of chronic urticaria are the challenges for the practitioners too.[8]

Lichen Planus

- Violaceous or hyperpigmented circular macules or plaques with raised borders may be associated with central atrophy.
- Convergence of multiple lichenoid violaceous or hyperpigmented, papular lesions in a circular fashion or an expansion of a papule or plaque with central involution and an advancing raised border give rise to annular lesions.
- Management is along the lines of treatment used for classical lichen planus including topical corticosteroids/tacrolimus and/or systemic corticosteroids/dapsone.

Erythema Multiforme

- Target lesion where papule or plaque expands in a circular fashion with necrotic center.
- It can be either be related to herpes simplex viral infection or can be drug-induced.
- Common differentials for EM include urticaria, Stevens–Johnson syndrome, fixed drug eruption, and bullous pemphigoid.
- Milder cases can be treated with symptomatic and/or supportive therapy. Patients with severe mucosal involvement may need hospitalization and management with systemic corticosteroids along with maintenance of fluid and electrolyte balance.[9]

COMMON CONDITIONS WITH INFREQUENT ANNULAR LESIONS

Bullous Impetigo

- Annular lesion with a thin crust and perilesional erythema which usually follows vesiculobullous lesion up to 5 cm in size, commonly seen on face, trunk, buttocks, perineum, axillae, and extremities **(Fig. 7)**.
- Patients can be treated with topical antibacterial such as fusidic acid, mupirocin, or retapamulin.

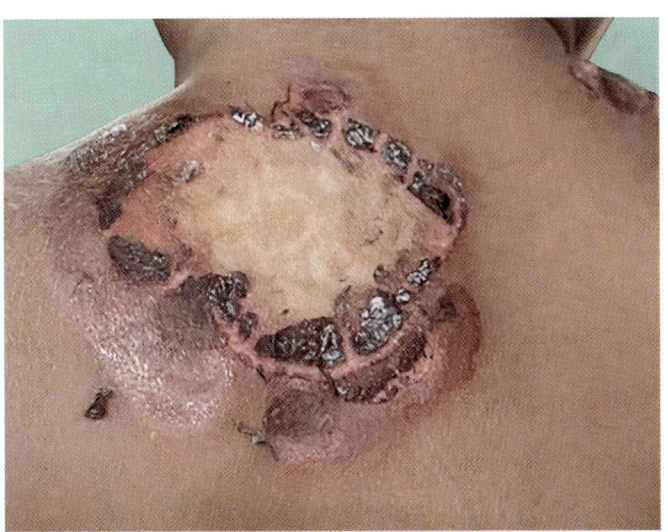

FIG. 7: Annular crusted lesion in bullous impetigo.

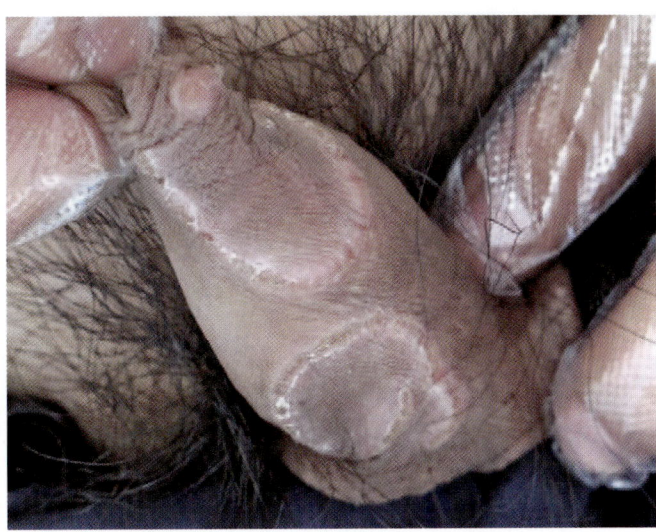

FIG. 8: Annular erythematous scaly lesions in a patient of secondary syphilis.
Courtesy: Dr Cai-Chou Zhao and Dr Jiu-Hong Li.[12]

- In infants/young children and adults with immunodeficiency or renal failure, exfoliative toxin may disseminate and cause staphylococcal scalded skin syndrome. Such patients require systemic antibiotics treatment.[10]

Nummular Eczema

- Coin-shaped eczematous lesions may have an annular pattern occasionally.
- Associated dry skin, emotional stress, stasis, or atopic dermatitis.
- External causes may contribute such as allergens (rubber chemicals, formaldehyde, neomycin, chrome, nickel, or dental amalgam), staphylococcal infection, seasonal variation, alcohol, and drugs (gold or isotretinoin).[11]

Secondary Syphilis

- Annular/arciform papules/plaques on palms and soles or genitals apart from generalized erythematous or coppery papulosquamous eruptions **(Fig. 8)**
- High-risk sexual behavior, clinical features, and serological findings diagnose the case.
- Screening for human immunodeficiency virus or any other sexually transmitted infection is a must.[12,13]

Fixed Drug Eruptions

- Single or multiple, hyperpigmented, usually ovoid lesions, but may be annular patches also followed by drug ingestion **(Fig. 9)**.
- Though it is easy to diagnose, identifying the culprit remains a challenge. Sulfonamides, metronidazole, doxycycline, phenobarbital, and ibuprofen are identified as common offenders.[14,15]
- It needs to be differentiated from lichen planus or postinflammatory hyperpigmentation.

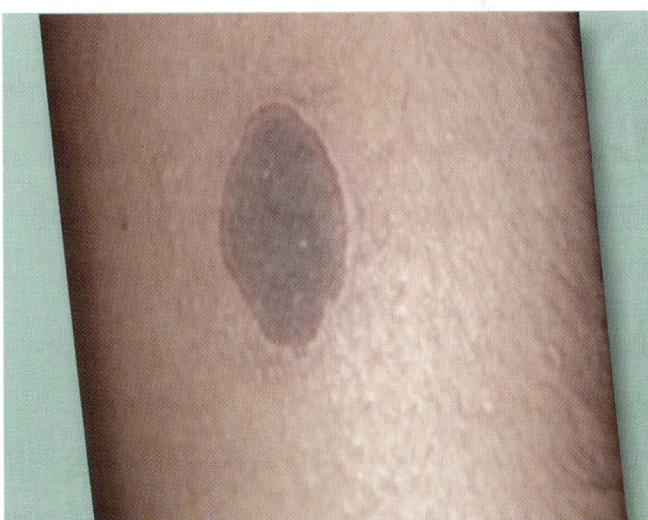

FIG. 9: Annular hyperpigmented patch in a patient of fixed drug eruption with doxycycline.

Lupus Erythematosus

- Discoid lupus erythematosus (DLE) or subacute cutaneous lupus erythematosus (SCLE) patients may present with annular lesions.
- Annular, erythematous, infiltrated, plaques with scaling at periphery and central clearing, which may be confluent, are seen in patients with DLE/SCLE. Lesions of DLE may heal with atrophy and depigmentation **(Figs. 10A and B)**.
- SCLE can be triggered by various drugs, such as hydrochlorothiazide, calcium channel blockers, angiotensin-converting enzyme (ACE) inhibitors, or terbinafine.

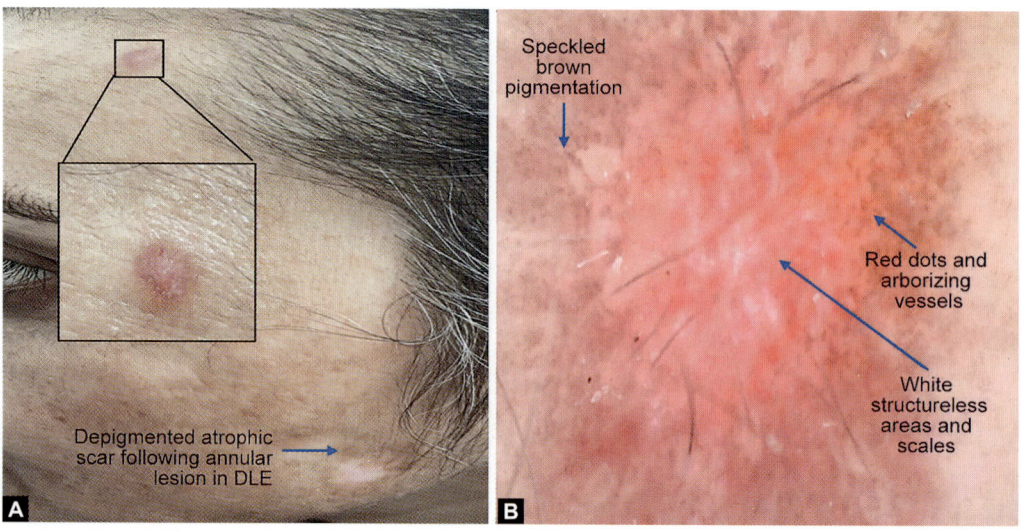

FIGS. 10A AND B: Showing clinical and dermoscopic findings in discoid lupus erythematosus with annular atrophic lesion.

- Anti-Ro/SSA or anti-La/SSB antibodies or both can be identified in such patients.
- Patients have a relapsing and recurring course of the illness. Some of the patients may develop milder form of systemic LE with SCLE.[16]

Few of the dermatoses that are not-so-common in clinical practice, present with classical annular lesions as a hallmark or as one of the clinical presentations **(Table 4)**.

UNCOMMON CONDITIONS WITH PREDOMINANTLY ANNULAR LESIONS

Granuloma Annulare

- Skin colored or slightly pink, asymptomatic, papular lesions coalescing to form annular plaques
- Clinical mimickers for granuloma annulare can be leprosy, psoriasis, annular lichen planus, or dermatophyte infections.
- Histopathology confirms the diagnosis by identifying classical palisading granuloma.[17]

Sarcoidosis

- Annular, infiltrated, erythematous, scaly plaques present more commonly on face.
- It is to be differentiated from leprosy, granuloma annulare, lupus vulgaris, and LE.
- Noncaseating, naked granuloma on histopathology is the key to diagnosis. This can be the marker of sarcoidosis which helps in early diagnosis and predicting systemic involvement mainly of lungs, lymph nodes, and eyes.[18]

Immunoglobulin A Pemphigus

- Flaccid, sterile pustules on scaly, erythematous plaques
- Immunoglobulin A (IgA) pemphigus can be associated with underlying malignancy, inflammatory bowel diseases, or rheumatoid arthritis.
- Differentials include impetigo (bacterial infection), dermatophytosis, psoriasis pustulosa, acute generalized exanthematous pustulosis, pemphigus foliaceus, and linear IgA dermatosis.
- Direct immunofluorescence (DIF) is needed to confirm the diagnosis.[19]

Urticarial Vasculitis

- When lesions of urticaria last for >24 hours and leave a residual transient hyperpigmentation, urticarial vasculitis should be suspected.
- It may be associated with fever, malaise, myalgia, and specific organ involvement.
- It may be recurrent, and may be present for months to years.
- It should be suspected in female patients with recurrent, uncontrolled urticaria accompanied by arthralgia or arthritis, respiratory distress, abdominal pain, and increased erythrocyte sedimentation rate (ESR).
- Systemic diseases associated with urticarial vasculitis include serum sickness, systemic LE, Sjögren's syndrome, hepatitis A/B/C or Epstein–Barr virus infection, neoplasia, IgG or immunoglobulin M (IgM) gammopathy, ultraviolet light or cold exposure, exercise, Wegener's granulomatosis, polyarteritis nodosa, Henoch–Schönlein purpura, adverse drug-reactions, and hereditary and acquired angioedema.[20]

Table 4: Salient features with diagnostic clue and preferred management for uncommon dermatoses with annular skin lesions.

Condition	History	Description of lesions	Key features	Diagnosis and management
Granuloma annulare	Asymptomatic, smooth, skin-colored annular skin lesions of varied duration	Smooth, skin-colored annular plaques and papules	• There will be no scaling or vesicles or pustules. More commonly occur on hands, feet, wrist, and ankles • Usually localized, but may be generalized	• Lesions may resolve with trauma caused by intralesional injections with innocuous agents such as lidocaine or normal saline or with therapeutic skin biopsy (reverse Koebner's phenomenon) • Intralesional corticosteroids or tacrolimus may be used for localized disorder
Sarcoidosis	Multiple varied types of asymptomatic skin lesions of 3 months to 2 years' duration	Asymptomatic, erythematous, indurated, annular plaques	Multisystem disorder with granulomatous infiltration predominantly involving lungs, skin, and eyes	• Biopsy is confirmatory. Needs thorough systemic evaluation • Immunomodulators such as corticosteroids, hydroxychloroquine/chloroquine, methotrexate, or thalidomide can be prescribed to control the disease
IgA pemphigus	Painful, pruritic, pustular lesions of few weeks' duration	Painful, pruritic, flaccid pustules on erythematous base, commonly in flexural area	• There may be an underlying associated conditions such as malignancy, infection, or irritable bowel syndrome • No mucosal involvement or constitutional symptoms	• There is massive neutrophilic infiltration with loss of keratinocyte cohesion as well as presence of IgA autoantibodies • Dapsone is the mainstay of the treatment • Corticosteroids may be used along with it
Urticarial vasculitis	Itchy, red skin lesions, lasting for longer than 24 hours, might be for 3–5 days	Urticarial lesions, having annular configuration of longer than 24 hours	• Represents small-vessel vasculitis • Underlying cause may be drugs, infections, malignancy, connective tissue disorders, or idiopathic	• Biopsy may show features of leukocytoclastic vasculitis • Patient responds well to oral antihistamines, oral corticosteroids, or colchicine along with the treatment of underlying cause
Subcorneal pustular dermatosis (Sneddon–Wilkinson disease)	Painful and/or itchy multiple pustular eruptions of acute onset commonly in flexures	Hypopyon (half-and-half) pustular eruptions with clear fluid on the top and pus at the bottom of the pustules on erythematous base, more commonly on trunk and flexural areas. It ruptures and gives rise to crust and scales arranged in an annular or circinate pattern	• It may be associated with pain and/or itching. Middle-aged females are commonly affected. Pustules are sterile in nature • It may be relapsing in nature	• In contrast to IgA pemphigus, no IgA deposition found on immunofluorescence • It may be associated with any of the systemic disorder such as connective tissue disorders, thyroid disorders, drugs, infections, or malignancies • Dapsone will be the drug of choice. Colchicine, oral retinoids, or systemic steroids can also be considered
Cutaneous T-cell lymphoma	Itchy, infiltrated, scaly skin lesions of varied duration of few months to years	Papule, plaques, tumors or erythrodermic, annular, arciform, or polycyclic lesions may be present	Having versatile presentation, it is challenging to diagnose the condition clinically	• Histopathology as well as genetic evidence confirms the diagnosis • Prognosis and treatment depend on the stage of the disease

Continued

Continued

Condition	History	Description of lesions	Key features	Diagnosis and management
Jessner's lymphocytic infiltration	Asymptomatic skin lesions more commonly on face, for few months, of an adult patient	Erythematous, annular or arciform papules and plaques, commonly on face and trunk	It needs to be differentiated from leprosy, photo lichenoid rash as well as T-cell lymphoma. It is a benign condition, having relapsing/remitting course	• Biopsy and immunohistochemistry confirm the diagnosis by lymphocytic infiltration with CD8+ T cells • Topical/intralesional corticosteroids can be effective • Immunomodulators can be used for severe cases
Urticarial bullous pemphigoid	Intensely pruritic, urticated papular eruptions of few months' duration	Tense bullous lesions which may present in an annular pattern	• Common in old age people • Mucosa is usually spared	• Subepidermal cleft will be identified with absence of acantholysis • Dapsone and systemic corticosteroids are the drugs of choice
Linear IgA dermatoses	Multiple fluid-filled lesions of acute onset, which may be asymptomatic or itchy, more on lower body parts	Multiple, tense bullous lesions with annular configuration, described as "strings of pearls" or "cluster of jewels," more on lower abdomen, thighs, and groin	Seen in pediatric group of patients. Also known as chronic bullous dermatosis of childhood	• Evident clinical diagnosis can be confirmed by histopathological and immunofluorescence findings • Drug of choice can be dapsone followed by systemic corticosteroids. Topical corticosteroids can be added to augment the response
Porokeratosis	Asymptomatic papule, slowly expanding outwards over a period of several weeks or months	Well-defined, circumscribed, hyperpigmented, annular plaque with central atrophy	Several clinical forms have been described	• Biopsy confirms the diagnosis by identifying coronoid lamella • Treatment targets elimination of the lesions due to cosmetic concern as well as risk of malignant transformation • Surgical excision (shaving), cryotherapy or LASER ablation may be helpful • 5-fluorouracil, imiquimod, or local retinoids can be tried

UNCOMMON CONDITIONS WITH INFREQUENT ANNULAR LESIONS

Neonatal Lupus Erythematosus
- Annular or papulosquamous, polycyclic lesions on face and scalp may be seen in a newborn with presence of maternal antibodies for LE.
- It is transient in nature, and resolves by the age of 6 months when maternal antibodies disappear.
- Cardiac involvement may lead to morbidity and mortality in such cases.[21]

Subcorneal Pustular Dermatosis (Sneddon–Wilkinson disease)
- Hypopyon or half-and-half pustules in a middle-aged female with annular or serpiginous pattern with central clearing and peripheral pustules
- Differentials such as pustular psoriasis or acute generalized exanthematous pustulosis should be considered.
  - Pustular psoriasis patients have preexisting psoriatic lesions and classical histopathological findings showing epidermal spongiform pustules, parakeratosis, and acanthosis.[22]
  - Acute generalized exanthematous pustulosis patients have precipitating drug history and histopathological changes.

Cutaneous T-cell Lymphoma
- Patients of cutaneous T-cell lymphoma (CTCL), when progressing from patch stage to plaque stage, may present with itchy, erythematous, infiltrated, elevated, scaly plaques forming annular lesions by coalescing.
- It may mimic tinea infection, psoriasis, or nummular dermatitis.
- It may progress to tumor stage over a period of few months to years.
- In progressive state, extracutaneous spread occurs by involving lymph nodes, lungs, spleen, liver, and gastrointestinal track.[23]

Jessner's Lymphocytic Infiltration
- Asymptomatic, erythematous, annular, or horseshoe-like papules and plaques, commonly found on face.
- Clinical differentials may include LE, polymorphic light eruptions, lymphocytoma cutis, leprosy, or granuloma annulare.
- Biopsy is the key to diagnose the condition which shows prominent dense, coat-sleeve-like, perivascular/periadnexal lymphocytic infiltrates that leave the epidermis untouched.[24]

Urticarial Bullous Pemphigoid
- Large, tense bullae on urticarial, erythematous, or normal skin
- Pruritic bullous eruption reappearing with several annular erythematous plaques may be indicative of atypical BP as a paraneoplastic phenomenon.
- The histological and DIF findings and the detection of circulating autoantibodies by indirect immunofluorescence or enzyme-linked immunosorbent assay leads to confirmation of diagnosis.[25]

Linear Immunoglobulin A Dermatoses
- Multiple, tense bullous lesions with annular configuration—string of pearls appearance
- Differentials include skin infections such as bullous impetigo and chickenpox or other vesiculobullous conditions such as dermatitis herpetiformis.
- Linear deposits of IgA along the basement membrane found on DIF are the confirmatory feature.[26]

Porokeratosis
- Porokeratosis of mibelli or disseminated superficial actinic porokeratosis present with asymptomatic or slightly pruritic, annular atrophic plaques with rimmed keratotic border **(Figs. 11A and B)**.
- The disease slowly progresses and may undergo malignant transformation into Bowen's disease, invasive squamous cell carcinoma, or basal cell carcinoma.[27]

Annular Erythemas
There are four "classic" figurate erythemas which present with annular, arciform, or polycyclic lesions. They are erythema migrans, erythema annulare centrifugum, erythema gyratum repens, and erythema marginatum. The etiology or trigger for figurate erythemas varies from infections (e.g., erythema migrans due to *Borrelia burgdorferi*) to neoplasms (e.g., erythema gyratum repens due to lung carcinoma) **(Table 5)**.

Erythema Migrans
- Oval or circular, slightly warm, erythematous patches with regular margins which may be itchy and/or painful are seen at the site of tick bite
- Early lesions of erythema migrans show growth rate of 20 cm^2/day spreading outward from the site of tick bite. The minimum diameter of skin lesion should exceed 5 cm in order to differentiate erythema migrans from other diseases.
- Shape of the lesions is partly determined by lines of skin tension like groin lesions may be oval along the horizontal axis or have an unusual configuration such as triangles may appear when spirochetes migrate over skin folds.
- Central vesicles may be observed which may be clear, cloudy, or hemorrhagic.
- Vesicular lesions need to be differentiated from bacterial cellulitis, arthropod bite, contact dermatitis, or even herpes simplex and varicella zoster virus infection.[28,29]

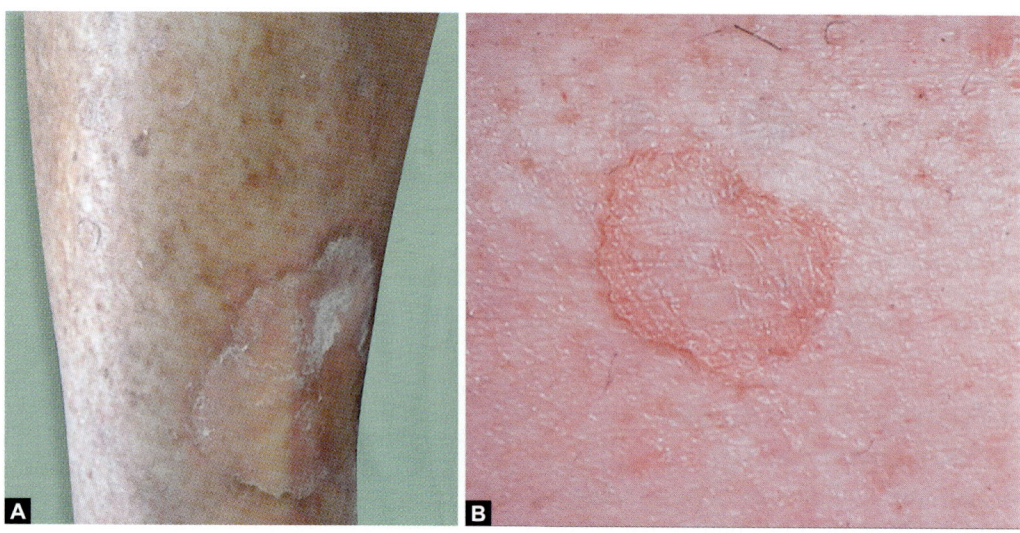

FIGS. 11A AND B: Annular well-defined plaques with keratotic borders in patients with porokeratosis.
Courtesy: Jean KANITAKIS.[27]

Table 5: Classic figurate type of erythema with annular lesions.			
Clinical condition	**Clinical features**	**Association**	**Treatment**
Erythema migrans	• Itchy, expanding red skin lesion at the site of bite, after 3–30 days of tick bite. • Annular, erythematous rash with/without central clearing	It may progress to involve extracutaneous organ system (cardiac, musculoskeletal, and neurologic) if not treated timely	Doxycycline/amoxicillin/cefuroxime can be prescribed effectively
Erythema annulare centrifugum	• Intensely pruritic, migrating, ring-shaped, scaly skin lesions with central clearing may be there. Expand slowly—2–3 mm/day. • Scaly (superficial) or nonscaly (deep), pruritic, annular erythematous eruptions more on trunk, buttocks, thigh, and legs	It is be a manifestation of underlying infection or malignancy	• Topical steroids and antihistamine for symptomatic relief. • Treatment of underlying condition augments the response
Erythema gyratum repens	Intensely pruritic, ring-shaped, annular lesions forming concentric figures in a wood-grain pattern. Expand rapidly—around 1 cm/day	Underlying malignancies of lung, breast, esophagus, stomach, or genitourinary tract	It resolves with treatment of underlying condition
Erythema marginatum	Asymptomatic, expanding red, nonscaly lesions, expanding in few hours to days	Rheumatic fever	The lesions will resolve with beta-lactam antibiotics to treat underlying streptococcal infection

Erythema Annulare Centrifugum

- Erythematous papules that migrate slowly (2–3 mm/day), flattening as they grow, forming annular or arciform lesions by clearing of a center.
- It may present as intensely pruritic superficial lesion with a peripheral desquamative border or an asymptomatic, non-scaly, deep lesion with infiltrated pronounced, cord-like border.
- It is most frequently associated with infection by *Candida albicans*, dermatophytes, Epstein–Barr virus, and poxvirus or malignancy such as leukemia and Hodgkin lymphoma.

Erythema Gyratum Repens

- Intensely pruritic, multiple, polycyclic, or annular erythematous lesions rapidly covering the body but sparing the face, hands, and feet seen with underlying malignancies of lung, breast, esophagus, stomach, or genitourinary tract.
- These lesions rapidly progress and grow by as much as 1 cm daily and form concentric figures in a wood-grain pattern, also mentioned as "knotty-cypress wood-grained" configuration, with scales on the advancing border.
- It resolves with treatment of underlying malignancy.[29]

> **Box 1: List of common conditions with annular lesions in pediatric age-group.**
>
> - Tinea corporis/tinea capitis
> - Pityriasis rosea
> - Bullous impetigo
> - Urticaria
> - Leprosy
> - Lupus erythematosus (neonatal/subacute cutaneous)
> - Granuloma annulare
> - Annular/figurate erythema:
>   ○ Erythema annulare centrifugum
>   ○ Erythema marginatum rheumatica
>   ○ Erythema gyratum repens

Erythema Marginatum Rheumatica

- Evanescent, transient (lasting from a few hours to a couple of days) asymptomatic erythema that appears during rheumatic fever.
- Papular plaques that extend peripherally to form annular or polycyclic plaques with central clearing but no desquamation or epidermal abnormalities, mainly on the trunk and proximal extremities.

- It is more common in children than in adults, a reflection of the higher prevalence of rheumatic fever in children.

ANNULAR LESIONS IN PEDIATRIC AGE-GROUP

Nearly one-third of pediatric patients present with dermatological problems.[30] Pediatricians must be competent enough to diagnose common dermatological disorders seen in children. The most frequent skin disorders presenting with annular lesions in children have been listed in **Box 1**.[31]

Annular lesions of the conditions such as tinea infection, psoriasis, or urticaria share similar types of lesions as in adults. It needs distinct approach to treat such cases considering their physiological state.

Patients with neonatal LE need periodical evaluation to offer early detection and treatment in case they develop LE or other autoimmune diseases during adulthood.[21]

It is important to distinguish between conditions which need our immediate attention and intervention to avoid mortality and morbidity (e.g., LE or urticaria) from milder self-limiting conditions (e.g., pityriasis alba) where only patient education and counseling along with conventional treatment helps in dealing with patients.

REFERENCES

1. Sharma A, Lambert PJ, Maghari A, Lambert WC. Arcuate, annular, and polycyclic inflammatory and infectious lesions. Clin Dermatol. 2011;29(2):140-50.
2. Toledo-Alberola F, Betlloch-Mas I. Eritemas anulares en la infancia [Annular erythema of infancy]. Actas Dermosifiliogr. 2010;101(6):473-84.
3. Trayes KP, Savage K, Studdiford JS. Annular lesions: Diagnosis and treatment. Am Fam Physician. 2018;98(5):283-91.
4. Leung AKC, Leong KF, Lam JM. Tinea imbricata: An overview. Curr Pediatr Rev. 2019;15(3):170-4.
5. Rengasamy M, Shenoy MM, Dogra S, Asokan N, Khurana A, Poojary S, et al. Indian Association of Dermatologists, Venereologists and Leprologists (IADVL) task force against recalcitrant tinea (ITART) consensus on the management of glabrous tinea (INTACT). Indian Dermatol Online J. 2020;11(4):502-19.
6. Nagarajan P, Thappa DM. Effect of an educational and psychological intervention on knowledge and quality of life among patients with psoriasis. Indian Dermatol Online J. 2018;9(1):27-32.
7. Stulberg DL, Wolfrey J. Pityriasis rosea. Am Fam Physician. 2004;69(1):87-91.
8. Khan S, Maitra A, Hissaria P, Roy S, Padukudru Anand M, Nag N, et al. Chronic urticaria: Indian context—challenges and treatment options. Dermatol Res Pract. 2013;2013: 651737.
9. Sokumbi O, Wetter DA. Clinical features, diagnosis, and treatment of erythema multiforme: a review for the practicing dermatologist. Int J Dermatol. 2012;51(8):889-902.
10. Hartman-Adams H, Banvard C, Juckett G. Impetigo: diagnosis and treatment. Am Fam Physician. 2014;90(4):229-35.
11. Jiamton S, Tangjaturonrusamee C, Kulthanan K. Clinical features and aggravating factors in nummular eczema in Thais. Asian Pac J Allergy Immunol. 2013;31(1):36-42.
12. Zhao CC, Zhang Z, Zheng S, Li JH. Annular secondary syphilis on the penis: A case report. Int J Dermatol Venereol. 2019;2(2): 118-9.
13. Parodi M, Ciccarese G, Drago F, Cozzani E, Buligan C, Turina M, et al. Annular and arciform lesions of the palms as unique manifestations of secondary syphilis. Int J STD AIDS. 2020;31(13):1323-6.
14. Kavoussi H, Rezaei M, Derakhshandeh K, Moradi A, Ebrahimi A, Rashidian H, et al. Clinical features and drug characteristics of patients with generalized fixed drug eruption in the West of Iran (2005-2014). Dermatol Res Pract. 2015;2015:236703.
15. Tan C, Zhu WY. Annular fixed drug eruption. J Dtsch Dermatol Ges. 2010;8(10):823-4.
16. Kuhn A, Ruzicka T. Classification of cutaneous lupus erythematosus. In: Cutaneous Lupus Erythematosus. Berlin, Heidelberg: Springer; 2005. pp. 53–7.
17. Naveen KN, Pai VV, Athanikar SB, Gupta G, Parshwanath HA. Remote reverse Koebner phenomenon in generalized

granuloma annulare. Indian Dermatol Online J. 2014;5(2): 219-21.
18. Mahajan VK, Sharma NL, Sharma RC, Sharma VC. Cutaneous sarcoidosis: clinical profile of 23 Indian patients. Indian J Dermatol Venereol Leprol. 2007;73(1):16-21.
19. Kiritsi D, Hoch M, Kern JS. Annular flaccid pustules on the trunk. JAMA Dermatol. 2017;153(9):921-2.
20. Kulthanan K, Cheepsomsong M, Jiamton S. Urticarial vasculitis: etiologies and clinical course. Asian Pac J Allergy Immunol. 2009;27(2-3):95-102.
21. Martin V, Lee LA, Askanase AD, Katholi M, Buyon JP. Long-term follow-up of children with neonatal lupus and their unaffected siblings. Arthritis Rheum. 2002;46(9):2377-83.
22. Adler DJ, Rower JM, Hashimoto K. Annular pustular psoriasis. Arch Dermatol. 1981;117(5):313-4.
23. Koh HK, Charif M, Weinstock MA. Epidemiology and clinical manifestations of cutaneous T-cell lymphoma. Hematol Oncol Clin North Am. 1995;9(5):943-60.
24. Poenitz N, Dippel E, Klemke CD, Qadoumi M, Goerdt S. Jessner's lymphocytic infiltration of the skin: a CD8+ polyclonal reactive skin condition. Dermatology. 2003;207(3):276-84.
25. Yu-Yang S, Chu-Sung Hu S, Yiao-Lin S. Bullous pemphigoid masquerading as erythema annulare centrifugum. Acta Dermatovenerol Croat. 2017;25(3):255-6.
26. Verma N, Pickles C, Khan MA. The "pearls" of multidisciplinary team: Conquering the uncommon rosette rash. Case Rep Pediatr. 2016;2016:5328603.
27. Kanitakis J. Porokeratoses: an update of clinical, aetiopathogenic and therapeutic features. Eur J Dermatol. 2014;24(5):533-44.
28. Nadelman RB. Erythema migrans. Infect Dis Clin North Am. 2015;29(2):211-39.
29. Boehner A, Neuhauser R, Zink A, Ring J. Figurate erythemas - update and diagnostic approach. J Dtsch Dermatol Ges. 2021; 19(7):963-72.
30. Sethuraman G, Bhari N. Common skin problems in children. Indian J Pediatr. 2014;81(4):381-90.
31. Narváez D, Di Martino Ortiz B, Rodríguez Masi M. Annular skin lesions in childhood: Review of the main differential diagnoses. Our Dermatol Online. 2017;8(1):75-80.

A Suspected Case of Panniculitis

Feroze Kaliyadan, Puravoor Jayasree

INTRODUCTION

Panniculitis is inflammation of the subcutaneous fat. The primary morphological presentation of panniculitis is in the form of deep plaques or subcutaneous nodules. There are many conditions which can present with panniculitis due to a wide range of causes **(Box 1)**. Getting the diagnosis right is important because some of the conditions presenting with panniculitis can be associated with a poor prognosis. Early diagnosis and appropriate treatment can help in patient outcomes.

APPROACH TO A CASE OF SUSPECTED PANNICULITIS

Clinical Aspects

Both history and examination **(Table 1)** as well as histopathological correlation help in clinching the diagnosis and underlying cause in cases of panniculitis.[1] Hence we need to make sure the pertinent points are covered in the history while evaluating a patient presenting with panniculitis.

Age of the patient, family history, evolution of the lesions (acute vs. chronic), site of the lesions (restricted to legs or other areas of the body), preceding complaints (sore throat), drug history [use of oral contraceptive pills (OCPs), injections] associated complaints (fever, photosensitivity, jaundice, joint pains, loss of weight, oral/genital ulcers, ophthalmological complaints, hair loss, neurological symptoms such as paresthesia, abdominal pain, back pain, altered bowel habits—diarrhea/constipation, bleeding tendencies) are all important pointers for further evaluation. Possibilities of sexually transmitted infection like syphilis have also to be considered.[1-3]

One of the first steps in dermatological examination, after history taking, is the identification of the primary lesion(s). In fact, dermatology, unlike other specialties like internal medicine, has the advantage of being able to plan and adapt your history taking process better, because the lesions are usually visible and generally primary differential diagnoses are already in the back of your mind. Primary lesions in a case of panniculitis are subcutaneous nodules because the inflammatory process is happening in the deeper layer of subcutaneous fat. But further qualifying features like tender or nontender, presence or absence of ulceration, distribution of the lesions further helps to differentiate the cause in a particular patient. Though most panniculitis lesions involve lower limbs and erythema nodosum is prototype of this category; lesions involving other sites might give us clue to etiology. Facial involvement is commonly seen with lupus panniculitis while lesions of erythema nodosum leprosum (ENL) **(Fig. 1)** can involve any site in the body including face. Other coexisting local findings are also important like presence of varicose veins point to a possibility of sclerosing panniculitis. Presence of ichthyotic changes on lower limb might suggest possibility of ENL **(Fig. 2)**. Absence of ulceration is helpful in differentiating from conditions like nodular vasculitis. Absence of associated skin features like livedo reticularis, cutaneous ulcers, and necrosis point against polyarteritis nodosa (PAN).

Thus, a short duration with acute presentation is more likely to be caused by an inflammatory and infective **(Fig. 3)** cause whereas slowly evolving lesions of chronic duration is more likely to be a neoplastic or deposition-associated presentation. The other issue is that some of the conditions might present with reactive conditions which can indicate the need to look for further underlying or associated conditions. For example, erythema nodosum can be triggered by a range of underlying factors—drugs, infections—mycobacterial

Box 1: Etiological classification of panniculitis.

Inflammatory
- Erythema nodosum
- Erythema nodosum migrans/subacute nodular migratory panniculitis/chronic erythema nodosum
- Lipodermatosclerosis (sclerosing panniculitis)
- Erythema induratum/nodular vasculitis
- Polyarteritis nodosa
- Superficial migratory thrombophlebitis
- Lupus panniculitis
- Deep morphea
- Necrobiosis lipoidica diabeticorum
- Rheumatoid nodule
- Subcutaneous granuloma annulare
- Leukocytoclastic vasculitis
- Subcutaneous sarcoidosis
- Erythema nodosum leprosum
- Poststeroid panniculitis
- Behçet's syndrome
- Erythema elevatum diutinum

Infection and infestation
- Infectious panniculitis—bacterial, mycobacterial, or fungal infections
- Parasites
- Arthropod bite

Trauma
- Cold panniculitis (popsicle panniculitis, equestrian panniculitis, sclerema neonatorum)
- Blunt trauma
- Factitial panniculitis (iatrogenic, accidental, or intentional injections)
- Postirradiation panniculitis
- Subcutaneous fat necrosis of the newborn

Enzymatic destruction
- Pancreatic panniculitis
- Alpha-1 antitrypsin deficiency

Malignancy
- Lymphoma
- Cytophagic histiocytic panniculitis
- Leukemia cutis/metastases

Deposition
- Gouty panniculitis
- Calciphylaxis
- Crystal storing histiocytosis
- Hyperoxaluria

infections, streptococcal infections, deep fungal infections, and human immunodeficiency virus (HIV) infection, lymphoma/leukemias, connective tissue disorders, and inflammatory bowel diseases.

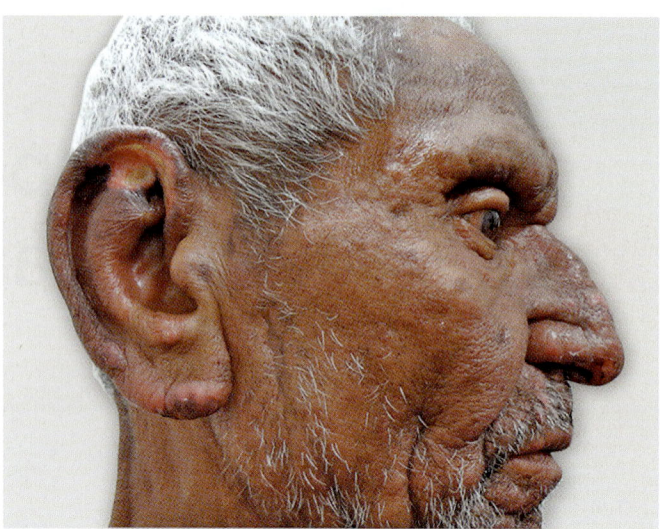

FIG. 1: Erythema nodosum leprosum necroticans on face in a case of lepromatous leprosy.
Courtesy: Dr Jigna Padhiyar.

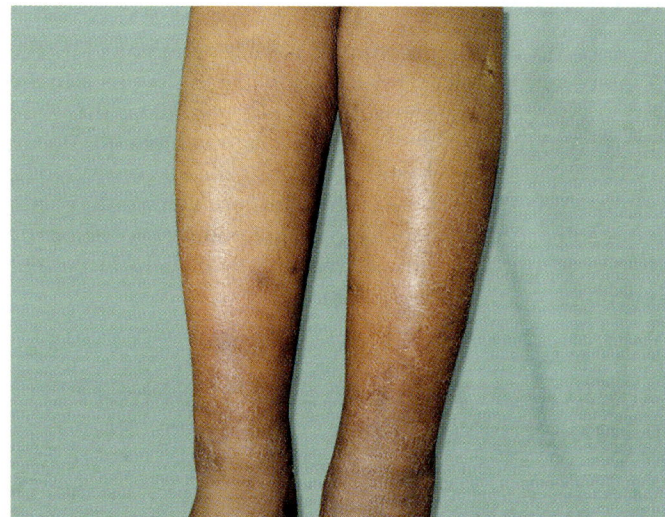

FIG. 2: Tender erythematous nodules of erythema nodosum leprosum with ichthyotic changes on bilateral lower limbs.
Courtesy: Dr Jigna Padhiyar.

So, what should our next step be?
- Confirm the subtype of panniculitis
- Rule out other possible diagnosis and other possible underlying causes

As mentioned, the morphological pattern of panniculitis is essentially a subcutaneous reaction pattern, which opens a wide range of differentials. In the case of panniculitis itself, it is more prudent to use a clinic-pathological approach. Normal subcutaneous tissue has lobules of adipocytes separated by fibrous septa. For suspected panniculitis always make it a point to take a deep biopsy, because the pathology is expected at the level of the panniculus.

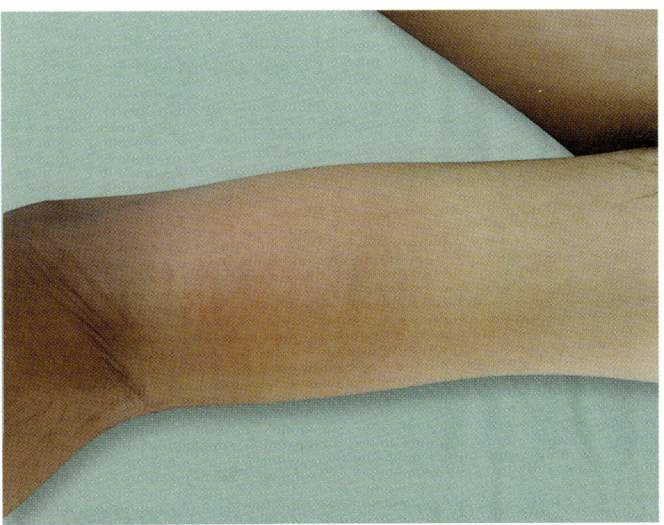

FIG. 3: Plaque of panniculitis over upper limb in a patient who had viral infection.

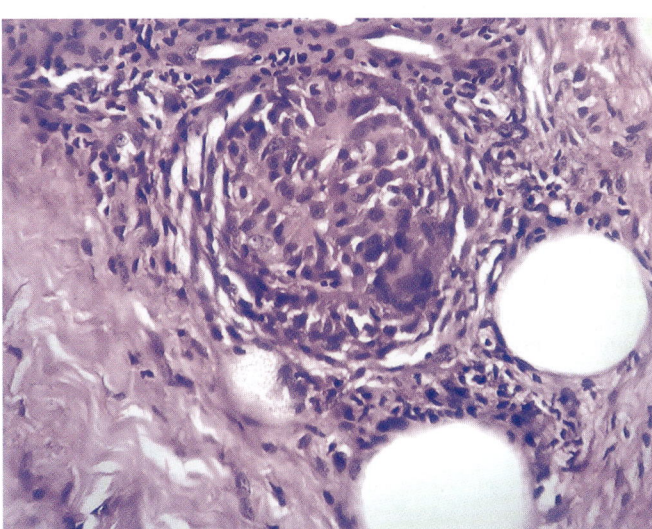

FIG. 5: Miescher's granuloma with central clefts in late stages of erythema nodosum.

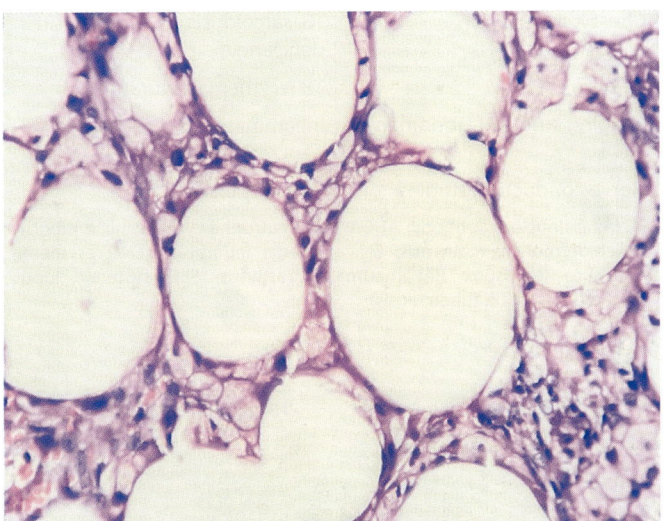

FIG. 4: Lipophagic necrosis of fat lobules.

Histopathology is key to identify the specific type of panniculitis. Key points to look for are whether the inflammation is primarily septal or lobular and the presence or absence of vasculitis. Even histopathology might not help to differentiate various disorders if the biopsy has been taken from very old lesions. End-stage finding like lipophagic appearance **(Fig. 4)** in a case of panniculitis is very much same for many disorders. Lipoatrophy can be a result of any inflammatory or autoimmune disorders as well as in cases of lipodystrophies. Membranous fat necrosis can be commonly seen in diseases associated with venous stasis, but it can be encountered as late stage finding in many other disorders. Cytophagic changes are usually observed in histiocytosis and malignancy involving subcutis. Hence, it is always important to take a new lesion for histopathological examination and note the duration of lesion for clinicopathological correlation.

For erythema nodosum, the histopathology essentially shows a septal panniculitis without vasculitis. The inflammation can vary from a primarily polymorphonuclear to granulomatous, depending on the stage **(Fig. 5)**.[6,7] **Table 2** summarizes the histological classification of panniculitis.

Table 1: Pointers in history, examination, and investigations in a suspected case of panniculitis.	
Point in history	**Clinical significance**
Age: • Newborn • Children	• Subcutaneous fat necrosis of newborn **(Fig. 6)**, sclerema neonatorum • Genetic causes—α-1 antitrypsin deficiency • Sudden withdrawal of high-dose steroids—post-steroid panniculitis
Exposure to cold	Cold panniculitis
Long-standing fever, evening rise of fever, night sweat	Possibility of TB, sarcoidosis, malignancy
Weight loss	Possibility of TB (etiology of EN, EI), malignancy
Drug history	Drug-induced EN
Previous injection site, substance abuse, psychiatric disorder	Factitious panniculitis

Continued

Continued

Point in history	Clinical significance
Radiation (breast cancer most commonly)	Postirradiation sclerodermatous panniculitis
Renal failure	Calciphylaxis
Early onset emphysema	Alpha-1 antitrypsin deficiency
Episodes of abdominal pain or jaundice, history of alcoholism	Pancreatic panniculitis
History of sexual exposure, genital ulcers	Syphilis
Associated complaints	*Significance*
Joint pain	Can be constitutional symptom of EN, connective tissue diseases—SLE, rheumatoid arthritis
Photosensitivity	SLE
Oral ulceration: • Painful • Painless	 • Behçet's disease • SLE
Breathlessness	Alpha-1 antitrypsin deficiency
Big toe involvement	Gout
Abdominal symptoms such as abdominal pain diarrhea and melena	EN associated with inflammatory bowel disease, pancreatic panniculitis
Immunosuppression	Infectious panniculitis
Neuropathy	Hansen disease
Local examination	*Significance*
Necrosis of nodules	Erythema induratum of Bazin/ nodular vasculitis, infectious panniculitis including ENL, α-1 antitrypsin deficiency, pancreatic panniculitis
Location: • Anterior lower legs • Posterior lower legs • Medial lower legs Abdomen, buttocks, flanks (more proximal)	 • Erythema nodosum **(Fig. 7)** • Erythema induratum • Lipodermatosclerosis **(Fig. 8)**/ stasis panniculitis • Pancreatic panniculitis, α-1 antitrypsin deficiency • Subcutaneous sarcoidosis
Face, breasts, upper torso, and limbs	Poststeroid panniculitis, popsicle panniculitis
Cheeks in children Face and breast	SLE **(Fig. 9)**
Livedo reticularis	Cutaneous polyarteritis nodosa
Telangiectasia, edema, varicose veins, thickened and hyperpigmented skin	Lipodermatosclerosis

Continued

Continued

Point in history	Clinical significance
Lymphadenopathy	Infections, sarcoidosis, malignancy
Investigations	*Interpretation*
Leukocytosis	Inflammatory and infectious causes
Atypical cells in peripheral smear	Hematological malignancy
RA factor	Rheumatoid arthritis panniculitis
ANCA	Polyarteritis nodosa
ANA	Systemic lupus erythematosus, dermatomyositis
Angiotensin-converting enzyme	Sarcoidosis
Serum lipase	Pancreatic panniculitis
Uric acid	Gout
Serum calcium	Calciphylaxis
Chest X-ray	TB, sarcoidosis, α-1 antitrypsin deficiency
Mantoux test	TB (erythema induratum)
Imaging studies—abdomen	Inflammatory Bowel disease, pancreatic diseases
Nerve conduction studies	Hansen's disease

(ANA: antinuclear antibody; ANCA: anti-neutrophil cytoplasmic antibody; EI: epidermolytic ichthyosis; EN: erythema induratum; ENL: erythema nodosum leprosum; RA: rheumatoid arthritis; SLE: systemic lupus erythematosus; TB: tuberculosis)

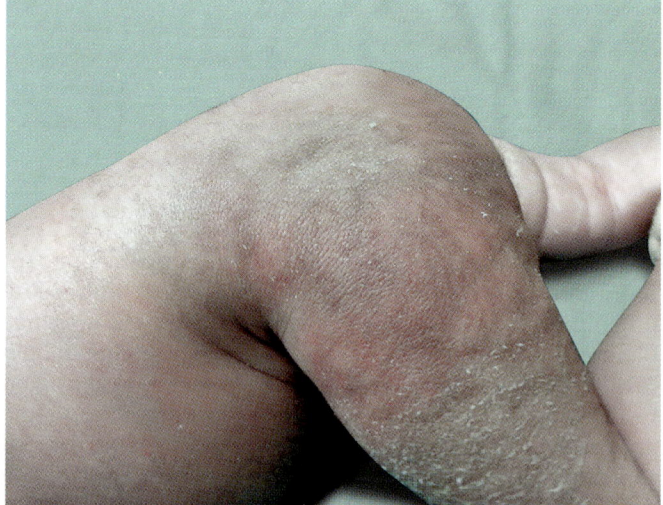

FIG. 6: Diffuse ill-defined erythematous plaque with pigmentary changes on thigh and leg of a newborn child.
Courtesy: Dr Nayan Patel.

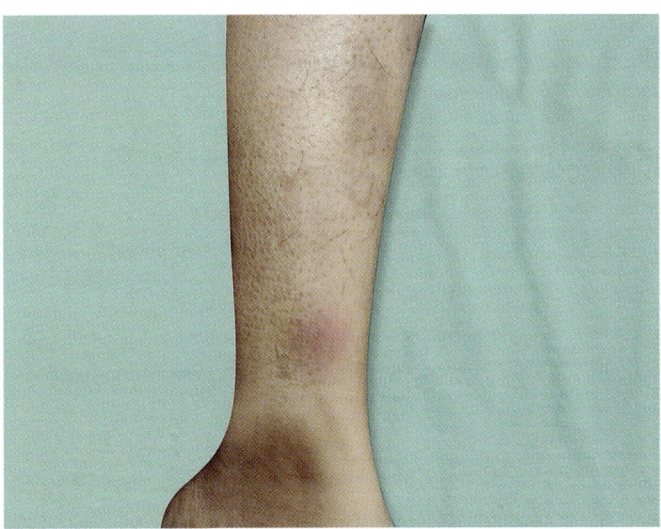

FIG. 7: Nodule of erythema nodosum on leg.

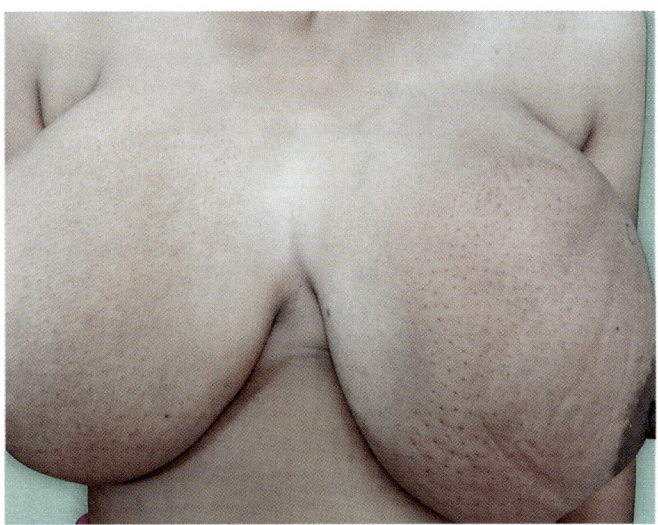

FIG. 9: Diffuse indurated plaque on left breast in a female with antinuclear antibody (ANA) and double-stranded deoxyribonucleic acid (dsDNA) antibody positivity.
Courtesy: Dr Jigna Padhiyar.

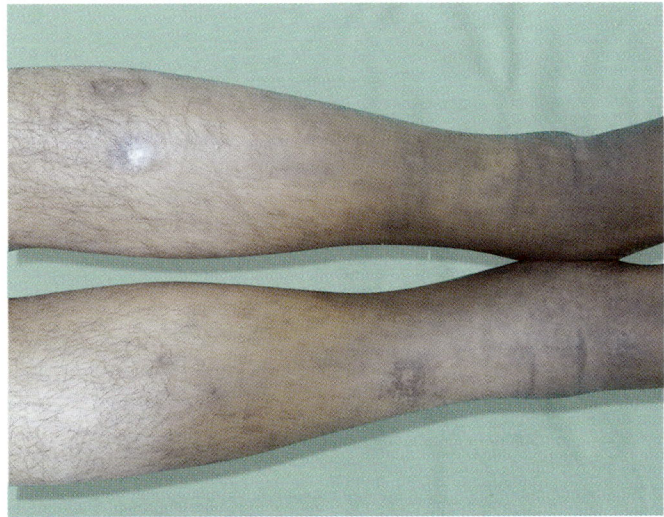

FIG. 8: Hyperpigmented nodule on leg with signs of venous stasis in a case of lipodermatosclerosis.
Courtesy: Dr Nayan Patel.

Once we have confirmed the diagnosis and narrowed down our differentials, further investigations would be to ensure that underlying/associated conditions are not missed. So essential tests indicated in all cases would include:[8-14]

- Complete blood count and peripheral smear (this would help in ruling out infections and leukemias)
- Radiology chest (to rule out tuberculosis/sarcoidosis—remember these are also differentials for subcutaneous nodules in general or can cause erythema nodosum like conditions as a reactive change)
- Antistreptolysin O (ASO)—titer/throat swab
- Antinuclear antibody (ANA) screen and ANA profile/anti-neutrophil cytoplasmic antibody (ANCA)/cyclic citrullinated peptide (CCP)/rheumatoid arthritis (RA) (to rule out connective tissue disorders-associated panniculitis/ANCA-positive vasculitis like PAN and RA)

Other investigations which can be considered if indicated include:

- Doppler ultrasound (USG) legs (to rule out a primary vascular condition like thrombophlebitis)
- HIV screen/venereal disease research laboratory (VDRL)
- Gastrointestinal (GI) endoscopy (to rule out associated/underlying inflammatory bowel disease)
- Bone marrow/lymph node biopsy

In **Table 1 and Flowchart 1**, we briefly cover these aspects to be covered in history, clinical examination, and other investigations.

Table 3 summarizes distinguished features of commonly encountered panniculitis in clinical practice and treatment options available. There are few vital features which help us to establish a diagnosis in a case of panniculitis. Knowing these features always help us to refine our differentials.

SOME OTHER LESS COMMON TYPES OF PANNICULITIDES

Factitial panniculitis associated with injection of various material into the skin like oils/paraffin shows lobular panniculitis, without vasculitis on histopathology. Usually seen in patients with associated psychiatric problems.[32]

Table 2: Histopathological classification of panniculitis.		
Pattern of subcutaneous tissue involvement	*Characteristic cellular infiltrate*	*Additional findings*
Predominantly septal panniculitis without vasculitis		
Erythema nodosum **(Fig. 10)**	Histiocytes, lymphocytes	Radial granulomas in septa
Necrobiotic xanthogranuloma	Histiocytes	Foamy histiocytes, cholesterol clefts
Subcutaneous granuloma annulare	Histiocytes	Mucin in the center of palisaded granuloma
Rheumatoid nodule	Histiocytes	Fibrin in the center of palisaded granuloma
Deep morphea, scleroderma	Lymphocytes and plasma cells	Collagenization in dermis, no granulomatous infiltrate
Necrobiosis lipoidica diabeticorum	Lymphocytes and plasma cells	Granulomatous infiltrate in septa, layered sandwich appearance, and necrobiosis
Predominantly septal panniculitis with vasculitis		
Cutaneous PAN	Neutrophils	Vasculitis involving large arteries
Superficial thrombophlebitis	Mixed	Vasculitis involving large veins
Predominantly lobular panniculitis without vasculitis		
Postirradiation panniculitis	Histiocytes	Sclerosis of the septa
Gout	Histiocytes	Uric acid crystals
Poststeroid panniculitis	Histiocytes	Needle-shaped crystals
Crystal storing histiocytosis	Histiocytes	Crystals
Fat necrosis of the newborn	Histiocytes	Needle-shaped crystals in radial fashion
Traumatic panniculitis	Histiocytes	No granulomas
Factitial panniculitis	Neutrophils	Foreign bodies
Pancreatic panniculitis	Neutrophils	Extensive fat necrosis with saponification of adipocytes
Infectious panniculitis **(Fig. 11)**	Neutrophils	Suppurative changes
Alpha-1 antitrypsin deficiency	Neutrophils	Neutrophils between collagen bundles
Lupus panniculitis **(Fig. 12)**	Lymphocytes and plasma cells	Lymphoid follicles, mucin deposition, hyalinization of fat and membranocystic change
Cold panniculitis	Lymphocytes	Superficial and deep perivascular infiltrate
Sclerema neonatorum	No inflammatory cells	Needle-shaped crystals
Oxalosis/calciphylaxis	No inflammatory cells	Vascular calcification, marked fibroblastic proliferation, radially arranged crystals in case of oxalosis
SPTCL (subcutaneous panniculitis like T-cell lymphoma)	Atypical lymphocytes	Rimming of atypical cell around adipocytes, cytophagic changes may be present.
Predominantly lobular panniculitis with vasculitis		
Lucio phenomenon, erythema nodosum leprosum **(Fig. 13)**	Foamy histiocytes/macrophage, neutrophils	Vasculitis of small vessels—venules, bacilli within lumen and wall of vessels in FF stain
Erythema induratum/nodular vasculitis	Predominantly lymphocytes	Vasculitis, well-formed granuloma with giant cells, lipophages, caseation necrosis
Rheumatoid arthritis-associated panniculitis	Neutrophils with occasional eosinophils	Leukocytoclastic vasculitis involving arterioles and venules, membranous change with cyst formation
(FF: Fite–Faraco; PAN: polyarteritis nodosa)		

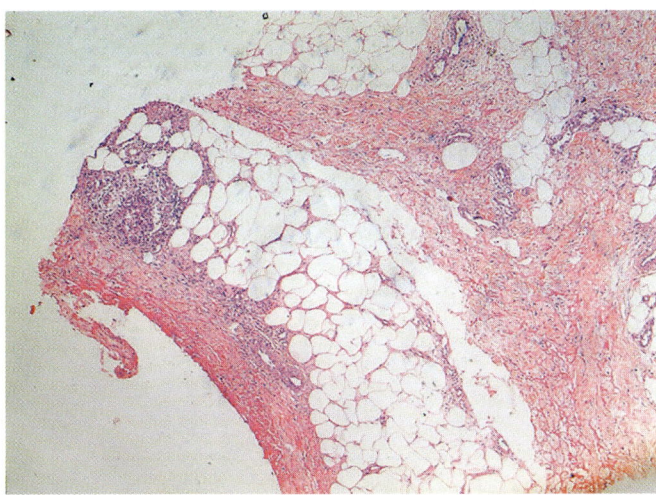

FIG. 10: Septal thickening with predominantly lymphocytic infiltrate in a case of erythema nodosum.

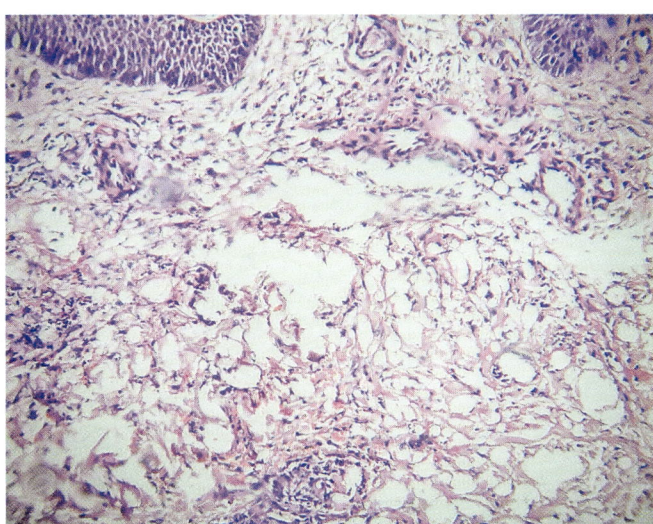

FIG. 12: Membranocystic changes with hyalinization changes in a case of lupus panniculitis.
Courtesy: Dr Jigna Padhiyar.

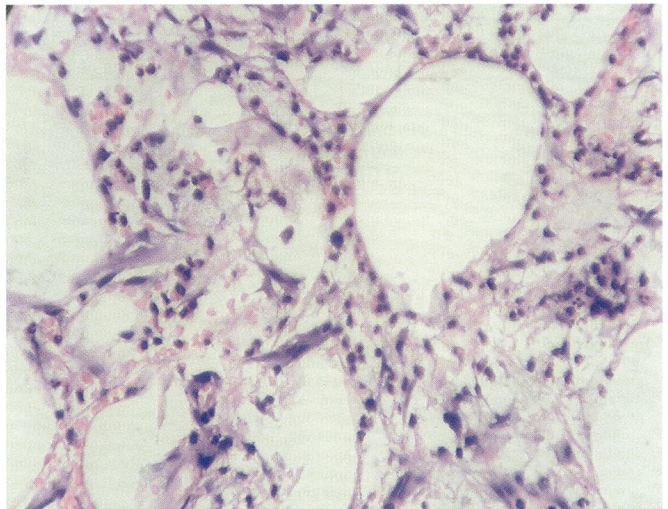

FIG. 11: Suppurative inflammation with neutrophils in a case of infective panniculitis.
Courtesy: Dr Nayan Patel.

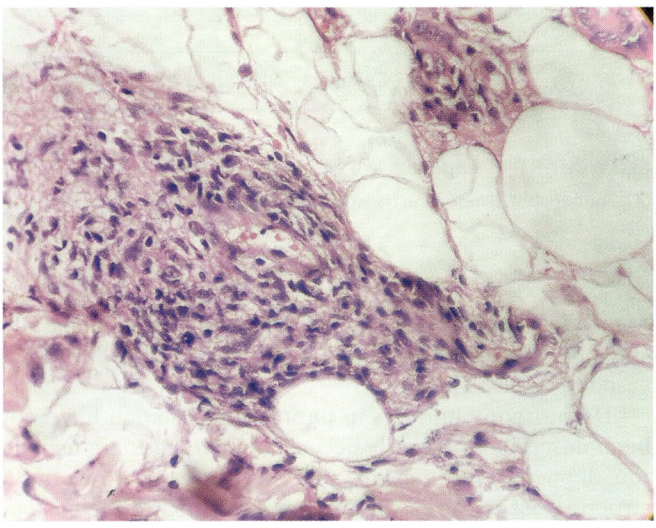

FIG. 13: Perivascular foamy histiocytes and neutrophils in a case of erythema nodosum leprosum.
Courtesy: Dr Jigna Padhiyar.

Dermatomyositis-associated panniculitis affects limbs and abdomen mainly. On pathological examination a mixed septal and lobular pattern is observed.[33]

Infectious/infective panniculitis can be associated with a wide variety or organisms and clinical presentation can be different according to the type of organism. Exposed sites like extremities and face are more commonly affected. Usually produces lobular inflammation and treatment depends on the causative organism.[34]

Erythema nodosum leprosum which is seen as part of type 2 reactions in leprosy. A previous history of leprosy helps to point toward the diagnosis. Lesions tend to be transient and more generalized as compared to differentials like erythema nodosum and leaves dull bluish pigmentation on healing. Dermoscopic findings such as milky-red areas along with brownish-yellow areas, white areas, and brown

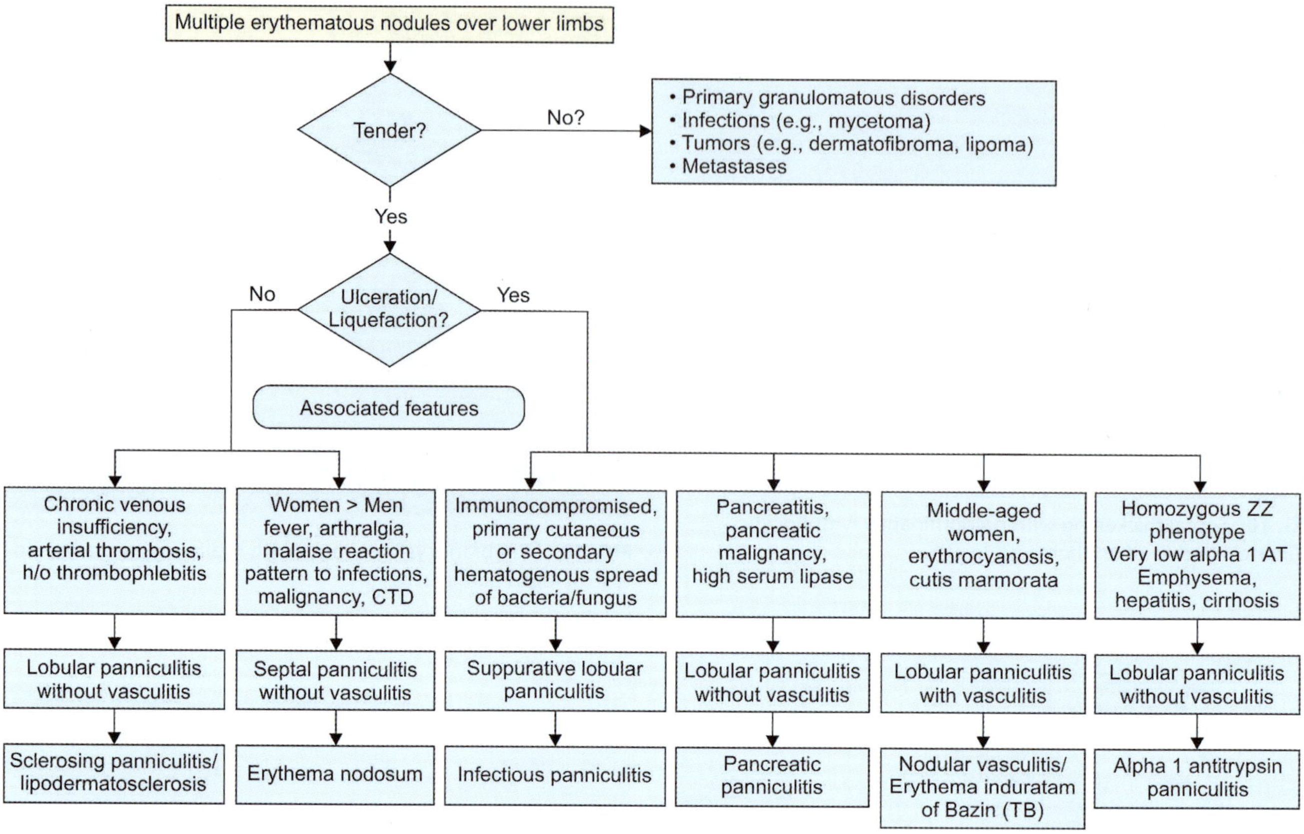

```
                    ┌─────────────────────────────────────┐
                    │ Multiple erythematous nodules over lower limbs │
                    └─────────────────────────────────────┘
                                    │
                                    ▼
                              ╱ Tender? ╲  ──No?──▶  • Primary granulomatous disorders
                              ╲         ╱            • Infections (e.g., mycetoma)
                                    │                • Tumors (e.g., dermatofibroma, lipoma)
                                   Yes               • Metastases
                                    ▼
                          ╱ Ulceration/ ╲
                      No ╱ Liquefaction? ╲ Yes
                                    │
                         Associated features
```

FLOWCHART 1: Approach in a case of panniculitis.
(AT: antitrypsin; CTD: creatine transporter deficiency)

Chronic venous insufficiency, arterial thrombosis, h/o thrombophlebitis	Women > Men fever, arthralgia, malaise reaction pattern to infections, malignancy, CTD	Immunocompromised, primary cutaneous or secondary hematogenous spread of bacteria/fungus	Pancreatitis, pancreatic malignancy, high serum lipase	Middle-aged women, erythrocyanosis, cutis marmorata	Homozygous ZZ phenotype Very low alpha 1 AT Emphysema, hepatitis, cirrhosis
Lobular panniculitis without vasculitis	Septal panniculitis without vasculitis	Suppurative lobular panniculitis	Lobular panniculitis without vasculitis	Lobular panniculitis with vasculitis	Lobular panniculitis without vasculitis
Sclerosing panniculitis/ lipodermatosclerosis	Erythema nodosum	Infectious panniculitis	Pancreatic panniculitis	Nodular vasculitis/ Erythema induratam of Bazin (TB)	Alpha 1 antitrypsin panniculitis

dots have been described. Histopathology will usually show the acid-fast bacilli and in many cases, neutrophilic vasculitis is also observed.[35]

Dermoscopy findings in panniculitis as such have not been described, primarily because the changes are usually too deep to produce any specific patterns. Ill-defined structureless red areas have been described in the case of erythema nodosum **(Fig. 14)**.[36]

Weber Christian panniculitis, also known as idiopathic lobular panniculitis, is a term used for nodular panniculitis associated with systemic signs/symptoms in which no specific diagnosis or cause can be found. It is basically a condition of exclusion.

To conclude we would like to emphasize the following points:
- Subcutaneous nodules in the skin open a wide range of differential diagnosis
- One of the differential diagnoses to be considered for acute onset, painful lesions is panniculitis.

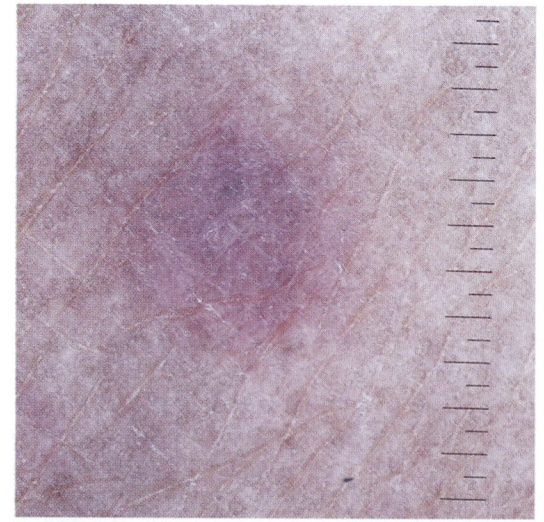

FIG. 14: Dermoscopy 10× polarized showing ill-defined structureless pink to red areas.

Table 3: Summary of the most common types of panniculitis.[1-6]

Diagnosis	Demographic features	Associated conditions	History and clinical course	Examination findings	Histopathology	Other investigations	Treatment	Key practice points
Erythema nodosum[4-14]	More common in females, second to fourth decade	• Can be associated with a multitude of underlying conditions including infections (tuberculosis, streptococcal, deep fungal, yersiniosis) • Connective tissue disorders, drugs (OCPs, minocycline), inflammatory bowel disease, sarcoidosis, malignancies	• Acute onset, tender erythematous nodules, most commonly over shins, can have associated fever, arthralgia, fatigue • Usually subsides over 6–8 weeks • Some patients have chronic erythema nodosum with lesions lasting or recurring for months	• Depends on the stage. Initial stage tender, erythematous nodules. No ulceration, atrophy or other surface changes • Resolves over 6–8 weeks • Over the course flattens, progresses through color changes like a bruise	• Septal panniculitis, without vasculitis • Initial stages inflammation is mainly polymorphonuclear. Later stages becomes granulomatous (Miescher granuloma)	To rule out underlying causes	• Treatment is essentially directed against underlying causes. Idiopathic cases show self-resolution over 6–8 weeks • Bed rest, NSAIDs, aspirin, colchicine, SSKI, systemic steroids are options which are used in the treatment	A detailed investigation to look for underlying/associated diseases is key in erythema nodosum
Erythema induratum[15,16]	Middle-aged women	Tuberculosis, Hepatitis virus B and C, obesity, venous insufficiency	Presentation similar to erythema nodosum initially – tender erythematous nodules mainly on legs. But unlike EN, calves affected frequently, and tendency to ulcerate and scar. Recurrences are common with each episode lasting for 3–6 weeks	Erythematous, tender, subcutaneous nodules, involving legs, including calves, with a tendency towards developing ulceration and scarring	Lobular panniculitis with 90% of the cases showing evidence of vasculitis. Early lesions show polymorphonuclear infiltrate and late lesions tend to be show histiocytic infiltrate, often with giant cells	To rule out underlying conditions	Treat underlying cause. Most important is to investigate for tuberculosis. Other treatment options, besides bed rest and compression include NSAIDs, oral corticosteroids, colchicine, SSKI and anti-malarials	The site (involvement of calves) and the ulceration are two key points which help to differentiate erythema induratum from erythema nodosum

Continued

Continued

Diagnosis	Demographic features	Associated conditions	History and clinical course	Examination findings	Histopathology	Other investigations	Treatment	Key practice points
Alpha-1 antitrypsin panniculitis[17,18]	Usually seen in the age group of 30–60 years	• Other conditions associated with α-1 antitrypsin deficiency (emphysema, hepatitis/cirrhosis/chronic pancreatitis) • Recently a SERPIN A1 gene mutation has been reported	• Initially starts as erythematous plaques/nodules over trunk and limbs which tend to ulcerate, releasing an oily material • Patient can have fever. Severe cases can be even fatal	• Erythematous plaque and nodules with ulceration/leakage of oily material • Common sites—trunk and proximal limbs, but can be generalized	Necrotic changes and liquefactive necrosis in fat lobules, with characteristic neutrophil splaying between collagen fibers	• Serum α-1 antitrypsin levels • Alpha-1 antitrypsin phenotype and genotyping • Investigations to assess for involvement of lungs, liver, and pancreas	• Avoid trauma • Avoid smoking and alcohol • Tetracyclines, dapsone, colchicine	• Look for other systemic features of α-1 antitrypsin deficiency (lungs, liver, and pancreas) • Liquefactive necrosis is quite characteristic
Pancreatic panniculitis[19,20]	More common in alcoholic men	• Pancreatic cancer and pancreatitis • Rarely other pancreatic disorders like pancreatic pseudocysts • Association with HIV infection	Tendency for recurrence depending on activity of underlying disease. Tendency to ulcerate and leave pigmentation and atrophic scarring Poor prognosis especially when associate with carcinoma pancreas, with a high mortality rate	Painful and tender subcutaneous nodules and plaques, coming in crops, most commonly over lower limbs. Lesions tend to break down releasing a brown, oily fluid (because of liquefaction of fat). Lesions are especially common over the shins and around the ankles Can have associated fever, abdominal pain and arthralgia	• Lobular panniculitis without vasculitis • Severe central lobular necrosis • Saponification, calcification, "ghost" adipocytes	Investigation for underlying pancreatic disease	Treatment of underlying condition, octreotide, plasmapheresis	Panniculitis associated with a pancreatic tumor can show a triad of eosinophilia, arthritis and panniculitis (referred to as the Schmid triad)

Continued

CHAPTER 7 A Suspected Case of Panniculitis 101

Continued

Diagnosis	Demographic features	Associated conditions	History and clinical course	Examination findings	Histopathology	Other investigations	Treatment	Key practice points
Lupus panniculitis[21,22]	Associated with lupus so more common in females	• Lupus erythematosus • Rarely with other connective tissue disorders	Can develop at any site. Resolve with depressions in the skin due to fat atrophy. Chronic with relapses	Long-lasting, subcutaneous nodules, with tenderness. Can affect any site of the body, but relative less common on lower legs	• Lobular panniculitis, without vasculitis, lymphoid follicles, hyaline fat necrosis • Vacuolar degeneration of basal cells, thickened basement membrane, mucin deposition, superficial and deep inflammatory infiltrate around blood vessels	Investigations for lupus	Treatment for underlying lupus erythematosus—hydroxychloroquine is first line Recently rituximab has been reported to be effective in the treatment of lupus panniculitis	A differential diagnosis to consider here would be subcutaneous panniculitis-like T-cell lymphoma (SPTCL). Lipocytes, surrounded by atypical lymphocytes and immunohistochemistry will help in differentiations. Focal erythrophagocytosis may also be present
Cytophagic histiocytic panniculitis[23,24]	Can be seen in all age groups	Hemophagocytic lymphohistiocytosis, Macrophage activation syndrome	• Course can vary, tends to start suddenly • Intermittent flares can be seen. In some patients can follow a fatal course	Erythematous or violaceous plaques and nodules most commonly over limbs and trunk	Lobular panniculitis without vasculitis. Significant necrosis can be seen. Typical finding is the bean bag cell (macrophage containing other cells like erythrocytes, platelets or leukocytes)	Bone marrow examination	Systemic steroids, cyclosporine	
Cold panniculitis[25-27]	Infants and young children, obese children are more prone	Cold exposure	• Lesions start within a few days of cold exposure • Tend to self-resolve over a few weeks	Firm, erythematous, nontender subcutaneous nodules	Lobular panniculitis, with fat necrosis, mixed inflammatory infiltrate and microcysts	None	Self-resolving. No specific treatment is required	In the case of lesions over the face in children a history of sucking popsicles is important as is the history of ice-packs

Continued

Continued

Diagnosis	Demographic features	Associated conditions	History and clinical course	Examination findings	Histopathology	Other investigations	Treatment	Key practice points
Traumatic fat necrosis[28]	More common in females	Trauma	Nodules similar to lipomas, after trauma, but history of trauma is sometimes not recalled by the patients.	Firm, mobile, subcutaneous nodules, most commonly seen on trunk and breasts of women	• Granulomatous lobular panniculitis. In later stages septal fibrosis is seen • Cystic changes, following trauma with hemorrhage into the lobules (myospherulosis/spherulocytosis)	None	No specific treatment is required	
Lipodermatosclerosis[29]	Obese, females, usually older than 40 years	Obesity, venous insufficiency, hypertension	Chronic, gradually develops and persists	Wooden, indurated plaques on lower legs (inverted champagne bottle appearance)	Lobular panniculitis without vasculitis, with evidence of changes related to stasis	Doppler studies, including the use of high frequency ultrasound which has been described recently	Compression, weight reduction, pentoxifylline, stanozolol	
Subcutaneous fat necrosis of newborn[30]	First 4 weeks of life, especially in preterm infants	• History of fetal distress, meconium aspiration, maternal narcotic usage • Associated hypoglycemia, hypercalcemia, lactic acidosis, and thrombocytopenia may be seen	Tend to resolve on its own, sometimes with fibrosis or calcification	Firm/rubbery erythematous nodules, mainly over trunk, buttocks, arms, thighs, and cheeks	Lobular panniculitis with granulomatous necrosis of adipocytes. Radially arranged needle-shaped clefts	Calcium levels are important as sometimes it can be associated with life-threatening hypercalcemia Radiological imaging helps in the diagnosis	Self-resolving. Treatment of associated hypercalcemia is important	
Sclerema neonatorum[31]	Premature, severely ill neonates	Hypothermia	Poor prognosis. Starts within first few days after birth, starting localized to one area like the buttocks and then spreading to involve the whole body	Dry, hard, board-like skin (skin cannot be pinched), color changes to yellowish white	Enlarged and necrotic adipocytes, filled with needle like clefts arranged in a radial fashion. Very little inflammation		Supportive treatment only. Exchange transfusion has been suggested to improve the condition	

(HIV: human immunodeficiency virus; OCPs: oral contraceptive pills)

- Different forms of panniculitis can usually be differentiated clinically—based on factors like demographic features, onset and course (acute vs. chronic/relapsing), symptoms (tender/nontender and systemic symptoms), site, morphology (especially presence or absence of ulceration/liquefaction), and associated/underlying systemic diseases. In most cases, a skin biopsy is indicated to confirm the specific diagnosis based on histopathological features like whether the panniculitis is essentially lobular or septal, the presence or absence of vasculitis, and the presence of specific histopathological clues.

Conflict of interest: No conflict of interest to declare.

REFERENCES

1. Amerson EH, Burgin S, Shinkai K. Fundamentals of clinical dermatology: morphology and special clinical considerations. In: Kang S, Amagai M, Bruckner AL, Enk AH, Margolis DJ, McMichael AJ, Orringer JS (Eds). Fitzpatrick's Dermatology, 9th edition. New York: McGraw Hill Education; 2019. pp. 1-17.
2. Lake EP, Worobek SM, Aronson IK. Panniculitis. In: Kang S, Amagai M, Bruckner AL, Enk AH, Margolis DJ, McMichael AJ, Orringer JS (Eds). Fitzpatrick's Dermatology, 9th edition. New York: McGraw Hill Education; 2019. pp. 1251-94.
3. James WD, Elston DM, Treat JR, Rosenbach MA, Neuhaus IM. Diseases of subcutaneous fat. In: James WD, Elston DM, Treat JR, Rosenbach MA, Neuhaus IM (Eds). Andrews' Diseases of the Skin: Clinical Dermatology, 13th edition. New York, NA: Elsevier; 2020. pp. 485-95.
4. Pérez-Garza DM, Chavez-Alvarez S, Ocampo-Candiani J, Gomez-Flores M. Erythema Nodosum: A Practical Approach and Diagnostic Algorithm. Am J Clin Dermatol. 2021;22(3):367-78.
5. Yi SW, Kim EH, Kang HY, Kim YC, Lee ES. Erythema nodosum: clinicopathologic correlations and their use in differential diagnosis. Yonsei Med J. 2007;48(4):601-8.
6. Sánchez Yus E, Sanz Vico MD, de Diego V. Miescher's radial granuloma. A characteristic marker of erythema nodosum. Am J Dermatopathol. 1989;11(5):434-42.
7. Requena L, Yus ES. Panniculitis. Part I. Mostly septal panniculitis. J Am Acad Dermatol. 2001;45(2):163-86.
8. Requena L, Sánchez Yus E. Erythema nodosum. Semin Cutan Med Surg. 2007;26(2):114-25.
9. Schwartz RA, Nervi SJ. Erythema nodosum: a sign of systemic disease. Am Fam Physician. 2007;75(5):695-700.
10. Garcia-Porrua C, Gonzalez-Gay MA, Vazquez-Caruncho M, Lopez-Lazaro L, Lueiro M, Fernandez ML, et al. Erythema nodosum: etiologic and predictive factors in a defined population. Arthritis Rheum. 2000;43(3):584-92.
11. Mert A, Ozaras R, Tabak F, Pekmezci S, Demirkesen C, Ozturk R. Erythema nodosum: an experience of 10 years. Scand J Infect Dis. 2004;36(6-7):424-7.
12. Cribier B, Caille A, Heid E, Grosshans E. Erythema nodosum and associated diseases: a study of 129 cases. Int J Dermatol. 1998;37(9):667-72.
13. Misago N, Tada Y, Koarada S, Narisawa Y. Erythema nodosum-like lesions in Behçet's disease: a clinicopathological study of 26 cases. Acta Derm Venereol. 2012;92(6):681-6.
14. Kim KS, Kim JS, Kim SS, Kim CW. Association between erythema nodosum/erythema induratum of Bazin and Mycobacterium tuberculosis infection in Koreans. Indian J Dermatol Venereol Leprol. 2021;2:1-5.
15. Irifune S, Yamamoto K, Ishijima S, Koike Y, Fukuoka J, Mukae H. Erythema induratum of Bazin-A subcutaneous granulomatous vasculitis that caused difficulty in walking. Int J Infect Dis. 2021;106:183-4.
16. Franciosi AN, Ralph J, O'Farrell NJ, Buckley C, Gulmann C, O'Kane M, et al. Alpha-1 antitrypsin deficiency-associated panniculitis. J Am Acad Dermatol. 2022 Oct;87(4):825-832.
17. Abdalla BMZ, Criado PR. Panniculitis as main clinical manifestation of alpha-1 antitrypsin deficiency revealing a SerpinA1 gene mutation. Australas J Dermatol. 2020;61(4):e470-e471.
18. Díaz-Alcázar MM, López-Hidalgo JL, Aneiros-Fernández J. Acute pancreatitis manifesting in the skin: Pancreatic panniculitis. Rev Gastroenterol Mex. 2021;86(3):309-10.
19. Miksch RC, Schiergens TS, Weniger M, Ilmer M, Kazmierczak PM, Guba MO, et al. Pancreatic panniculitis and elevated serum lipase in metastasized acinar cell carcinoma of the pancreas: A case report and review of literature. World J Clin Cases. 2020;8(21):5304-12.
20. Gupta P, Dhanawat A, Mohanty I, Padhan P. Refractory lupus panniculitis treated successfully with rituximab: Two cases. Ann Afr Med. 2020;19(3):207-10.
21. Musick SR, Lynch DT. Subcutaneous Panniculitis Like T-cell Lymphoma. In: StatPearls [Internet]. Treasure Island (FL): StatPearls Publishing; 2022.
22. Kimura R, Sugita K, Goto H, Yamamoto O. Cytophagic Histiocytic Panniculitis Associated with Myelodysplastic Syndrome. Acta Derm Venereol. 2019;99(1):97-8.
23. Pasqualini C, Jorini M, Carloni I, Giangiacomi M, Cetica V, Aricò M, et al. Cytophagic histiocytic panniculitis, hemophagocytic lymphohistiocytosis and undetermined autoimmune disorder: reconciling the puzzle. Ital J Pediatr. 2014;40(1):17.
24. Saenz Ibarra B, Meeker J, Jalali O, Lynch MC. Cold-Induced Dermatoses: Case Report and Review of Literature. Am J Dermatopathol. 2018;40(4):291-4.
25. Kluger N, Marty L, Bourseau-Quetier C, Blum M, Camus M. Perniosis/cold panniculitis in French equestrians: four cases. Int J Dermatol. 2016;55(12):e618-e620.
26. Adachi A, Masaki S, Akiyama M. Equestrian cold panniculitis in a cold-storage-room worker. J Dermatol. 2019;46(7):e245-e246.
27. Akyol M, Kayali A, Yildirim N. Traumatic fat necrosis of male breast. Clin Imaging. 2013;37(5):954-6.
28. Woźniak W, Danowska A, Mlosek RK. The use of high-frequency skin ultrasound in the diagnosis of lipodermatosclerosis. J Ultrason. 2021;20(83):e284-e290.
29. Velasquez JH, Mendez MD. Newborn Subcutaneous Fat Necrosis. In: StatPearls [Internet]. Treasure Island (FL): StatPearls Publishing; 2022.
30. Nakalema G, Egesa WI, Kumbakulu PK, Nduwimana M, Anaya AD, Kizito MS, et al. Sclerema Neonatorum in a Term Infant: A Case Report and Literature Review. Case Rep Pediatr. 2020;2020:8837064.
31. Yanes AF, Owen JL, Colavincenzo ML. Factitial panniculitis as a manifestation of self-imposed factitious disorder. Dermatol Online J. 2019;25(5):13030/qt9dx484qq.

32. Santos-Briz A, Calle A, Linos K, Semans B, Carlson A, Sangüeza OP, et al. Dermatomyositis panniculitis: a clinicopathological and immunohistochemical study of 18 cases. J Eur Acad Dermatol Venereol. 2018;32(8):1352-9.
33. Young TK, Gutierrez D, Meehan SA, Pellett Madan R, Oza VS. Neutrophilic panniculitis arising from hematogenous spread of methicillin-resistant Staphylococcus aureus. Pediatr Dermatol. 2020;37(3):531-3.
34. Chopra A, Mitra D, Agarwal R, Saraswat N, Talukdar K, Solanki A. Correlation of Dermoscopic and Histopathologic Patterns in Leprosy—A Pilot Study. Indian Dermatol Online J. 2019;10(6):663-8.
35. Chuh A, Zawar V, Fölster-Holst R. The first application of epiluminescence dermoscopy in erythema nodosum. Our Dermatol Online. 2018;9(3):282-4.
36. Rotondo C, Corrado A, Mansueto N, Cici D, Corsi F, Pennella A, et al. Pfeifer-Weber-Christian Disease: A Case Report and Review of Literature on Visceral Involvements and Treatment Choices. Clin Med Insights Case Rep. 2020;13:1179547620917958.

8
A Patient of Facial Melanosis

Chirag Ashwin Desai, Nandita Krishnagopal Patel

PART 1: A PATIENT OF FACIAL HYPERMELANOSIS

INTRODUCTION

Facial hypermelanosis (FH) is one of the most common presentation of cosmetic concern in Indian patients predominantly involving the face and the neck.[1] It forms a group of heterogeneous entities, many of which share common clinical features and thus pose a diagnostic dilemma sometimes. Darker races, especially of the Asian and the Eastern descent, are genetically more prone to FH.

There are both internal and external factors which play a role in the pathogenesis of FH, these include endocrine hormones, sunlight, artificial light sources, photosensitive chemicals, etc.[1] Photodynamic chemicals play a pivotal role in occupational FH (cosmetics) as well as photocontact dermatitis (Riehl melanosis) and erythromelanosis and poikiloderma of Civatte. Lack of proper knowledge with regards to sun-protective measures leads to exacerbation of FH.

Based on the location of melanin (epidermal/dermal), as identified clinically by color of lesion, diagnostically by accentuation on woods lamp and histologically, hypermelanosis can be classified as mentioned in **Tables 1 and 2**.

For ease of description, we will be describing various entities under FH as given in **Table 3**.

MELASMA

Melasma, also known as chloasma in pregnancy, is the most common acquired FH characterized by symmetrical, hyperpigmented macules coalescing to form patches with no associated symptoms. It is derived from the Greek word ""melas" meaning black.

Table 1: Classification of hypermelanosis on basis of etiology and pathogenesis.		
Epidermal/ brown hypermelanosis	Etiology	• Pigment accentuated under Wood's lamp • Excess melanin in basal and suprabasal layer
	Pathogenesis	• *Melanotic hypermelanosis*: Due to increased melanin production by normal number of melanocytes • *Melanocytic hypermelanosis*: Due to increased number of melanocytes
Dermal/blue hypermelanosis/ ceruloderma	Etiology	• Pigment not accentuated under wood's lamp • Excess melanin in dermis
	Pathogenesis	• *Pigment incontinence*: Increased transfer of melanin to dermis from epidermis • *Binding of melanin*: To exogenous pigment in dermis • *Production of melanin*: By dendritic dermal melanocytes
Mixed hypermelanosis	Etiology	Due to increase epidermal and dermal melanin

Table 2: Location of melanin.		
	Pigment	*Margins*
Epidermal	Brown	Well-defined
Dermal	Gray-brown	Poorly defined
Mixed	Features of both epidermal and dermal melasma	

Table 3: Causes of hyperpigmentation and hypopigmentation.		
	Hyperpigmentation	*Hypopigmentation*
Congenital	• Nevus of Ota (NOO) • Giant melanocytic nevus • Laugier–Hunziker syndrome • Peutz–Jeghers syndrome	• Albinism • Piebaldism • Ash leaf macules
Acquired	*Autoimmune*: Lichen planus pigmentosus	*Autoimmune*: • Vitiligo • Sarcoidosis • Lichen sclerosis et atrophicus
	Chemical: • Riehl melanosis • Ashy dermatosis • Exogenous ochronosis • Poikiloderma of Civatte • Erythromelanosis peribuccal pigmentation of Brocq	*Infections*: • Fungal (pityriasis versicolor) • Bacterial (leprosy and syphilis) • Protozoal (PKDL)
	Drugs: • NSAIDs • Phenytoin • Antimalarials • Amiodarone • Antipsychotics • Cytotoxic • Tetracyclines	Chemical leukoderma
	Idiopathic: • Melasma • Periorbital hyperpigmentation • Frictional melanosis • Postinflammatory hyperpigmentation • Freckles • Chronic actinic dermatitis • Sun-tan • Sebomelanosis • Pigmentary demarcation line	*Malignancy*: Hypopigmented mycosis fungoides

Continued

	Hyperpigmentation	*Hypopigmentation*
	Endocrine: Acanthosis nigricans	*PIH*: • Inflammatory (atopic, lichen striatus) • Infections (fungal and viral) • Procedures (cryotherapy and dermabrasion) • Burns

(NSAID: nonsteroidal anti-inflammatory drug; PIH: postinflammatory hyperpigmentation; PKDL: post-Kala-azar dermal leishmaniasis)

Table 4: Area involved.		
	Frequency	*Area*
Centrofacial	Most frequent (63%)	• Cheeks • Forehead • Upper lip • Nose • Chin
Malar	21%	• Cheeks • Nose
Mandibular	Least common (16%)	Ramus of mandible

Clinical Features

Melasma is characterized by bilaterally symmetrical, hyperpigmented macules coalescing to form patches on the face. Rarely, it can also involve the V area of the neck and dorsal aspect of the hands. Melasma can be classified depending on the location of pigment **(Table 2)** and area involved **(Table 4)**.

POSTINFLAMMATORY HYPERPIGMENTATION[2]

Postinflammatory hyperpigmentation (PIH) is commonly acquired skin pigmentary disorder occurring as a result of inflammatory reaction, induced by preceding cutaneous insults such as acne, dermatitis (atopic, irritant, allergic), impetigo, psoriasis, lichen planus, phototoxic reactions, physical injury, or trauma (burns, insect bite) as well as complications secondary to laser therapy.

Clinical Features

Postinflammatory hyperpigmentation clinically presents as hyperpigmented macules, which coalesce to form patches on the site affected previously with inflammation. The exact location of pigment in the skin determines its discoloration. While epidermal pigmentation appears as brown or tan colored, dermal one shows bluish-gray discoloration.

Postinflammatory hyperpigmentation (depending on the level of insult) can last from weeks to years. It can significantly impair quality of life of affected individual. The severity of PIH is less with short-term acute inflammation when compared to long-term chronic inflammation.

PERIORBITAL HYPERPIGMENTATION[3]

Periorbital hyperpigmentation is also known as periorbital melanosis, dark circles, or periorbital hyperpigmentation that presents as bilaterally symmetrical, round, or semicircular brown or dark brown pigmented macules in periocular area **(Table 5)**. It affects the patient psychosocially, thus influencing their quality of life. It is a worldwide problem, challenging to treat with complex pathogenesis and lacking straightforward treatment. The probable causative factors are listed in **Table 6**.

Classification

On the basis of clinical pattern of vasculature and pigmentation, progressive osseous heteroplasia (POH) can be classified on the basis of clinical pattern of vasculature and pigmentation **(Table 5)**.

Clinical Features

Progressive osseous heteroplasia is diagnosed clinically and presents as hyperpigmentation around eyes giving a tired look to the patient. Manual stretching of lower skin can help to differentiate between apparent pigmentation and shadowing effect, former retaining its appearance with stretching.

Table 5: Progressive osseous heteroplasia (POH) classification.		
Type	**Color**	**Associating features**
Pigmented	Brownish hue	None
Vascular	Blue/pink/purple hue	+/– Periorbital puffiness
Structural	Skin color	• Infraorbital palpable bags • Blepharoptosis • Loss of fat with bony prominence
Mixed (two or three of the above appearances)	• Pigmented—vascular • Pigmented—structural • Vascular—structural • Combination of three	

EPHELIDES/FRECKLES[1]

Actinic lentigines, also called as solar lentigines, are light brown, even colored, or reticulated macules occurring mainly in sun-exposed areas. Actinic freckles are considered to be clinical sign of photoaging and frequency increases with age.

Clinical Features

Single/multiple, well-defined, brown macules with clear edges present on sun-exposed sites such as dorsal aspect of hands, face, extensor flexors, and upper trunk.

LICHEN PLANUS PIGMENTOSUS[4]

Lichen planus pigmentosus (LPP) was first reported in 1974 in India by Bhutani et al. It is characterized by asymptomatic and persistent slate-gray pigmentation, predominantly on the face and rarely on flexors in light-skinned individual. This disease of unknown origin runs a prolonged and insidious course and is usually characterized by dark brown macules on sun-exposed areas and is sometimes associated with pruritus.

Table 6: Probable causative factors in periorbital pigmentation.		
Exogenous	PIH secondary to atopy, allergy, and contact dermatitis	
	Shadowing effect	Due to skin laxity and tear trough with aging
Endogenous	Genetic/hereditary	Appears early in the childhood and increases with age, with no improvement
	Periorbital edema	Due to excessive sponginess in the lower eyelid region leads to fluid accumulation, which worsens in morning and after salty food consumption. The cause may be systemic or local
	Tear trough depression	An anatomical location that becomes depressed with age, occurring due to loss of subcutaneous fat
	Excessive vascularity	Superficial location of vasculature and thin skin over orbicularis oculi gives violaceous hue on lower lid due to pooling of blood. The lower lid when stretched manually results in deepening of violaceous hue

Clinical Features

The disease starts usually on face and neck followed by upper extremities and trunk (photo distributed area), rarely involving oral mucosa and folds (groin, axilla, and inframammary). Initial physical examination reveals small, brown macules with diffuse borders and merge later on to become well-defined, symmetrical, hyperpigmented patches. The pigmentation can be blotchy, reticulate, diffuse, or perifollicular. Generally, the patches are symmetrical in distribution, but rarely can be zosteriform, segmental, or blaschkoid pattern.

Variants

- LPP inversus
- Localized
- Zosteriform
- Segmental
- Linear
- Along line of Blaschko
- Oral mucosa

Associations

- Scarring alopecia with circular ANA
- Frontal fibrosing alopecia
- Nephrotic syndrome
- Hepatitis C infection
- Acrokeratosis of Bazex

RIEHL'S MELANOSIS[1,5]

Riehl's melanosis also called as pigmented cosmetic/contact dermatitis is attributable to phototoxic reaction due to textile or cosmetic antigens. It is predominately seen in Asians with striking dark brown to grayish brown pigmentation on temples, forehead, and zygomatic regions of face.

Clinical Features

It is found most commonly in middle-aged women, presenting as brown-gray pigmentation developing rapidly over the face (especially over forehead and temples and rarely on neck, chest, forearm, and hands). Clinically, RM is characterized by patchy/diffuse/reticulate macules and follicular hyperkeratosis, sometimes preceded by mild erythema. Identification and avoidance of causative contact are must for treatment.

ASHY DERMATOSIS OF RAMIREZ[6]

Ashy dermatosis of Ramirez, also known as erythema dyschromicum perstans (EDP), is a pigmented dermatosis of unknown origin, with anecdotal reports incriminating exposure to radiographic contrast dye, ammonium nitrite, cobalt allergy, intestinal whipworm infestation, and human immunodeficiency virus (HIV) infection. It is sometimes associated with genetic susceptibility to HLA-DR4. It is a controversial entity which is considered as a variant of LPP by some authors.

It usually presents as symmetrical, asymptomatic, multiple, erythematous macules with elevated dusky border which gradually increases in number and size to form a hyperpigmented patch involving face, trunk, and limb. Mucosal involvement is rarely seen.

EXOGENOUS OCHRONOSIS[7]

First described by Beddard and Plumtrein in 1912, exogenous ochronosis (EO) is a rare complication of HQ, phenol, resorcinol, and oral antimalarials. It occurs due to inhibition of homogentisic oxidase and accumulation of acid in superficial dermis. The pigmentation is generally present in HQ treated sun-exposed areas, sparing systemic involvement.

Three clinical stages are as follow:
1. Erythema and mild hyperpigmentation
2. Caviar-like pigmented colloid milium
3. Papulonodular lesions

NEVUS OF OTA

The term ceruloderma was first described in 1980. Nevus of Ota (NOO) or "nevus fuscocaeruleus ophthalmomaxillaris" consists of unilateral hyperpigmentation of face and mucous in distribution of the maxillary, ophthalmic, and, occasionally, the mandibular divisions of facial nerve.

Clinical Features

Nevus of Ota is characterized by bluish, nonhairy, confluent, flat, pigmented patches with poorly defined margins on areas supplied by first and second division of trigeminal nerve, affecting periorbital region, temples, and forehead. It can affect the mucosal surface such as oral cavity, nasal mucosa, EAC, tympanic membrane, meninges, orbital fissures, and brain. Morphologically, it is generally macular but can rarely presents as papules or nodules with patchy brown/slate blue/gray black pigmentation.

Exogenous factors such as fatigue, emotional excitement, insomnia, hormonal fluctuations (irregular menstruation, menopause), and temperature variations (cold or warm weather) can cause darkening of pigmentation.

Tanino classified NOO into four types based on the extent and distribution of the lesion **(Table 7)**.

Giant Melanocytic Nevus

The CAMN, i.e., common acquired melanocytic nevus, is a benign proliferation of nevi cells. Genetic factors are strongly associated with development of the nevus and

Table 7: Classification of nevus of Ota.		
Type I	IA: Mild orbital type	Distribution over the upper and lower eyelids, periocular, and temple region
	IB: Mild zygomatic type	Pigmentation is found in the intrapalpebral fold, nasolabial fold, and the zygomatic region
	IC: Mild forehead type	Involvement of the forehead alone
	ID	Involvement of ala nasi alone
Type II	Moderate type	Distribution over the upper and lower eyelids, periocular, zygomatic, cheek, and temple regions
Type III		The lesion involves the scalp, forehead, eyebrow, and nose
Type IV	Bilateral type	Both sides are involved

can be aggravated by environmental factors. Males are more affected than females. The nevus cells originate from pluripotent cells; which migrate from neural crest to skin via peripheral nerves. They are terminally differentiated once they reach dermis or epidermis. They are well-circumscribed nevi, round to oval in shape with well-defined borders. Though diagnosed clinically, CAMN can be classified into different categories, based on dermoscopic features: Globular, reticular, starburst, and homogenous. Depending on the location of the lesion, they can be classified as junctional, dermal, and compound. Excision of the nevi is the gold standard treatment.

LAUGIER–HUNZIKER SYNDROME

Laugier–Hunziker syndrome (LHS) is an acquired pigmentary disorder of skin that is usually benign and involves oral cavity, including lips. It is usually associated with longitudinal melanonychia of nails. Rarely, extended mucocutaneous pigmentation can be seen on neck, abdomen, palms, and soles. The pigmentation is well-defined brown, black, or slate-colored macules and smooth surfaced. Differential includes Peutz–Jeghers syndrome, Addison disease, McCune–Albright syndrome, and LEOPARD syndrome. Treatment is mainly for cosmetic purpose and includes strict sun protection and Nd:YaG or Q-switched alexandrite laser therapy.

PEUTZ–JEGHERS SYNDROME

Peutz–Jeghers syndrome is a genetic syndrome characterized by mucocutaneous macules and gastrointestinal (GI) polyps, with predisposition to cancers such as GI (colorectal, gastric, and pancreatic), breast, uterine, cervical, lunch, ovaries, and testicles. The clinical course manifests when germ line STK11 mutation occurs. It is a rare syndrome with incidence of about 1 in 25,000–30,000 births and affects males and females equally. Hyperpigmented dark blue, brown to black macules are present on skin and mucous membrane (lips, buccal mucosa, nostrils, perianal, and perioral areas). Treatment includes strict surveillance of GI tract and non-GI organs for malignancy.

DRUG INDUCED

Drug-induced pigmentation of skin accounts for 10–20% of all the cases of acquired hyperpigmentation.[8] Skin pigmentation may be induced by wide variety of drugs; the main one includes **(Table 8)**.

ERYTHROSE PERIBUCCALE PIGMENTATION OF BROCQ[1]

It occurs predominately in middle-aged females. Photodynamic chemical in cosmetic plays very pivotal role in development of EPPB. It is characterized by symmetrically arranged diffuse, brownish red colored pigmentation develops around mouth, and sparing perioral ring. Erythema may fluctuate but pigmentation is permanent. Rarely, the pigmentation may fade of slowly once the cause is eliminated.

Table 8: Drugs causing hyperpigmentation.	
Drugs	Sites affected
Nonsteroidal anti-inflammatory drugs (NSAIDs)	• Face • Extremities • Genitals
Phenytoin	• Face • Neck
Antimalarials	• Bluish-gray pigmentation on face, neck, and sometimes lower legs and forearms • Nail beds and corneal and retinal changes may also develop
Amiodarone	• Blue-grey pigmentation in sun-exposed areas (face and hands) • Photosensitivity
Antipsychotic drugs	Bluish-gray pigmentation, especially in sun-exposed areas
Cytotoxic drugs	• Busulfan, cyclophosphamide, bleomycin, and adriamycin have all produced hyperpigmentation to some degree • Often involves nails
Tetracyclines	• Bluish pigmentation, especially in scars • May affect nails and skin

POIKILODERMA OF CIVATTE[1]

Poikiloderma of Civatte, also known as erythromelanosis interfollicularis colli, is rarely reported, milder disease occurring due to photodynamic substance in cosmetics, predominately in middle-aged women. Postmenopausal Caucasian women are generally affected, but rarely is seen in individuals with skin of color.

It presents as mottled pigmentation (telangiectasia, atrophy, and hyper- or hypopigmentation) on the convexities of cheeks and side of neck, and upper aspect of chest. Generally, submandibular and submental areas are spared, indicating sunlight as the possible aggravating factor.

SEBORRHEIC MELANOSIS

A term broadly used by Indian doctors to describe the localized hyperpigmentation on seborrheic areas such as alar groves, labiomental crease, and angle of mouth. It is more common in women but is seen in males too.

Clinical examination initially reveals localized faint erythema which further progresses to develop darkish pigmentation on the alar grooves. Mild yellowish flaking is often associated with chronic cases. In addition, there is shadowing effect from the outer pouting of lower lip that accentuates the pigmentation.

PIGMENTARY DEMARCATION LINES

Also referred to as Voigt's line, pigmentary demarcation lines (PDL) are differential areas of pigmentation due to differences in melanocyte distribution that may be influenced by various factors. Facial PDL presents as bilaterally symmetrical, homogenous, hyperpigmentation involving nose, forehead, lateral orbit, and angle of lip.

PERIORAL PIGMENTATION

Perioral areas are known to have darker pigmentation in Indian skin. Thus, pigmentation of these areas is often referred to as physiological or constitutional. Many authors believe that this pigmentation is often genetically determined and is accentuated by physiological factors such as hormonal changes and sun exposure.

Pigmentation involved the chin and upper lips and is laterally limited by nasolabial folds and mentolabial folds. Such pigmentary patch has been found to be oriented laterally downward.

FRICTIONAL MELANOSIS

Frictional melanosis (FM) is an acquired hyperpigmented disorder affecting mainly young individual. It is believed that repeated frictional trauma due to scrub pads or clothing against the underlying bony protuberance. Avoidance can be the causative factor aids in the treatment.

This hyperpigmented disorders can be differentiated on the basis of history, cutaneous examination, and investigations.

Other causes of hyperpigmentation need to be added.

Try to find and incorporate if you find any literature on perioral pigmentation which again is a very common presentation in India. Try to incorporate in approach section.

History

Past History to be Considered for Facial Hyperpigmentation

- Uncontrolled diabetes mellitus, weight gain, and obesity are the common features of acanthosis nigricans.
- Occupation is the important factor to consider in facial hypermelanosis. Sun tan, melasma, freckles, and chronic actinic dermatosis are commonly seen in patients with history of excessive exposure to heat like: Outdoor workers like farmers, construction workers, airlines and sailors and indoor workers like cooks and office workers
- Frequent application of cosmetic or fragrances causes EO, Riehl melanosis, ashy dermatosis, poikiloderma of Civatte, erythromelanosis peribuccal pigmentation of Brocq
- Past history of trauma points to PIH.
- Past history of consumption of offending agent indicates drug-induced melanosis.
- Genetic factor needs to be considered for perioral pigmentation.
- Pregnancy may accentuate PDLs.
- History of sudden or chronic skin dermatosis such as atopic dermatosis, psoriasis, immune-bullous disease, lichen planus, Stevens–Johnson syndrome, etc., points to PIH.
- Constant friction due to wiping of sweat in a case of hyperhidrosis also contributes to frictional melanosis.

Characteristic Sites of Involvement in FH

- Linear pigmentation on forehead and temporal area is seen in acanthosis nigricans.
- The butterfly area of face (malar and nose) is the common site for melasma and freckles **(Figs. 1 and 2)**.
- Periorbital area is involved in AN and POH **(Fig. 2)**.
- Diffuse pigmentation is seen in LPP, EO, chronic actinic dermatosis, and sun tanning **(Figs. 3 and 4)**.
- Ear pinna is involved in chronic actinic dermatosis.
- Temples are predominately involved in Riehl's melanosis and ashy dermatosis.
- Cheek involvement indicates possibility toward poikiloderma of Civatte and erythromelanosis peribuccal pigmentation of Brocq

CHAPTER 8 A Patient of Facial Melanosis

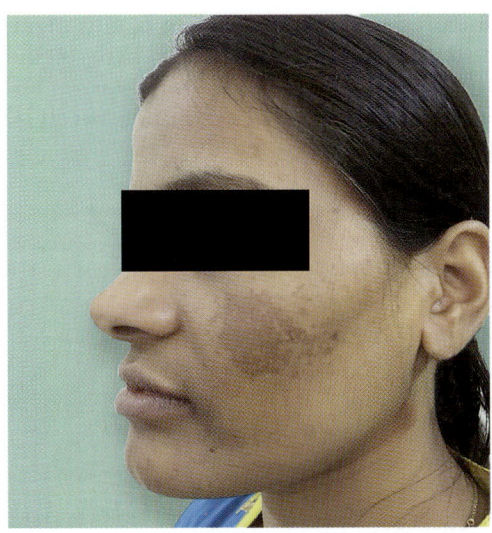

FIG. 1: Brownish macular coalescing lesion on cheeks (melasma).

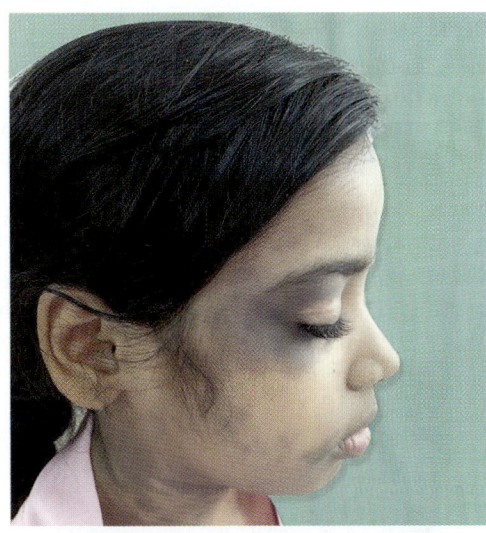

FIG. 3: Violaceous macular diffuse pigmentation of lichen planus pigmentosus.

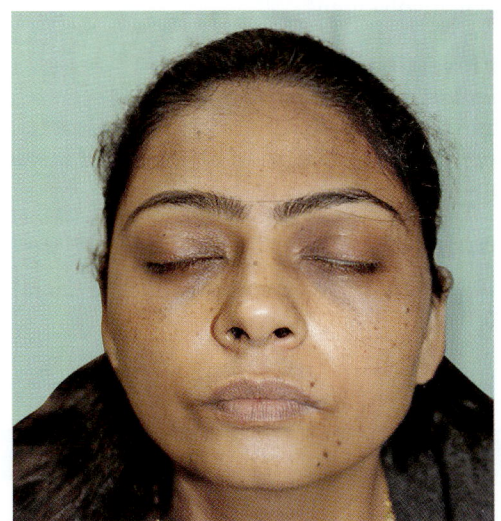

FIG. 2: Hyperpigmentation in periorbital region with multiple freckles on both cheeks.

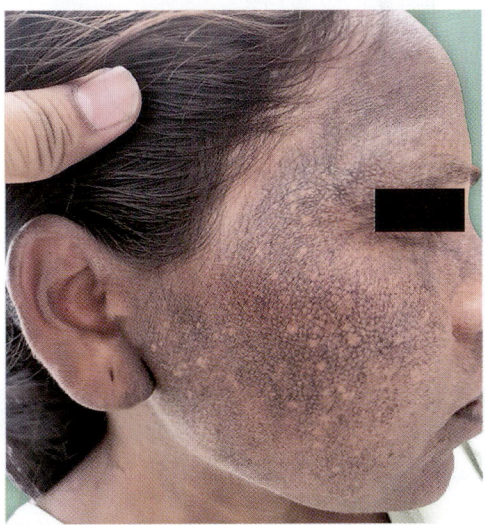

FIG. 4: Mottled/reticulate pattern of pigmentation in exogenous ochronosis.
Courtesy: Dr Vijay Raut, Assistant Professor, Government Medical College, Kolhapur, Maharashtra, India.

- Alar grooves, angles of mouth, and labiomental crease (seborrheic areas of face) are pigmented in Seborrheic melanosis.
- "V"-shaped (type F) or "W"-shaped (type G) area of hyperpigmentation between the temple and the malar area and hyperpigmented band between the angle of mouth and lateral aspect of chin (type H) are the typical locations of facial PDLs.
- Upper lip and chin are involved in perioral pigmentation.
- NOO is seen unilaterally (rarely bilateral) on upper face and is present at birth **(Fig. 5)**.

Cutaneous Examination
Color of Pigment
- Dark brown to grayish pigmentation is seen in LPP, EO, Riehl's melanosis, and EPPS

- Bluish gray pigmentation usually points to ashy dermatosis.
- Brown to dark brown macules are seen in melasma, POH, PIH, AN, chronic actinic dermatosis, seborrheic melanosis, and perioral pigmentation.
- Brownish pigmentation is seen in sun tan, freckles, and PDL.
- Slat grayish pigmentation is seen after amiodarone intake.
- Coppery red color is seen due to clofazimine.
- Bluish black hues may be seen after minocycline consumption.

Associated Cutaneous Findings in FH

- Papules, nodules, and wrinkles are associated with chronic actinic dermatosis.
- Skin tags, acne, and hirsutism are associated with AN.
- Pigmentary linea alba, scars, and pregnancy are seen with chloasma.
- Nail pigmentation can be associated with various drugs such as minocycline and antivirals agents.
- Extrafacial pigmentation is seen in melasma (neck and chest) and EO (neck). Extrafacial pigmentation can also be present in cases of lichen planus pigmentosus, ashy dermatosis and drug induced hyperpigmentation. Involvement of other flexural area favors acanthosis nigricans. Involvement of ear cartilages can be clue to endogenous ochronosis and drug-induced pigmentation.

Investigations (Table 9)

Algorithmic Approach to FH

History
- *Onset*: Birth/middle age/pregnancy/old age
- *Course*: Rapid/slow
- Occupation
- *Progress*: Self-limited/progressive
- Trauma/drug history

Salient Features
- *General examination*: DM uncontrolled: AN
- *Cutaneous examination*: Site, color, additional lesions, and nail involvement

Specific Investigations
- *Woods lamp*: Epidermal/dermal/mixed
- Dermoscopy
- *Histopathology*: Location of pigment and melanocytes, number of melanocytes

Treatment

Table 10 enlists treatment modalities in facial hyperpigmentation.

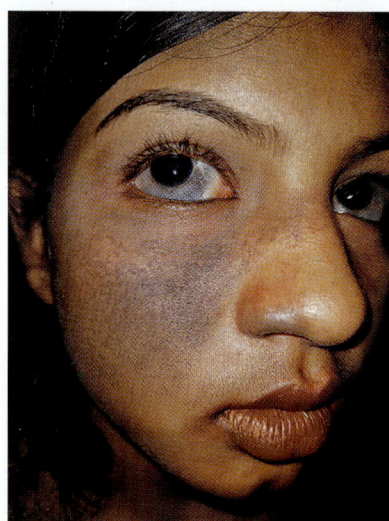

FIG. 5: Nevus of Ota.
Courtesy: Dr Shikha Mandloi Jain, Choithram Hospital and Research Centre, Indore, Madhya Pradesh, India.

Table 9: Investigations for hyperpigmentation.			
Disease	**Woods lamp**	**Histopathology**	**Dermoscopy**
Melasma	• *Epidermal*: Pigment accentuated under Wood's lamp • *Dermal*: Pigment not accentuated under Wood's lamp	Biopsy is rarely done for diagnosis of melasma. Usual findings include increased melanin in the basal layer of epidermis, without an increase in number of melanocytes. Melanocytes are slightly larger with increased number of dendrites. Dermis shows a sparse superficial perivascular lymphohistiocytic infiltrate with mild dilatation of vessels	Diffuse light to dark brown pigmented background with dark brown dots/blotches/granules/globules with perifollicular sparing. The pattern may be reticular or pseudoreticular
POH	Same as melasma	Biopsy findings are usually nonspecific and usually clinical correlation is necessary	POH is characterized by bilateral homogenous, hyperchromic macules, and patches
Freckles		Normal epidermis with increased melanization of the basal layer without an increase in number of melanocytes	Faint pigmented network or finger print-like structures
LPP		Epidermis may slight atrophy with basket weave hyperkeratosis. Basal layer shows focal vacuolar degeneration with pigment incontinence. Occasional colloid bodies may be seen close to the dermoepidermal junction. Dermis shows patchy lichenoid and superficial perivascular lymphohistiocytic infiltrate with scattered melanophages	Exaggeration of normal pseudoreticular pigment network, brown dots, or globules

Continued

Continued

Disease	Woods lamp	Histopathology	Dermoscopy
RM		Biopsy shows features similar to lichen planus pigmentosus. Slight focal spongiosis in the epidermis is noted by some workers. Some workers do not differentiate between lichen planus pigmentosus, ashy dermatosis, and pigmented contact dermatitis, as they consider it the same entity	Pseudonetwork and gray dots/granules are most suggestive of RM
Ashy dermatosis of Ramirez		Histology is similar to lichen planus pigmentosus	Brown gray dots/globules
Exogenous ochronosis		EO classically shows banana-shaped deposits in papillary dermis, popularly called as "banana bodies" with degeneration of collagen. The epidermis is unremarkable	Dark brown globules on diffuse brownish pigmentation
NOO		Shows pigmented melanocytes in dermis, which are spindle-shaped or dendritic in shape	Brown and gray structureless areas with patchy distribution and scattered brown-gray dots, terminal hairs, perifollicular hypopigmentation
Poikiloderma of Civatte		Telangiectasia in superficial dermis along with fibrosis and melanophages. Mild epidermal atrophy may sometimes be present, particularly in chronic lesions	
Seborrheic melanosis		Acute stage shows spongiosis and in the chronic form, psoriasiform hyperplasia is prominent feature along with mild spongiosis	A light pink background with focus of linear and arborizing vessels was seen along with prominent hyperpigmented pseudonetwork. The presence of whitish yellow sebum along the shaft of vellus hairs was the common feature
PDL		Melanophages are seen in upper dermis	

(EO: exogenous ochronosis; NOO: Nevus of Ota; PDL: pigmentary demarcation lines; PIH: postinflammatory hyperpigmentation; POH: progressive osseous heteroplasia; RM: Riehl's melanosis)

Table 10: Line of treatment for hyperpigmentation.[9]

	First line	Second line	Miscellaneous/off label
Melasma	Oral: Antioxidants Topical (main agents): • Photoprotection • Hydroquinone • Triple combination Topical (alternative agent): • Azelaic acid • Kojic acid • Glycolic acid • Lactic acid • Mequinol • Arbutin • Ascorbic acid • Niacinamide • Flavonoids	Oral: Tranexamic acid 500 mg/day Supportive: • Lasers • Chemical peel	Topical: N-acetyl-4-S-cysteaminylphenol

Continued

Continued

	First line	**Second line**	**Miscellaneous/off label**
PIH	*Topical (main agents):* • Hydroquinone (4%) • Topical retinoids • Sunscreen • Combination therapy *Topical (alternative agent):* • Azelaic acid • Kojic acid • Glycolic acid • Lactic acid • Mequinol • Arbutin • Ascorbic acid • Niacinamide • Flavonoids	• Chemical peels (glycolic acid, trichloroacetic acid, and Jessner's solution) • Laser therapy	
POH	• *Hyperpigmentation:* Topical hydroquinone • *Vascular:* Lasers • *Lax skin:* Fillers	*Hyperpigmentation:* • Chemical peels • Lasers	
Freckles	• *Topical:* Hydroquinone • Retinoids • Chemical peels • Lasers	Cryotherapy	
LPP	*Topical:* • Sun protection • Steroids • Tacrolimus *Systemic:* • Steroids • Dapsone • Colchicine • Hydroxychloroquine	Lasers	
Riehl melanosis	*Topical:* • Photoprotection • Hydroquinone • Steroids • Retinoids • Azelaic acid	• Cosmetic camouflage makeup • Chemical peels • Lasers	
Ashy dermatosis	*Topical:* Steroids *Oral:* • Clofazimine • Pigmentary lasers	*Oral:* • Dapsone • Griseofulvin • Hydroxychloroquine • Isoniazid	
Exogenous ochronosis	Primary preventive measures stopping the offending agent	Lasers	• Photobiomodulation • Photodynamic therapy

Continued

Continued

	First line	**Second line**	**Miscellaneous/off label**
NOO	Lasers		
Giant melanocytic nevus	No arbitrary guidelines can be provided for treatment. Multiple treatment interventions includes skin graft, dermabrasions, lasers, curettage		
Laugier–Hunziker syndrome	Lasers	Cryotherapy	
Peutz–Jeghers syndrome	Lasers		
Drug induced	*Topical:* • Hydroquinone (4%) • Topical retinoids • Sunscreen • Combination therapy *Topical:* • Azelaic acid • Kojic acid • Glycolic acid • Lactic acid • Mequinol • Arbutin • Ascorbic acid	Chemical peels	
Erythrose peribuccal pigmentation of Brocq (EPPB)	No main line treatment options are available for EPPB. Topical anti-inflammatory agents have been tried		
Poikiloderma of Civatte	• Avoiding offending agent • Sun protection • Lasers (PDL, IPL < Nd:YAG)		
Seborrheic melanosis	Topical and oral antifungals	• Depigmenting agents • Chemical peels	
Pigmentary demarcation line	Kligman formula or hydroquinone alone topically with sun protection is preferred as first-line therapy in PDL	Chemical peels	
Perioral pigmentation	Bleaching agents such as hydroquinone and retinoids as main therapy	Chemical peels	
Frictional melanosis	• Preventive measures such as avoiding friction, using photo block • Depigmenting topical agents	Chemical peels	

(IPL: intense pulsed light; LPP: lichen planus pigmentosus; Nd:YAG: neodymium-doped yttrium aluminum garnet; NOO: Nevus of Ota; PDL: pigmentary demarcation lines; PIH: postinflammatory hyperpigmentation; POH: progressive osseous heteroplasia)

PART 2: A PATIENT WITH FACIAL HYPOMELANOSIS

INTRODUCTION

Hypopigmented lesions on face are among the most common skin disorders for which patients seek medical attention. Hypopigmentation means decreased pigmentation of the affected skin due to reduced melanin content, while depigmentation means complete absence of melanin in the affected skin.

Hypopigmented lesions are mostly acquired, seldom congenital.[10]

CONGENITAL DISORDERS

- Albinism (AR)
- Piebaldism (AD)
- Nevus depigmentosus
- Ash leaf macules of tuberous sclerosis

ACQUIRED DISORDERS

Commonly seen acquired disorders characterized by hypopigmentation are enlisted in **Table 11**.

ALBINISM[11]

Clinical Features

All types of OCA have similar features, including congenital nystagmus, iris translucency, reduced retinal pigmentation, refractive errors, reduced visual acuity, and sometimes color visual impairment. The characteristic finding is optic nerve misrouting, especially at optic chiasma, resulting in strabismus.

The degree of skin and hair pigmentation varies with types of albinism:

- In OCA1A, hair and skin are white and do not tan. Iris are fully translucent and light blue in color. Amelanotic nevus may be present with intense photophobia.
- In OCA1B, hair and skin may gradually develop pigment till 3 years of age, and blue-colored iris may change to brown/green. Temperature sensitive variant can manifest as depigmented hair on body with pigmented hair on the hands and the feet due to lower body temperature.
- In OCA2, amount of cutaneous pigmentation varies. Nevi and ephelides are common features. Iris color varies in this variant.
- In OCA3, individuals have red hair and reddish-brown skin because the hypopigmentation is not sufficient to alter skin development.
- OCA4 cannot be distinguished from OCA2 clinically.

Differential Diagnosis

Albinism is part of multiple syndromes as listed in **Table 12**, which can be differentiated on the basis of clinical presentation and biochemical criteria.

Table 11: Causes of acquired hypopigmented lesions.	
Autoimmune	• Vitiligo • Sarcoidosis • Extragenital LSA
Infections	• Fungal (pityriasis versicolor) • Bacterial (leprosy and syphilis) • Protozoal (PKDL)
Chemicals	• Lead • Hydroquinone
Malignancy	Hypopigmented mycosis fungoides
PIH	• Inflammatory (atopic, lichen striatus) • Infections (fungal, viral) • Procedures (cryotherapy, dermabrasion) • Burns

(LSA: lichen sclerosus et atrophicus; PIH: postinflammatory hyperpigmentation; PKDL; post-Kala-azar dermal leishmaniasis)

Table 12: Differential diagnosis of albinism.	
Hermansky–Pudlak syndrome	• Rare disorder, except in Puerto Rico (1:1,800) • Autosomal recessive *Cutaneous:* • Hypopigmentation • Ceroid deposition in tissue throughout the body *Systemic:* • Interstitial lung fibrosis • Granulomatous colitis • Bleeding tendencies *Immunology:* Neutropenia
Chediak–Higashi syndrome	• Rare disorder • Autosomal recessive *Cutaneous:* • Skin, hair, and eye pigmentation are diluted resulting in hypopigmentation • Increased susceptibility to infections *Systemic:* • Prolonged bleeding time • Easy bruisability • Peripheral neuropathy
Griscelli syndrome	• Rare autosomal recessive disorder with immune impairment or neurological deficit • Hypopigmentation of skin and hair • Presence of large clumps of pigment in hair shafts

PIEBALDISM

Piebaldism is a rare autosomal dominant disorder affecting skin and hair due to mutation of c-kit gene, located on chromosome 4q12 (affects differentiation and migration of melanoblasts), characterized by congenital absence of melanocytes. A white forelock is the classical presentation at birth. The incidence is estimated to be <1:20,000, with equal prevalence in males and females.

Clinical Features

At birth, affected individuals present with relatively stable depigmentation of hair and skin. In number of patients, regimentation (partial or complete) can occur spontaneously after an injury.

A white forelock of hair, a triangular, diamond-shaped depigmented macule presenting on forehead, is the most common manifestation in piebaldism seen in 80–90% affected individuals. Eyebrows and eyelashes may sometimes be affected. The characteristic distribution of patch is forehead, extending up to chest and anterior abdomen, lateral trunk (sparing dorsal spine), mid arms, and legs (sparing hands and feet). The depigmented macules have symmetrical distribution and can be rectangular, rhomboid in shape. Islands of hyperpigmentation are present typically on the border of patch or in the middle. Histologically, melanocytes are considerably reduced or absent in depigmented area and absolutely normal in number and function in hyperpigmented area.

NEVUS DEPIGMENTOSUS

A localized hypomelanosis in children visible since birth is nevus depigmentosus that occurs due to pigmentary mosaicism as postulated by Happle. It is often confused with childhood vitiligo and can be differentiated using wood's lamp examination. Some authors have divided it in three categories, i.e., isolated, segmental, and blaschkoid form. The closest differential to nevus depigmentosus is nevus anemicus which is because of the vascular malformation and can be differentiated using diascopy.

ASH LEAF MACULES

Seen in tuberous sclerosus, an autosomal dominant condition causing hypoplasia of mesodermal and ectodermal cells. It is a multisystem rare genetic disorder involving skin, heart, kidney, lungs, and eyes. Skin shows hypopigmented oval macules on body and confetti-like lesions. Rarely, these lesions may also be seen on face.

VITILIGO

Vitiligo is an ancient term and its earliest authentic reference can be traced back to period of Aushooryan (2200 BC), in classic Tarikh-e-Tib-e-Iran (Fig. 6). Vitiligo occurs all over the globe; world literature if filled with references to condition and different aspects of the etiology audits therapy. Vitiligo is derived from Latin word "vitium," meaning "defect."

Vitiligo is an acquired, idiopathic discoloration of skin, characterized by well-circumscribed, ivory, or milky white macules, devoid of identifiable melanocytes. The macules are flushed to the surface of the skin. The hair in the existing lesion can be normal or white (poliosis).[12] In contract to vitiligo, leukoderma refers to hypopigmented macules with known underlying cause.

Epidemiology

It affects 1% of world's population and 3–4% of Indians approximately.[13] However, across country its incidence ranges from 0.1 to >8.8. The highest incidence of vitiligo has been recorded in Indians, followed by Mexico and Japan. The difference in the incidence can be because of higher reporting of vitiligo in population, where stigma of color attached to condition may force them to seek early consultation.

The most common site of involvement being face (24.5%), followed by neck (18.8%) and scalp (11.2%).[14] Adults and children are affected equally of both the sexes, although females are reported in greater number due to social consequences to girls affected by vitiligo. Majority of the cases are reported during the active growth phase, half

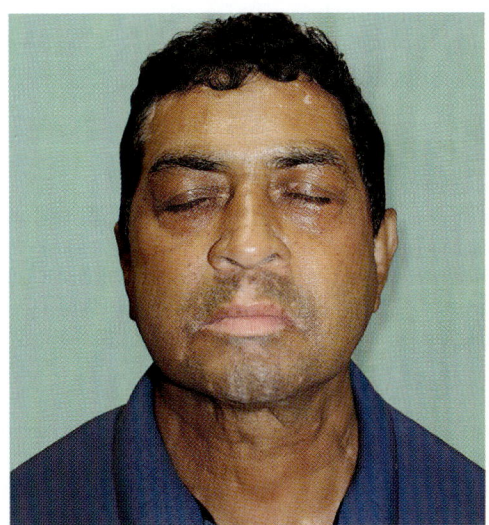

FIG. 6: Hypo- to depigmented macular lesions of vitiligo.

of them presents before the age of 20 years. The mode of transmission of vitiligo is polygenic with variable penetrance. In India, the proportion of patient with positive history varies from 6.25 to 18%, with as high as 40% in few studies.[15]

Precipitating Factors
- Genetic
- Stress
- Trauma (Koebner's phenomenon)
- Infections
- Drugs

Clinical Features[16-18]
Vitiligo is a slow and progressive disease, characterized by appearance of discoloration of typical milky white macules coalescing to form patches. The macules are oval to round in shape with well-defined borders affecting skin and mucous membrane. The lesions are generally asymptomatic but can be sometimes associated with burning or itching.

Morphological Variations
- *Trichrome vitiligo*: A narrow band of color between vitiligo macule and normal pigmented surrounding skin
- *Quadrichrome vitiligo*: A fourth color in vitiligo lesions, usually seen in dark skin type. A marginal hyper pigmentation or perifollicular macules denotes regimenting disease.
- *Penta chrome*: There is a sequential color display of tan, white, blue-gray, brown pigmentation with normal skin.
- *Blue vitiligo*: Vitiligo occurring at the site of postinflammatory hypermelanosis.
- *Inflammatory vitiligo*: Erythematous, raised border in depigmented macule

Classification
It is classified as:
- *Focal*: A rare form with hypopigmented macules restricted in a small area
- *Segmental*: It is commonly seen in children with poor prognosis. The lesions present with sharp midline restriction or appears along the line of Blaschko's.
- *Mucosal*: It affects mucous membrane of mouth or genitals.
- *Lip tip vitiligo*: Commonly seen in adults with patches on finger tips and lips.
- *Generalized*: Most common form of vitiligo with patches appearing in various places on body
- *Universal*: More than 80% of the skin lacks pigment.

Associations
Along with cutaneous side effects, vitiligo is also associated with ocular and systemic complications.

HYPOPIGMENTED SARCOIDOSIS
This variant is mostly seen in Negros. Clinically, lesions can range from hypochromic to shiny macules, papules, or plaques extensively seen on trunk and extremities and rarely on face.

EXTRAGENITAL LICHEN SCLEROSIS ET ATROPHICANS
Lichen sclerosus et atrophicus (LSA), also known as Csillag disease, is an autoimmune disease with unknown etiology. It is characterized by porcelain white and sclerosis occurs on genitals and anal area. Extragenital LSA develops on neck and limbs and rarely on face. Most commonly associated diseases are vitiligo, thyroid, alopecia areata, morphea, lichen planus, and pernicious anemia.

INFECTIONS
Fungal Infection
Pityriasis Versicolor
Tinea versicolor or pityriasis versicolor is a superficial fungal infection caused by *Malassezia furfur*. It is a chronically recurring fungal infection involving the stratum corneum, presenting clinically as scaly, well-defined, hypopigmented macules on trunk and extremities and rarely on face. Malassezia is a yeast, a dimorphic fungus (mycelial phase) is responsible for lesions of pityriasis versicolor. It is a member of physiological skin flora, which under favorable environment transforms into filamentous pathogenic form. Lesions are asymptomatic and the patient seeks medical attention for hypopigmented patches. The organism can easily be identified on 10% KOH (spaghetti and meatball appearance).

Bacterial Infection
Leprosy
The earliest presentation of leprosy is often in the form of ill-defined, hypopigmented patches. The color, however, varies within same individual depending on the skin type. The lesions are erythematous in fair-skinned individual and coppery brown in dark-skinned person. The initial presentation of leprosy is called as indeterminate leprosy and is generally observed as first sign of disease. Hypoesthesia is not prominent with negative slit skin smear. Histopathology may not show classical features. Prognosis is good with treatment, without any reactions or neurological sequelae.

Syphilis
Leukoderma syphiliticum, also known as leukoderma colli, syphilide pigmentaire, and syphilitic vitiligo, is a rare

manifestation of secondary syphilis. Very few cases have ever been described in literature. Lesions present as round to oval, nonscaling, well-demarcated, hypochromic patches on trunk, abdomen, and face. Also called as "syphilitic ring" in literature slowly regresses postbenzathine penicillin G treatment.

Post-kala-azar Dermal Leishmaniasis

It is the late sequel of visceral leishmaniasis, occurring 1–3 years after manifestation of systemic symptoms. It is thought to be the cutaneous immunological reaction to attenuated parasite (post-treatment) in dermis. Polymorphic cutaneous lesions seen on face, trunk, and limbs include hypopigmented macules, papules, and nodules. On histopathology, nodules show dense lymphohistiocytic infiltrate with plasma cells in upper dermis. Follicular plugging is prominent in facial lesions. Sodium stibogluconate 20 mg/kg is given for 4 months with fair results.

CHEMICALS

Chemical vitiligo (leukoderma) is an acquired hypomelanosis induced by repeated exposure to specific chemical compounds. It remains an underdiagnosed entity. Contact dermatitis is a prerequisite for chemical leukoderma, characterized by presence of multiple hypopigmented confetti or pea-sized macules. The most common chemicals include:
- p-tertiary butylphenol (*bindi* dermatitis)
- Hydroquinone (bleaching agent)
- p-phenylenediamine (*henna* and hair dyes)

MYCOSIS FUNGOIDES

Hypopigmented mycosis fungoides (HMF) rarely occurs on face. Usually, it presents as single or multiple hypopigmented patches on trunk and extremities. Majority of reported cases are in children and young adults. Clinical differentials of HMF include vitiligo, leprosy, and pityriasis versicolor. Topical antifungals for 4–6 weeks are used for mild infection, while oral itraconazole and fluconazole are reserved for extensive infection.

Hypopigmented lesions can be differentiated on the basis of history, cutaneous examination, and investigations.[19]

History

Past History in Facial Hypopigmented Lesions

Table 13 enlists important points that needs to be elicited in past history.

Cutaneous Examination (Table 14)

Characteristic Lesions

Size, shape, and color of the lesion (hypopigmented or depigmented); unilateral/bilateral; well-defined/ill-defined; stable/progressive; coalescing/noncoalescing; scaly/non scaly.

Other Cutaneous Findings

- Forelock patch is seen in piebaldism.
- Beige's sign is seen in syphilis.
- Besnier's sign is seen in PV.
- Satellite lesions are characteristic of leprosy and vitiligo.
- Leukotrichia is classically seen in vitiligo.
- Papules or nodules are seen in sarcoidosis, PKDL, and leprosy.
- Decreased/loss of sensations is associated with leprosy.

Investigation

Table 15 outlines investigations to be done.

Treatment

Table 16 enlists the treatment modalities for certain hypopigmentary disorders.

Table 13: Relevance of past history in hypopigmented lesions.	
History	**Relevance**
Where the lesions present since birth or did it appear after birth?	To differentiated vitiligo and ash leaf macules from childhood vitiligo
If acquired, was it sudden or gradual and did it appear before adolescence or after	Childhood vitiligo is generally seen before puberty
Other autoimmune diseases such as thyroid or cholesterol and rheumatic arthritis	LSA and vitiligo
Prior inflammation or chemical exposure	Leukoderma or bindi dermatitis
Is the lesions itchy/painful?	Fungal or bacterial infection
Ulceration on genitals	Syphilis
Promiscuous behavior	Syphilis
Decrease in power, muscle wasting, and loss of sensations	Leprosy
(LSA: lichen sclerosus et atrophicus)	

Table 14: Cutaneous investigations for hypopigmented lesions.

	Hypo or depigmented	Any specific location	Surface changes	Size and shape	Associated features
Albinism	Depigmented	Along with hair and skin; iris is also affected	Leukotrichia	Generalized	
Piebaldism	Depigmented	White forelock of hair	Leukotrichia	Triangular, diamond-shaped lesion	Islands of hyperpigmentation on the border of patch
Ash leaf macules	Hypopigmented	• Trunk • Lower extremities	Leukotrichia	Ash leaf/oval-shaped, confetti like, thumb print shaped	• Facial angiofibromas • Shagreen patches • Subungual fibromas • Hypomelanotic macules • Benign fibromas in heart, kidney, brain, and lungs
Nevus depigmentosus	Hypopigmented	Trunk	None	Irregular round or polygonal macules	
Vitiligo	Depigmented (chalk white color)	Lip tip vitiligo	Leukotrichia	Localized or generalized	Leukotrichia mucosal involvement
Sarcoidosis	Hypopigmented	Nose, trunk	Increased vascularity on face lesions	• Macules • Papules • Plaques • Nodular	Macules, papules or plaques seen extensively on trunk and extremities
Extragenital LSA	Depigmented	Trunk	• Sclerosis • Prominent keratin plug	Irregular shaped	Occasional pruritus
Pityriasis versicolor	Hypopigmented	Neck, upper chest, and back	Scaling	Macule coalescing to form patch	Itching
Leprosy	Hypopigmented	Trunk	Loss of hair, dry skin	Well-defined to ill-defined macules, plaques, and nodules	Loss of sensations, decreased power
Syphilis	Hypopigmented	Genitals	Syphilitic chancre on face	Well-defined	History of oral and genital ulcers
Post-Kala-azar leishmaniasis	Hypopigmented	Trunk	None	Ill-defined	
Mycosis fungicides	Hypopigmented	Trunk and extremities	Scaling	Plaque stage can affect face and scalp with annular or horseshoe-shaped infiltrated plaques	Pruritus

(LSA: lichen sclerosus et atrophicus)

Table 15: Investigations for hypopigmentation.

Disease	Wood's lamp	Histopathology	Dermoscopy
Vitiligo	Depigmented lesions (e.g., vitiligo) and hypopigmented lesions with decreased melanin production are markedly enhanced, appear bright white, whereas hypopigmented lesions with normal melanin (PMH) are not accentuated	Complete absence of melanocytes in association with a total loss of epidermal pigmentation. Superficial perivascular and perifollicular lymphocytic infiltrates may be observed at the margin of vitiliginous lesions	While perifollicular depigmentation (PFD) was predictive of stable vitiligo, perifollicular pigmentation (PFP) was characteristic of active disease. Starburst appearance, altered pigment network, and comet tail appearance can also be noted, and these were typical of progressive vitiligo. A new dermoscopic feature, the "tapioca sago" appearance (sabudana) can be observed in the skin adjacent to the vitiligo lesion only in patients with progressive vitiligo

Continued

CHAPTER 8 A Patient of Facial Melanosis

Continued

Disease	Wood's lamp	Histopathology	Dermoscopy
Sarcoidosis		The presence of multiple well-formed, noncaseating granulomas, which are compact clusters of epithelioid cells and multinucleated giant cells with minimal to no central necrosis. The granulomas are often surrounded by lymphocytes. Several types of inclusions may be seen in the granulomas, such as Schaumann bodies, asteroid bodies, Hamazaki–Wesenberg bodies, and calcium oxalate crystals	Translucent orange globules with linear and branching vessels. White scar-like areas appearing as white patches or lines are also seen
LSA		Vacuolar interface dermatitis with dermal sclerosis is the characteristic feature of LSA	Inflammatory lesions show white structureless areas, comedo-like openings, linear telangiectasia with variable diameter, and peppered arrangement of gray-blue and brown dots which correspond to the dermal fibrosis, follicular plugs, capillary dilatation and epidermal as well as dermal melanophages, respectively
Pityriasis versicolor		Spores and hyphae are seen in thickened stratum corneum, described as "Spaghetti and meatballs" appearance. Dermis shows sparse perivascular infiltrate	Dermoscopy of pityriasis versicolor shows diffuse white scales which are more prominent in skin cleavage lines and focal white areas. Double-edged scales are seen due stretching of lesion
Leprosy		<ul><li>Tuberculoid; primary polar tuberculoid leprosy has large and compact epithelioid cell granulomas along the neurovascular bundles with lymphocytes. Langhans giant cells are typically scanty or absent</li><li>*Borderline leprosy*: The epithelioid granulomas of BT do not invade into the epidermis and have less lymphocytes in comparison to TT. The granulomas are arranged in a curvilinear pattern along the neurovascular bundle. Nerve erosion by the granuloma is typical, and AFB are scanty</li></ul>	Dermoscopy of flat hypopigmented lesion of leprosy shows focal white areas, broken hairs and pigtail hairs, and subtle pigment network within the lesion
Syphilis		The histopathologic pictures of all lesions, irrespective of classification, are essentially identical. The cellular infiltrate consists primarily of lymphocytes, plasma cells, macrophages, some polymorphonuclear leukocytes, epithelioid cells, and occasional giant cells. The areas involved are the cutis, the lower portion of the rete malpighii, and in certain instances, the cuticular appendages. The vessels around the lesions typically show inflammatory proliferative changes and cellular infiltrates in their walls, along with various degrees of dilatation	
PKDL		The epidermis in these biopsies was atrophic and the dermal adnexa were either caught up in the infiltrate or were displaced downward. Compact epithelioid granulomas are seen more frequently in the nodules than in the macules or papules. Leishman–Donovan (LD) bodies are the characteristic feature	Advanced hypopigmented lesions show central erosion, white starburst pattern, and peripheral vascular pattern like comma-shaped vessels, dotted vessels, and hairpin vessels

Continued

Continued

Disease	Wood's lamp	Histopathology	Dermoscopy
MF		Increased number of mononuclear cells distributed singly or in small collections within an epidermis devoid of spongiotic microvesiculation. Other important features are lacunae surrounding intraepidermal mononuclear cells which give them the appearance of "haloed cells"	Rosettes and geometric white lines are unique to MF
(AFB: acid-fast bacillus; BT: borderline tuberculoid; LSA: lichen sclerosus et atrophicus; MF: mycosis fungoides; PKDL: post-Kala-azar dermal leishmaniasis; PMH: progressive macular hypomelanosis; TT: tuberculoid)			

Table 16: Line of treatment for hypopigmentation.[19]

	First line	Second line
Vitiligo	Topical: • L-phenylalanine • Topical steroids alone or in combination with topical vitamin D3 analog Systemic: Steroids	NBUVB alone or in combination with topical calcineurin inhibitors Systemic: • NBUVB with systemic steroids • NBUVB with polypodium leucotomos • UVA with psoralens • UVA with systemic steroids Supportive: • Excimer laser • Surgery
Sarcoidosis	Topical: • Steroids • Intralesional steroids Systemic: • Hydroxychloroquine 200–400 mg daily • Mepacrine 100 mg alternate days	Systemic: • Methotrexate 15–25 mg/week • Azathioprine 1–3 mg/kg/day • MMF 1–3 g/day With or without hydroxychloroquine
Extragenital LSA	Topical: • Steroids • Calcineurin inhibitors	
Pityriasis versicolor	Topical antifungal	Systemic: Fluconazole
Leprosy	Topical: Emollients Systemic: MB-MDT	Systemic: • Ofloxacin/moxifloxacin • Clarithromycin • Minocycline Along with rifampicin
Syphilis	Benzathine penicillin G	Erythromycin
Post-Kala-azar leishmaniasis	Miltefosine	
Mycosis fungicides	Early stage: • Topical corticosteroids • Heliotherapy • Radiation therapy Advanced stage: • Oral doxorubicin • Oral gemcitabine	Early stage: • Topical chemotherapy (mechlorethamine or carmustine) • Low dose oral methotrexate Advanced stage: • Chlorambucil • Cyclophosphamide • Etoposide • High-dose methotrexate
(LSA: lichen sclerosus et atrophicus; MB-MDT: multibacillary-multi-drug treatment; MMF: mycophenolate mofetil; NBUVB: narrow-band ultraviolet B)		

REFERENCES

1. Khanna N, Rasool S. Facial melanoses: Indian perspective. Indian J Dermatol Venereol Leprol. 2011;77(5):552-64.
2. Lee AY. Recent progress in melasma pathogenesis. Pigment Cell Melanoma Res. 2015;28(6):648-60.
3. Davis EC, Callender VD. Postinflammatory hyperpigmentation: A review of the epidemiology, clinical features, and treatment options in skin of color. J Clin Aesthet Dermatol. 2010;3(7):20-31.
4. Sarkar R, Ranjan R, Garg S, Garg V, Sonthalia S, Bansal S. Periorbital hyperpigmentation: a comprehensive review. J Clin Aesthet Dermatol. 2016;9(1):49-55.
5. Wolff M, Sabzevari N, Gropper C, Hoffman C. A case of lichen planus pigmentosus with facial dyspigmentation responsive to combination therapy with chemical peels and topical retinoids. J Clin Aesthet Dermatol. 2016;9(11):44-50.
6. Yim JH, Kang IH, Shin MK, Lee MH. Differences among dermoscopic findings in Riehl's melanosis of the cheek and neck. Ann Dermatol. 2019;31(4):460-3.
7. Chakrabarti N, Chattopadhyay C. Ashy dermatosis: A controversial entity. Indian J Dermatol. 2012;57(1):61-2.
8. Bhattar PA, Zawar VP, Godse KV, Patil SP, Nadkarni NJ, Gautam MM. Exogenous ochronosis. Indian J Dermatol. 2015;60(6):537-43.
9. Ghosh A, Das A, Sarkar R. Diffuse hyperpigmentation: A comprehensive approach. Pigment Int. 2018;5(1):4-13.
10. Kumari R, Thappa DM. Familial nevus of ota. Indian J Dermatol. 2006;51(3):198-9.
11. Kar HK, Gupta L. 1064 nm Q switched Nd:YAG laser treatment of nevus of Ota: An Indian open label prospective study of 50 patients. Indian J Dermatol Venereol Leprol. 2011;77(5):565-70.
12. Dereure O. Drug-induced skin pigmentation. Epidemiology, diagnosis and treatment. Am J Clin Dermatol. 2001;2(4):253-62.
13. Madireddy S, Crane JS. Hypopigmented macules. In: StatPearls [Internet]. Treasure Island (FL): StatPearls Publishing; 2021.
14. Grønskov K, Ek J, Brondum-Nielsen K. Oculocutaneous albinism. Orphanet J Rare Dis. 2007;2:43.
15. Sehgal VN. Vitiligo. Textbook of clinical Dermatology, 4th edition. New Delhi: Jaypee Brothers Medical Publishers; 2004. pp. 99-101.
16. Song MS, Hann SK, Ahn PS, Im S, Park YK. Clinical study of vitiligo: Comparative study of type A and B vitiligo. Ann Dermatol. 1994;6:22-30.
17. Lerner AB. Vitiligo. J Invest Dermatol. 1959;32(2 Part 2):285-310.
18. Palit A, Inamadar AC. Childhood vitiligo. Indian J Dermatol Venereol Leprol. 2012;78(1):30-41.
19. Sehgal VN, Srivastava G. Vitiligo: Compendium of clinico-epidemiological features. Indian J Dermatol Venereol Leprol. 2007;73(3):149-56.

Part 2: Disorders of Nail and Hair

9

Trachyonychia

Shravya Rimmalapudi, Bhushan Madke

INTRODUCTION

Trachyonychia is derived from a Greek word "trakos" which means rough.[1]

It is an acquired benign inflammatory disease of the proximal nail matrix producing characteristic nail plate surface abnormalities.[2] It is usually insidious in onset and self-limiting. The symptoms may take years to resolve.

It is also known as "sandpaper nails". Any number of nails can be involved and the involvement of all the twenty nails is called as "twenty nail dystrophy" but is usually nonscarring and only rarely there is nail destruction.[3] The reason for this is, to cause complete destruction of nail plate there must be total involvement of proximal nail matrix and nail fold; however, in trachyonychia, there is focal rather nonuniform levels of inflammatory activity which is either constant or interspersed with normal nail matrix function. Hence, it does not cause permanent scarring unlike other nail matrix disorders.[1] The cuticle is usually ragged, thickened, and hyperkeratotic.[4] Trachyonychia can be idiopathic or associated with various dermatological or systemic diseases.

ETIOPATHOGENESIS[4]

The various causes of trachyonychia are idiopathic which is more common or can be associated with various diseases given in **Table 1**.

It can be inherited as autosomal dominant disorder.

Any kind of alteration to the nail plate is a direct reflection of the damage to the proximal matrix and this can be mild or severe.

Damage to the nail matrix keratinocytes impairs the differentiation and maturation without interrupting the

Table 1: Etiology of trachyonychia.[1]	
Idiopathic	
Dermatological disorders	• Alopecia areata • Lichen planus • Psoriasis • Ichthyosis vulgaris • Vitiligo • Atopic dermatitis • Pemphigus • Sarcoidosis • Congenital cutaneous candidiasis • Nail patella syndrome • Pachyonychia congenita • Koilonychia • Incontinentia pigmenti
Nondermatological disorders	• Primary biliary cirrhosis • Reflex sympathetic dystrophy • Hematological abnormalities (e.g., idiopathic thrombocytopenia) • Immunoglobulin A deficiency • Autoimmune hemolytic anemia • Graft-versus-host rejection reaction
Syndromes	• Bart syndrome • Brauer–Buschke–Fischer syndrome • Clouston syndrome
Drugs	• *Chemotherapeutics*: Vincristine • *Kinase inhibitors*: Imatinib • *Retinoids*: Acitretin
Trauma	

Table 2: Pathogenesis involved with different variants of trachyonychia.

Types	Pathogenesis	Appearance
Opaque: Most common type	Severe and persistent inflammation where the whole nail plate is thin and abnormal because of diffuse damage to the nail matrix	Rough, lusterless, sandpaper like nails with diffuse ridging
Shiny: Less common type	A milder and more intermittent inflammation where the nail matrix damage is multifocal rather than diffuse	Uniform opalescent nails with numerous superficial pits which reflect light giving shiny appearance

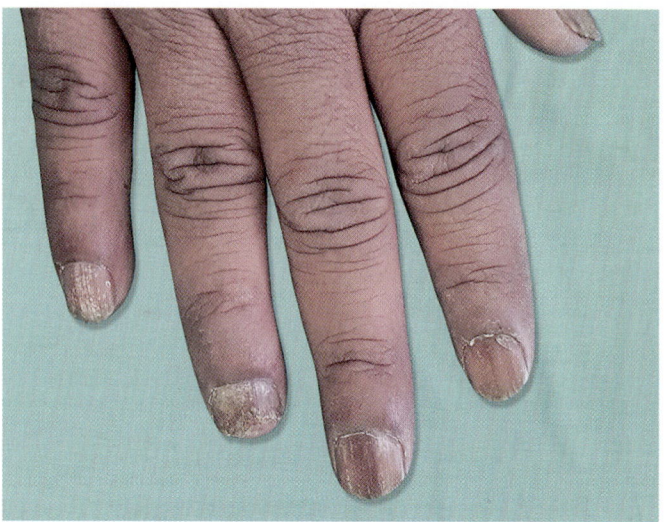

FIG. 1: Opaque variant with excessive longitudinal ridging, onychoschizia and discoloration.

mitotic activity giving rise to trachyonychia. The extent of the nail plate abnormalities depends on the course of inflammatory process. The pathogenesis involved with different variants of trachyonychia is mentioned in **Table 2**.

In all these diseases mentioned earlier that might show trachyonychia, there is abnormal keratinization of nail matrix onychocytes followed by retention of nuclei and thus instead of maturing to form a compact layer of tightly adherent flat cells. The nail matrix produces a stratum corneum like layer that easily desquamates.

There are two variants **(Figs. 1 and 2)** of trachyonychia which may coexist in a single patient. The two variants are described in **Table 2**.

DEMOGRAPHY

It is more common in children **(Fig. 3)** with peak age being 3–12 years although it can occur at any age.[1]

The exact prevalence is not known. Females and males are equally affected.[5] 3.65% of patients with alopecia areata and 10% of patients with lichen planus can have trachyonychia.[1,6] 60% of patients with psoriasis show nail changes in general not necessarily trachyonychia.[7]

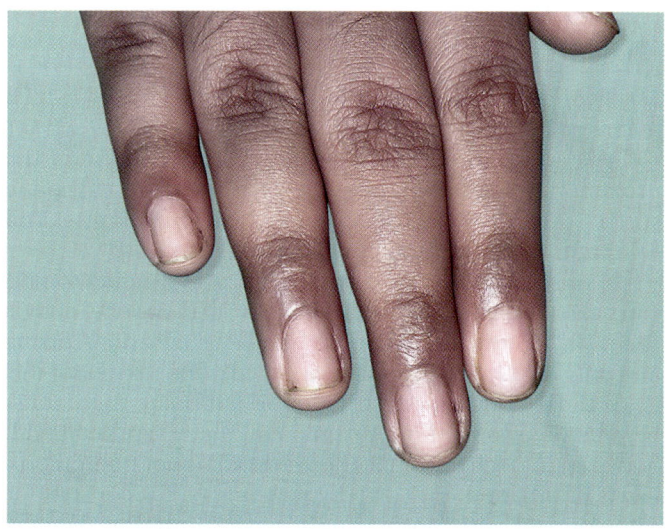

FIG. 2: Shiny nails of trachyonychia in a case of diffuse alopecia areata, also notice ragged cuticles.
Courtesy: Dr Jigna Padhiyar.

CLINICAL FEATURES

History

- Patient complains of rough, lusterless nails with thinning
- It is usually insidious onset initially involving one or two nails **(Fig. 3)** and gradually progressive to involve few or all nails over a span of months to years.
- The number of nails affected may vary in different patients and trachyonychia often involves a few nails or only one
- Fingernails are affected more frequently than toenails.

- *Points to ask in history to rule out associated disorders*:
  ○ History of age of onset—to rule out congenital syndromes
  ○ History of pre-existing skin lesions on other parts of the body—to rule out trachyonychia associated with dermatological diseases like lichen planus, psoriasis, ichthyosis, etc.
  ○ History of pigmentary lesions—incontinentia pigmenti, lichen planus
  ○ History of oral lesions such as ulceration, patterned pigmentation—to rule out lichen planus
  ○ History of joint pains—to rule out psoriasis
  ○ History of atopy/atopic diathesis such as pruritus and flexural/extensors if toddlers and infants for chronic lesions—to rule out atopic dermatitis

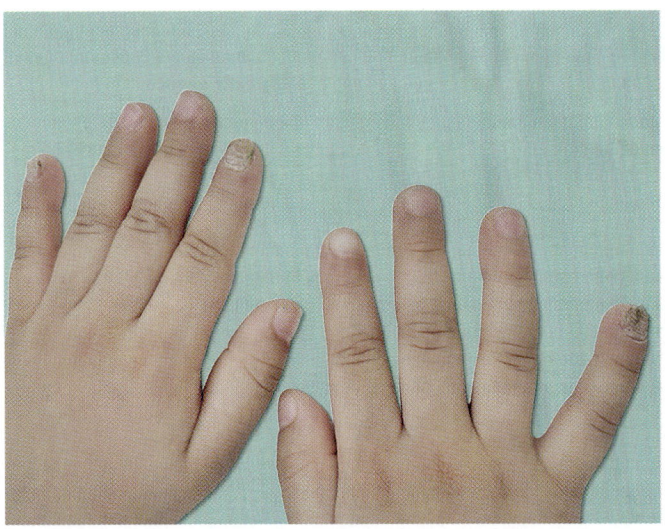

FIG. 3: Only few nails showing changes of trachyonychia in a child with a history of atopic diathesis.
Courtesy: Dr Jigna Padhiyar.

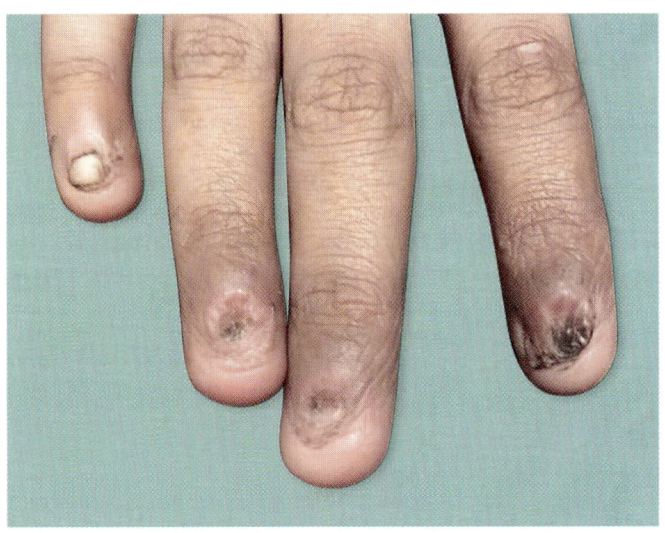

FIG. 4: Dystrophic/absent nail plates because of lichen planus.
Courtesy: Dr Jigna Padhiyar.

- History of patchy or diffuse hair loss—for considering alopecia areata as possibility
- History of purpuric/petechial lesions—to rule out idiopathic thrombocytopenic purpura
- History of trauma—to differentiate it from traumatic dystrophies and changes
- History of prior drug intake—to rule out drug-induced cause
- History of swelling, redness, pain around nails—to rule out paronychia
- History of nail discoloration—to rule out onychomycosis, melanonychia, etc
- History of malaise, shortness of breath—to rule out hemolytic anemia
- Family history to look for genetic associations
- History of:
  - Thyroid disorders or other autoimmune diseases
  - Food allergies

EXAMINATION[1]

- *General examination*: Look for
  - Icterus—to rule out primary biliary cirrhosis
  - Koilonychia—can be associated with trachyonychia
  - Pallor—to rule out iron deficiency or autoimmune hemolytic anemia
- *Cutaneous examination*:
  - *Nail findings*:
    - One, several, or all digits may be involved with nail plate surface showing excessive longitudinal ridging or fissuring (opaque nails) as shown in **Figure 1**.
    - In some, the nail plate is shiny with myriad miniscule superficial punctate depressions arranged in longitudinal line (shiny nails—**Fig. 2**)
    - These nail plate surface abnormalities are monomorphous and regularly distributed on nail plate.
    - Nail roughness is a prominent sign of severe cases.
    - There can be nail thinning, fragility, onychorrhexis, onychoschizia, and distal chipping of the nail plates.
    - A yellowish thickening of the thumb nails and great toe nails may be present.
    - Presence of dystrophy **(Fig. 4)** is strongly suggestive of lichen planus affecting nails and dystrophy is never found in cases of trachyonychia.
    - Examine the overall skin to rule out associated dermatological disorders:
      - Face, flexors—for atopic dermatitis
      - Scalp, extensors—for psoriasis
      - Oral—for lichen planus, pemphigus vulgaris
      - Hair, beard, eyebrows—for alopecia areata
      - Overall body—for ichthyosis

DIFFERENTIAL DIAGNOSIS

- Alopecia areata
- Psoriasis
- Lichen planus
- Brittle nails
- Senile nails
- Onychomycosis

Table 3: Trachyonychia associated with psoriasis, lichen planus, and alopecia areata.[8]			
	Psoriasis	**Lichen planus**	**Alopecia areata**
Clinical findings	• *Nail plate*—pitting (irregular and randomly placed), Beau's lines • *Nail bed*—salmon patch, onycholysis, splinter hemorrhages, subungual hyperkeratosis, nail discoloration	Longitudinal fissures, pterygium, nail plate thinning, or atrophy	Geometrical, superficial, regularly arranged small pits
Histopathology	Focal parakeratosis, hyperkeratosis, acanthosis, accumulations of polymorphonucleocytes with neutrophils, nail bed, and plate show granular layer	Hyperkeratosis, hypergranulosis, acanthosis in ventral portion of proximal nail fold and also nail matrix, superficial dermis show band-like lymphocytic infiltrate, vacuolar alteration in basal layer	Lymphocytes can be present in nail matrix

Clinical and histopathological differences between trachyonychia associated with psoriasis, lichen planus, and alopecia areata is given in **Table 3**.[8]

Blood Investigations

- Complete blood count with peripheral smear—rule out hematological abnormalities
- Liver function test, antimitochondrial antibody—to rule out primary biliary cirrhosis, graft versus host reaction
- Direct Coombs test—to rule out autoimmune hemolytic anemia

Microscopy and Culture

Nail scrapping and clippings can be dissolved in 20-40% potassium hydroxide to look for fungal elements in microscopy and it can be cultured in sabouraud dextrose agar to rule out onychomycosis.

Dermoscopy Findings

In trachyonychia, nail plate shows multiple fine and superficial longitudinal fissures usually associated with mild scaling **(Fig. 5)**. The shiny variant however shows superficial ridging and small geometrical pits **(Fig. 6)**.[9,10] Nail dermoscopy features to differentiate nail psoriasis and lichen planus is given in the **Table 4**.

Histopathology Findings

Invasive procedure like nail biopsy can be done to establish definite diagnosis but is not really required in trachyonychia since it does not cause permanent scarring including cases of trachyonychia caused by lichen planus and it has a benign outcome. If nail destruction occurs the diagnosis is purely lichen planus **(Figs. 4 and 7)**.[11]

The most common findings are spongiosis and exocytosis of inflammatory cells into the epithelium of nail which are seen in idiopathic and in trachyonychia associated with alopecia areata. The histopathological findings of associated disorders such as alopecia areata, lichen planus, and psoriasis are given in the **Table 3**.

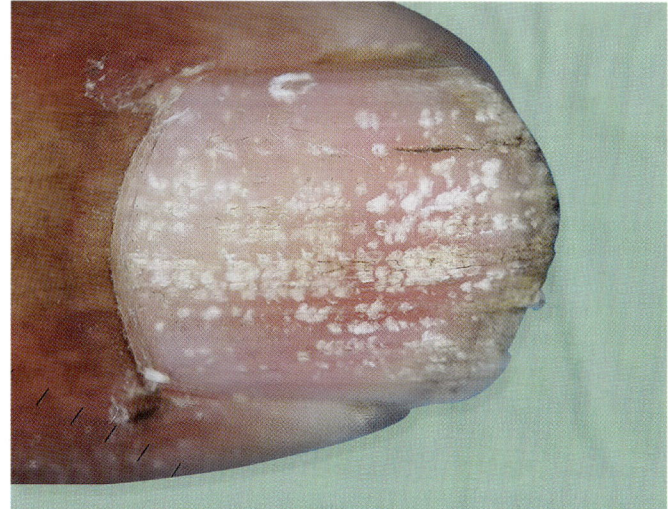

FIG. 5: Multiple deep longitudinal fissures with distal splitting of the nail plate.

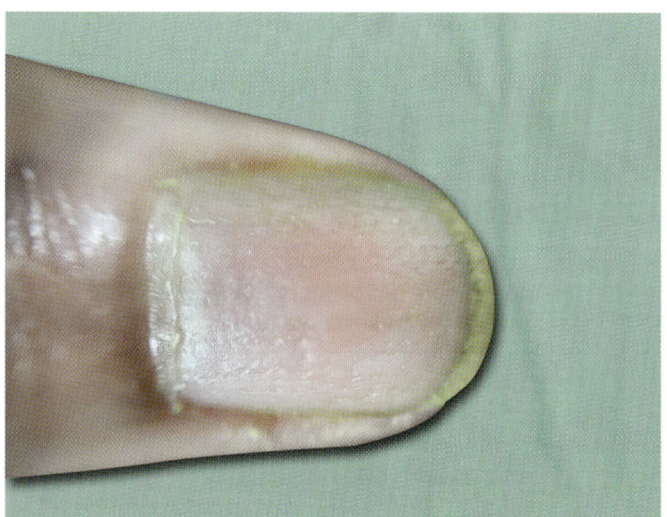

FIG. 6: Shiny nails dermoscopic findings showing ridging and geographical arrangement of pits.
Courtesy: Dr Jigna Padhiyar.

	Lichen planus	Psoriasis	Alopecia areata	Onychomycosis
Nail fold	Dorsal pterygium is formed by skin and is continuous with the skin of proximal nail fold pink-red in early lesions with elongated capillaries and white in chronic cases due to fibrosis	Can show capillary as red dots and scaling	Scally, cuticle, and lateral nail folds	–
Nail plate: Longitudinal fissures	Multiple deep fissure until the distal part of the nail along with absence of the nail plate, melanonychia, longitudinal split in nail plate	Longitudinal or transverse ridges may be seen	Lamellar splitting	Irregular opaque white areas
Pits	Rarely very fine pits can be seen in early stage changes	Pits are large, deep and irregular in shape, size, and distribution surrounded by whitish halo usually covered with large scales	Pits are regular, superficial, and homogenously distributed along geometrical lines	
Nail bed: Discoloration	–	Circular translucent yellow-red area of discoloration representing salmon patch	–	• Distal subungual—white-yellow longitudinal striae with bands of fading color • Dermatophytoma—round yellow-orange patch in mid nail bed connected by narrow channel to distal edge of nail plate representing subungual accumulation of hyphae and scales
Splinter hemorrhages	–	Seen as longitudinal orientation of red lines	–	Seen as longitudinal orientation of red lines
Onycholysis	–	Erythematous border surrounding the distal edge of detachment appears as bright yellow with slightly dented margin of detachment	–	Detachment is along the horny layer of nail bed hence the ragged border with jagged edge and sharp structures
Subungual hyperkeratosis	–	seen	–	Seen

Table 4: Dermoscopy findings of nail psoriasis, lichen planus, and onychomycosis.

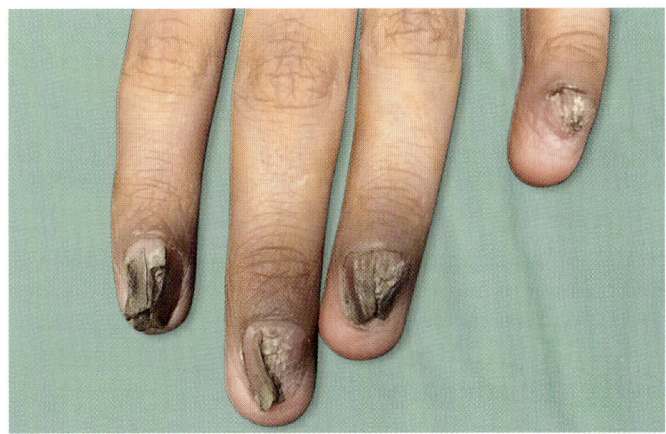

FIG. 7: Pterygium formation splitting the nails longitudinally giving pup-tent appearance in a case of nail lichen planus.
Courtesy: Dr Jigna Padhiyar.

DIAGNOSTIC APPROACH

The diagnostic approach has been depicted in **Flowchart 1**.

TREATMENT

Trachyonychia is a chronic benign self-limiting condition which is nonscarring and nonpainful. Hence, counseling regarding the minimal long-term risk and reassurance is required. Children have comparatively shorter duration than adults.[12] In about 50% patients, it resolves within 5–6 years. There is no specific treatment for trachyonychia currently but treatment is offered either for cosmetic reason or if the patient feels their nail functioning is hampered. The treatment is based on regulating the keratinocyte

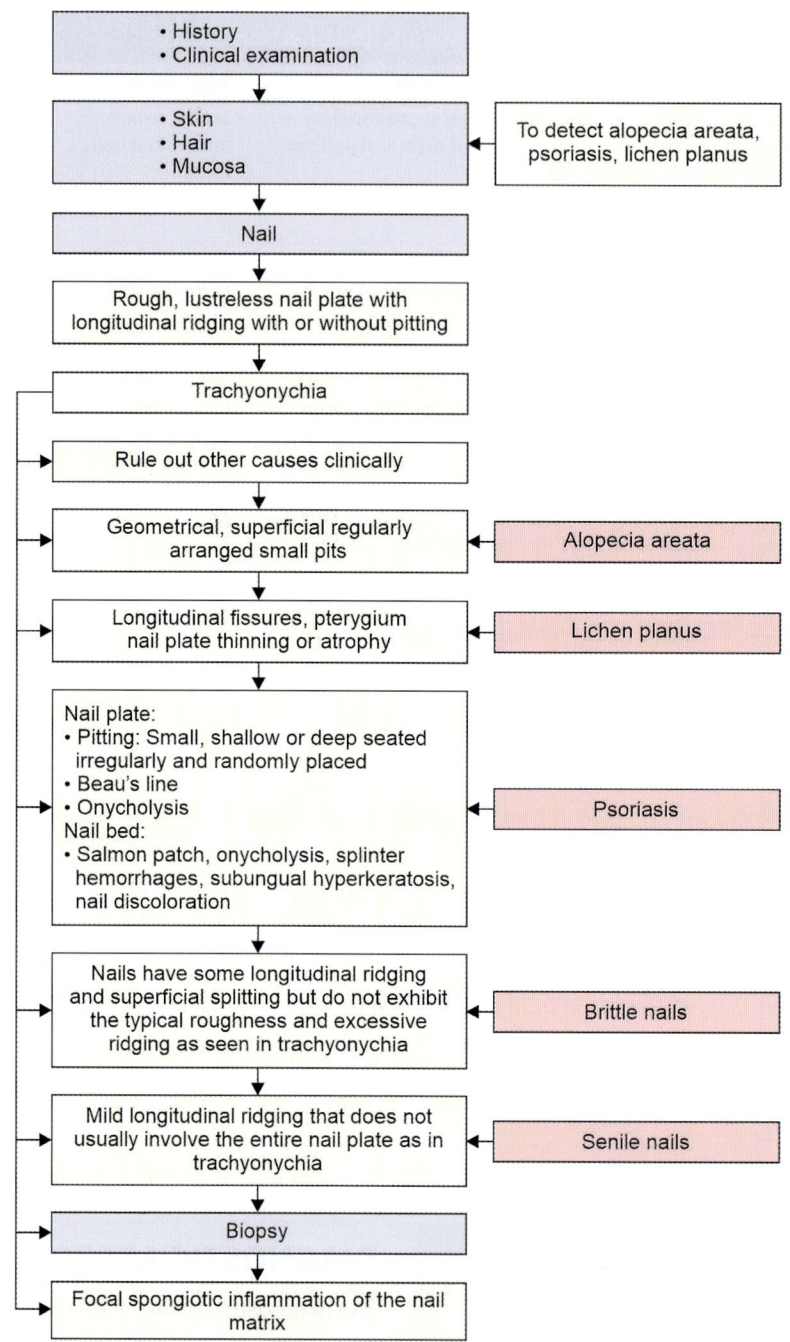

FLOWCHART 1: Diagnostic approach of trachyonychia.

differentiation or decreasing the inflammation in nail fold or matrix.

Topical Treatments

Topical treatments (mentioned in **Table 5**) are generally used for mild disease in nail psoriasis if it is limited to one or two digits or if it the only manifestation of the disease and in children. Systemic treatment can be started according to patient's preference to target the underlying disease, involvement of many nails and should be carefully decided in regard to risk factors.

Systemic Therapy[1,2,13-16]

Systemic therapy can be used for severe involvement and in those associated with underlying diseases such as psoriasis or lichen planus. It is given in **Table 6**.

Table 5: Topical treatments.[1,7]		
Drug	*Frequency and dose*	**Duration**
Calcipotriol/betamethasone dipropionate ointment	Once daily to the proximal nail fold	6 months
Topical Psoralen plus Psoralen plus ultraviolet A (PUVA)	0.7–1.4 J/cm^2 three times a week	7 months
Topical 5-fluorouracil 5% cream	Short contact application from alternate day to once a week	2–3 months
Topical tazarotene 1% gel	HS	3 months
Nail plate dressing*	Weekly	3–6 months
Emollients and camouflage with nail polish		
Intralesional triamcinolone acetonide	2.5–10 mg/mL weekly (intramatricial) into the proximal nail fold	2–3 months
Intralesional methotrexate	2.5 mg/mL intramatricial in each affected nail once a month	3 months

* Ultrathin adhesive bandage with lactic acid, silicon dioxide, aluminum acetylacetonate, azelaic acid, and copolymer of vinyl acetate with acrylic acid.

Table 6: Systemic therapy.		
Drug	*Frequency and dose*	**Duration**
Cyclosporine	2.5–3 mg/kg/day	8–24 months
Betamethasone	4 mg twice a week	1–2 months
Acitretin	0.3 mg/kg oral	3 months
Biotin	20 mg/day	
Methotrexate	5 mg/week then 7.5–25 mg	3 months
Chloroquine phosphate	250 mg twice a day	6 months
Triamcinolone acetonide	0.5–1 mg/kg/month intramuscular	4 months
Vitamin A	30,000 units/day	4 months
Tofacitinib	5 mg twice daily	10 months

REFERENCES

1. Gordon KA, Vega JM, Tosti A. Trachyonychia: A comprehensive review. Indian J Dermatol Venereol Leprol. 2011;77:640-5.
2. Tosti A, Piraccini BM, Iorizzo, M. Trachyonychia and related disorders: evaluation and treatment plans. Dermatol Ther. 2002;15(2):121-5.
3. Scheinfeld NS. Trachyonychia: a case report and review of manifestations, associations, and treatments. Cutis. 2003;71(4):299-302.
4. Leung AKC, Leong KF, Barankin B. Trachyonychia. J Pediatr. 2020;216:239-9.
5. Sehgal VN. Twenty nail dystrophy trachyonychia: an overview. J Dermatol. 2007;34(6):361-6.
6. Jacobsen AA, Tosti A. Trachyonychia. In: Rubin AI, Jellinek NJ, Daniel CR, Scher RK (Eds). Scher and Daniel's Nails: Diagnosis, Surgery, Therapy. Switzerland: Springer, Cham; 2018. pp. 145-51.
7. Jacobsen AA, Tosti A. Trachyonychia and Twenty-Nail Dystrophy: A Comprehensive Review and Discussion of Diagnostic Accuracy. Skin Appendage Disord. 2016;2:7-13.
8. Alessandrini A, Starace M, Piraccini BM. Dermoscopy in the Evaluation of Nail Disorders. Skin Appendage Disord. 2047;3(2):70-82.
9. Grover C, Jakhar D. Onychoscopy: A practical guide. Indian J Dermatol Venereol Leprol. 2017;83:536-49.
10. Anggowarsito JL, Kandou RT. (2014). Trachyonychia associated with alopecia areata and secondary onychomycosis. J Biomedik. 2014;6(1):50-9.
11. Haber JS, Chairatchaneeboon M, Rubin AI. Trachyonychia: Review and Update on Clinical Aspects, Histology, and Therapy. Skin Appendage Disord. 2017;2(3-4):109-15.
12. Ferreira SB, Scheinberg M, Steiner D, Steiner T, Bedin GL, Ferreira RB. Remarkable Improvement of Nail Changes in Alopecia Areata Universalis with 10 Months of Treatment with Tofacitinib: A Case Report. Case Rep Dermatol. 2016;8:262-6.
13. Kumar MG, Ciliberto H, Bayliss SJ. Long-term follow-up of pediatric trachyonychia. Pediatr Dermatol. 2015;32(2):198-200.
14. McClanahan DR, English JC 3rd. Therapeutics for Adult Nail Psoriasis and Nail Lichen Planus: A Guide for Clinicians. Am J Clin Dermatol. 2018;19:559-84.
15. Sarıcaoglu H, Oz A, Turan H. Nail psoriasis successfully treated with intralesional methotrexate: case report. Dermatology. 2011;222(1):5-7.
16. Mokni S, Ameur K, Ghariani N, Sriha B, Belajouza V, Denguezli M, et al. A Case of Nail Psoriasis Successfully Treated with Intralesional Methotrexate. Dermatol Ther (Heidelb). 2018;8(4):647-51.

10

A Case of Hirsutism

Vidya Kuntoji, Jagadish P

INTRODUCTION

Hirsutism is a common clinical condition characterized by presence of terminal hair at body sites under androgenic influence. These sites include face, chest, abdomen, upper thigh, back, and areole. The prevalence of hirsutism in among reproductive-age women in the general population is 5–10%.[1,2] It can be cosmetically and socially embarrassing and can cause significant psychological distress. The term "patient important hirsutism" refers to hair growth that causes distress in the absence of an abnormal hirsutism score. It emphasizes the patient's perception of the severity of the condition and the importance of taking patient preference into consideration when decision is made to initiate treatment.[2] Hirsutism differs from hypertrichosis in that excessive hair growth, terminal or vellus hair is seen in nonandrogen-dependent areas of the body.

ETIOPATHOGENESIS

The interaction between the circulating androgens and the apparent sensitivity of the hair follicle to androgens plays a vital role in the causation of hirsutism.

Androgens majorly influence the type and pattern of distribution of hair over the human body. During puberty, the physiological increase in androgen levels induces vellus follicles in sex-specific areas to develop into terminal hairs, which are larger and more heavily pigmented. They also act on pilosebaceous unit and cause increase in sebum secretion and thereby increased oiliness of skin and hair. Their paradoxical effects on body and scalp hair include prolongation of anagen phase in the former and shortening in the latter.[3-5]

Excess androgen levels from ovarian and/or adrenal disorders and/or increased sensitivity of hair follicle to the circulating androgens lead to increased terminal hair growth in most androgen-sensitive sites. The sensitivity of the hair follicle is determined in part by the local metabolism of androgens, particularly by conversion of testosterone to dihydrotestosterone (DHT) by the enzyme 5α-reductase and subsequent binding of these molecules to the androgen receptor. Although androgen excess is seen in most cases of hirsutism, due to variability in the pilosebaceous unit androgen metabolism and expression of androgen receptor, there is a lack of clear correlation between serum androgens and hirsutism.[3,6]

CAUSES (TABLES 1 AND 2)[3,7-18]

Table 1: Causes of hirsutism.	
Ovarian	- Polycystic ovarian syndrome - Stromal hyperthecosis - Ovarian tumors (thecal cell tumors, Leydig cell tumors, luteoma of pregnancy, hilar cell tumors, arrhenoblastomas)
Adrenal	*Congenital adrenal hyperplasia*: - Classical (early onset) - Nonclassical (late onset) *Cushing's syndrome* *Adrenal tumors*: - Adenoma - Carcinoma
Idiopathic	
Iatrogenic	*Cyclosporine*: - Testosterone injections, creams, patches - Progestins - Diazoxide - Danazol - Glucocorticoids - Anabolic steroids
Others	- Pituitary adenoma - Acromegaly - Hyperprolactinemia - Thyroid disorders - HAIR-AN syndrome
(HAIR-AN: hyperandrogenic insulin-resistant-acanthosis nigricans)	

Table 2: Causes explained with diagnostic workup.		
Causes of hirsutism	**Important points in history taking and examination**	**Laboratory workup**
PCOS (70% cases) Diagnostic criteria as per revised Rotterdam criteria 2003 (two out of three required): 1. Clinical and/or biochemical hyperandrogenism 2. Oligo-/amenorrhea, anovulation	- Menstrual dysfunction - Infertility - Pelvic pain - Hirsutism - Obesity - Family history of PCOS	- Normal or slightly elevated androgen levels - Fasting glucose, insulin may be elevated, lipid profile may be deranged - Polycystic ovarian morphology on USG Polycystic ovarian morphology on ultrasonography (USG). Features include: 1. *Increased follicle number per ovary (FNPO)*: Usually ≥20 (as per the recent international PCOS consensus statement. The initial Rotterdam recommendation was ≥12 follicles per ovary) 2. Individual follicles are generally similar in size and measure 2–9 mm in diameter 3. Peripheral distribution of follicles; this can give a "string of pearls" appearance 4. Background ovarian enlargement (volume >10 mL) 5. Central stromal brightness +/- prominence [increased ovarian stromal area to total ovarian area (S/A) ratio]

Continued

Continued

Causes of hirsutism	Important points in history taking and examination	Laboratory workup
		• Transvaginal USG is considered the gold standard. The features may affect either one or both ovaries. If a dominant follicle (>10 mm) or corpus luteum is detected, the scan should be repeated during the next cycle
3. Polycystic ovaries appearance on ultrasound (USG) 4. Phenotypes of PCOS (explained in **Table 3**)	• Acanthosis nigricans • Skin tags • Acne • Female pattern hair loss	• *Increase in serum anti-Mullerian hormone (AMH)*: AMH, a member of transforming growth factor (TGF) β family, is expressed by preantral and small antral follicles in the ovaries. Its levels correlate with the number of antral follicles. The levels of AMH are 2–4 times higher in women with PCOS. A serum AMH threshold to diagnose PCOS is not yet defined, but a value of 35 pmol/L or 4.9 ng/mL using the enzyme immunoassay (AMH-EIA) has been proposed
• Idiopathic hirsutism • Increased sensitivity of pilosebaceous unit to circulating androgens, overactive 5α-reductase activity is implicated	• Hirsutism • Normal menstrual cycle • No other symptoms and signs	Normal androgen levels, normal ovarian morphology
Nonclassic or late onset congenital adrenal hyperplasia (21-hydroxylase deficient)	• High-risk ethnic group (Ashkenazi Jews, Mediterranean, Middle Eastern, Indian populations) • Family history of adrenal hyperplasia • Infertility • Menstrual dysfunction • Androgenetic alopecia	• Screening for congenital adrenal hyperplasia should be done in hirsute patients with a positive family history, member of a high-risk ethnic group by measuring early morning 17-hydroxyprogesterone levels in the follicular phase or on a random day for those with amenorrhea or infrequent menses • Elevated 17-hydroxyprogesterone level before and after corticotropin stimulation test
Androgen-secreting tumors	• Palpable abdominal or pelvic mass • Progression of hirsutism despite treatment • Rapid onset of hirsutism • Indolent course if there are small masses • Virilization (clitoromegaly, increases muscularity, deepened voice)	• Elevated testosterone and DHEAS • Ultrasound and MRI for ovarian imaging; CT and MRI for adrenal imaging
Iatrogenic hirsutism	• History of anabolic-androgenic steroid use • Use of topical testosterone in a partner (testosterone gels offer an invisible and convenient mode of transdermal testosterone therapy for men. The recommended application sites are abdomen, shoulders, upper arms, and inner thighs) • Use of valproic acid	Elevated testosterone
Cushing syndrome	• Acne • Central obesity • Hypertension • Moon facies • Proximal muscle weakness • Purple skin striae	• Elevated 24-hour urine free cortisol level • Impaired glucose tolerance

Continued

Causes of hirsutism	Important points in history taking and examination	Laboratory workup
Hyperprolactinemia	• Amenorrhea • Galactorrhea	Elevated prolactin levels
Thyroid disorders	• Menstrual dysfunction • Hypothyroidism • Weight gain, fatigue, cold intolerance, difficulty concentration, dry skin, hair loss, myxedema	Elevated TSH levels
Acromegaly	• Coarse facial features • Deepened voice • Enlargement of nose and ears • Frontal bossing • Hyperhidrosis • Increased hand and foot size • Mandibular enlargement with increased interdental spacing	Elevated IGF-1 levels
Hyperandrogenic insulin-resistant acanthosis nigricans (HAIR-AN)	• Acanthosis nigricans • Obesity • Hypertension • Hyperlipidemia • Diabetes • Hirsutism	Elevated fasting glucose and fasting insulin, deranged lipid profile

(CT: computed tomography; DHEAS: dehydroepiandrosterone sulfate; IGF-1: insulin-like growth factor 1; MRI: magnetic resonance imaging; PCOS: polycystic ovary syndrome; TSH: thyroid-stimulating hormone)

Table 3: Phenotypes of PCOS.[19,20]

Type	Description
Frank or classic polycystic ovary syndrome (PCOS) (Phenotype A)	Chronic anovulation, hyperandrogenism, polycystic ovaries
Classic non-PCOS (Phenotype B)	Chronic anovulation, hyperandrogenism, normal ovaries
Nonclassic ovulatory PCOS (Phenotype C)	Regular menstrual cycles, hyperandrogenism, polycystic ovaries
Nonclassic mild or normoandrogenic PCOS (Phenotype D)	Chronic anovulation, normal androgens, polycystic ovaries

CLINICAL FEATURES (FIGS. 1A AND B)[2,5,7]

Hirsutism is a clinical diagnosis. Modified Ferriman Gallwey score is the standard method used in the assessment of hirsutism. Increased hair growth is assessed at nine sites (upper lip, chin, chest, upper back, lower back, upper abdomen, lower abdomen, arms, and thighs). Each area is graded from 0 to 4. Minimum score is zero and maximum is 36. A score of 8 or greater is considered as hirsutism; however, there is ethnic variation (2–7 or greater is considered hirsute in Asian women depending on ethnicity, and 9–10 or greater in Hispanic and Middle eastern women). The severity of hirsutism is graded as follows: mild 8–16, moderate 17–25, and severe >25.

Drawbacks of the Score
- Variation in hair growth between different ethnic groups
- Failure to account for regional hirsutism
- Prior use of cosmetic measures such as chemical depilatories, electrolysis, and laser is not considered.

EVALUATION

The main aim of evaluation is to identify the cause of hirsutism and to recommend the right treatment based on the etiological factor.

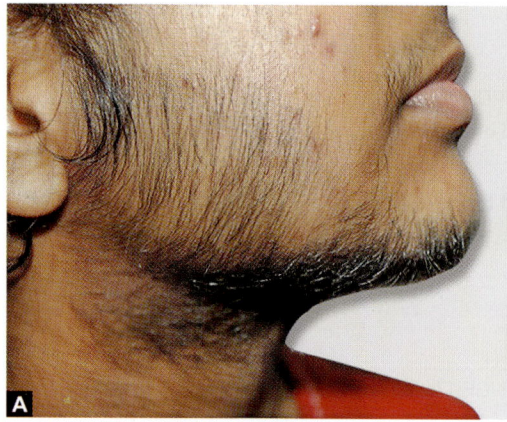
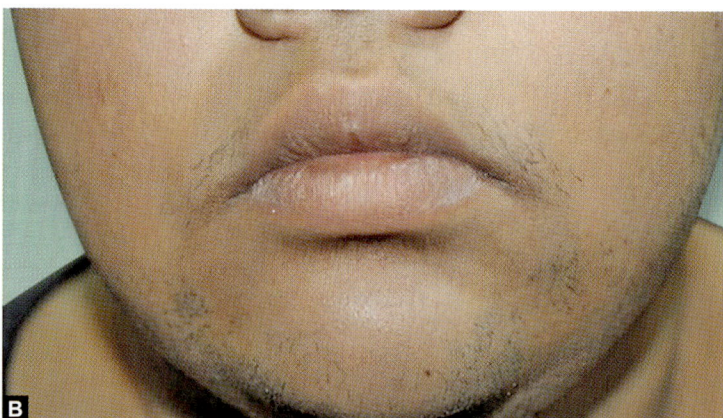

FIGS. 1A AND B: Hirsutism.

History (Table 4)[1,13]

Table 4: Points to be noted in history taking and their relevance.	
Age of onset	Age younger than 35 years increases the relative probability of PCOS, whereas age older than 35 years slightly increases tumor risk
Duration and rate of onset of symptoms and progression	Recent onset, rapid development of hirsutism, onset later in life rather than near puberty, progression despite therapy indicate androgen secreting tumor
Menstrual history—frequency and duration	Oligomenorrhea is usually seen in PCOS, nonclassic adrenal hyperplasia, hyperprolactinemia, hypothyroidism, acromegaly
Symptoms or signs of virilization—deepening of voice, acne, increased muscle mass, infrequent menstruation, male pattern hair loss, loss of breast tissue or loss of female body contour, increased libido, clitoromegaly	Suspect androgen secreting tumors
Timing and progression of weight gain in cases of obesity, history of diabetes mellitus, hypertension	To evaluate for metabolic syndrome
Medication use	• Off label use of anabolic or androgenic steroids especially among athletes, patients with endometriosis, sexual dysfunction, use of topical testosterone gel by partner • Use of anticonvulsants like valproic acid (raises plasma testosterone levels)

Continued

Continued

History of shaving, laser hair removal/electrolysis, and medical treatment of hirsutism	For the assessment of severity (grading) of hirsutism
History of hirsutism, acne, polycystic ovary syndrome (PCOS), obesity, infertility in family members	

PHYSICAL EXAMINATION (TABLE 5)[1,12,13]

Table 5: Points to be noted in physical examination and their relevance.	
Distribution of hair: Ascertain whether the coarse hairs are localized in male distribution or there is generalized increase in growth of the hair on all of the body	To differentiate between hirsutism and hypertrichosis
Calculation of body mass index (BMI)	Evaluation of associated cardiovascular risk factors, hypothyroidism, Cushing syndrome
Measurement of blood pressure	Evaluation of associated cardiovascular risk factors, Cushing syndrome
Acne, hirsutism, seborrhea, acne, female pattern hair loss	Cutaneous signs of hyperandrogenism
Hypertension, obesity, centripetal fat distribution, skin tags, acanthosis nigricans	Signs of insulin resistance
Thinning of skin, rounding of face, dorsal fat pad, abdominal striae, easy bruising	Features of Cushing's syndrome
Increased muscle mass, male pattern hair loss, loss of breast tissue, loss of female body contour, clitoromegaly	Features of virilization, virilizing tumors
Abdominal and pelvic examination	Pelvic mass (tumors)

BIOCHEMICAL TESTS[3,7]

Preliminary Tests

- *Total testosterone*: Testosterone is the key androgen to measure because it is the major circulating androgen. Levels >200 ng/dL is suggestive of tumor.
- *Free testosterone*: It is more specific marker than total testosterone as its levels can be elevated in conditions with normal total testosterone with equivocal or severe hyperandrogenism.
- Luteinizing hormone/follicle-stimulating hormone (LH/FSH) ratio >3 is indicative of PCOS.
- *Thyroid-stimulating hormone (TSH)*: It is tested in all potential cases of PCOS. Levels >4.5 mU/L suggests hypothyroidism. Hypophyseal hypothyroidism can act as a cofactor in hirsutism causing raised TSH.
- *Prolactin*: It is done in all potential cases of PCOS. Levels >20 ng/mL suggests hyperprolactinemia. Prolactin would be raised in hyperprolactinemia due to hypothalamic disease or a pituitary tumor.
- *17-hydroxyprogesterone*: A basal 17-hydroxyprogesterone value of 200 ng/dL is approximately 95% sensitive and 90% specific for nonclassic congenital adrenal hyperplasia (NCCAH). Mildly increased levels between 300 and 1,000 ng/dL require an adrenocorticotropic hormone (ACTH) stimulation test. Cosyntropin (synthetic ACTH), 250 µg, is administered intravenously, and levels of 17-hydroxyprogesterone are measured before and 1 hour after the injection. Poststimulation values (>1,000 ng/dL) constitute a positive test.
- Dehydroepiandrosterone sulfate (DHEAS) severe elevation (>700 µg/dL) suggests possible tumor. Imaging is advised in postmenopausal women with levels >400 µg/dL.
- *Lipid profile*: Total cholesterol, high-density lipoprotein (HDL), low-density lipoprotein (LDL), and triglycerides and oral glucose tolerance test. They are tested to assess associated metabolic risk.

Additional Tests

- *Sex hormone-binding globulin (SHBG)*: Low levels suggest hyperandrogenemia. The test is indicated in conditions with normal total testosterone with either equivocal or severe clinical hyperandrogenism. Low SHBG itself is a useful marker for the insulin resistance that underlies the metabolic risks common in PCOS.
- *Luteal phase—progesterone*: It is tested to detect anovulation in potential eumenorrheic cases of PCOS.
- *Androstenedione*: It may be a more sensitive indicator of PCOS-related androgen excess than total testosterone.
- Cushing syndrome test (24-h urine cortisol, late night salivary cortisol, or dexamethasone suppression test).
- *Urine testosterone/epitestosterone ratio*: It is indicated in exogenous testosterone use. Levels >6 is strongly suggestive.
- *Insulin-like growth factor 1 (IGF-1)*: Elevated levels suggest acromegaly.

IMAGING[5]

- Pelvic ultrasonography for diagnosis of PCOS
- Ovarian and adrenal imaging in the evaluation of tumors. A pelvic ultrasound is indicated in women with a suspected ovarian androgen-secreting tumor. Ultrasound and magnetic resonance imaging (MRI) for ovarian imaging; computed tomography (CT), and MRI for adrenal imaging. CT of the adrenals is recommended for women with a suspected adrenal tumor with significant elevation in testosterone levels.

TREATMENT[4,13,21-23]

Hirsutism can impact the psyche of the patient; counseling plays a pivotal role. Mild or moderate hirsutism does not always require treatment. However, the treatment should be tailor made and given due consideration for treatment in case of "patient-important hirsutism". Patient should be educated about the cause of the disorder and the available treatment options and the long duration of treatment. It should be emphasized that the response of the treatment will be seen after several months. Regular follow-up with Ferriman–Gallwey score and photographic documentation should be done at successive visits.

Treatment Guidelines

- For women with mild hirsutism and no evidence of an endocrine disorder, either pharmacologic therapy or direct hair removal method is suggested as initial therapy.
- For patient important hirsutism, treatment should be started with pharmacologic therapy. Direct hair removal methods are suggested for those who desire additional cosmetic benefits.
- Lifestyle changes are recommended for hirsute women with obesity including those with PCOS.
- A trial of at least 6 months is suggested for all pharmacologic therapies for hirsutism before making changes in dose, switching to a new medication, or adding medication.
- Oral contraceptive pills are the first line of pharmacologic treatment in women who are not planning for pregnancy.
- For women with hirsutism at higher risk for venous thromboembolism, oral contraceptive pill containing lowest effective dose of ethinylestradiol (EE) (usually 20 mg) and low-risk progestin is suggested.

- Considering the teratogenic potential, antiandrogen monotherapy is best avoided as initial treatment. It should be considered in the following scenarios: patient is not sexually active, have undergone permanent sterilization, or using long-acting reversible contraception.

The mainstay of treatment includes lifestyle modifications, cosmetic methods of temporary hair removal, permanent methods of hair reduction (laser treatment, electrolysis), and medical therapy.

Lifestyle Modifications

Lifestyle modifications form the cornerstone in the treatment of PCOS. These include moderate exercise, dietary modification, avoidance of psychosocial stressors, cessation of smoking, moderation in caffeine, and alcohol consumption. Decrease in body weight in obese women regulates the menstrual cycle, improves fertility, reduces insulin and testosterone levels, decreases the degree of acne and hirsutism, and benefits psychological wellbeing.

Cosmetic Methods of Temporary Hair Removal

These include shaving, waxing, use of depilatory creams, plucking, threading, bleaching, and use of depilatory creams. Each method helps to get rid of unwanted hair, the effect lasting for a variable duration. The side effect profile includes irritation, discomfort/pain, itching, folliculitis, irritant dermatitis, and hyperpigmentation.

Permanent Methods of Hair Reduction

Permanent hair reduction is defined as attaining at least a 30% reduction of terminal hairs and sustaining this reduction for a period longer than the complete growth cycle of hair follicles (4–12 months, depending on body site). Laser treatment and electrolysis are the two methods of permanent methods of hair reduction.

Laser and Light Treatment

A thorough evaluation should be done through detailed history, clinical examination, and hormonal profile before starting treatment with lasers. An ideal patient for conventional laser hair removal is one who has thick, dark terminal hairs, light skin, and normal hormonal status.

Various lasers used in the treatment of hirsutism include Ruby (694 nm), alexandrite (755 nm), diode (800–1,000 nm), Q-switched and long-pulsed neodymium; yttrium-aluminum-garnet (Nd: YAG;1064 nm), and intense pulsed light sources (550–1,200 nm). Long-pulsed Nd: YAG laser is preferred as safe treatment option for dark skinned individuals with the Fitzpatrick skin type III-VI.

Side effects: Burns, blistering, hyperpigmentation, hypopigmentation, and/or scarring, paradoxical hypertrichosis.

Electrolysis

It is the most effective and permanent method of hair removal. There are three types: galvanic (direct current) electrolysis, thermolysis (alternating current) and combination/blend method and the procedure involves placing a fine needle into the hair follicle and dermal papilla and applying the electric current to destroy and prevent regrowth of hair follicles. Each follicle is treated individually.

The disadvantage of electrolysis is difficult to treat large areas like hair on the chest or upper back and it can be time consuming.

Side effects: Pain, scarring/keloid formation in susceptible patients, post inflammatory hypopigmentation or hyperpigmentation.

Pharmacologic Treatment

Oral Contraceptives

Combined oral contraceptives should be used as initial therapy for hirsutism in women who are not planning for pregnancy. The estrogen most used is EE, while the progestin component varies.

Mechanism of action

- Suppression of LH secretion, thereby suppressing ovarian androgen secretion
- Stimulation of hepatic production of SHBG, thereby increasing androgen binding in serum and reducing circulating free testosterone and subsequent activation of androgen receptors
- Inhibition of 5α-reductase activity in the pilosebaceous unit, thereby decreasing peripheral conversion of testosterone to the more potent androgen DHT

Dosage: EE0.035 mg, CPA 2 mg, EE0.03 mg-drospirenone 3 mg, EE0.035 mg-norgestimate 0.25 mg, EE0.02 mg-desogestrel 0.15 mg.

Side effects: Nausea, vomiting, bloating, breast tenderness, spotting between menstrual periods, weight gain, and increased risk of thromboembolism.

Spironolactone

Spironolactone is a synthetic mineralocorticoid and aldosterone receptor antagonist.

Mechanism of action

- It competes with testosterone and DHT for androgen receptor binding
- Spironolactone also destroys a cofactor of cytochrome p450 necessary for testosterone synthesis
- It increases SHBG levels, and reduces 5α-reductase activity

Dosage: 50 mg twice a day, which is then increased to 100 mg twice daily if needed.

Side effects: Spironolactone is generally well-tolerated; side effects are dose related.
- Menstrual irregularities
- Breast tenderness
- Decreased libido in women
- Diuresis, headache, and dizziness
- Hyperkalemia and hyponatremia because it is a potassium-sparing diuretic.

Spironolactone should not be given to women who are currently or planning to become pregnant because of its potential risk of feminization of a male fetus.

Finasteride

Finasteride is a 5α-reductase inhibitor that prevents the conversion of testosterone to DHT. Finasteride competitively inhibits 5α-reductase isoenzyme type II, which is found in reproductive tissues.

Dosage: 5 mg/day, although few studies suggest 7.5 mg/day may be more effective.

Side effects: Headaches, depression, nausea, hot flashes, decreased libido, and reduced intensity of orgasm.

Finasteride is contraindicated in women who are currently pregnant or trying to conceive.

Flutamide

Flutamide is a nonsteroidal antiandrogen. It antagonizes the androgen receptor to which testosterone and DHT bind.

Dosage: It varies from 250 to 750 mg per day, 500 mg/day being the most common dose. Studies have also shown doses as low as 62.5–250 mg may also be effective in the management of hirsutism.

Side effects: It is associated with hepatotoxicity, which may be dose dependent. It is not recommended as first-line therapy and the lowest effective dose should be used with careful monitoring of liver function.

Cyproterone Acetate

It is derivative of 17-hydroxyprogesterone acetate and has strong progestogenic effects. *Mechanism of action*: It mainly inhibits androgen receptor and to a lesser degree inhibits 5α-reductase activity. It also suppresses serum gonadotropin (LH), thereby leading to decrease in circulating androgens.

Dosage: It is used at a low dose of 2 mg as the progestin part of combination oral contraceptives, or at a higher dose of 12.5–100 mg/day as monotherapy.

Insulin Sensitizers

Reducing insulin levels pharmacologically attenuates hyperandrogenemia. Metformin, an insulin lowering drug, has been used in women with PCOS, including hirsutism. It is considered an insulin sensitizer since it lowers glucose levels without increasing insulin secretion. In women with PCOS, metformin administered at doses of up to 1500 mg/day decreases insulin, testosterone and LH levels and it also appears to favor some weight loss. Thiazolidinediones are other less commonly used insulin sensitizers compared to Metformin. In the absence of metabolic disturbances, the role of insulin sensitizers is controversial.

Gonadotropin-releasing Hormone Agonists

They are mainly used in women with severe forms of hyperandrogenemia such as ovarian hyperthecosis, who have a suboptimal response to oral contraceptives and antiandrogens inhibit gonadotropins and decrease ovarian androgen production leading to decreased hirsutism but also lower estrogen levels. They are usually used in conjunction with low-dose estrogen progestin pills to eliminate the effects of estrogen deficiency.

Dose: Leuprolide injection 3.75 mg monthly

Side effects: Menopausal symptoms (hot flashes, bone loss)

Steroids

Glucocorticoids are usually used long term in women with classic adrenal hyperplasia due to 21-hydroxylase deficiency. They suppress adrenal androgen production and control hirsutism, while maintaining ovulatory cycles.

In NCCAH, the mainstay of treatment includes oral contraceptives and/or antiandrogens. Glucocorticoids are used for ovulation induction and not very effective in the management of hirsutism, although they are used when there is suboptimal response or intolerance to oral contraceptives and antiandrogens.

Dosage: In the management of hirsutism, 4–6 mg daily. For ovulation induction, 5–7.5 mg is used.

Side effects: Weight gain, increased blood pressure, cushingoid striae, adrenal atrophy, and decreased bone mineral density.

Topical Treatment

Eflornithine hydrochloride 13.9% is a topical preparation that inhibits hair growth by irreversibly inhibiting ornithine decarboxylase. It does not remove hair, but rather slows hair growth. It can be used alone or in conjunction with other therapies in women who desire a more rapid initial response.

Side effects: Irritation, itching, and folliculitis.

REFERENCES

1. Chhabra S, Gautam RK, Kulshreshtha B, Prasad A, Sharma N. Hirsutism. A Clinico-investigative Study. Int J Trichology. 2012; 4(4):246-50.
2. Mimoto MS, Oyler JL, Davis AM. Evaluation and Treatment of Hirsutism in Premenopausal Women. JAMA. 2018;319(15): 1613-4.
3. Screening and Management of the Hyperandrogenic Adolescent: ACOG Committee Opinion, Number 789. Obstet Gynecol. 2019;134(4):e106-e114.
4. Martin KA, Anderson RR, Chang RJ, Ehrmann DA, Lobo RA, Murad MH, et al. Evaluation and Treatment of Hirsutism in Premenopausal Women: An Endocrine Society Clinical Practice Guideline. J Clin Endocrinol Metab. 2018;103(4):1233-57.
5. Mihailidis J, Dermesropian R, Taxel P, Luthra P, Grant-Kels JM. Endocrine evaluation of hirsutism. Int J Womens Dermatol. 2015;1(2):90-4.
6. Schmidt TH, Shinkai K. Evidence-based approach to cutaneous hyperandrogenism in women. J Am Acad Dermatol. 2015;73(4): 672-90.
7. Mahajan VK, Chauhan PS, Chandel M, Mehta KS, Singh VK, Sharma A, et al. Clinico-investigative attributes of 122 patients with hirsutism: A 5-year retrospective study from India. Int J Womens Dermatol. 2020;7(3):237-42.
8. Ilagan MKCC, Paz-Pacheco E, Totesora DZ, Clemente-Chua LR, Jalique JRK. The Modified Ferriman-Gallwey Score and Hirsutism among Filipino Women. Endocrinol Metab (Seoul). 2019;34(4):374-81.
9. Moolhuijsen LM, Visser JA. AMH in PCOS: Controlling the ovary, placenta, or brain? Curr Opin Endocr Metab Res. 2020;12:91-7.
10. Toosy S, Sodi R, Pappachan JM. Lean polycystic ovary syndrome (PCOS): an evidence-based practical approach. J Diabetes Metab Disord. 2018;17(2):277-85.
11. Cuhaci N, Aydın C, Yesilyurt A, Pınarlı FA, Ersoy R, Cakir B. Nonclassical Congenital Adrenal Hyperplasia and Pregnancy. Case Rep Endocrinol. 2015;2015:296924.
12. Curran DR, Moore C, Huber T. Clinical inquiries. What is the best approach to the evaluation of hirsutism? J Fam Pract. 2005;54(5):465-7.
13. Matheson E, Bain J. Hirsutism in Women. Am Fam Physician. 2019;100(3):168-75.
14. de Ronde W. Hyperandrogenism after transfer of topical testosterone gel: case report and review of published and unpublished studies. Hum Reprod. 2009;24(2):425-8.
15. Teede H, Misso M, Costello M, Dokras A, Laven J, et al. International evidence based guideline for the assessment and management of polycystic ovary syndrome. Melbourne. Updated Feb 2018. Available from: PCOS_Evidence-Based-Guidelines_20181009.pdf (monash.edu)
16. Barber TM, Alvey C, Greenslade T, Gooding M, Barber D, Smith R, et al. Patterns of Ovarian Morphology in Polycystic Ovary Syndrome: A Study Utilising Magnetic Resonance Imaging. Eur Radiol. 2010;20(5):1207-13.
17. Fulghesu A, Canu E, Casula L, Melis F, Gambineri A. Polycystic Ovarian Morphology in Normocyclic Non-Hyperandrogenic Adolescents. J Pediatr Adolesc Gynecol. 2021;34(5):610-6.
18. Radswiki T, Weerakkody Y, Knipe H, et al. Polycystic ovaries. Reference article, Radiopaedia.org (Accessed on 23 Nov 2022) https://doi.org/10.53347/rID-14971.
19. El Hayek S, Bitar L, Hamdar LH, Mirza FG, Daoud G. Poly Cystic Ovarian Syndrome: An Updated Overview. Front Physiol. 2016;7:124.
20. Mumusoglu S, Yildiz BO. Polycystic ovary syndrome phenotypes and prevalence: Differential impact of diagnostic criteria and clinical versus unselected population. Curr Opin Endocr and Metab Res. 2020;12:66-71.
21. Bhat YJ, Bashir S, Nabi N, Hassan I. Laser Treatment in Hirsutism: An Update. Dermatology practical and conceptual. 2020;10(2), e2020048. https://doi.org/10.5826/dpc.1002a48.
22. Azarchi S, Bienenfeld A, Lo Sicco K, Marchbein S, Shapiro J, Nagler AR. Androgens in women: Hormone-modulating therapies for skin disease. J Am Acad Dermatol. 2019;6: 1509-21.
23. Kang CN, Shah M, Lynde C, Fleming P. Hair Removal Practices: A Literature Review. Skin Therapy Lett. 2021;26(5):6-11.

A Patient with Diffuse Hair Loss

Smita Nagpal, Neha Sharma

INTRODUCTION

Hair is an integral part of one's external appearance and is essentially important for self-confidence in terms of an individual's esthetic appeal. Diffuse hair loss is seen affecting majority of the scalp for most of the patients. In today's times, especially since coronavirus disease 2019 (COVID-19) hit our lives, there has been a significant surge in the number of cases with diffuse hair loss. As a dermatologist, we should be able to diagnose the patients clinically, and if needed, we should not hesitate from advising investigations, so that we can help our patients in the best possible way. **Box 1** shows the possible differential diagnoses of diffuse hair loss.

APPROACH TO A PATIENT WITH DIFFUSE HAIR LOSS

The outcome of the patient's visit to the doctor depends upon the protocols that a physician follows regarding the management of the case of diffuse hair loss. Ideally, the focus should be upon establishing a diagnosis after a thorough clinical examination aided by few bedside tests and laboratory investigations. This should be followed by treatment targeted toward the etiological factors apart from a relevant lifestyle modification.

TELOGEN EFFLUVIUM

A diffuse, nonscarring shedding of hair is the most prominent characteristic of telogen effluvium.[2] It is very frequently encountered by the dermatologists in their clinical practice. It could be triggered by various chemical, physical, and mental causes.[3] One can classify this kind of hair loss as acute or chronic telogen effluvium (CTE). A hair shedding continuously for <6 months signifies acute type. After the trigger exposure, hair fall starts in 2–3 months. In approximately one-third of the cases, the reason is still unknown.[4] Overall, in Indian set up, nutritional deficiency remains major cause of telogen effluvium or diffuse hair loss in females closely followed by female pattern hair loss (FPHL). While in males other causes prevail. The detailed causes of telogen effluvium are enumerated in **Table 1**.

ANAGEN EFFLUVIUM

Anagen effluvium is the sudden loss of hair that are in their growth phase as a result of a trigger that hampers the mitotic or multiplying potential of the hair follicle.[7] It is frequently encountered in radiotherapy patients treated for head and neck cancers or chemotherapy with drugs such as antimetabolites, alkylating agents, and mitotic inhibitors.[3,8] Such drugs can damage or halt the anagen cycle and lead to follicle dystrophy. As majority of scalp hair are in the anagen phase, a huge number of hair start to shed. Patients with

---

Box 1: Differential diagnosis of diffuse hair loss.[1]

- Telogen effluvium (TE)
- Diffuse type of female pattern hair loss (FPHL)
- Chronic telogen effluvium (CTE)
- Anagen effluvium/loose anagen syndrome
- Diffuse type of alopecia areata
- Congenital atrichia
- Congenital hypotrichosis
- Hair shaft abnormalities

Table 1: Possible etiologies of acute and chronic telogen effluvium.			
Telogen effluvium			
Acute telogen effluvium (6 months duration)[5]			Chronic telogen effluvium (>6 months duration)
Physiological causes	***Pathological causes***		• No attributable causes/illnesses
Hair shedding in the new born	• Post febrile • Endocrinopathies • Severe infection • Stress • Severe chronic illness • Drugs • Severe prolonged psychological stress • Deficiency of iron, riboflavin, folate, vitamin B12, biotin • Postsurgical • Ultraviolet rays		• The disorder mostly affects middle-aged women, having a prolonged fluctuating course. The examination of the scalp shows hair having normal thickness with signs of shorter regrowing hair in the frontal and bitemporal areas
Postpartum hair shedding—telogen gravidarum occurs approximately 3 months after childbirth[6]			

Table 2: Chemotherapeutic agents associated with anagen effluvium.	
Common dystrophic anagen effluvium	
Chemotherapy induced	
Commonly associated cytotoxic agents:	Uncommonly associated cytotoxic agents:
• Doxorubicin • Daunorubicin • Paclitaxel • Docetaxel • Cyclophosphamide • Etoposide • Ifosphamide • Bleomycin • Mechlorethamine	• Vincristine • Vinblastine • 5-fluorouracil • Hydroxyurea • Thiotepa

roughly one-tenth of their hair remaining after an insult are pretty much the cases of anagen effluvium.

For the purpose of classification, the anagen effluvium can be divided into common dystrophic anagen effluvium and loose anagen hair syndrome (LAHS).[9] The detailed causes are shown in **Table 2**.

Anagen effluvium is frequently encountered with chemotherapy and radiation to the head and neck[10,11] and less frequently with other triggers such as severe protein energy malnutrition, pemphigus vulgaris,[12] alopecia areata (AA),[13] and exposure to toxic agents like mercury,[14] boron,[15] thallium,[16] etc. Rare reasons behind anagen effluvium are bismuth, levodopa, colchicine, and cyclosporine. Systemic disorders such as systemic lupus erythematosus and secondary syphilis can cause anagen arrest by causing peribulbar inflammation.

LOOSE ANAGEN HAIR SYNDROME

The LAHS is a rare sporadic or autosomal dominant disorder with incomplete penetrance characterized by loosely anchored anagen hairs that can be comfortably and painlessly pulled from the roots. It is commonly observed in light-haired children, with a preponderance for females, with females affected six times more than the males in terms of number of patients. Occasionally, the disease could target adults.[17-19]

DIFFUSE ALOPECIA AREATA

Alopecia areata is a common cause of nonscarring hair loss that generally causes round patches of baldness on the scalp, or the whole scalp, or the entire body. In some patients, however, AA is characterized by a diffuse hair loss, commonly misdiagnosed as telogen effluvium or androgenetic alopecia. The two most common variants of nonpatchy AA are alopecia areata incognita (AAI) and diffuse alopecia areata (DAA). DAA is described as a unique AA that lacks the characteristic patches of AA and instead, demonstrates widespread scalp hair thinning.[20] This type of AA can at times be difficult to diagnose as it can easily be confused with other forms of nonscarring alopecia. However, mechanism leading to this abrupt and diffuse type of hair loss remains unclear. Both the types have been commonly reported in young females with later being more common. AAI is more commonly associated with androgenic alopecia. AAI involves occipital and parietal region while DAA involves anterior temporal and parietal region. Presence of pigtail sign on dermoscopy suggests diagnosis of AAI.[21,22]

DIFFUSE FEMALE PATTERN HAIR LOSS

Female pattern hair loss is a gradual onset, slowly progressive nonscarring alopecia, which can be seen any time after menarche, but is most common in females aged 20–40 years. It results from a progressive reduction of successive hair cycle time leading to miniaturization of hair follicles. These changes are mediated through interaction between androgens, their respective receptors and enzymes such as 5α reductase and p450 aromatase.[23,24] Androgens definitely take part in the pathogenesis of the androgenetic alopecia in males, but their role in female alopecia is less certain and needs further investigation.

Three types of FPHL patterns have been described **(Table 3)**.[25] The first two types are common and the third type is seen infrequently. The first type is often confused with CTE.

Total testosterone levels >200 ng/dL or dehydroepiandrosterone sulfate (DHEAS) (>2 × normal or >700 µg/dL in premenopausal and >400 µg/dL in menopausal women) should alert the physician about the possibility of androgen secreting tumor.[26]

HISTORY TAKING AND EXAMINATION

There are various clues in the history taking and examination that can guide us toward the final diagnosis. If these points are kept in mind, there is negligible chance of one missing the correct diagnosis.

The different points in history taking should include age and sex predilection, onset, duration and progress of the hair fall, associated symptoms, associated comorbidities, general examination, and local examination **(Tables 4 to 7)**.

Table 3: Types of female pattern hair loss.

Ludwig's type	Olsen type/frontal accentuation	Hamilton type
• Diffuse central thinning • Mild (stage I), moderate (stage II), or severe, that is, near-complete baldness of the crown (stage III) • Intact frontal hair line	Widening of central parting line and thereafter to Christmas-tree pattern	Frontotemporal recession/vertex loss

Table 4: Onset and progress of hair fall.

Acute telogen effluvium	Abrupt onset after 2–3 months triggering event, self-limiting within 6 months
Chronic telogen effluvium	Abrupt onset with no identifiable trigger, prolonged course of >6 months
Anagen effluvium	Abrupt onset 1–3 weeks after the inciting event, regrowth occurs after 2–3 months
Loose anagen syndrome	Gradually visible, in neonates and infants, improves during adulthood
Diffuse alopecia areata	Gradual onset, prolonged course
Alopecia areata incognito	Abrupt within weeks, unpredictable course
Diffuse female pattern hair loss	Gradual onset

Table 5: Associated findings/comorbidities in history taking.

Positive family history of hair loss	Female pattern hair loss, alopecia areata, male pattern baldness
History of thyroid disorders, chronic illness, weakness suggestive of anemia	Chronic telogen effluvium (CTE)/alopecia areata
Personal/family history of ischemic heart disease of prostrate cancer	Androgenetic alopecia in men
History of atopy and rough nails	Alopecia areata
Features of hyperandrogenism/metabolic syndrome, menstrual irregularities, hirsutism, acanthosis nigricans, weight gain	Female pattern hair loss
Recent chemotherapy in drug history	Anagen effluvium
Recent physical and emotional stress, any major medical or surgical illness	Telogen effluvium
Chronic illness, weakness suggestive of anemia	Telogen effluvium /CTE
Oral retinoids, especially etretinate and acitretin, high-dose contraceptive pills (OCPs) or hormone replacement therapy (HRT), antithyroids, anticoagulants (especially heparin), and anticonvulsants, hypolipidemic drugs, heavy metals in drug history	Telogen effluvium/anagen effluvium rarely
Dietary history suggestive of crash dieting	Telogen effluvium
Fever, joint pain, photosensitivity suggestive of autoimmune connective tissue disorders	Telogen effluvium/alopecia areata

Table 6: General examination findings.

Fever	Autoimmune connective tissue disorder (AICTD)	Telogen effluvium
Tachycardia	Anemia	Telogen effluvium
Hypertension	Cardiovascular disorders	Alopecia areata
Icterus	Hemolytic anemia, viral hepatitis	Telogen effluvium
Pallor	Anemia	Telogen effluvium
Pedal edema	Anemia	Telogen effluvium
Lymphadenopathy	Malignancy	Anagen effluvium
Malar rash	AICTD	Telogen effluvium
Terminal facial hair in females, acanthosis nigricans	Polycystic ovary syndrome (PCOS)	Female pattern hair loss
Neck swelling, excessive sleeping, dryness of skin, weight gain in hypothyroidism and weight loss in hyperthyroidism	Thyroid dysfunction	Telogen effluvium/Chronic telogen effluvium (CTE)

Table 7: Local examination of the scalp.

Etiology of diffuse hair loss	Site of involvement and type of hair loss	Number of hairs shed	Vellus hair	Hair pull test	Trichogram
Acute telogen effluvium	Diffuse thinning, hair coming out by roots	>100	<10%	+ throughout scalp	>25% telogen hair
Chronic telogen effluvium	Diffuse thinning, hair coming out by roots	<100	<10%	+ in active phase	Reduced A:T ratio
Anagen effluvium	Excessive shedding/hair breaking at scalp, affects a large percentage of the scalp with major thinning and hair loss	>80% hair are lost very quickly	<10%	+ in active phase	Anagen hair without sheath, bulb is often misshapen, ruffled cuticle
Loose anagen syndrome	Short blonde hair or sparse hair that does not grow long and have patches of dull, unruly, or matted hair	Loss of hair with painless traction	<10%	Traumatic painless pull +	>50% hair with misshapen bulbs, absent root sheaths, and ruffled cuticles
Diffuse alopecia areata	Irregularly diffuse hair loss mainly in parietal and anterior temporal region, graying of hair	Hair are lost very quickly in a diffuse pattern	<10%	+ in active areas	Variable, telogen hair and miniature or dystrophic anagen follicles
Alopecia areata incognito	Irregularly diffuse hair loss mainly in occipital-parietal region, graying of hair	Acute hair loss is not observed in huge numbers	<10%	+ in active areas	Variable, telogen hair and miniature or dystrophic anagen follicles
Diffuse female pattern hair loss	Irregularly diffuse hair loss, marked thinning visible in frontal and parietal scalp	>20%	>10%	-/in active phase rarely positive in central scalp	A:T ratio is normal or slightly reduced

Age and Sex Predilection

Except loose anagen syndrome which begins in childhood and FPHL which begins at puberty rest all diffuse hair loss affects middle-aged to elderly women. All etiology of diffuse hair loss are overall more common in females.

Important Findings in History

Taking a patient's history thoroughly goes a long way in coming to a conclusive diagnosis clinically. So, one should always be alert about the important points to be emphasized upon while taking patient's history.

General Examination Findings

While doing a general examination for a hair fall patient, there are certain clues that guide us toward the etiology of the hair loss.

Local Examination of the Scalp

Giving a focus on the scalp minutely gives us additional points about the possible reasons behind the hair loss.

BEDSIDE TESTS (BOX 2)
Global Photography

It is a significant help in managing hair patients in the clinical practice. It helps the dermatologist as well as the patient to assess scalp appearance in general and certain areas of hair thinning or bald patches. Scalp photographs must be clicked of every hair patient at their initial visit to the clinic or before starting any new treatment modality. Improvement can be assessed when photographs are taken at subsequent visits.

Modified Wash Test and Hair Loss Count

It helps in diagnosing telogen effluvium or androgenetic alopecia, and in assessing the severity of disease. It is performed after 5 days of no shampooing. The patients are asked to wash and rinse their hair in a sink covered by gauze, collect the hair, let them dry, and put them in an envelope. Later on, the collected hair are counted along with the proportion of vellus hair.

Hair Pull Test

For hair pull test, obtain a sample 3 cm above the auricle. Tightly grasp approximately 60 hair between thumb and forefinger, exert a slow, constant traction to slightly tent the scalp and slide the fingers up the hair shaft. There should be fewer than six club hairs extracted. Repeat the count on the opposite side of the head and two other areas.

Trichogram

It involves pulling out of 40–60 hair in a restricted area of scalp. It is a painful technique involving abrupt extraction of hair from scalp with the help of a rubber tipped needle holder. Excess hair, 1 cm from the roots, are cut and examined on a wet microscope slide.

Phototrichogram and TrichoScan®

It includes shaving the hair of a 2 cm² area of scalp, pictures of the same area clicked on multiple days throughout the treatment, and then assessing in terms of hair density, hair growth, and rate of shedding. As just the anagen hair would grow, it contributes in the assessment of the ratio of anagen: telogen hair.

A TrichoScan is a fully computerized phototrichogram. It is a simplified, less intervening, reliable, and more sensitive tool in comparison with the conventional trichogram and is very helpful in the diagnosis of hair loss.

Videodermoscopy

In the case of acute telogen effluvium, videodermoscopy will show numerous tiny hair popping out of the scalp with consistent density **(Table 8)**.

Part Width

Make a coronal part with a comb over the vertex. Note the part width. Make a series of parallel parts over the vertex and visually compare the part diameter. Do the same over the occipital and temporal scalp. Visually compare the part diameters in different anatomical scalp areas. Hair density is greatest in the childhood and decreases with age. Hair is less dense in vertex for both genders. And thinning increases with age.

Unit Area Trichogram

It is a better version of trichogram technique and involves pulling out hair in a well circumscribed zone (mostly >30 mm²) and helps in finding out hair density.

As videodermoscopy and phototrichogram help with figuring out the hair thickness, density and ratio between anagen and telogen hair, trichograms should be used only in certain circumstances that challenge us as encountered with loose anagen syndrome or DAA.

The procedure involves suffering a transient painful experience which leads to a tiny well-defined zone of

> **Box 2: Bedside tests.**
> - Global photography
> - Modified wash test and hair loss counts
> - Unit area trichogram/hair growth window
> - Tug test
> - Gentle hair pull test
> - Hair card test
> - Trichoscopy
> - Computerized trichometric analysis
> - Wood's lamp examination
> - Part width
> - Clip test

baldness that recovers in weeks and also staying away from hair shampooing for 5 days is a bit too overwhelming for a few patients.

Contrast Paper Method

It must be performed in all the hair fall patients. A contrast paper (white in patients with dark hair and black in patients with light/white hair) needs to be placed perpendicular to the scalp in the background of hair and one can spot the hair with tapering tips as the new growth of hair and the cut hair as broken hair.

Bag Sign

When the patients come to the dermatologist with their fallen hair in a bag, those hair should be examined thoroughly to see their roots, which if bulbous, can be indicative of telogen effluvium.

Trichoscopy Findings (Table 8)

It is a recent advance in diagnostic techniques available for common diseases pertaining to scalp and hair. Being a painless, simple and noninvasive technique, it is very frequently used by dermatologists in their clinics. It involves dermoscopic imaging of the scalp and hair.

LABORATORY INVESTIGATIONS (TABLE 9)

There are many commonly done blood tests, histopathological tests (Table 10) and microbiological tests which further aid in finding the etiology for hair loss patients which makes the dermatologist more equipped when it comes to prescribing the medication (Table 11).

HISTOPATHOLOGICAL FINDINGS (TABLE 10)

Radiological Tests

Ultrasonography of abdomen and pelvis: To rule out polycystic ovary syndrome (PCOS).

TREATMENT MODALITIES FOR DIFFUSE HAIR LOSS WITH PROPOSED MECHANISMS OF ACTION

A broad approach in the management of diffuse hair loss is given in **Table 11**.

Table 8: Trichoscopy findings.					
Differential diagnosis	Telogen effluvium	Anagen effluvium	Diffuse alopecia areata	Alopecia areata incognito (AAI)	Diffuse female pattern hair loss
Trichoscopy findings	• Trichoscopy is not specific • Short regrowing hair may be seen in acute and chronic cases	• Broken hairs • Black dots • Yellow dots • Dystrophic hairs	Polycyclic yellow dots[27-29] and tapered,[30,31] short, regrowing terminal hairs	Most frequent patterns of AAI have empty yellow dots, yellow dots with vellus hair, small hair in regrowth, and pigtail hair	• Presence of hair diameter variability >20%. Moreover, it may show yellow dots that are indicative of empty follicles, small areas of focal atrichia and peripilar hyperpigmentation • Follicular ostia are usually preserved[32]

Table 9: Laboratory investigations.	
Baseline investigations	**Additional investigations**
• Complete hemogram with ESR • Serum TSH • Serum vitamin B12 • Serum vitamin D3 • Serum iron, ferritin, TIBC	• Scalp biopsy for histopathology • Fungal culture, KOH examination • Serum free testosterone, LH, FSH, DHEAS, ANA titer, LFT
(ANA: antinuclear antibody; DHEAS: dehydroepiandrosterone sulfate; ESR: erythrocyte sedimentation rate; FSH: follicle-stimulating hormone; LFT: liver function test; LH: luteinizing hormone; TIBC: total iron-binding capacity; TSH: thyroid-stimulating hormone)	

Table 10: Histopathological findings.					
Differential diagnosis	Telogen effluvium	Anagen effluvium	Lichen planopilaris	Diffuse alopecia areata	Diffuse female pattern hair loss
Histopathological findings	Normal total number of hairs • Normal number of terminal (large) hairs • Increase in the telogen count to >20% (>15% is suggestive; telogen count seldom exceeds 50%; >80% is inconsistent with telogen effluvium • Absence of inflammation and scarring	• <15% follicles in the telogen phase. A normal anagen-to-telogen ratio in a patient with hair loss is characteristic of anagen effluvium • Follicles show no signs of inflammation, dystrophy of the inner sheath, or traction, which are helpful in the distinction of anagen effluvium from AA, androgenetic alopecia, and traction alopecia	• Band-like mononuclear cell infiltrate obscuring the interface between follicular epithelium and dermis; vacuolar alteration at the interface and hypergranulosis within affected infundibula is typical • Colloid or Civatte bodies are occasionally found as part of the interface alteration • Inflammation affects the upper portion of the follicle (infundibulum and isthmus) most severely • Occasionally, epidermal changes of lichen planus are found • Over time, perifollicular fibrosis becomes prominent and the lymphocytic infiltrate seems to "back away" from the follicle • An artifactual cleft between epithelium and stroma is often found, with epithelium "floating" within the cleft (Max–Joseph spaces) • Grouped globular immunofluorescence (usually IgM) adjacent to the follicular epithelium is the characteristic pattern	Early, progressive disease ("acute" and "subacute") • Normal total number of hairs • Peribulbar mononuclear cell infiltrate (with occasional eosinophils), predominantly affecting terminal anagen and catagen hair bulbs • Occasional exocytosis of inflammatory cells into bulbar epithelium • Degenerative changes of hair matrix • Increased number of terminal catagen and telogen hairs • Increased number of miniaturized hairs • Trichomalacia and marked narrowing of hair shafts longstanding and stable disease ("chronic") • Majority of hairs in catagen or telogen phases • Numerous miniaturized, "arrested", rapidly cycling hairs, referred to as nanogen hair • Mild peribulbar mononuclear cell infiltrate around those nanogen hair possessing anagen-like or catagen-like bulbs	Normal total number of follicles and no significant inflammation • Increased number and percentage of vellus hairs • Numerous fibrous "streamers" • Slightly increased telogen count • Uninvolved scalp (e.g., occiput) appears normal

(AA: alopecia areata; IgM: immunoglobulin M)

Table 11: A broad approach in the management of diffuse hair loss.				
Type of diffuse hair loss	**Conservative/medical management**			**Physical/interventional treatments**
	First-line treatment	*Second-line treatment*	*Third-line treatment*	
Telogen effluvium	• Elimination of the precipitating cause • Reassurance and counseling	Iron supplementation	• Topical corticosteroids • CNPDA	• Low level laser therapy • Microneedling • Fractional lasers • Platelet-rich plasma therapy • Hair transplant
Anagen effluvium	• Reassurance and counseling • Hair piece or wig temporarily	Scalp tourniquet[30-32]/ scalp hypothermia	AS101[33-35]/minoxidil	
Alopecia areata	Systemic steroids (intramuscular/oral)[35-37]	Topical immunotherapy	• JAK/STAT inhibitors • PUVA • Biologics	
Female pattern hair loss	Topical minoxidil	• Oral contraceptives • Spironolactone • Finasteride • Dutasteride	Topical tretinoin, procapil, capixyl	

[AS101: ammonium-trichloro (0,0' dioxyethylene) tellurate; CNPDA: caffeine, niacinamide, panthenol, dimethicone, and an acrylate polymer; JAK: Janus kinase; PUVA: psoralen plus ultraviolet A; STAT: signal transducers and activators of transcription]

REFERENCES

1. Shrivastava SB. Diffuse hair loss in an adult female: Approach to diagnosis and management. Indian J Dermatol Venereol Leprol. 2009;75:20-8.
2. Grover C, Khurana A. Telogen efflfluvium. Indian J Dermatol Venereol Leprol. 2013;79:591-603.
3. Tosti A, Pazzaglia M. Drug reactions affecting hair: diagnosis. Dermatol Clin. 2007;25:223-31.
4. Headington JT. Telogen effluvium: new concepts and review. Arch Dermatol. 1993;129:356-63.
5. Whiting DA. Chronic telogen effluvium: increased scalp hair shedding in middle-aged women. J Am Acad Dermatol. 1996;35:899-906.
6. Kligman AM. Pathologic dynamics of human hair loss: I. Telogen effluvium. Arch Dermatol. 1961;83:175-98.
7. Trüeb RM. Diffuse hair loss. In: Blume-Peytavi U, Tosti A, Whiting DA, Trüeb RM (Eds). Hair Growth and Disorders. Berlin: Springer; 2008. pp. 259-72.
8. Sperling LC. Hair and systemic disease. Dermatol Clin. 2001;19:711-26.
9. Paus R, Olsen EA, Messenger AG. Hair Growth Disorders. In: Wolff K, Goldsmith LA, Katz SI, Gilchrest BA, Zller AS, Leffell DJ (Eds). Fitzpatrick's Dermatology in General Medicine, 7th edition. New York: McGraw-Hill; 2008. pp. 753-77.
10. Trüeb R. Chemotherapy-induced Hair Loss. Skin Therapy Lett. 2010;15:5-7.
11. Sinclair R, Grossman KL, Kvedar JC. Anagen hair loss, in Disorders of Hair Growth: Diagnosis and Treatment. In: Olsen EA (Ed). New York: McGraw-Hill; 2002. p. 275.
12. Delmonte S, Semino MT, Parodi A, Rebora A. Normal anagen effluvium: A sign of pemphigus vulgaris. Br J Dermatol. 2000;142:1244-5.
13. Quercetani R, Rebora AE, Fedi MC, Carelli G, Mei S, Chelli A, et al. Patients with profuse hair shedding may reveal anagen hair dystrophy: A diagnostic clue of alopecia areata incognita. J Eur Acad Dermatol Venereol. 2011;25:808-10.
14. Elhassani SB. The many faces of methyl mercury poisoning. J Toxicol Clin Toxicol. 1982;19:875-906.
15. Stein KM, Odom RB, Justice GR, Martin GC. Toxic alopecia from ingestion of boric acid. Arch Dermatol. 1973;108:95-7.
16. Bank WJ, Pleasure DE, Suzuki K, Nigro M, Katz R. Thallium poisoning. Arch Neurol. 1972;26:456-64.
17. Price VH, Gummer CL. Loose anagen syndrome. J Am Acad Dermatol. 1989;20:249-56.
18. Hamm H, Traupe H. Loose anagen hair of childhood: The phenomenon of easily pluckable hair. J Am Acad Dermatol. 1989;20 (2 Pt 1):242-8.
19. Tosti A, Piraccini BM. Loose anagen hair syndrome and loose anagen hair. Arch Dermatol. 2002;138:521-2.
20. Dinh QQ, Chong AH. A case of widespread non-pigmented hair regrowth in diffuse alopecia areata. Australas J Dermatol. 2007;48:221-3.
21. Rebora A. Alopecia areata incognita: a hypothesis. Dermatologica. 1987;174(5):214-8.
22. Molina L, Donati A, Valente NS, Romiti R. Alopecia areata incognita. Clinics (Sao Paulo). 2011;66(3):513-5.
23. Pringle T. The relationship between thyroxin, estradiol and postnatal alopecia, with relevance to womenís health in general. Med Hypothesis. 2000;55:44-9.
24. Dallob AL, Sadick NS, Unger W, Lipert S, Geissler LA, Gregoire SL, et al. The effect of finestride, a 5a-reductase inhibitor, on scalp skin testosterone and dihydro-testosterone concentrations in patients with male pattern baldness. J Clin Endocrinol Metab. 1994;79:703-6.

25. Sawaya MF, Price VH. Different levels of 5a-reductase type I and type II, aromatase, and androgen receptor in hair follicles of women and men with androgenetic alopecia. J Invest Dermatol. 1997;109:296-300.
26. Futterweit MD, Dunaif A, Yeh HC, Kingslay P. The prevalence of hyperandrogenism in 109 consecutive female patients with diffuse alopecia. J Am Acad Dermatol. 1988;19:831-6.
27. Ross EK, Vincenzi C, Tosti A. Videodermoscopy in the evaluation of hair and scalp disorders. J Am Acad Dermatol. 2006;55:799-806.
28. Mane M, Nath AK, Thappa DM. Utility of dermoscopy in alopecia areata. Indian J Dermatol. 2011;56:407-11.
29. Karadag Köse Ö, Güleç AT. Clinical evaluation of alopecias using a handheld dermatoscope. J Am Acad Dermatol. 2012;67:206-14.
30. Wang J, Lu Z, Au JL. Protection against chemotherapy-induced alopecia. Pharm Res. 2006;23:2505-14.
31. Hussein AM. Chemotherapy-induced alopecia: New developments. South Med J. 1993;86:489-96.
32. Cline BW. Prevention of chemotherapy-induced alopecia: A review of the literature. Cancer Nurs. 1984;7:221-8.
33. Sredni B, Xu RH, Albeck M, Gafter U, Gal R, Shani A, et al. The protective role of the immunomodulator AS101 against chemotherapy-induced alopecia studies on human and animal models. Int J Cancer. 1996;65:97-103.
34. Rodriguez R, Machiavelli M, Leone B, Romero A, Cuevas MA, Langhi M, et al. Minoxidil (Mx) as a prophylaxis of doxorubicin-induced alopecia. Ann Oncol. 1994;5:769-70.
35. Friedli A, Labarthe MP, Engelhardt E, Feldmann R, Salomon D, Saurat JH. Pulse methylprednisolone therapy for severe alopecia areata: An open prospective study of 45 patients. J Am Acad Dermatol. 1998;39:597-602.
36. Kar BR, Handa S, Dogra S, Kumar B. Placebo-controlled oral pulse prednisolone therapy in alopecia areata. J Am Acad Dermatol. 2005;52:287-90.
37. Kurosawa M, Nakagawa S, Mizuashi M, Sasaki Y, Kawamura M, Saito M, et al. A comparison of the efficacy, relapse rate and side effects among three modalities of systemic corticosteroid therapy for alopecia areata. Dermatology. 2006;212:361-5.

12

A Patient with Cicatricial Alopecia

Ranjan Raval, Nishi Trivedi

DEFINITION

Cicatricial alopecia is the loss of hair with scarring. It is caused by a diverse group of disorders that destroy the hair follicle and replace it with scar tissue leading to permanent hair loss **(Table 1)**.

Table 1: Differential diagnosis of a patient presenting with cicatricial alopecia.	
Primary Preferential damage to hair follicle due to its inflammation with relative sparing of interfollicular reticular dermis	Secondary Hair follicle damage due to surrounding inflammation of interfollicular dermis
• Chronic cutaneous lupus erythematosus (CCLE) • Lichen planopilaris (LPP) • Pseudopelade of Brocq • Central centrifugal cicatricial alopecia • Follicular mucinosis • Keratosis follicularis spinulosa decalvans • Folliculitis decalvans • Dissecting cellulitis • Acne keloidalis • Acne necrotica • Erosive pustular dermatosis of the scalp • Idiopathic scarring alopecia • Aplasia cutis congenita	*Traumatic:* • Mechanical trauma • Postoperative • Burns • Toxic/corrosive substances (acid/alkali burns) • Radiation • Traction (trichotillomania)
	Infections: • Bacterial (folliculitis, carbuncle) • Fungal (kerion, flavus) • Viral (HIV, herpes simplex, varicella) • Protozoal (leishmaniasis) • Treponemal (syphilis) • Mycobacterial (tuberculosis)

Continued

• Incontinentia pigmenti • Darier's disease • Ichthyosis • Epidermal nevus • Epidermolysis bullosa • Conradi–Hünermann–Happle syndrome • Ectodermal dysplasia • Marie–Unna hereditary hypotrichosis (MUHH)	*Autoimmune disorders:* • Morphea • Scleroderma (en coup de sabre) • Lichen sclerosus • Chronic GVHD • Cicatricial pemphigoid
	Granulomatous disorders: • Infectious granuloma • Sarcoidosis • Necrobiosis lipoidica
	Inflammatory diseases: • Psoriasis • Pityriasis amiantacea
	Deposition dermatoses: • Amyloidosis • Mucinosis
	Neoplastic: • Benign tumors (e.g., cylindroma) • Primary malignancy (BCC, SCC, CTCL) • Metastases

(BCC: basal cell carcinoma; CTCL: cutaneous T-cell lymphoma; GVHD: graft-versus-host disease; HIV: human immunodeficiency virus; SCC: squamous cell carcinoma)

APPROACH TO A CASE

History

- *Age of onset*:
  - *At birth*: Aplasia cutis, incontinentia pigmenti, lamellar ichthyosis
  - *Child*: Tinea capitis

- *Adults*: Lichen planopilaris (LPP), chronic cutaneous lupus erythematosus (CCLE), folliculitis decalvans
- *Elderly*: Erosive pustular dermatosis, malignancy
- Gender:
  - *Female predilection*: LPP, frontal fibrosing alopecia (FFA), CCLE
  - *Male predilection*: Acne keloidalis
- *Duration of complain*:
  - *Acute course*: Infective (tinea capitis, bacterial folliculitis) or traumatic cause (mechanical injury, burns)
  - *Chronic course*: LPP, FFA, CCLE
- Progression of existing lesions/new lesions—important to know about current disease activity; whether disease is active or stable.
- *Active hair loss*: Diffuse or localized to alopecic patch—important to know about disease activity
- *First episode or recurrent*:
  - First episodes—more likely to be due to traumatic or infective cause
  - Recurrent episodes—autoimmune conditions
- *Associated symptoms*:
  - *Pruritus*: LPP, tinea capitis, folliculitis
  - *Tenderness/dysesthesia*: LPP, CCLE
  - *Asymptomatic*: FFA, pseudopelade of Brocq
  - *Fever, weight loss, fatigue*: LE, malignancy
- Associated diseases—systemic or cutaneous **(Table 2)**
- *Hair loss in other parts of body*:
  - *Axilla, groin*: Graham-Little-Piccardi-Lasseur syndrome
  - *Axilla, beard, pubis*: Folliculitis decalvans
  - Eyebrows, eyelashes, truncal hair thinning—FFA
  - *Eyebrow hair loss*: Alopecia mucinosa
  - Eyebrows, pubis: Trichotillomania
- *Cosmetic history or hairstyling habits*:
  - *Traction*: Turban wearing in Sikhs, occupational or recreational wearing of helmets or hats
  - Chemical or physical straightening products or procedures
- *Obstetric history*: Menopause (alopecias like FFA occur in postmenopausal women)
- *Drug history*: Intralesional steroid
- History of mental or physical stress
- *Family history*: Aplasia cutis and Marie–Unna hereditary hypotrichosis (MUHH) are autosomal dominant

Examination

General examination: Pallor can be present due to anemia in patients of lupus erythematosus (LE), lymph node enlargement can provide a clue to infectious cause such as tinea capitis or bacterial folliculitis.

Local examination:
- *Site of involvement*:
  - *Frontal hairline recession*: FFA
  - *Occipital area*: Acne keloidalis nuchae
  - *Vertex*: Pseudopelade of Brocq
  - *All hair margins involved*: Traction alopecia
- *Pattern of involvement*:
  - *Footprints in snow*: In pseudopelade of Brocq due to coalescing of small oval or round patches of alopecia
  - *Receding frontal hairline in a straight manner*: FFA
  - *Linear scarring alopecia extending from the forehead*: En coup de sabre morphea
  - *Male pattern baldness in child*: MUHH
  - *Whorled pattern of scarring alopecia*: Incontinentia pigmenti
- *Extent of alopecia*:
  - *Single patch*: Mechanical or infective cause
  - *Few small patches*: Pseudopelade of Brocq, bacterial folliculitis
  - *Diffuse reduction in hair density*: Early stage of LPP
- *Signs of scarring alopecia*:
  - Increased wrinkling
  - Thin, shiny, depressed skin
  - Absent follicular ostia

Table 2: Associated cutaneous/systemic disease with cicatricial alopecia.	
Cicatricial alopecia suspected	*Associated cutaneous/systemic disease*
Tinea capitis	Dermatophytosis on body elsewhere
LPP	Lichen planus on body elsewhere, oral mucosa may show white streaks in a reticular pattern over violaceous patches. Nail changes may include nail plate thinning, longitudinal ridges, dorsal pterygium, etc.
CCLE	CCLE lesions on rest of body—erythematous indurated scaly plaques, sparse eyebrows with erythema, atrophic/hypertrophic/cribriform/acneiform scarring representative of old healed lesions, dyspigmentation, patient can have other systemic symptoms of LE such as fever, joint pain, painless oral ulcers, Raynaud's phenomenon, etc.
Graham–Little–Piccardi—Lasseur syndrome, keratosis follicularis spinulosa decalvans (KFSD)	Keratosis pilaris
Alopecia mucinosa	Cutaneous T-cell lymphoma (CTCL)
Trichotillomania	Psychiatric illness—anxiety/depressive disorders, obsessive compulsive disorders[1]
Acne, hidradenitis suppurativa	Can be part of follicular occlusion syndrome
(CCLE: chronic cutaneous lupus erythematosus; LE: lupus erythematosus; LPP: lichen planopilaris)	

- Overlying telangiectasias
- Periphery shows twisted hair and standing on end "lonely hairs"
- *Cutaneous examination on scalp*:
  - *Peripheral hyperpigmentation and central depigmentation*: Discoid lupus erythematosus (DLE)
  - *Violaceous erythematous follicular papules*: LPP
  - *Boggy swelling studded with pustules*: Tinea capitis
  - *Pinpoint follicular pustules with crusting*: Folliculitis decalvans
  - *Erosions/ulcers*: Aplasia cutis
  - *No signs of inflammation*: Pseudopelade of Brocq or end stage/burnt out stage of any cicatricial alopecia
- *Hair pull test*: To evaluate intensity and activity of hair loss
  - Positive in tinea capitis, dissecting cellulitis of scalp at the site of alopecia. In LPP, can be positive in peripheral margins of patch of cicatricial alopecia in active disease (positive if >2 hairs per 50–60 hairs bundle are removed)[2]
  - Negative in trichotillomania and end-stage scarring alopecia of any cause.
- *Trichoscopy*: To differentiate scarring alopecia from nonscarring and to select the best site for scalp biopsy. Scarring hair loss will have prominent loss of follicular ostia. Honeycomb pigment network, peripilar erythema and scales, white areas, red dots, simple or arborizing red loops, and crust favor scarring alopecia.[3] Specific features are described elsewhere in the chapter.
- *Trichogram*: In MUHH, twists, kinks, bands, and dystrophic anagen hairs may be seen.
- *Other hair-bearing sites examination*: Eyebrows/eyelashes/axilla/groin/body hairs
  Eyebrows, eyelashes, and other body hair are sparse or lost in FFA, sparseness or absent hair are seen in axillae, groin in Graham–Little–Piccardi–Lasseur syndrome. Beard hair may also have follicular pustules with scarring alopecia in folliculitis decalvans. Loss of eyebrow hair is possible in alopecia mucinosa. Eyebrows and pubic alopecia may be involved in trichotillomania.
- *Other cutaneous lesions:* Refer **Table 3**
- *Mucous membrane examination*:
  - *Cheilitis, painless oral ulcers (s/o LE)*: CCLE
  - *Oral erosions, violaceous patches with whitish lacy streaks (s/o oral LP)*: LPP
  - *Symblepharon, keratitis, trichiasis, entropion*: Cicatricial pemphigoid
  - *Conjunctival blistering, corneal ulceration, symblepharon formation, blepharitis, ectropion, nasolacrimal duct obstruction, vision disturbance*:[4] Dystrophic epidermolysis bullosa
- *Nail examination*:
  - *Nail plate thinning, longitudinal ridging, trachyonychia, dorsal pterygium, onycholysis, subungual hyperkeratosis[5] (s/o nail LP)*: LPP
  - Focal lesions of CCLE occurring over the nail fold can produce nail plate dystrophy with longitudinal ridging. Punctate or striate leukonychia, nail pitting or ridging, onycholysis, nail fold erythema, red lunulae, nail fold hyperkeratosis with ragged cuticles and splinter hemorrhages can all be seen with varying frequency. Nail fold capillary microscopy can show tortuous and corkscrew-shaped capillary loops.[6]

Table 3: Examination findings on skin leading to specific cicatricial alopecia to be suspected.

Cutaneous lesions	Cicatricial alopecia to be suspected
Violaceous, pruritic, plane topped papules (lichen planus)	LPP
Well defined, annular or polycyclic scaly erythematous plaques (dermatophytosis)	Tinea capitis
Well defined erythematous/centrally depigmented with peripheral hyperpigmentation indurated plaques over face, rest of body. Cribriform scarring over face	CCLE
Follicular hyperkeratotic papules (keratosis pilaris)	Graham–Little–Piccardi–Lasseur syndrome, KFSD
Ill-defined erythematous patches, perifollicular papules and discrete plaques (mycosis fungoides)	Alopecia mucinosa

(CCLE: chronic cutaneous lupus erythematosus; KFSD: keratosis follicularis spinulosa decalvans; LE: lupus erythematosus; LPP: lichen planopilaris)

Developmental Causes

Developmental causes are elucidated in **Table 4**.

Traumatic Causes

- *Tractional alopecia* is an important cause, most commonly seen in Sikhs in India due to turban wearing and tight hairstyles. It is present circumferentially (in all hair lines not just anterior or posterior hair line).
- *Mechanical trauma*: Scalp injuries, such as accidents and machinery with pulling of hair and laceration, sometimes leading to descalpation.
- *Third-degree burns* can lead to scarring alopecia. Usually other body parts are affected as well. Temperatures above 60°C can lead to third-degree burns within a few minutes.
- *In postoperative pressure-induced alopecia*, tenderness, swelling, erythema, and also exudation are typical in the initial stages. Hair loss occurs 1–4 weeks after the event. If scarring has occurred, the lesion usually presents as an oval hairless patch on the occipital scalp. Frequent intra- and postoperative repositioning of the head can prevent pressure-induced alopecia.
- *Chemical injury* from acids, alkalis, and metallic salts may cause irreversible scalp damage, depending on their concentration and the duration of exposure. There are reports of scarring alopecia due to improper application of hairstyling substances, such as bleaching or perm

Table 4: Salient features of developmental cicatricial alopecia.			
Disease	**Inheritance**	**Age of presentation**	**Salient points**
Aplasia cutis congenita[7]	Autosomal dominant	• At birth—ulcer or erosion • Early childhood—scarring alopecia	• There is focal absence of skin mostly limited to scalp • Lesions are noninflammatory and well circumscribed • Classified into nine types based on associated anomalies
Incontinentia pigmenti[8]	X-linked dominant	• At birth or in infancy—along with other features • In adults—whorled scarring alopecia may be the only sign	Multisystem disorder, which affects ectodermal structures. An initial inflammatory or vesiculobullous eruption is followed by a verrucous phase, leading to hyperpigmented and finally an atrophic stage
Epidermolysis bullosa[9]	Autosomal recessive	At birth or in infancy	In dystrophic and junctional types—alopecia ranges from circumscribed to diffuse, and coin-sized patches to complete baldness. Associated with skin fragility and generalized blistering
Keratosis follicularis spinulosa decalvans	Usually X-linked recessive	Childhood	Cicatricial alopecia of scalp and eyebrows along with keratosis pilaris like lesions beginning from the face. Ocular abnormalities may occur
Ichthyosis	• Nonbullous congenital ichthyosiform erythroderma and lamellar ichthyosis—autosomal recessive • X-linked ichthyosis—X-linked recessive	Infancy or childhood	• Inflammatory and lead to loss of follicles causing large areas of cicatricial alopecia • After collodion membrane peels, scales with flexural involvement occur or erythroderma may present
Conradi–Hünermann–Happle syndrome	X-linked dominant	• Infancy—ichthyosiform erythroderma • Childhood—alopecia with other cutaneous features	Follicular atrophoderma, short stature, limb shortening are associated. Cicatricial alopecia may be patchy
Marie–Unna hereditary hypotrichosis (MUHH)	Autosomal dominant	After puberty	Sparse scalp hair at birth is replaced by coarse, flat, twisted hair followed by progressive scarring alopecia after puberty. In child, presents like male pattern baldness pattern

preparations. Early neutralization of the chemical is crucial. Once scarred areas have developed, they are usually sharply demarcated and irregularly shaped.
- *Radiation therapy* with X-rays and ionizing rays has been used to treat intracranial and skull tumors. There are differing data on the threshold above which permanent alopecia can develop. The degree of alopecia correlates with the dose per follicle. Clinically, poikilodermatous features such as telangiectasia, pigment changes, and atrophy can be present.
- *Trichotillomania* is the repetitive pulling out of one's own hair leading to hair loss. Clinically, it presents with alopecic patches of bizarre shape and size, more likely over the parietal and occipital area. Patches are not completely bald, but appear irregularly covered by broken hair **(Fig. 1)**. Long standing and severe cases lead to scarring.[10] Trichoscopy will reveal black dots, broken hair of varying lengths, fraying of hair, longitudinally split hair, signs of scratching, and bleeding.

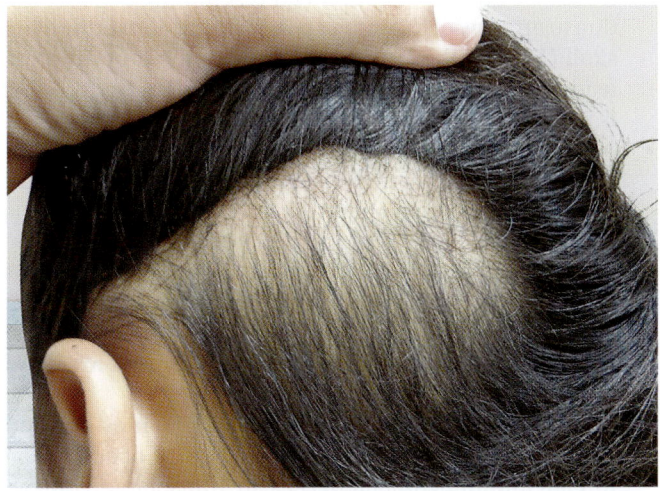

FIG. 1: Trichotillomania: Irregular patch of cicatricial alopecia with overlying broken hairs.

Infectious Causes

- *Furuncle/carbuncle* due to confluence of staphylococcal folliculitides may heal with scarring. Microbiologic culture usually reveals *Staphylococcus aureus*. Topical and occasionally oral antibiotics are necessary while a surgical intervention is required if there is an abscess.
- *In tertiary syphilis*, formation of gummas occurs. They evolve in the skin or underlying bone and often affect the scalp. Sharply demarcated necrotic ulcerations heal with polycyclic scars leading to scarring alopecia.
- *Cutaneous tuberculosis* mainly occurs through endogenous reinfection from lymph nodes or bone or hematogenous spreading from other organs, affecting the head and neck and frequently involving the scalp. Red and beige granulomatous tumors initially cause alopecia and heal with a scar.
- *Varicella* typically affects the scalp in the form of multiple vesicles and usually does not heal with scars. Scarring can develop from scratching of the itchy lesions, superinfection, or when keloids result which will cause patchy cicatricial alopecia. A severe form of segmental herpes zoster (segments V1, C2/3) may also cause scarring alopecia, as well as artifactual excoriation due to dysesthesia.
- *Tinea capitis* is a fungal scalp infection that can lead to scarring if it is chronic or highly inflammatory. Kerion is a deep, highly inflammatory fungal infection of the scalp. Boggy, nodular deep folliculitis is its characteristic. Favus is a chronic superficial dermatophyte infection characterized by sulfuric-yellow crusts; in severe cases leading to central atrophy with centrifugal spreading.

Autoimmune Disorders

- *In en coup de sabre morphea*, a yellow-ivory discoloration develops into a linear depression with minimal inflammation and a shiny surface. It extends from the frontal scalp over the forehead resembling a sabre cut, due to atrophy of the galea aponeurotica, and underlying skull **(Fig. 2)**. The hair is shed early in the process, then leading to sclerotic alopecia. Antinuclear antibody (ANA) is positive in a number of cases.
- *In lichen sclerosus*, there are reports of scalp involvement with alopecia. Initially, porcelain white papules expand and then develop into atrophic plaques. Pruritic lesions can cause extensive scarring alopecia.
- *Cicatricial pemphigoid* is a chronic autoimmune bullous disorder that predominantly affects the mucosae. When the scalp is affected, recurrent, tense, or flaccid bullae and erosions are usually present in a limited area and lead to cicatricial alopecia.
- *Chronic graft-versus-host disease (GVHD)* may develop de novo or progress from the acute type. It occurs when foreign immunocompetent cells are transplanted into an immunoincompetent host. Clinically, lichenoid papules are followed by scleroderma-like lesions, resulting in cicatricial alopecia.

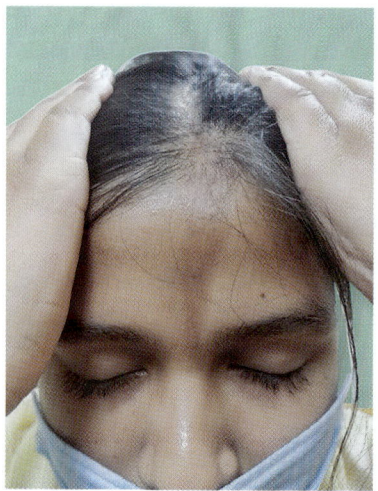

FIG. 2: En coup de sabre morphea: Linear depressed and hyperpigmented plaque extending from forehead to frontal scalp with loss of hair localized to the plaque.

Inflammatory Disorders

- *Psoriasis* frequently affects the scalp but there have been only a few reports of a permanent psoriatic alopecia.
- *Pityriasis amiantacea* is a massively scaly scalp condition and can result in permanent alopecia, most likely in combination with mechanical manipulation when the scales are removed. Clinically, mica-like adherent white scales extend onto the hair shafts. It represents a morphologic reaction pattern of the scalp in chronic irritation, such as seborrheic dermatitis and contact dermatitis.

Others

- *Sarcoidosis* is a systemic disease. Cicatricial alopecia has been reported to result from scalp involvement but also in the beard area. Small orange-brown or livid-red confluent papules are typical, often extending from the hairline. On pathology, scattered superficial and deep "naked" sarcoidal granulomas can be found.
- *Necrobiosis lipoidica* occurs in a few patients with diabetes mellitus. Yellow atrophic plaques with telangiectasias are typical which on scalp can cause cicatricial alopecia.
- *Alopecia mucinosa or follicular mucinosis* is characterized by pruritic erythematous scaly plaques with firm erythematous follicular papules with adherent scales. Nonspecific intrafollicular mucin deposition causes nonscarring alopecia but in very rare cases there may be scarring. The histologic characteristic of alopecia mucinosa is the accumulation of mucin in the follicular epithelium and sebocytes of the affected pilosebaceous apparatus. A nonspecific inflammatory cell infiltrate, predominantly of lymphocytes, is seen in a follicular, perifollicular, and perivascular location.[11] It has a strong association with cutaneous T-cell lymphoma.[12]

Table 5: Differences between the most commonly encountered primary cicatricial alopecia (PCA).

	Discoid lupus erythematosus (DLE)[13]	Classic lichen planopilaris (LPP)	Frontal fibrosing alopecia (FFA)	Graham–Little–Piccardi–Lasseur syndrome	Pseudopelade of Brocq
Age and sex	20–40 years, F > M	30–50 years, F > M	Postmenopausal women	30–70 years, F > M	Mostly adults, F > M
Clinical features	Erythematous scaly plaques with hyperkeratotic adherent follicular plugs at periphery of plaque, central atrophy and depigmentation with peripheral hyperpigmentation **(Fig. 3)**	Alopecic patches with violaceous or erythematous papules, spinous follicular hyperkeratosis. Atrophic smooth alopecic patches mark end stage **(Fig. 4)**	Recession of frontal hairline with perifollicular erythema at periphery. Gradual, slowly progressive course **(Fig. 7)**	Triad of: • Patchy cicatricial alopecia of scalp • Noncicatricial alopecia of axilla and groin • Keratosis pilaris elsewhere **(Fig. 8)**	• Irregular shaped and confluent patches of alopecia • "Footprints in snow appearance" **(Fig. 9)** • In early lesions—perifollicular erythema at periphery
Associated symptoms	Itching, tenderness, burning or asymptomatic	Itching, tenderness	Asymptomatic, itching, dysesthesia, increased scalp sweating	Itching, tenderness on scalp	Asymptomatic
Sites	Scalp (vertex), face, neck or disseminated lesions	Scalp (vertex), axillae, inguinal folds	Frontal hairline + posterior hairline occasionally	Scalp, axillae, pubis	Vertex initially
Associated conditions	Cutaneous LE lesions, nonspecific LE lesions, Raynaud's phenomenon, lupus pernio, periungual nail changes	LP elsewhere on skin, mucosae or nails	Loss of eyebrows, scarring alopecia of facial vellus hair follicles (facial papules), LP elsewhere, "lonely hairs", glabellar red dots, depression of frontal veins	LP may coexist	–

Trichoscopy	• Follicular white scales
	• Perifollicular erythema
	• Red spider in yellow dot
	  ○ Thick, arborizing vessels
	  ○ Large yellow dots
	In long inactive cases, lack of follicular orifices and structureless milky white areas[14]
		• Tubular follicular casts
		• Elongated concentric blood vessels
		• White dots
		• Blue gray dots around the follicle "target pattern" **(Fig. 5)**
			• Same as LPP
			• Eyebrows: Red or gray dots
				Same as LPP	Nonspecific features:
					• Loss of follicular ostia
					• Ivory white colored areas
					• Solitary dystrophic hairs

Continued

Continued

	Discoid lupus erythematosus (DLE)[13]	Classic lichen planopilaris (LPP)	Frontal fibrosing alopecia (FFA)	Graham–Little–Piccardi–Lasseur syndrome	Pseudopelade of Brocq
Histopathology	• Thinning of epidermis • Hypogranulosis • Follicular horny plugs • Thickened BMZ with band-like infiltrate • Perivascular lymphocytic infiltrate	• Infundibular hyperkeratosis • Hypergranulosis • Saw toothed rete ridges • Band-like infiltrate of lymphocytes • Perifollicular inflammation **(Fig. 6)**	Same as LPP	Same as LPP	• Normal epidermis • Absent marked inflammation—variably dense perifollicular lymphocytic infiltrate in early stage • Prominent perifollicular fibrosis • Loss of sebaceous glands **(Fig. 10)**
DIF	Linear IgG, IgM, C3 > IgA in BMZ	IgM, fibrinogen in upper dermis, C3 in BMZ	Same as LPP	Same as LPP	Negative or weak IgM in sun exposed areas
Treatment	Photoprotection, potent topical corticosteroid, intralesional corticosteroid, antimalarials • For flare ups: systemic corticosteroids pulse or short term	• Potent topical corticosteroid, intralesional corticosteroid ± hydroxychloroquine/oral retinoids/oral tetracyclines/cyclosporine/mycophenolate mofetil/azathioprine • For flare ups: + systemic corticosteroids	• Same as LPP • Finasteride, topical calcineurin inhibitors	Same as LPP	Counseling. No satisfactory treatment. Potent topical corticosteroid. Hair transplant if inactive disease

(BMZ: basement membrane zone; DIF: direct immunofluorescence; IgG: immunoglobulin G; LE: lupus erythematosus; LP: lichen planus)

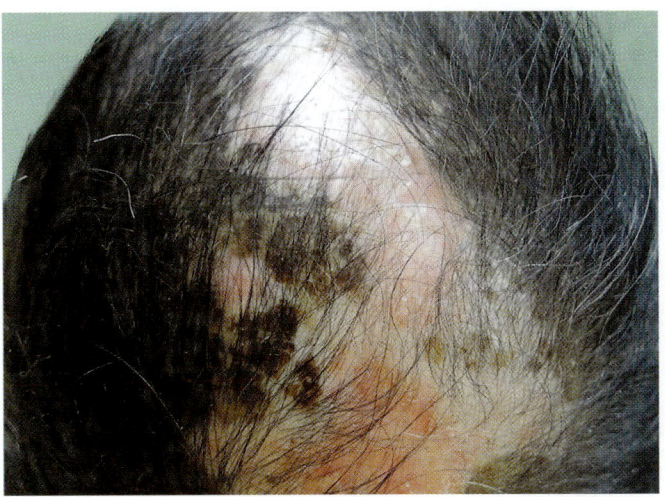

FIG. 3: Chronic cutaneous lupus erythematosus—depigmented, scaly atrophic plaque of cicatricial alopecia with peripheral hyperpigmentation.

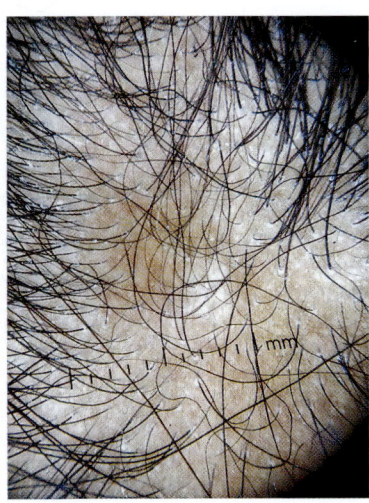

FIG. 5: Trichoscopic features of lichen planopilaris (LPP)—white dots with perifollicular tubular casts.

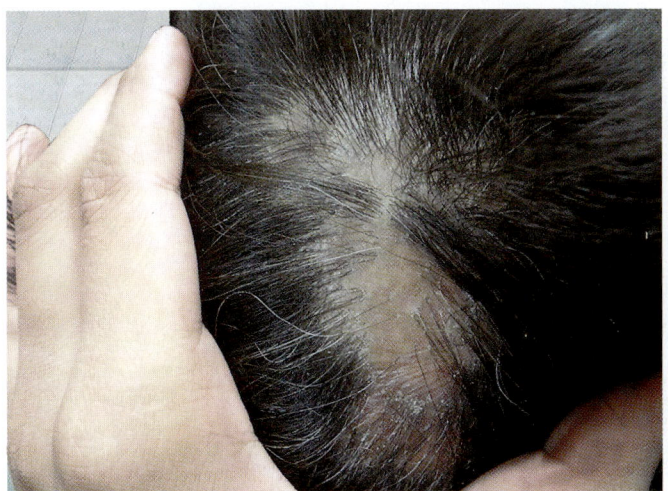

FIG. 4: Lichen planopilaris: Cicatricial alopecia with perifollicular scaling and violaceous pigmentation.

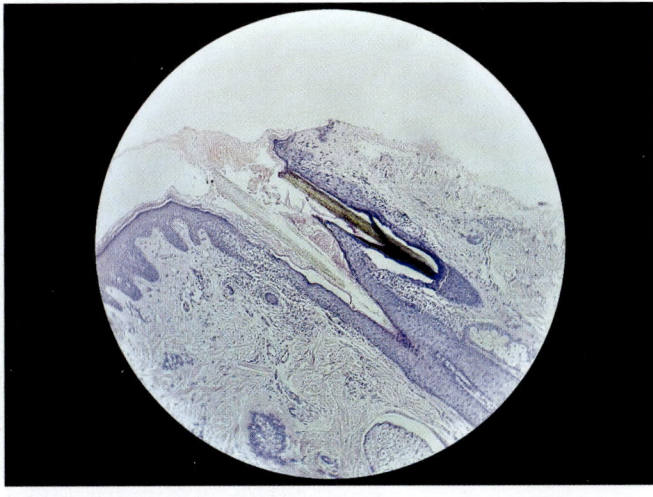

FIG. 6: Histopathological examination (HPE) of lichen planopilaris (LPP) (10×)—basal cell vacuolization with interface dermatitis in infundibular region of hair follicle.

PRIMARY CICATRICIAL ALOPECIAS (TABLE 5)

- *Central centrifugal cicatricial alopecia* presents with scarring at the vertex or crown of the scalp that tends to spread centrifugally. It is more common in women of African descent due to their practice of using hot combs to tame their hair and symptoms can range from pruritus, dysesthesia to none at all.[15] Trichoscopic findings include perifollicular gray-white halo and >1 hair emerging out of a single ostium. Histology shows lamellar fibroplasias and lymphocytic infiltration surrounding the follicle at level of isthmus leading to follicular destruction and fibrous tract formation.

Table 6 shows differential diagnosis of patch of hair loss with pustules.

INVESTIGATING A CASE OF CICATRICIAL ALOPECIA

In some cases, history, clinical diagnosis, and trichoscopy are sufficient to clinch the etiology of disease. In other

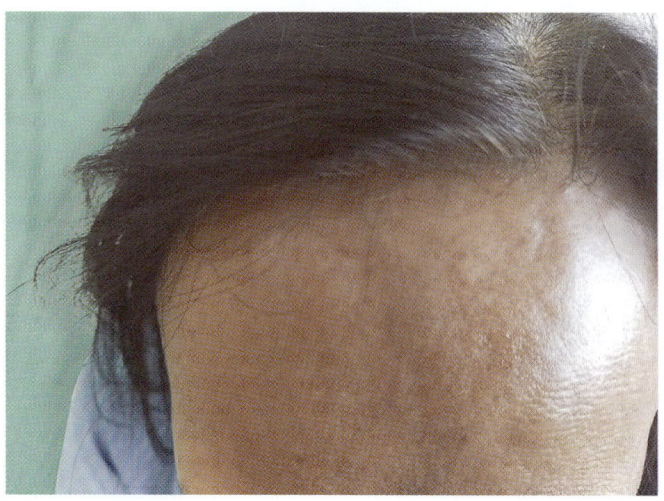

FIG. 7: Frontal fibrosing alopecia (FFA)—frontal recession in postmenopausal female.

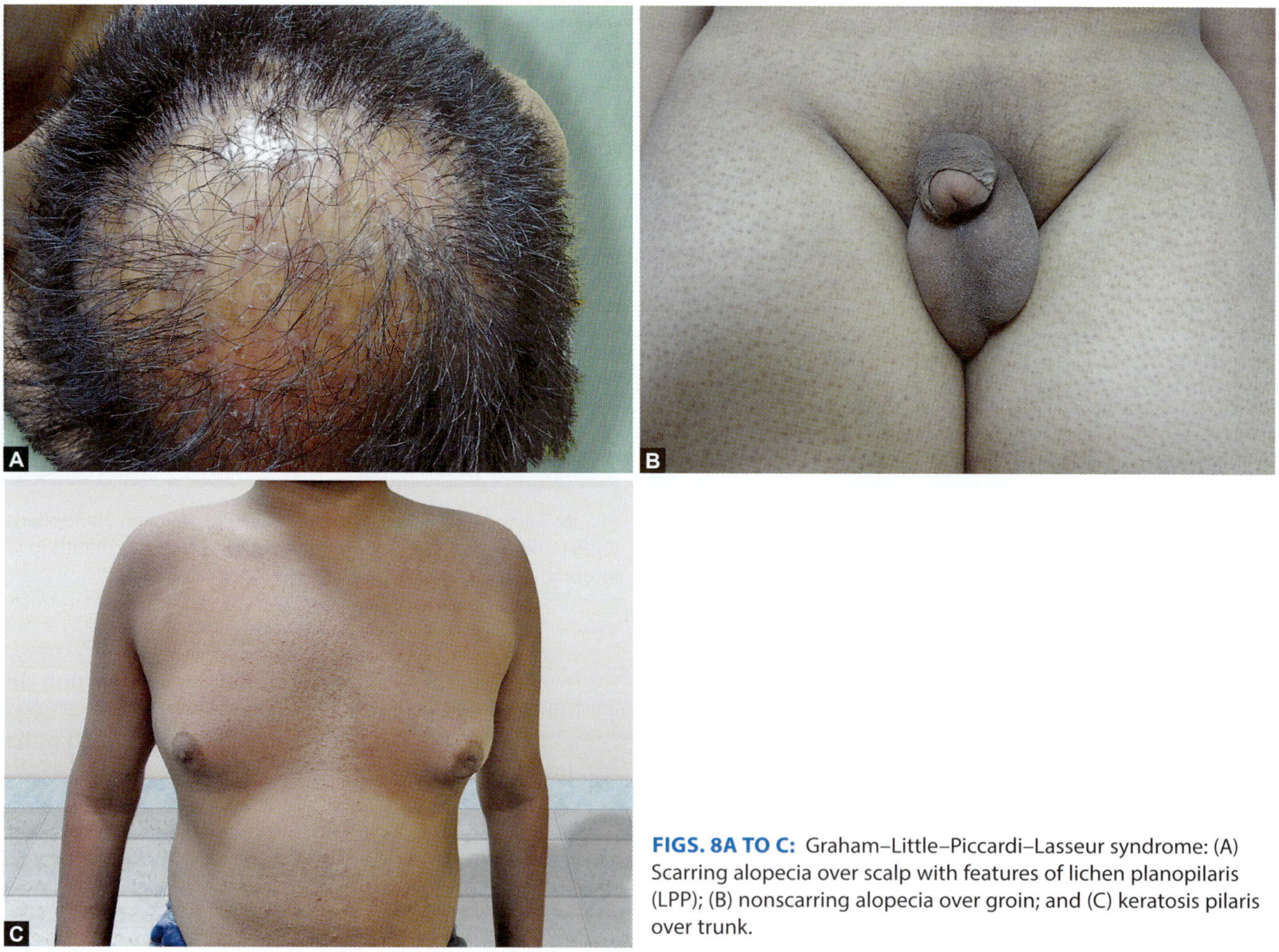

FIGS. 8A TO C: Graham–Little–Piccardi–Lasseur syndrome: (A) Scarring alopecia over scalp with features of lichen planopilaris (LPP); (B) nonscarring alopecia over groin; and (C) keratosis pilaris over trunk.

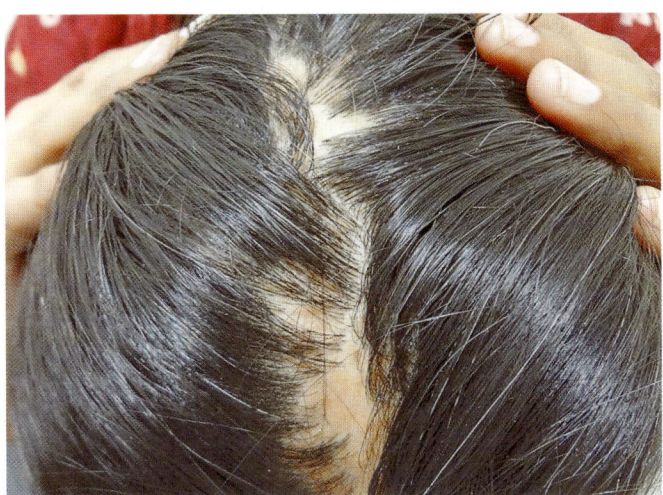

FIG. 9: Pseudopelade of Brocq: Multiple well defined coin-shaped patches of alopecia forming "footprints in snow" appearance.

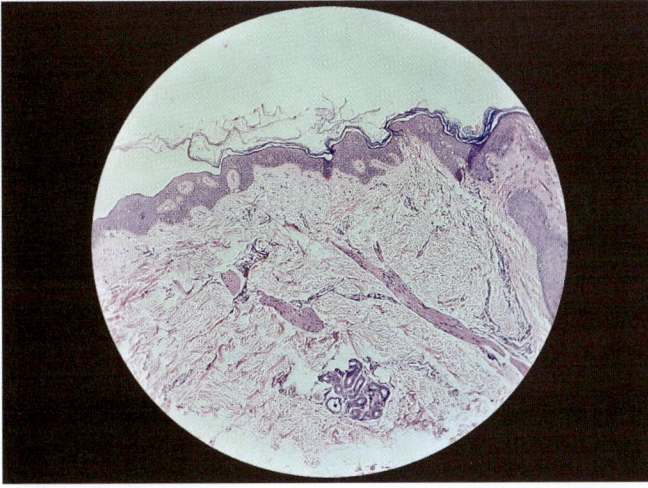

FIG. 10: Histopathological examination (HPE) of pseudopelade of Brocq (10×)—hair follicle density decreased. Subtle lymphocytic infiltrate with dermal atrophy.

cases, diagnosing the cause of cicatricial alopecia might be a dilemma and skin biopsy may be required. Investigations for diagnosis and as screening before starting systemic therapy should be performed. Clinical history should guide the investigations ordered.

1. Complete blood count ⎫
2. Liver function tests ⎬ Screening for systemic therapy mainly
3. Renal function tests ⎭
4. Thyroid function tests (thyroid disease is associated with LPP)
5. Bacterial or fungal cultures of pus or hair (for infective cause)
6. KOH examination (for tinea capitis—Kerion)
7. ANA by IF (in patients of DLE)
8. Skin biopsy
9. Direct immunofluorescence (DIF)

Importance of Skin Biopsy

Histopathology of scalp is an essential tool in distinguishing cicatricial alopecia from noncicatricial alopecia. It is also useful in diagnosing the different primary cicatricial alopecia (PCA) depending upon the inflammatory infiltrate. Trichoscopy can guide the site of biopsy. For an accurate histopathological diagnosis of PCA, multiple biopsy samples are required from active sites that must be sectioned both vertically and transversely. Transverse sections enable both qualitative (e.g., inflammatory change, fibrosis) and quantitative (e.g., hair follicle numbers, size, phase of hair cycle) examination of scalp biopsy samples.[25] The "HoVert" technique, a processing technique that produces horizontal and vertical sections from a single biopsy can be used to avoid taking multiple biopsies.[26] Based upon the predominant inflammatory infiltrate, PCAs are classified as mentioned in **Table 7**.

MANAGEMENT

The treatment of every case is unique to the underlying cause of cicatricial alopecia. It is often a challenge to the treating dermatologist and patient counseling should be the first step to management. Individual treatment options have been discussed in the text. Main aims of treatment should be symptomatic relief and halting the progression of disease. A general rule followed is to treat lymphocyte-mediated PCA with immunosuppression and neutrophil-mediated PCA with antimicrobials. Regrowth of hair in scarred areas cannot be expected and this should be clearly communicated to the patient in order to maintain realistic expectations during planned treatment.

Surgical options can be considered in stable cases such as those secondary to isolated events such as trauma, infection, surgeries and PCA which have not progressed for 1–2 years. There are other factors to be considered before planning surgery such as possibility of development of future androgenetic alopecia, the availability of donor hair, scalp laxity, the patient's healing characteristics, vascular supply, and the location of the subsequent scar. Options include alopecia reduction by surgical excision or hair transplantation.[27]

In advanced stages that are not amenable to treatment or when surgery is not an alternative, camouflage is the only option aside from psychological support. Camouflage techniques can include changing hairstyle in order to cover the area involved, braided and unbraided lace wigs, partial hairpieces, tattooing the scar to mimic hair, and temporary coloring agent to alopecic patch.[28]

Table 6: Differential diagnosis of patch of hair loss with pustules.

	Tinea capitis (inflammatory type)	Bacterial folliculitis	Folliculitis decalvans[16]	Dissecting cellulitis of scalp	Acne keloidalis nuchae	Erosive pustular dermatosis
Age and sex	Children, F = M	Any age, F = M	Young adults, M > F	Young males	Young males	Elderly females
Etiology	Microsporum canis, Trichophyton violaceum, Trichophyton tonsurans[17]	Staphylococcus aureus	Uncertain, excessive inflammatory response to staphylococcal antigens	Follicular hyperkeratosis leading to retention of follicular products due to occlusion[18]	Unclear; triggers—close shave, trauma, friction, humidity, infection, autoimmunity, excess androgens	Unclear; autoimmune response toward the hair follicles induced by trauma
Clinical features	• Highly suppurative, boggy nodular deep folliculitis and pus secretion from several openings • Lymphadenopathy+	Follicular pustules coalescing to form carbuncle which may heal with scarring	Crops of pinhead-sized follicular pustules followed by round patches of scarring hair loss. Dolly hair+	Multiple, firm, dome shaped, violaceous papules coalescing to form plaques and nodules leading to scarring alopecia	Follicular papules and pustules causing patchy scarring hair loss. Some lesions coalesce to form painful keloids with tufted hairs	Sterile pustules, erosions, and crusted lesions of the scalp leading to skin atrophy and scarring alopecia[19]
Symptoms	Itching, pain	Itching, pain	Hemorrhagic crusts, erosions, induration, itching, hyperesthesia, trichodynia	Itching, pain, pus discharge	Itching, pain or asymptomatic	Asymptomatic
Site	Scalp (vertex)	Scalp	Scalp (vertex, occiput), beard, neck, axillae, pubis	Scalp (vertex, occiput)	Scalp (occiput), neck	Scalp (vertex, frontal, parietal, temporal)
Associated conditions	Dermatophytosis elsewhere on the body	—	—	Arthritis, keratitis, acne conglobata, hidradenitis suppurativa, pyoderma gangrenosum, keratitis-ichthyosis-deafness syndrome, pilonidal cysts, and osteomyelitis	Pseudofolliculitis barbae, chronic scalp folliculitis, metabolic syndrome[20]	Rheumatoid arthritis, autoimmune hepatitis, Hashimoto's thyroiditis, Takayasu's arteritis

Continued

Continued

	Tinea capitis (inflammatory type)	Bacterial folliculitis	Folliculitis decalvans[16]	Dissecting cellulitis of scalp	Acne keloidalis nuchae	Erosive pustular dermatosis
Trichoscopy (specific findings)	• Broken hairs • Black dots • Perifollicular and diffuse scaling • Comma hairs • Corkscrew hairs • Morse code-like hairs • Zigzag hairs[21]	Not described. Only nonspecific findings	• Tufted hairs • Perifollicular white-yellowish scales with collar like widening distally "dolly hair"	• "3-D" yellow dots • Large brown dots • Inter and perifollicular erythema • Polytrichia[22]	• Black dots • Peripilar scales and casts • Elongated vessels • Crusts and pustules	• Severe skin atrophy • Follicular crusts • Visualization of the hair follicle bulbs
Histopathology findings	Perifollicular lymphocytic infiltrate with dermal fibrosis. PAS stain shows fungal spores and hyphae in hair follicles	Neutrophilic perifollicular abscess formation	Acneiform dilatation with perifollicular neutrophilic inflammation round the upper follicle. Follicular rupture then causes foreign body giant cell granuloma (Fig. 11)	Infundibular acneiform distension with intra- and perifollicular neutrophilic infiltration. In later stages, abscesses become partially lined by squamous epithelium forming sinus tracts	Peri- and intrafollicular lymphoplasmacytic infiltrate at level of sebaceous glands	Nonspecific, variable degree of epidermal erosions, atrophy, acanthosis, parakeratosis, and subcorneal pustules. Dermis shows mixed chronic inflammatory infiltrate with absent hair follicles
Management	Oral, topical antifungals	Oral, topical antibiotics	Oral (clindamycin, rifampicin) and topical antibiotics, isotretinoin, cyclosporine, surgical removal of tufted hair	Isotretinoin, intralesional steroid, oral and topical antibiotics, low dose oral steroids, colchicine, dapsone, excision, and skin grafting[23]	Potent topical steroids, oral antibiotics, intralesional steroids, surgical excision, CO_2 laser, isotretinoin[24]	Topical steroids, topical immunomodulators, oral steroids, isotretinoin

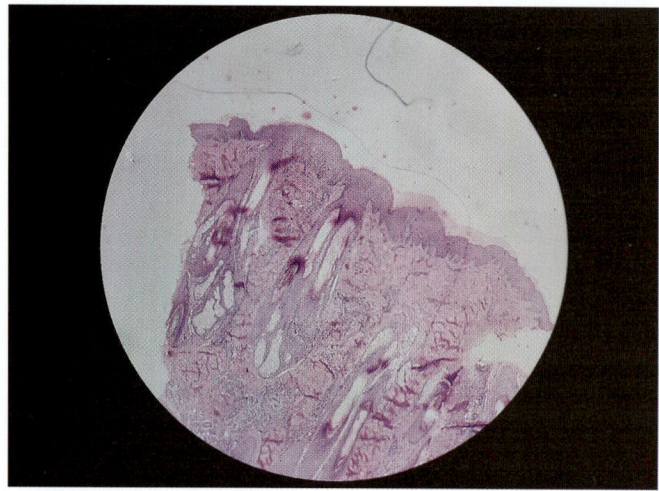

FIG. 11: Histopathological examination (HPE) of folliculitis decalvans (10×)—perifollicular neutrophilic inflammatory infiltrate visible.

CONCLUSION

- Cicatricial alopecia is a distressing condition cosmetically as well as an important dermatological disease. We must evaluate the patient for underlying systemic and cutaneous conditions as required.
- Clinical examination, trichoscopy, and histopathology are all essential tools to clinch the diagnosis.
- The progress of the alopecia decides the prognosis of the disease.
- Early diagnosis and appropriate medical treatment can halt progress and further damage to hair follicles.

Table 7: Classification of primary cicatricial alopecia proposed by the North American Hair Research Society.

Inflammatory infiltrate	Diagnosis

Lymphocytic infiltrate	• Chronic cutaneous lupus erythematosus of scalp
	• Lichen planopilaris:
	  ○ Classic LPP
	  ○ Frontal fibrosing alopecia (FFA)
	  ○ Graham–Little–Piccardi–Lasseur syndrome
	• Pseudopelade of Brocq
	• Central centrifugal cicatricial alopecia
	• Follicular mucinosis
	• Keratosis follicularis spinulosa decalvans

Neutrophilic infiltrate	• Folliculitis decalvans • Dissecting cellulitis of scalp/perifolliculitis capitis abscedens et suffodiens
Mixed cell infiltrate	• Acne keloidalis • Acne necrotica • Erosive pustular dermatosis of the scalp
Nonspecific infiltrate	End stage scarring alopecia

- Surgical intervention in the form of hair transplantation or cosmetic camouflage can be the last hope for some patients.

REFERENCES

1. Grant JE, Dougherty DD, Chamberlain SR. Prevalence, gender correlates, and co-morbidity of trichotillomania. Psychiatry Res. 2020;288:112948.
2. McDonald KA, Shelley AJ, Colantonio S, Beecker J. Hair pull test: evidence-based update and revision of guidelines. J Am Acad Dermatol. 2017;76(3):472-7.
3. Chiramel M, Sharma V, Khandpur S, Sreenivas V. Relevance of trichoscopy in the differential diagnosis of alopecia: a cross-sectional study from North India. Indian J Dermatol Venereol Leprol. 2016;82(6):651-8.
4. Mohapatra SS, Das D, Bhattacharjee H. Ocular involvement in a case of dystrophic epidermolysis bullosa with conjunctival blistering without eyelid or corneal disease: A rare case report. TNOA J Ophthalmic Sci Res. 2021;59(2):169-71.
5. Yesudian PD, de Berker DA. Inflammatory nail conditions. Part 2: nail changes in lichen planus and alopecia areata. ClinI Exp Dermatol. 2021;46(1):16-20.
6. Trüeb RM. Hair and nail involvement in lupus erythematosus. Clin Dermatol. 2004;22(2):139-47.
7. Finner AM, Otberg N, Shapiro J. Secondary cicatricial and other permanent alopecias. Dermatol Ther. 2008;21(4):279-94.
8. Popli U, Yesudian PD. Whorled scarring alopecia—The only adult marker of incontinentia pigmenti. Int J Trichology. 2018;10(1):24-5.
9. Xie D, Bilgic-Temel A, Abu Alrub N, Murrell DF. Pathogenesis and clinical features of alopecia in epidermolysis bullosa: A systematic review. Pediatr Dermatol. 2019;36(4):430-6.
10. Alessandrini A, Bruni F, Piraccini BM, Starace M. Common causes of hair loss—clinical manifestations, trichoscopy and therapy. J Eur Acad Dermatol Venereol. 2021;35(3):629-40.
11. Anderson BE, Mackley CL, Helm KF. Alopecia mucinosa: report of a case and review. J Cutan Med Surg. 2003;7(2):124-8.
12. Kreutzer KM, Effendy I. Cicatricial Alopecia Related to Folliculotropic Mycosis Fungoides. Dermatol Ther (Heidelb). 2020;10(5):1175-80.
13. Concha JS, Werth VP. Alopecias in lupus erythematosus. Lupus Sci Med. 2018;5(1):e000291.

14. Kanti V, Röwert-Huber J, Vogt A, Blume-Peytavi U. Cicatricial alopecia. J Dtsch Dermatol Ges. 2018;16(4):435-61.
15. Dlova NC, Salkey KS, Callender VD, McMichael AJ. Central centrifugal cicatricial alopecia: new insights and a call for action. J Investig Dermatol Symp Proc. 2017;18(2):S54-S56.
16. Rambhia PH, Conic RR, Murad A, Atanaskova-Mesinkovska N, Piliang M, Bergfeld W. Updates in therapeutics for folliculitis decalvans: a systematic review with evidence-based analysis. J Am Acad Dermatol. 2019;80(3):794-801.
17. Rodríguez-Cerdeira C, Martínez-Herrera E, Szepietowski JC, Pinto-Almazán R, Frías-De-León MG, Espinosa-Hernández VM, et al. A systematic review of worldwide data on tinea capitis: analysis of the last 20 years. J Eur Acad Dermatol Venereol. 2021;35(4):844-83.
18. Syed TA, Asad ZU, Salem G, Garg K, Rubin E, Agudelo N. Dissecting Cellulitis of the Scalp: A Rare Dermatological Manifestation of Crohn's Disease. ACG Case Rep J. 2018;5:e8.
19. Starace M, Loi C, Bruni F, Alessandrini A, Misciali C, Patrizi A, et al. Erosive pustular dermatosis of the scalp: clinical, trichoscopic, and histopathologic features of 20 cases. J Am Acad Dermatol. 2017;76(6):1109-14.e2.
20. East-Innis AD, Stylianou K, Paolino A, Ho JD. Acne keloidalis nuchae: risk factors and associated disorders—a retrospective study. Int J Dermatol. 2017;56(8):828-32.
21. Waśkiel-Burnat A, Rakowska A, Sikora M, Ciechanowicz P, Olszewska M, Rudnicka L. Trichoscopy of tinea capitis: a systematic review. Dermatol Ther (Heidelb). 2020;10(1):43-52.
22. Melo DF, Slaibi EB, Siqueira TM, Tortelly VD. Trichoscopy findings in dissecting cellulitis. An Bras Dermatol. 2019;94(5): 608–11.
23. Dogra S, Sarangal R. What's new in cicatricial alopecia? Indian J Dermatol Venereol Leprol. 2013;79(5):576-90.
24. Maranda EL, Simmons BJ, Nguyen AH, Lim VM, Keri JE. Treatment of acne keloidalis nuchae: a systematic review of the literature. Dermatol Ther (Heidelb). 2016;6(3):363-78.
25. Tan E, Martinka M, Ball N, Shapiro J. Primary cicatricial alopecias: clinicopathology of 112 cases. J Am Acad Dermatol. 2004;50(1):25-32.
26. Nguyen JV, Hudacek K, Whitten JA, Rubin AI, Seykora JT. The HoVert technique: a novel method for the sectioning of alopecia biopsies. J Cutan Pathol. 2011;38(5):401-6.
27. Unger W, Unger R, Wesley C. The surgical treatment of cicatricial alopecia. Dermatol Ther. 2008;21(4):295-311.
28. Agor A, Ward KH. Camouflaging techniques for patients with central centrifugal cicatricial alopecia. Int J Womens Dermatol. 2020;7(2):180-3.

A Patient with Premature Graying of Hair

Sujata Mehta Ambalal

"My hair is grey, but not with years, Nor grew it white in a single night, As men's have grown from sudden fears."
—**Lord Byron (from "The Prisoner of Chillon")**

INTRODUCTION

Graying of hair is the most visible manifestation of aging. The word canities (Latin, pronounced kə-ˈnish-ē-ˌēz) is sometimes used for grayness of hair. It is a process of gradual, progressive reduction of melanin pigment in the hair shaft. The perception of a mixture of depigmented white, silver, or amelanotic hair, lightly pigmented, gray or hypomelanotic hair and normally pigmented, dark or eumelanotic hair together on the scalp gives the appearance of gray color. The end of the process results in complete whitening of all the hair.

Poliosis refers to a local, circumscribed depigmented hair as seen in piebaldism, vitiligo, alopecia areata, post-trauma, etc.[1]

CAUSES OF PREMATURE GRAYING

Premature graying is associated with various congenital disorders, nutritional deficiencies, autoimmune, and lifestyle diseases **(Table 1)**. Sometimes combinations of factors are responsible for premature hair graying and patients must be thoroughly evaluated **(Fig. 1)**. Many studies have found a correlation between atopic diathesis and premature graying **(Fig. 2)**.

Drugs have been reported to induce hair color changes. The underlying mechanisms of drug-induced hair color changes are not clear and the relationship between drug intake and color modification is often difficult to prove. Various drugs implicated are chloroquine, hydroxychloroquine, mephenesin (a muscle relaxant), dixyrazine (an

Table 1: Causes of premature graying.[4-6]	
Inherited/genetic	• Progeria • Down's syndrome • Werner syndrome/pangeria • Vogt–Koyanagi–Harada syndrome • Congenital fibrosis of extraocular muscles with juvenile canities • Moyamoya syndrome • Waardenburg syndrome • Book's syndrome • Cri du chat syndrome • Ataxia-telangiectasia • Seckel syndrome • Fisch syndrome • Dystrophia myotonica
Nutritional deficiencies	• Iron • Folic acid • Vitamin D • Vitamin B12 • Protein • Copper • Zinc
Lifestyle factors	• Stress • Low sun exposure • Tobacco • Smoking • Alcohol • Vegetarianism

Continued

CHAPTER 13 A Patient with Premature Graying of Hair

Continued

Atopic diathesis	
Autoimmune disorders	• Thyroid disorders • Pernicious anemia
Chronic diseases	• Human immunodeficiency virus (HIV) • Cystic fibrosis • Hodgkin's lymphoma

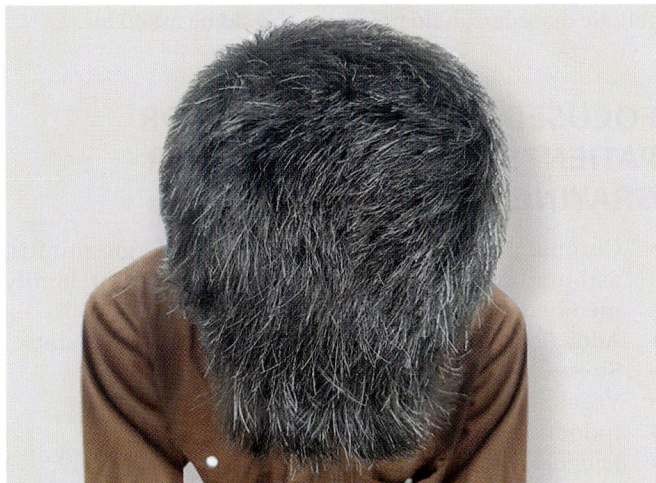

FIG. 1: Premature graying in a 22-year-old male with tobacco addiction. Patient was a vegetarian who reports excessive intake of junk food. Investigations showed low levels of vitamin B12 and D and elevated low-density lipoprotein (LDL) levels.

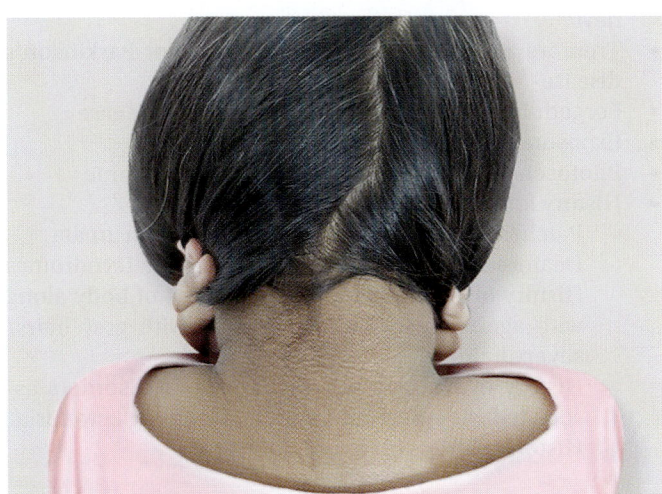

FIG. 2: Premature graying and atopic "dirty neck" in a 7-year-old female with iron deficiency and raised immunoglobulin E (IgE) level.

antipsychotic), tyrosine kinase inhibitors such as imatinib (known to cause both depigmentation and repigmentation of hair), interferon α; anticonvulsants such as valproic acid, phenytoin, phenobarbital; and topicals such as medicated oils, resorcin, and prostaglandin F2α analogs.[2,3]

HAIR PIGMENTATION AND MECHANISM OF GRAYING[4,7,8]

The bulge and hair germ region harbors two stem cell populations—epithelial-derived Hair Follicle Stem Cells (HFSCs) and neural crest-derived melanocyte stem cells (MeSCs). Both are activated concurrently during early anagen to regenerate a new hair follicle and produce mature melanocyte respectively. Mature melanocytes are destroyed during catagen phase, leaving only the MeSCs that will initiate new rounds of melanogenesis in future cycles.[9] It is thought that, as we age, these melanocyte stem cells lose the ability to self-maintain and proliferate to replace old melanocytes.

Studies have revealed that pigment synthesis pathways were significantly impaired in gray versus black hair in same individual, with a significantly decreased expression of multiple key genes crucial for the stability, trafficking and proliferation of melanocytes.[10] Intraindividual and inter-follicular heterogeneity strongly argues against a solely genetic pathobiology of graying. This is perhaps most evident in so-called steel/salt and pepper-headed individuals, which can remain a life-long feature.[11]

HAIR AGING AND RISK FACTORS FOR PREMATURE GRAYING

Similar to skin, hair aging comprises both intrinsic aging, which includes the natural physiological changes that occur with time, and extrinsic aging, changes associated with environmental exposures and physical stress. The most well-recognized sign of intrinsic aging is graying of the hair. Early onset of gray hair does not necessarily correlate with rapid progression.[12] The onset and progression of graying or canities correlate very closely with chronological aging (but not with photoaging) and occur in varying degrees in all individuals eventually, regardless of gender or race. Scalp hair graying first appears usually at the temples and spreads to the vertex and then the remainder of the scalp, affecting the occiput last. Beard and body hair are usually affected later.[13]

Most of the vitamins and minerals as well as a balanced redox state in the dopa oxidase positive melanocytes are needed for optimum melanogenesis. Chemical straightening of hair has been reported to cause graying of hair shaft possibly because of alkaline pH of chemicals used to break disulfide bonds of cortex.[1,14] Oxidative stress causes free radical induced melanocyte damage.

Stressful stimuli activate the sympathetic nervous system, increasing noradrenaline release in hair follicles. Noradrenaline causes complete conversion of MeSCs into melanocytes. The hair follicle is depleted of MeSCs that would have differentiated to replace these melanocytes. This results in mass migration of melanocytes away from the bulge, and leaves no remaining stem cells.[15] Cases of seemingly overnight or sudden graying of hair, also known as canities subita, ascribed to severe stress or trauma, have been reported in history.

HISTORY POINTS IN PREMATURE GRAYING OF HAIR

A patient presenting with premature graying warrants a detailed history, examination, and investigations to rule out reversible factors contributing to it. Age of onset, onset after any major physical or mental stressor event, and rate of progression should be inquired.

RELEVANCE OF AGE

The average age of onset of hair graying appears to be mid- to late 40s; however, this varies with race, with the average age for Caucasians being mid-30s, that for Asians being late 30s, and that for Africans being mid-40s. Graying hair is considered premature if it occurs before the ages of 20 years in Caucasians, 25 years in Asians, and 30 years in Africans, respectively.[16] The average age of graying of hairs in the Indian population has been observed to be beyond 30 years of age. Although many studies use an arbitrary age of 25 years, the actual cut off age to define graying as premature has not been formally studied.

A community-based study of young adults (15 to 30 years age group) in North India pegged prevalence of premature graying at 27.4% with only 1% having severe graying. Mean age of participants with gray hair was 23.7 ± 4.5 years.[5] Some studies have found a male preponderance.

Congenital disorders with premature aging will also show premature graying of hair, such as progeria or Down's syndrome. Sparse gray hair is seen from 2 years of age in progeria while from adolescence to as young as 8 years of age in pangeria.[4]

RecQ helicase is an enzyme involved in deoxyribonucleic acid (DNA) maintenance and its deficiency is implicated in some premature aging syndromes like Werner syndrome, Vogt–Koyanagi–Harada syndrome, congenital fibrosis of extraocular muscles with juvenile canities, Moyamoya syndrome, Waardenburg syndrome, etc. Carriers of telomerase reverse transcriptase (TERT) mutation have younger onset of gray hair compared to noncarriers.[17] Book's syndrome and cri du chat syndrome are also associated with premature graying.

An increasing number of animal and human studies have identified gray hair as an age-independent predictor of serious extracutaneous pathology, including Alzheimer's disease, Parkinson's disease, and cardiovascular disease. There are possible associations with osteopenia and hearing loss, raising suspicion that hair graying may indeed act as an important indicator of systemic aging-associated pathology.[11]

IMPORTANCE OF FAMILY HISTORY OF PREMATURE HAIR GRAYING

Genetic factors are considered to play a major role. Heritability in hair graying ranges from 27 to 90% in various analyses. Family history of early graying of hair, atopy, genetic disorders, halo nevi, etc., should be asked for.

FOCUSED HISTORY POINTS FOR PATIENTS OF PREMATURE HAIR GRAYING

- Chronic pruritus, childhood eczema, allergic rhinitis, asthma, allergic conjunctivitis in patient or family members: Atopic diathesis
- Addiction:[18] Smoking, alcoholism, and substance abuse
- Stress
- Vegetarian diet, crash dieting, and junk food
- Indoor and sedentary lifestyle
- Fatigue: Nutritional deficiency
- Alterations in weight, sleep patterns, bowel movements, skin pigmentary changes on face and bony prominences, menstrual disturbances in females and hair loss: for thyroid or nutritional disturbances, and malignancies
- Chemical straightening of hair
- Vitiligo or depigmentation surrounding melanocytic nevi[19]
- Tremors and involuntary movements: For Parkinson's disease
- Forgetfulness: For early onset Alzheimer's disease
- Exposure to ultraviolet (UV) light
- Photosensitivity: Rothmund–Thomson syndrome
- History for ruling out similar conditions:
  - Patches of hair loss on scalp—for alopecia areata
  - Deafness—for ruling out various congenital syndromes
  - History of silvery hairs on other parts of body along with age of onset—for syndromes with gray hairs/silvery hairs
  - History of black urine—for metabolic disorders associated with pigment dilution like phenylketonuria
  - History of drugs like chemotherapy

EXAMINATION POINTS TO BE CONSIDERED AND THEIR RELEVANCE

Examination is important to rule out etiology and various differential diagnosis. Examination points and their significance are summarized in **Table 2**.

Alternating areas of pigment presence or absence on individual hair shaft indicate partial or intermittent melanocyte activity. Serial photographs would help document improvement or worsening. Keeping in mind the hair cycle, a time frame of weeks or even months should be allowed before seeing a reduction in rate of hair graying.

Table 2: Examination points and their significance.	
Woods lamp examination	To rule out vitiligo/leukoderma (Fig. 3)
Cutaneous changes such as dry skin, eczema, and various signs of atopic dermatitis	Atopic dermatitis, hypothyroidism
Pallor, knuckle pigmentation, cheilitis, and koilonychia	Nutritional deficiency
Patches of hair loss, nail pitting	Alopecia areata (Fig. 3)
Graying of hair on other parts	Pigment dilution related to metabolic disorders and syndromes associated with silvery hairs [Griscelli syndrome (Fig. 4), Chediak–Higashi syndrome, and Elejalde syndrome]
Skin wrinkling and aging changes such as freckling and milia	Premature aging syndrome
Body mass index (BMI) and blood pressure	Metabolic disorders
Auscultation of heart sounds	For ruling out associated cardiac disorders
Wide spaced eyes with Mongolian slant and sandal gap	Down's syndrome
Myotonia	Dystrophia myotonica

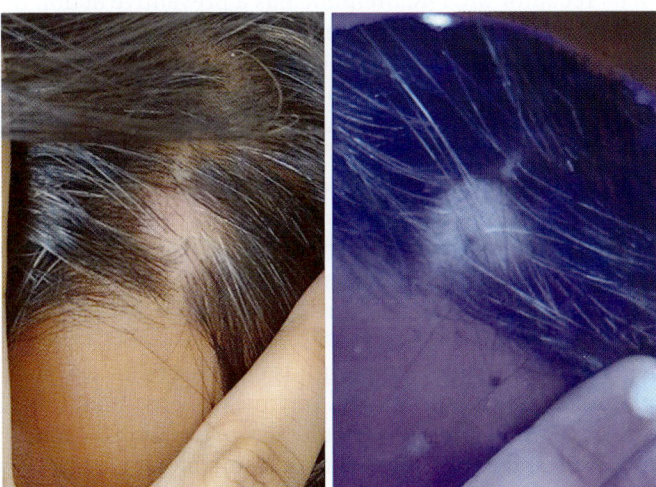

FIG. 3: Wood's lamp examination of patient presenting with "premature gray hair" and "patchy hair loss" of alopecia areata showing concurrent vitiligo.

SCORING SYSTEM

Various scoring systems have been used for evaluation of premature graying including hair whitening score (HWS) and graying severity score (GSS). HWS was used on older patients and may not be specific for the younger population. GSS is calculated by photographing and counting gray hair in 1 cm² areas from five different zones of the scalp. It has been developed specifically for premature canities.[20] In a busy, non-research set up, simple photographic records repeated every 3 months may help gauge the progress of graying and response to treatment.

Investigations **(Table 3)**: Complete blood count (CBC), thyroid-stimulating hormone (TSH), serum vitamin D, vitamin B12, serum iron/ferritin (not accurate in chronic diseases), and serum lipid profile.

Additional investigations: Serum folic acid, zinc, copper, biotin, calcium, protein, and serum immunoglobulin E (IgE).

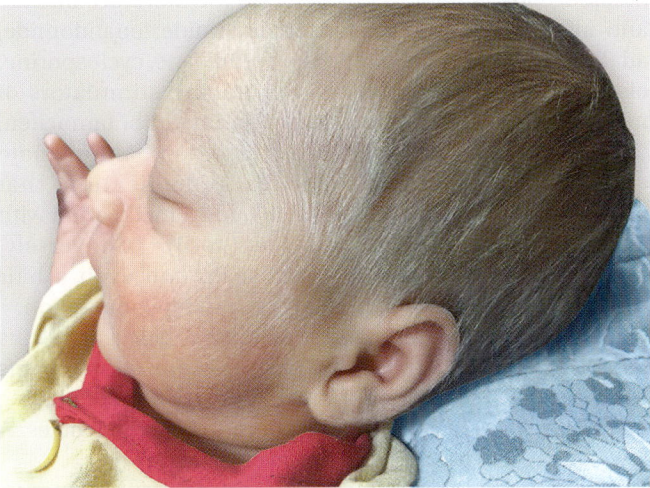

FIG. 4: Silvery hair in a neonate with Griscelli syndrome.
Courtesy: Dr Jigna Padhiyar.

Table 3: Routine and additional investigations.	
Routine investigations	• CBC: Hb for anemia, WBC count, and ESR for chronic infections • TSH: Screening for thyroid disorders • Serum vitamin D, vitamin B12, serum iron—for diagnosing common deficiencies • Serum lipid profile—for dyslipidemia
Additional investigations	• Serum folic acid, zinc, copper, biotin, calcium, protein—for diagnosing deficiencies • IgE—for suspected atopy

(CBC: complete blood count; ESR: erythrocyte sedimentation rate; IgE: immunoglobulin E; TSH: thyroid-stimulating hormone; WBC: white blood cell)

MANAGEMENT

Repigmentation of Gray Hair

An optimal therapy would permanently reverse the gray back to its original hair color, without causing damage to the hair shaft or scalp irritation. In a quest for development of this type of therapy, anecdotal reports of medications associated with hair repigmentation have been described. Unfortunately, little is understood about the pathophysiology behind hair repigmentation. The lack of replicability of these drugs in leading to repigmentation, or side effects in a setting outside the original intended use, prevent them from finding their place as a routine treatment for premature graying. There is low-quality evidence that some vitamin B complex supplementation can promote gray hair darkening. Conditions occasionally associated with darkening of hair color include Addison's disease, neurodermatitis, porphyria cutanea tarda, and inflammatory scalp conditions. Diffuse repigmentation of gray hair can be induced by certain medications that inhibit inflammation or stimulate melanogenesis. Medications noted in the literature include anti-inflammatory medications (thalidomide, lenalidomide, adalimumab, acitretin, etretinate, prednisone, cyclosporine, cisplatinum, interferon-α, and psoralen); stimulators of melanogenesis (latanoprost, erlotinib, imatinib, tamoxifen, and levodopa); and supplements (calcium pantothenate and para-amino benzoic acid), a medication that accumulates in tissues (clofazimine), and a medication with an undetermined mechanism (captopril).[21] Conversely, inflammatory dermatoses of the scalp and even a hair transplant have been reported to result in repigmentation.

Patients can be prescribed supplements based on results of investigations. In the author's observation, supplements can help slow down or even halt the progression of graying in younger patients with significant nutrient deficiencies. A few patients have even reported reversal of gray hair.

Cases have been reported of iron, B12 supplements, peptides, minoxidil, latanoprost, etc., reversing premature graying. However, most publications of reversal of premature graying are case reports, and large-scale clinical trials showing reproducible, long-term results of any one therapy are lacking. Therapy with a combination of biotin, zinc, and calcium pantothenate showed no significant efficacy.[22] The paramount therapeutic challenge for future antigraying strategies is to halt graying early, and to capture the, relatively wide, window of therapeutic opportunity in which the late, irreversible stage of graying has not yet been reached.[11]

Hair Color (Table 4)

Hair color or dye offers the only solution for premature canities which cannot be reversed by treatment. Hair dying systems may be temporary, semipermanent, demipermanent, and permanent. Details about each are given in **Table 4**.

Temporary and semipermanent products are direct dyes relying on van der Waals forces for adhesion; hence, they do not require chemical reactions to impart color. Permanent dyes are actually colorless precursors and contain hydrogen peroxide (as oxidizing agents) and ammonia (as alkalizer).[26] Airborne contact dermatitis, irritant contact dermatitis, photocontact dermatitis, periorbital eczema, hand eczema, lichenoid lesions, and lichen planus pigmentosus-like pigmentary changes were the commonly observed clinical patterns of hair dye dermatitis. Paraphenylenediamine (PPD) is the major culprit responsible for most of the adverse effects. Contact leukoderma, contact urticaria, lymphomatoid papulosis, erythema multiforme-like or prurigo nodularis-like lesions, and anaphylaxis have also occurred with PPD. PPD intoxication results in multisystem involvement and can cause rhabdomyolysis and acute kidney injury, flaccid paralysis, severe gastrointestinal manifestations, cardiotoxicity, and arrhythmias.[25] Paratoluidine diamine sulfate (PTDS) may be tolerated by 50% patients allergic to PPD. Early exposure to chemicals of hair colors may have long-term implications. Hair color, especially permanent hair color has been associated with various cancers such as breast cancer, leukemia, and possibly bladder cancer.[27-29]

CURRENTLY AVAILABLE AND POSSIBLE FUTURE THERAPIES (TABLE 5)

Melitane, a biomimetic peptide agonist of α-melanocyte-stimulating hormone (α-MSH), stimulates melanin synthesis, inducing skin pigmentation via the activation of its receptor MC1-R. Melitane has a preventive action on DNA damage induced by UV radiations. It is recommended for premature canities between 8 and 25 years of age only. Various topical preparations containing phytic acid, amino acids, peptides and acetyl hexapeptide-1, capixyl, pea proteins, etc., are available in market. It usually takes a minimum of 3 months of continuous application for a visible change. On discontinuation however, premature canities will most likely restart and be visible again after 4–6 weeks. Hence, prolonged treatment would be necessary. Further studies are required for validation of these products.[1]

Topical antiaging compounds such as green tea polyphenols, selenium, copper, phytoestrogens, melatonin, and as yet unidentified substances from traditional Chinese medicine and Ayurvedic medicine, L-methionine and a new type of compounds called SkQs [Sk for penetrating cation

Table 4: Hair colors, their composition and characteristics.[23-25]

Hair color	Nonoxidative (no bleaching agent)		Oxidative (with bleaching agent)	
Type	Temporary	Semipermanent	Demi-permanent	Permanent
Duration	Removed on first wash	3–6 washes	Up to 20 washes	Till new hair grows out
Composition, molecular size and penetration	• Anionic, acid dyes combined for desired natural color • High molecular weight so do not penetrate cortex	• Cationic, basic dyes which may be mixed with nitroaniline dyes. Gradual coloring agents are made of metallic (lead, bismuth, and silver) or vegetable (henna, tea, coffee, walnut, indigo, etc.) derivatives. • Low molecular size, high affinity for keratin, slight penetration of cortex	Similar to semi-permanent or permanent	Contain benzene derivative para dyes such as para phenyl-enediamine (PPD) or para-aminophenol (PAP), oxidizer, alkalizer, coupler (react with para dye to give different colors). Small dye molecules penetrate cuticle and form large molecules in presence of hydrogen peroxide and ammonia, which get trapped inside
Ammonia or other alkaline agents (to open cuticle) and oxidizing agents (to bleach natural melanin)	No	No	Monoethanolamine instead of ammonia as alkalizer. Lower concentration (2%) H_2O_2 so lower bleaching of melanin	Ammonia, 6% H_2O_2
Additional information	• Available as powders, sprays, shampoos, or crayons • Anionic and hence highly water soluble • Suitable for only small quantity of white hair	Available as lotions, shampoos, mousses, and emulsions. Applied to freshly shampooed hair and allowed to remain on the hair for approximately 10–40 minutes then hair rinsed with water. Metallic and vegetable colors require repeated applications till desired color is reached. Metals may give different, even unexpected colors on interaction with other chemicals or sulfur in keratin	• Precursor (para dye and alkalizer) and developer (oxidizer) available in separate containers to be mixed before application • Patch test recommended • Patients sensitive to PPD may cross react with local anesthetics, sulfa drugs, azo dyes used as food and medicine colorants, and PABA used in cosmetics	

(PABA: para-aminobenzoic acid; PPD: paraphenylenediamine)

Table 5: Currently available and possible future therapies.

Minoxidil, latanoprost (prostaglandin), nutrient supplements	
Peptides	Melitane, phytic acid, amino acids, peptides and acetyl hexapeptide-1, capixyl, pea proteins, and L-methionine
Topical anti-aging compounds	Green tea polyphenols, selenium, copper, phytoestrogens, and melatonin
SkQ's, hormonal anti-aging protocols, recombinant human growth hormone	
Nanotechnology derived compounds	Synthetic melanin

("Skulachev ion") and Q for plastoquinone] are being tried. Use of hormonal antiaging protocols containing recombinant human growth hormone has resulted in darkening of hair in some cases.

With the rapid expansion of nanotechnology, novel creative approaches can now be exploited for the design of new hair dyes. Human hair dyeing using synthetic melanin has been explored recently.[30]

Premature graying of hair as a condition is not fully understood and an effective and reliable treatment still eludes us. Having ruled out reversible causes such as deficiencies or thyroid disorders, the clinician can offer empathetic counseling with a focus on healthy diet and lifestyle **(Flowchart 1)**. Patients and their parents are often unaware of side effects of hair color, especially its carcinogenic potential, hence they can be educated to make an informed choice about using it.

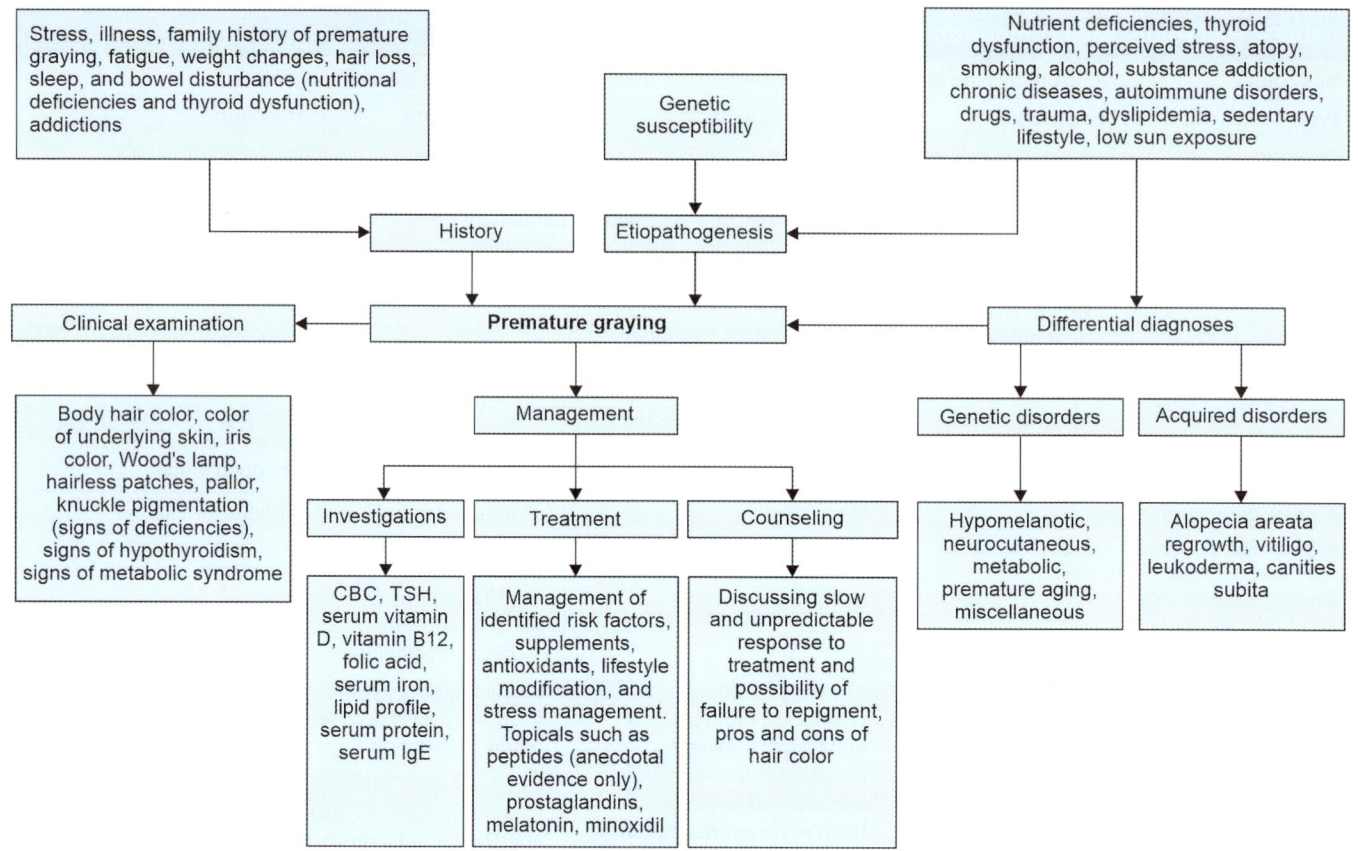

FLOWCHART 1: Mind map of approach to a patient of premature graying.
(CBC: complete blood count; IgE: immunoglobulin E; TSH: thyroid-stimulating hormone)

REFERENCES

1. Sehrawat M, Sinha S, Meena N, Sharma PK. Biology of hair pigmentation and its role in premature canities. Pigment Int. 2017;4:7-1.
2. Majid I, Mubashir S. Canities and Pigment Anomalies of Hair. In: Chandrashekar BS, Madura C (Eds). IADVL Textbook of Trichology. New Delhi: Jaypee Brothers Medical Publishers (p) Ltd.; 2018. p. 331.
3. Ricci F, De Simone C, Del Regno L, Peris K. Drug-induced hair colour changes. Eur J Dermatol. 2016;26(6):531-6.
4. Pandhi D, Khanna D. Premature greying of hair. Indian J Dermatol Venereol Leprol. 2013;79:641-53.
5. Nath B, Gupta V, Kumari R. A community based study to estimate prevalence and determine correlates of premature greying of hair among young adults in Srinagar, Uttarakhand, India. Int J Trichol. 2020;12:206-12.
6. Acer E, Kaya Erdoğan H, İğrek A, Parlak H, Saraçoğlu ZN, Bilgin M. Relationship between diet, atopy, family history, and premature hair greying. J Cosmet Dermatol. 2019;18(2):665-70.
7. Maymone MBC, Laughter M, Pollock S, Khan I, Marques T, Abdat R, et al. Hair Aging in Different Races and Ethnicities. J Clin Aesthet Dermatol. 2021;14(1):38-44.
8. Tobin DJ, Paus R. Greying: Gerontobiology of the hair follicle pigmentary unit. Exp Gerontol. 2001;36:29-54.
9. Zhang B, Ma S, Rachmin I, He M, Baral P, Choi S, et al. Hyperactivation of sympathetic nerves drives depletion of melanocyte stem cells. Nature. 2020;577(7792):676-81.
10. Bian Y, Wei G, Song X, Yuan L, Chen H, Ni T, et al. Global downregulation of pigmentation-associated genes in human premature hair greying. Exp Ther Med. 2019;18:1155-63.
11. O'Sullivan JD, Nicu C, Picard M, Chéret J, Bedogni B, Tobin DJ, et al. The biology of human hair greying. Biological Reviews. 2021;96(1):107-28.
12. Jo SJ, Paik SH, Choi JW, Lee JH, Cho S, Kim KH, et al. Hair greying pattern depends on gender, onset age and smoking habits. Acta Derm Venereol. 2012;92(2):160-1.
13. Tobin DJ. Aging of the hair follicle pigmentation system. Int J Trichology. 2009;1(2):83-93.
14. Paik SH, Jang S, Joh HK, Lim CS, Cho B, Kwon O, et al. Association Between Premature Hair Greying and Metabolic Risk Factors: A Cross-sectional Study. Acta Dermato-venereologica. 2018;98(8):748-52.
15. Clark SA, Deppmann CD. How the stress of fight or flight turns hair white. Nature. 2020;577(7792):623-4.
16. Keogh EV, Walsh RJ. Rate of greying of human hair. Nature. 1965;207(999):877-8.

17. Mahendiratta S, Sarma P, Kaur H, Kaur S, Kaur H, Bansal S, et al. Premature greying of hair: Risk factors, co-morbid conditions, pharmacotherapy and reversal-A systematic review and meta-analysis. Dermatol Ther. 2020;33(6):e13990.
18. Reece AS. Hair greying in substance addiction. Arch Dermatol. 2007;143(1):116-8.
19. Ezzedine K, Diallo A, Léauté-Labrèze C, Seneschal J, Mossalayi D, AlGhamdi K, et al. Halo nevi association in nonsegmental vitiligo affects age at onset and depigmentation pattern. Arch Dermatol. 2012;148(4):497-502.
20. Singal A, Daulatabad D, Grover C. Greying severity score: A useful tool for evaluation of premature canities. Indian Dermatol Online J. 2016;7(3):164-7.
21. Yale K, Juhasz M, Mesinkovska NA. Medication-induced repigmentation of grey hair: a systematic review. Skin Appendage Disord. 2020;6(1):1-10.
22. Pavani P, Madhavi Latha M, Praveena T. The study of premature canities and its association in tertiary care hospital. MedPulse Int J Med. 2020;16(3):90-4.
23. Da França SA, Dario MF, Esteves VB, Baby AR, Velasco MVR. Types of Hair Dye and Their Mechanisms of Action. Cosmetics. 2015;2(2):110-26.
24. Madnani N, Khan K. Hair cosmetics. Indian J Dermatol Venereol Leprol. 2013;79:654-67.
25. George NM, Potlapati A. Hair colouring: what a dermatologist should know? Int J Res Dermatol. 2021;7:496-502.
26. Kim KH, Kabir E, Jahan SA. The use of personal hair dye and its implications for human health. Environ Int. 2016;89-90:222-7.
27. Eberle CE, Sandler DP, Taylor KW, White AJ. Hair dye and chemical straightener use and breast cancer risk in a large US population of black and white women. Int J Cancer. 2020; 147(2):383-91.
28. Towle KM, Grespin ME, Monnot AD. Personal use of hair dyes and risk of leukemia: a systematic literature review and meta-analysis. Cancer Med. 2017;6(10):2471-86.
29. Gago-Dominguez M, Castelao JE, Yuan JM, Yu MC, Ross RK. Use of permanent hair dyes and bladder-cancer risk. Int J Cancer. 2001;91(4):575-9.
30. Battistella C, McCallum NC, Gnanasekaran K, Zhou X, Caponetti V, Montalti M, et al. Mimicking natural human hair pigmentation with synthetic melanin. ACS central science. 2020;6(7): 1179-88.

Part 3: Involvement of Specific Site

A Patient with Leg Ulcer

Nainesh P Bhatt, Yogesh U Patel

INTRODUCTION

Ulcers of skin can result from complete loss of the epidermis and often portions of the dermis and even subcutaneous fat.[1] Chronic leg ulcer **(Fig. 1)** is defined as a defect in the skin below the level of knee persisting for >6 weeks and shows no tendency to heal after 3 or more months.[2] Ulcers related to venous insufficiency constitute 70%, arterial disease 10%, and ulcers of mixed etiology 15% of leg ulcer presentations.[3] So more emphasis would be given on these two types. In diabetic patients, mixed etiologies may be responsible for chronic leg ulcers. **Table 1** shows classification of leg ulcers.

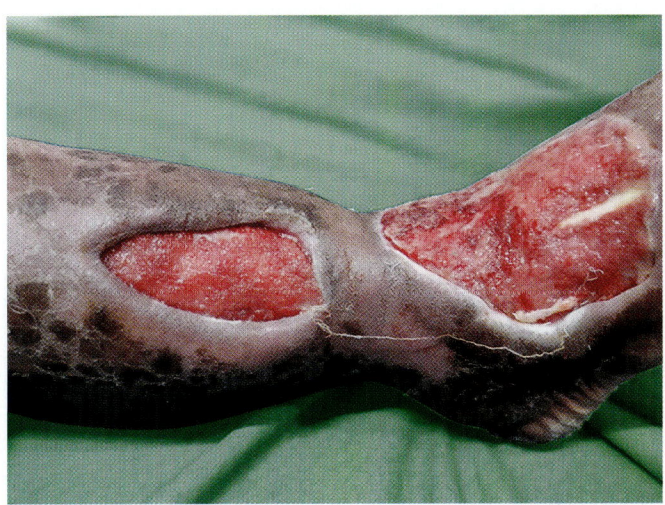

FIG. 1: Deep leg ulcer with healthy granulation tissue.

Table 1: Causes of leg ulcers.[4]	
Types of ulcer	**Causes of ulcer**
Vascular	• Venous insufficiency **(Fig. 2)** • Peripheral arterial diseases • Mixed venous and arterial • Raynaud's phenomenon
Vasculitis ulcers and autoimmune disease	• Leukocytoclastic vasculitis **(Fig. 3)** • Cryoglobulinemic vasculitis • Granulomatosis with polyangiitis • Rheumatoid arthritis • Systemic lupus erythematosus • Systemic sclerosis • Polyarteritis nodosa • Pyoderma gangrenosum
Vasculopathies	• Livedoid vasculopathy • Occlusive vasculopathies (calciphylaxis, cholesterol embolie, cryofibrinogenemia) • Hypercoagulable states (factor V leiden, antiphospholipid antibody syndrome, protein C, protein S deficiency, antithrombin III deficiency, hyperhomocysteinemia, G20210A mutation, etc.) • Thromboangiitis obliterans (Buerger's disease)
Neuropathic[5]	• Leprosy **(Fig. 4)** • Diabetes **(Fig. 5)** • Alcoholic neuropathy • Syringomyelia • Tabes dorsalis

Continued

Continued

Types of ulcer	Causes of ulcer
Metabolic	• Diabetes • Gout • Calcinosis cutis • Prolidase deficiencies
Hematological[5,6]	• Sickle cell disease • Thalassemia • Polycythemia rubra vera • Leukemia • Hereditary spherocytosis • Thrombotic thrombocytopenic purpura • Granulocytopenia • Polyclonal dysproteinemia • Cryoglobulinemia
Trauma	• Pressure • Thermal injury • Radiation injury • Factitious
Tumors	• Basal cell carcinoma • Squamous cell carcinoma • Lymphoma • Kaposi's sarcoma • Melanoma
Infections	*Bacterial* **(Fig. 6)**: • Atypical mycobacteria • Cutaneous tuberculosis • Leprosy *Fungal infections:* • Mycetoma • Sporotrichosis • Chromoblastomycosis • Blastomycosis • Zygomycosis (rarely histoplasmosis, lobomycosis, invasive candidiasis) *Parasitic:* • Leishmaniasis
Panniculitis	• Necrobiosis lipoidica • Fat necrosis • Erythema induratum • Pancreatitis associated panniculitis
Other	• Pyoderma gangrenosum • Chronic kidney disease (CKD) • Drug induced
Contributing factors along with other causes[7] which might delay wound healing	• Malnutrition • Deficiencies of vitamins • Deficiencies of minerals such as zinc

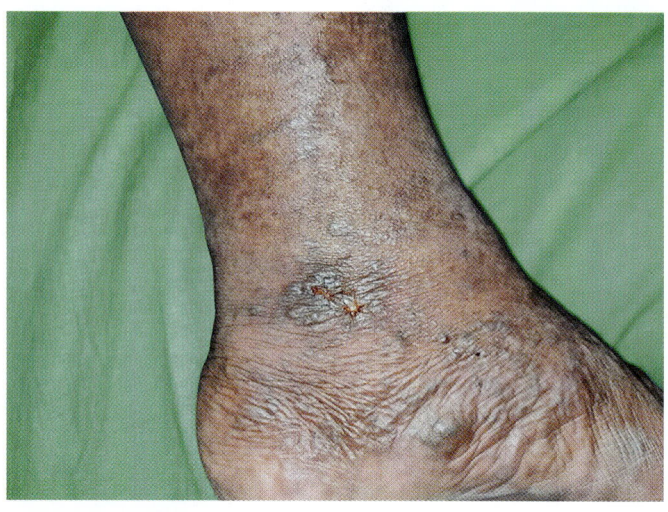

FIG. 2: Venous leg ulcer with varicose vein.

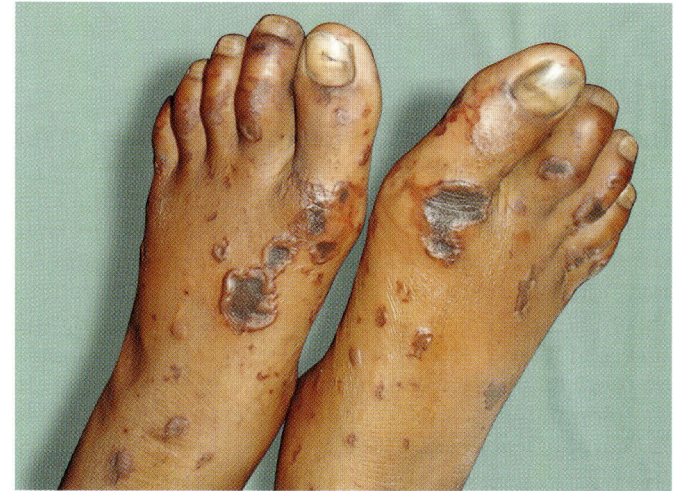

FIG. 3: Lesion of vasculitis impending to ulcerate.

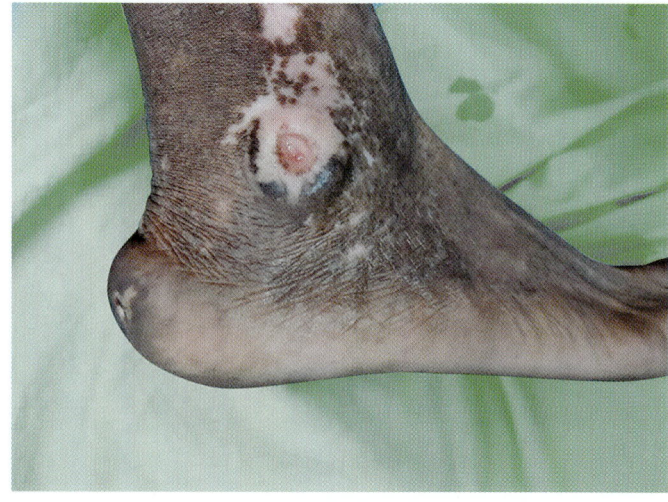

FIG. 4: Trophic ulcer in patient having leprosy.

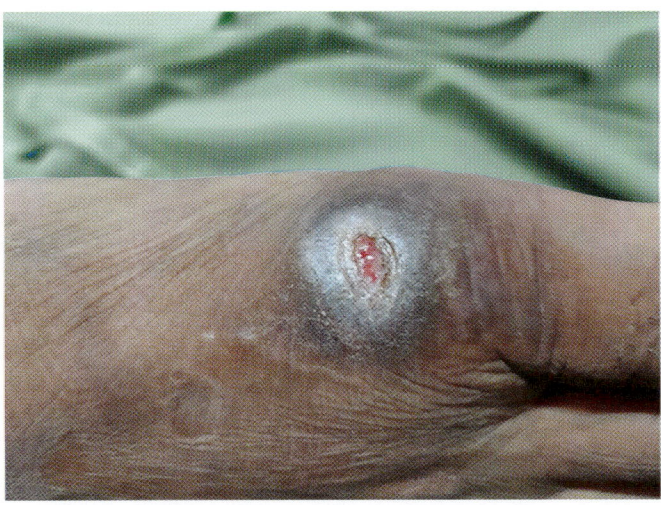

FIG. 5: Ulcer over head of metatarsal in diabetic patient.

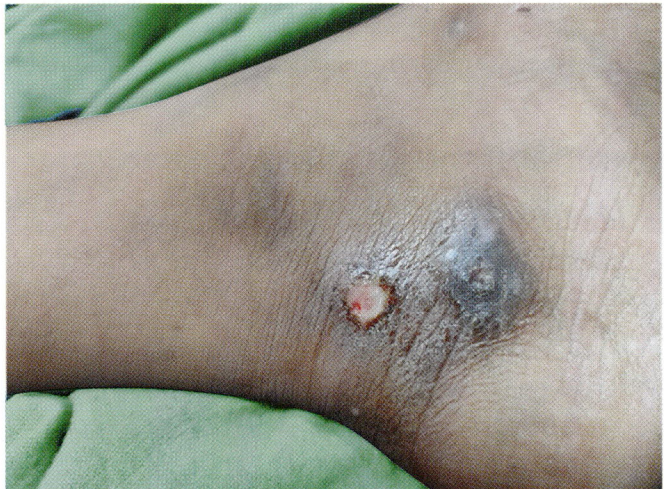

FIG. 6: Leg ulcer following bacterial infection.

CLINICAL ASSESSMENT OF LEG ULCERS

History Points

- *Age*: Chances of venous ulcer increases with age. Arterial ulcers affect male >50 years of age while in females it affects patients of >65 years.
- *Sex*: Chronic ulcers associated with autoimmune disorders are more common in females. Livedoid vasculopathy are more common in females while arterial disorders associated ulcers are more common in males. Female preponderance has been observed in pyoderma gangrenosum (PG).
- *Duration*:
  - *Rapid onset*: Ulcers of infectious origin and pyoderma gangrenosum are of rapid onset to start with then eventually becomes chronic. Arterial ulcers and vasculopathic ulcers are also of rapid onset.
  - *Gradual onset*: Venous ulcers and neuropathic ulcers are of gradual onset.
- *Initiating factors/precipitating factors*:
  - *Immobility*: This could be initiating factors in cases of patients with hypercoagulable state and pressure ulcers.
  - *Trauma*: This could be evaluated in cases where neuropathic ulcers, pyoderma gangrenosum, and infections like atypical mycobacterial as well as deep fungal infection.
  - *Postures*: Prolonged standing or sitting pertaining to various occupations might exacerbate or precipitate venous ulcers.
  - *Smoking*: Aggravates attacks of thromboangiitis obliterans and may precipitate the same.
- *Progression of ulcers*: In livedoid vasculopathy to start with livedoid purpura occurs which ulcerates and heals with porcelain white scarring. In vasculitis, palpable purpura vesiculates and ruptures. Classic PG begins as an inflammatory pustule with a surrounding halo that enlarges and ulcerates.
- *Drug history*: History of drugs which can cause chronic ulcers as mentioned in **Table 1**. Immunosuppressive drugs may be responsible for development of chronic infectious leg ulcers. Oral contraceptive pills may induce hypercoagulable state in females.
- *Addiction*: Alcoholism may be contributing factor for neuropathy.
- *Nature of pain*:
  - Most ulcers are painful except neuropathic ulcers. Though tuberculous ulcers and deep fungal infections are usually painless, sometimes they can be painful also.
  - Burning pain precedes development of ulcers in livedoid vasculopathy which is a clue to its diagnosis.
  - Pain may be severe, excruciating, penetrating, sharp, and stinging in nature in sickle cell disease.
  - *Aggravating/alleviating factors of pain*:
    - Venous leg ulcer: Throbbing, aching, and heavy feeling in legs on dependent posture, while improve with elevation and rest.
    - Arterial leg ulcer: Intermittent claudication and can be worse at night and rest, while improve with dependency.
- *Associated history*:
  - *Intermittent claudication*: Arterial ulcer
  - *Pedal edema*: Venous ulcer
  - *Paresthesia*: Neuropathic ulcer
  - *Burning and bluish discoloration on cold exposure*: Raynaud's phenomenon.
  - *Fever*: Connective tissue disease (CTD), panniculitis, evening rise fever in tuberculosis and atypical mycobacterial ulcers, infective chronic ulcers in patients of immunosuppression, erythema nodosum leprosum (ENL) necroticans, Lucio phenomenon
  - *Loss of footwear*: Neuropathies
  - *Weight loss*: Tuberculosis, malignancy

- *History of associated disorders/conditions*:
  - *Diabetes mellitus*: It can cause microvascular abnormality and sensory neuropathy predispose to neuropathic or metabolic ulcer or arterial ulcer.
  - *Coronary artery disease*: It is mostly associated with hypercholesterolemia and atherosclerosis which is predisposing factor for arterial ulcer or occlusive vasculopathy because of emboli.
  - *Previous major surgery*: Might lead to immobility and hence deep vein thrombosis and pressure ulcers.
  - *History of major bone fracture*: To rule out fat embolism.
  - *Pregnancy*: Can cause venous hypertension and lead to venous ulcer as well as pregnancy itself is a hypercoagulable state.
  - *History of genital ulcers*: For tertiary syphilis
  - *History of viral hepatitis*: For cryoglobulinemia.
  - Family history of coagulopathies.

Examination Points (Tables 2 and 3)

- *Site of ulcers*: Ulcers in cases of livedoid vasculopathy involves mainly dorsa of feet and ankle areas of skin. Pretibial and malleolar regions are involved in cases of systemic lupus erythematosus (SLE).
- *Size of ulcers*: Venous ulcers are usually large in size compared to arterial ulcers.
- *Shape of ulcers*: Venous ulcers are usually longitudinally oval. Ulcers in vasculopathies could be of bizarre shape.
- *Borders of ulcers*: Undermined borders are described with tuberculous ulcers and pyoderma gangrenosum, with later having purplish tinge to it.

Table 4 shows major distinguishing features between neuropathic ulcer from pressure ulcer.

CHARACTERISTIC OF RARE CAUSES OF CHRONIC ULCER

Tropical Ulcer

The lesion first appears as a small papule on the lower leg, usually at the site of trauma. The ulcer then spreads rapidly, forms a blister and undergoes necrosis, which is associated with pain, fever, and malaise. Within a few weeks the ulcer enlarges to 10–12 cm and a superficial, necrotic, malodorous,

Table 2: Major differentiating points on examination among lower limb ulcers of venous, arterial, and neuropathic cause.[8]

	Venous ulcer	*Arterial ulcer*	*Neuropathic ulcer*
Site	Gaiter area of leg, above medial or lateral malleolus	Lateral malleolus, tibial area, toes or shin or over pressure points	Sole of foot or pressure points
Size and shape	Large and shallow, oval	Small, rounded or stellate shape	Deep, small/large
Borders	Shallow with irregular flat	Punched out	Well demarcated
Ulcer bed	• Slough at the base with granulation tissue • Moderate to heavy exudate	• No granulation tissue, necrotic tissue or fixed slough • Low exudate	Granulation tissue normal
Changes surrounding skin			
Pigmentation	Hyperpigmented with eczematous changes	Shiny and thin	Normal pigmentation
Scarring	Atrophie blanche of previous lesion	Absent	Absent
Induration	• Present • Thickening and fibrosis or crusty, dry hyperkeratotic with eczematous skin, "inverted champagne bottle appearance"	• Absent • Thin, shiny dry skin with reduced or no hair	Callosity of surrounding skin
Temperature	Warm	Cool	Warm
Pedal pulse	Normal	Absent or weak	Normal
Edema	Present	Absent	Absent
Varicosity	Present	Absent	Absent
Capillary refill time	<3 seconds	>3 seconds	<3 seconds
Sensory evaluation for fine touch	Normal	Normal	Decreased or absent
Ankle-brachial pressure index (ABPI) (by Doppler flow meter)	>0.95	• >0.8–0.95—mild arterial disease • >0.5–0.8—moderate arterial disease • >0.3–0.5—severe arterial disease	>0.95

Table 3: Additional examination findings for various etiology.	
Body built	• Cachexic in nutritional deficiency/malnutrition, HIV, tuberculosis • Obesity might be associated with venous ulcers and pressure ulcers
Anemia, jaundice, hepatosplenomegaly	Hematological disorders
Lymphadenopathy	Tuberculosis, malignancy
Sensation loss	Neuropathic ulcers, typically gloves and stocking pattern in cases of leprosy, and diabetic neuropathy
Palpable purpura	Vasculitis
Irregular bizarre, shaped purpura	Vasculopathy especially APLA
Retiform purpura	Livedoid vasculopathy, PAN, occlusive microvasculopathy, SLE, cryofibrinogenemia
Atrophie blanche	Livedoid vasculopathy and rarely in other vasculopathies
Cribriform scaring	Pyoderma gangrenosum
Nodules and indurated plaques	Panniculitis as mentioned in **Table 1**, rheumatoid nodules, PAN
Varicosities and lipodermatosclerosis	Venous ulcers
Gangrenous changes on toes (dry)	Arterial disorders and Lucio phenomenon
Petechial lesions	Hematological disorders and malignancy
Bluish discoloration on cold test	Raynaud's phenomenon, CTD, rheumatoid arthritis
Whitish material discharge from ulcer	Calcinosis cutis
Yellow oily material discharge from ulcer	Panniculitis
Muscle wasting	Can be associated findings in cases of neuropathy
Arthritis	Vasculitis, rheumatoid arthritis, gout
Priapism and pulmonary hypertension	Sickle cell disease
Fragile skin, saddle nose, small chin, protruded jaw and wide set eyes	Prolidase deficiency

(APLA: antiphospholipid antibody; CTD: connective tissue disease; HIV: human immunodeficiency virus; PAN: polyarteritis nodosa; SLE: systemic lupus erythematosus)

Table 4: Characteristics of neuropathic and pressure ulcer.[9]			
Ulcer type	**General characteristics**	**Pathophysiology**	**Site of ulcer**
Neuropathic	• Associated with diabetes mellitus • Leprosy • Alcoholic neuropathy	Underlying nerve damage causing loss of sensation, motor weakness causing anatomical deformity, autonomic nervous dysfunction with associated vascular compromise. Trauma, prolonged pressure	On plantar aspect of feet
Pressure	In patients with limited mobility	Tissue ischemia and necrosis secondary to prolonged pressure	Located over bony prominences, heels and ankles

purulent, hemorrhagic black coating develops. After 3–4 weeks, the edge becomes flatter, and the swelling and pain decrease.

Atypical Mycobacteria especially *Mycobacterium ulcerans*

Buruli ulcer usually starts as a small nodule which ulcerates. Thickening and darkening of the skin surrounding the lesion can be observed.

Leprosy infection causes neuropathic ulceration due to sensory neuropathy. Rarely Lucio phenomenon in cases of diffuse leprosy gives rise to vasculopathic ulcers.

Cutaneous Tuberculosis

Tuberculous chancre results from the direct entry of the organism into the skin of a nonsensitized individual. The lesion begins as red-brown papule or nodule that evolves into a painless, shallow, and undermined ulcer with a granulomatous base, most commonly affecting the face or extremities. Size of the lesion rarely exceeds 5 cm ulcer heals with scarring. Infection can be identified by swabs and biopsy samples sent for microscopy and culture.

Fungal

They are usually asymmetrical and are located over trauma-prone areas of the legs and affects people of temperate and humid climate. Characteristically triad of swelling, draining sinuses, and extrusion of colonial grains in the exudates are seen though it may not be seen with all the organisms. Ulcers are mostly recurrent. The causative fungus in them may either be identified through smears/histopathologic sections or on culture.

Protozoal: Leishmaniasis

The skin lesion begins as a nontender, firm, red papule several centimeters in size at the site of the sandfly bite. In time, the lesion becomes darker, widens with central ulceration, serous crusting, and granuloma formation. The border often has a raised erythematous rim. Lesions heal with scarring.

Necrobiosis Lipoidica

Patients usually present shiny brown-yellow patches affecting shins. Lesions have a red advancing indurated border and central atrophy with a shiny, waxy surface, and telangiectasias. Ulcerations appear in around 30% of patients. Comorbidities and cofactors included diabetes mellitus, arterial hypertension, obesity, hypercholesterolaemia, renal insufficiency, respiratory diseases, smoking, and neoplasia.

Fat Necrosis

Post-traumatic fat necrosis of the subcutaneous fat tissue can occur following a fall, blunt injury, surgery, and minor procedures such as injections. It is more prevalent in women. Usually a hematoma develops at the site of injury to be followed by a deeper induration that may rarely ulcerate.

Pyoderma Gangrenosum

It is an autoimmune inflammatory disease associated with few systemic disorders. Ulcers are rapidly progressive, large, and painful with wide margin and undermined necrotic edge. Pathergy test might be positive. It is a diagnosis of exclusion.

Chronic Kidney Disease

Calciphylaxis is a rare complication of chronic kidney disease which presents as nodular subcutaneous calcification and necrosis which often results in ulceration.

Certain laboratory investigations may be helpful:
- *Screening tests*:
  - *Complete blood count*: Raised WBC count suggest possible infection
  - *Erythrocyte sedimentation rate (ESR)*: Elevated ESR may be marker of tuberculous infection (e.g., tuberculous ulcer)
  - *Blood glucose*: Poor glycemic control is risk factor for development of diabetic neuropathy as well as vasculopathy.
  - *Serum albumin*: Hypoproteinemia may associated with delayed wound healing
  - *Serum transferring, serum iron, zinc*: Deficiency is associated with delayed wound healing
- *Additional tests—which can be ordered as per history points*:
  - Lipid profile, renal function tests, and liver function tests
  - Serum antinuclear antibody (ANA)
  - Lupus anticoagulant
  - Antithrombin III
  - Protein C, protein S
  - Cryoglobulin
  - Cryofibrinogen
  - Rheumatoid arthritis (RA) factor
  - Screening for hepatitis B virus (HBV), hepatitis C virus (HCV)
  - Rapid plasma reagin (RPR) test
  - Blood culture in severely ill
  - Infected individuals
- The ankle-brachial pressure index (ABPI) using a handheld Doppler ultrasound and sphygmomanometer to assess arterial perfusion[10]
- The leg ulcer measurement tool (LUMT) is a validated tool that has been used to quantify leg ulcer assessment and can be used to track change in wound status over time.[11]
- The plain radiography of the foot along with CT and MRI should be done to rule out osteomyelitis and malignancy.
- *Laboratory screening tests for vasculitis*: Urine analysis for proteinuria, hematuria, cylindruria, routine and immunohistopathology of skin biopsies, antinuclear antibodies, rheumatoid factor, complement C4, circulating immune complexes, paraproteins, immunoglobulin fractions, antineutrophil cytoplasmic antibodies, serological tests, and cultures for underlying infections.[12]
- Venography may be performed as an investigational procedure prior to valvular surgery. Lower extremities arteriography is indicated in patients with ischemia.[6]
- Color duplex ultrasound scanning which is becoming the de facto standard for evaluation of venous obstruction is also used to assess the location and extent of reflux in venous ulcers.[13]

- Plethysmography and venous pressure data are important in determining the need for surgical bypass or valve replacement.
- A quantitative bacterial culture is more specific and should be performed once wound infection is suspected.[5]
- Ulcer biopsy is important in making a correct diagnosis and to rule out malignancy.[14,15]

MANAGEMENT OF LEG ULCERS

Treatment depends on the cause of ulcer.

Venous Ulcers

General Measures

- Avoidance of smoking and adequate nutrition
- Avoid sitting with legs crossed and standing for prolonged period
- Avoid constricting clothes
- Exercise the feet and ankles when legs are elevated.
- Use compression therapy every morning before rising

Compression Therapy

- It forms the mainstay of therapy and prevents venous hypertension, reduces edema, promotes ulcer healing, prevents recurrence
- Aim is to achieve external ankle pressure of 35–40 mm Hg
- Arterial disease must be ruled out before starting compression therapy.
- *Compression can be achieved by:*
  - Nonelastic bandages
  - Multilayered elastic bandages
  - Elastic bandages
  - Elastic support stockings

Topical Therapy

- *Wound dressing*: A moist wound environment prevents wound infection and promotes faster re-epithelialization. Selection of dressing depends on exudate **(Table 5)**.
- *Topical antibiotics and steroids*: Topical antibiotics are usually not indicated unless there are signs of infection. Cadexomer iodine and controlled released silver ion preparations are preferred topical antiseptic. Topical steroids may be used if stasis dermatitis or allergic contact dermatitis develops in the surrounding skin.

Table 5: Types of dressings.[16]	
Ulcer characteristic	**Dressing**
Heavy exudate	Foams, alginates
Moderate exudate	Hydrocolloids, foams
Mild exudate	Hydrogels, hydrocolloids

- *Systemic therapy*: Pentoxifylline (400 mg tds), aspirin (75 mg od), cilostazol, and stanozolol are particularly useful in patients having lipodermatosclerosis.

Surgical Therapy

Vein surgery: Useful in preventing recurrences in those patients who cannot tolerate or are not compliant with compression therapy.

Indication: Isolated superficial venous reflux or segmental deep reflux

Skin grafts: Pinch grafts
- Split thickness grafts
- Composite grafts
- Cultured keratinocyte grafts

Factors predictive of delayed wound healing:
- Original area ≥5 cm^2
- ≥1 year duration
- ≤40% of ulcer healing by third week
- Presence of fibrin over 50% wound bed
- Previous hip/knee replacement
- ABPI ≤0.8

Arterial Ulcers

General Measures

- Avoidance of smoking and cold exposure
- Avoidance of constricting clothing
- Ambulation as tolerated
- Regular exercise

Consultation with a vascular surgeon is necessary.
Patient can be given tablet aspirin.
Tablet pentoxifylline or cilostazol helps in reducing the symptoms of claudication.
Local wound care should be performed with moist dressing.

Neuropathic Ulcers

General Measures

- Perform daily foot care (inspect the feet, wash and dry well between the toes, wear clean socks that wick away moisture from the skin, socks should not have seams or mended areas)
- Apply good quality moisturizer (avoid in toe webs)
- Avoid soaking of feet and wearing shoes without socks or stockings
- Avoid sandals with thongs between the toes
- Avoid crossing the legs
- Reduce the pressure on bony prominences by wearing soft pads
- Avoid extreme temperatures
- Avoid smoking

- Keep diabetes under control
- Avoid over-the-counter medicines for corns, calluses, antiseptic lotions, adhesive tapes

Specific Therapy

- *Debridement*: Aggressive removal of all calluses, nonviable tissues
- Mechanical offloading by total contact casts
- Moist wound dressing
- *Vascular control*: If vascular compromise is present, revascularization may be necessary.
- Infection control
- *Adjunctive therapy*:
  - *Growth factors*: Becaplermin, a platelet-derived growth factor
  - Tissue engineered skin
  - Topical tretinoin

Treatment for leg ulcers due to other causes: General measures along with specific therapy pertaining to etiology like antitubercular therapy for tuberculosis, immunomodulators for autoimmune disorders and vasculitis, anticoagulants for coagulative disorders, and antifungal for fungal infections.

REFERENCES

1. van Gent WB, Wilschut ED, Wittens C. Management of venous ulcer disease. BMJ. 2010;341(7782):1092-6.
2. Kahle B, Hermanns HJ, Gallenkemper G. Evidence-based treatment of chronic leg ulcers. Dtsch Arztebl Int. 2011;108(14):231-7.
3. Casey G. Causes and management of leg and foot ulcers. Nurs Stand. 2004;18(45):57-8, 60, 62 passim.
4. Sarkar PK, Ballantyne S. Management of leg ulcers. Postgrad Med J. 2000;76(901):674-82.
5. Rayner R, Carville K, Keaton J, Prentice J, Santamaria XN. Leg ulcers: atypical presentations and associated co-morbidities. Wound Pract Res. 2009;17(4):168-85.
6. London NJ, Donnelly R. ABC of arterial and venous disease. Ulcerated lower limb. BMJ. 2000;320(7249):1589-91.
7. Amir O, Liu A, Chang ALS. Stratification of highest-risk patients with chronic skin ulcers in a Stanford retrospective cohort includes diabetes, need for systemic antibiotics, and albumin levels. Ulcers. 2012;2012:767861.
8. Newton H. Leg ulcers: differences between venous and arterial. Wounds Essentials. 2011;6(1):20-8.
9. Aydin A, Shenbagamurthi S, Brem H. Lower extremity ulcers: venous, arterial, or diabetic? Emerg Med. 2009;41(8):18-24.
10. Grey JE, Harding KG, Enoch S. Venous and arterial leg ulcers. BMJ. 2006;332(7537):347-50.
11. Burrows C. Leg ulcers. Wound Care Can. 2008;8(2):16-8.
12. Mekkes JR, Loots MA, Van Der Wal AC, Bos JD. Causes, investigation and treatment of leg ulceration. Br J Dermatol. 2003;148(3):388-401.
13. Siddiqui AR, Bernstein JM. Chronic wound infection: facts and controversies. Clin Dermatol. 2010;28(5):519-26.
14. Ghauri AS, Nyamekye IK. Leg ulceration: the importance of treating the underlying pathophysiology. Phlebology. 2010;25, Suppl 1:42-51.
15. Agale SV, Kulkarni DR, Valand AG, Zode RR, Grover S Marjolin's ulcer—a diagnostic dilemma. J Assoc Physicians India. 2009;57(8):593-94.
16. Paddle-Ledinek JE, Nasa Z, Cleland HJ. Effect of different wound dressings on cell viability and proliferation. Plast Reconstr Surg. 2006;117:110S-118S.

15. A Patient with Chronic and Recurrent Oral Ulcers or Erosions

Jigna Padhiyar

INTRODUCTION

Gingiva, hard palate, and dorsal surface of tongue are keratinized surface in oral cavity. Rest of the parts have nonkeratinized mucosa.

In routine dermatology outpatient consultation, one of the most challenging parts is to diagnose and treat a patient with chronic, recurrent oral ulcers, and stomatitis. They can be painful as well as affects chewing, swallowing, and speech.

Chronic oral ulcers are defined as ulcers persisting beyond 14 days.[1] Recurrent oral ulcers are defined as episodes of ulcers with intermitting remission periods. When in cases of recurrent oral ulcers, no systemic causes are found; they are termed as recurrent aphthous stomatitis (RAS) **(Fig. 1)**.[2] While, in case of associated disease, they are termed aphthous-like ulcers.

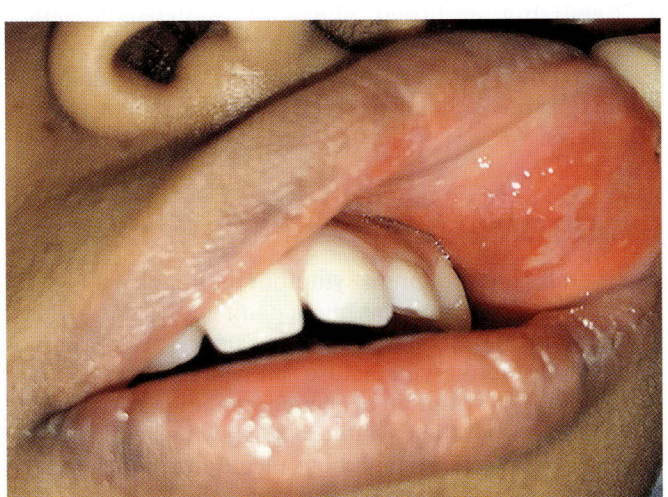

FIG. 1: Minor aphthous ulcer with surrounding erythematous hallo involving buccal mucosa.

Acute oral ulcers and gingivostomatitis are mainly due to viral and bacterial infections and are associated with prodromal symptoms. Herpes virus can remain latent and may be responsible for recurrent ulcers. Similarly, cytomegalovirus has also been responsible for chronic and recurrent oral ulcers in immunocompromised state. Rarely few fungi can also cause chronic oral lesions most commonly in immunocompromised state. Acute oral ulcers and stomatitis is not included in this chapter.

DIFFERENTIAL DIAGNOSIS OF CHRONIC AND RECURRENT ORAL ULCERS INCLUDES[1,3-5]

- Aphthous ulcers (though this is most common cause, not all chronic and recurrent oral ulcers are aphthous ulcers)
- Persistent traumatic ulcer (most common cause in adults, trauma could be in form of thermal, mechanical, electrical, or chemical)
- *Infectious causes*: Tuberculosis (TB), syphilitic gumma, blastomycosis, mucormycosis, recurrent herpes stomatitis, and cytomegalovirus-associated recurrent oral ulcers
- Erosive/ulcerative oral lichen planus (LP)
- Vesiculobullous disorders (most commonly oral pemphigus vulgaris and mucous membrane pemphigoid, rarely others)
- Behçet's syndrome
- *Autoinflammatory syndromes*: PFAPA syndrome (periodic fever, aphthous stomatitis, pharyngitis, and adenitis syndrome), FMF (familial Mediterranean fever), HID (hyperimmunoglobulinemia D), and PAPA (pyogenic sterile arthritis, pyoderma gangrenosum, and acne)

- *Rarely*: Epidermolysis bullosa, malignancy, radiation, and drugs
- Systemic diseases **(Table 1)**

AGE OF THE PATIENT[1-5]

Age of the patient might help us to shorten down the list of differential diagnosis in a particular patient. Aphthous and autoinflammatory syndrome usually present in early childhood to adolescent period while cyclical neutropenia can present in infancy **(Table 2)**.

Table 1: Systemic disorders associated with chronic and recurrent oral ulcers.	
Nutritional deficiency	Iron, folic acid, and vitamin B12 deficiency (including pernicious anemia)
Gastrointestinal disorders	Malabsorption state in pernicious anemia, celiac disease, Crohn's disease, and ulcerative colitis
Endocrine disorders	Luteal phase of menstrual cycle, pregnancy, puberty, OCP
Hematological disorders	Anemia, leukemia, neutropenia, and blood dyscrasia
Rheumatological disorders	Lupus erythematosus, sweet syndrome, reactive arthritis
Drugs	Antibiotics, NSAIDs, chemotherapeutic agents, radiotherapy, nicorandil, alendronate, and drugs causing erythema multiforme and FDR
Malignancy	SCC, glucagonoma
Disorders of uncertain pathogenesis	Hypereosinophilic syndrome, eosinophilic ulcer (rarely chronic)
Miscellaneous	Certain foods, cessation of smoking, GVHD, vasculitis, monoclonal plasmacytic ulcerative stomatitis

(FDR: fixed-drug reaction; GVHD: graft-versus-host disease; NSAIDs: nonsteroidal anti-inflammatory drugs; SCC: squamous cell carcinoma)

Table 2: Relevance of age in case of oral ulcers.	
Infancy	Cyclical neutropenia, rarely FMF
Childhood to adolescence	Starting age for aphthous ulcers, autoinflammatory syndrome
>40 years of age	Necrotizing sialometaplasia, eosinophilic ulcers, SCC
>50–60 years	BP, MMP, LAD
20–40 years	Recurrent EM, Behçet's disease

(BP: bullous pemphigoid; EM: erythema multiforme; FMF: familial Mediterranean fever; LAD: linear immunoglobulin A dermatosis; MMP: mucous membrane pemphigoid; SCC: squamous cell carcinoma)

GENDER PREDILECTION[1-6]

Male predominance: Traumatic ulcer, SCC, TB, and recurrent herpes.

Female predominance: LP, linear immunoglobulin A dermatosis (LAD), RAS, and connective tissue disorder (CTD). In general, autoimmune disease associated oral ulcers affect females more compared to males.

No predilection: Eosinophilic ulcer, Behçet's disease, and inflammatory bowel disease (IBD).

DURATION OF LESIONS

Sutton's disease takes approximately 6 weeks to heal while minor and herpetiform RAS takes 2 weeks and 4 weeks respectively.

Cyclical neutropenia: Lesions heal in 3–6 days.

Necrotizing sialometaplasia: It might heal over a long time with range of duration being 2–20 weeks.

Eosinophilic ulcer: It might heal within 2–3 weeks but may take as long as 1 year.

Traumatic ulcer: Usually heals within 10 days. Beyond that it is known as persistent or chronic traumatic ulcers.

Chemotherapy-related oral mucositis and ulcers: It appears 7–10 days after starting chemotherapy and heals after 2–4 weeks of completion of regimen.

Period of Normalcy in Between

All recurrent ulcers might have a period of normalcy in between, but exact duration of normalcy is not defined for every recurrent oral ulcer. Recurrence of herpes simplex can be affected by immunosuppression and associated medical conditions.
- Recurring every 21 days—cyclical neutropenia
- Recurring in luteal phase of menstrual cycle—progesterone-induced recurrent ulcers

Progress of lesions:[7,8] History regarding progression of lesions **(Table 3)** helps us to differentiate similar looking oral ulcers.

SYMPTOMS[1-8]

- Overall, most common symptom of oral ulcers is pain, but few other symptoms might point toward the etiology.
- Asymptomatic ulcers are characteristic feature of systemic lupus erythematosus and malignancy.
- Burning is a symptom of allergic stomatitis as well as LP. This is a prodromal symptom along with slight swelling in cases of recurrent aphthous ulcers and herpes.
- Numbness could be a symptom of malignancy.
- Loose tooth and nonhealing socket of tooth extraction is a symptom of malignancy.

Table 3: Progression of oral ulcers and their significance.

Progression of lesion	Relevance
Burning → swelling → ulcer → may coalesce with surrounding hallo	Aphthous ulcers
Red patches → irregular slit-like ulcers → occasional scaring	SLE
Red patches → irregular ulcers with white border	DLE
Bullae → rapidly ruptures → large, painful → irregular ulcers	Pemphigus
Vesicles or bullae which does not rupture rapidly and could be hemorrhagic	Pemphigoid group of disorders
Ulcers → thick sanguineous crusts	Drug-induced erythema multiforme
Erythema → burning sensation → edema and ulceration → deep painful ulcers → heals without scar	Chemotherapy (most common are doxorubicin, methotrexate, bleomycin, fluorouracil, cisplatin) induced mucositis and oral ulcers

(DLE: discoid lupus erythematosus; SLE: systemic lupus erythematosus)

EXACERBATING/RELIEVING FACTORS[9,10]

- Identifying traumatic agent (ill-fitting denture, mechanical/thermal/chemical irritants) and eliminating it will help in faster healing of persistent traumatic ulcer.
- Identifying contact allergen (dental, oral hygiene and food products, flavoring agents, preservatives, etc.) might help in improving stomatitis and ulcers which might not respond to standard treatments until allergens are eliminated.
- Stress might exacerbate or precipitate RAS.
- Smoking and tobacco might relieve/improve RAS and Behçet's syndrome but at the same time they increase the chances of oral malignancy.

Focused history points: Dental procedure and hygiene products, sexual and TB exposure history, drug history, and smoking and alcohol history can be asked separately apart from the associated symptoms mentioned in **Table 4**.

Family history of same lesions: Cyclical neutropenia[11] is inherited as autosomal dominant pattern and family history might help in ruling out same. RAS also sometimes affects few members of family simultaneously and role of genetic polymorphism has been found responsible for it.[12]

Table 4: Associated symptoms and their relevance to various disorders.

Associated symptoms/signs	Relevance	Investigations which can be ordered as per symptoms or signs
Weakness, tiredness, glossitis, angular cheilitis	Nutritional deficiency	CBC, serum vitamin B12
Abdominal pain, cramping, bloating, gas, diarrhea and/or constipation	Irritable Bowel syndrome	Colonoscopy, endoscopy, lactose intolerance test, breath test, stool tests
Ulcers at other sites (genital), photophobia, lesions on skin	Behçet's disease, reactive arthritis, Sweet's syndrome	Pathergy tests, biopsy, serological tests for various organisms
Erosions at other sites (genital), whitish reticular pattern	Lichen planus	Biopsy, hepatitis C
Fever, pharyngitis	Antibiotics, infections, autoinflammatory syndromes (PFAPA, FMF, HIDS, NOMID), cyclic neutropenia	CBC, inflammatory markers
Fever, joint pain, photosensitivity	LE and other CTD	CBC, RFT, ANA, biopsy, DIF
Recurrent diarrhea, infections	Immune deficiency—acquired or primary	HIV testing, genetic analysis, specific tests as per symptoms of infectious disease
Bullae on skin, other mucosal involvement, gingivostomatitis	Pemphigus and pemphigoid group of disorders	Biopsy, DIF, ELISA for specific antibodies, antigen mapping
Targetoid lesions on skin	Herpes or drugs associated EM, FDR	HSV serology, history of drugs and scores for temporal association, drug rechallenge (rarely done because of risks associated with it)
Lymphadenopathy, dysphagia, weight loss	Malignancy	Biopsy, imaging studies, peripheral blood smear, CBC

(ANA: antinuclear antibody; CBC: complete blood count; CTD: connective tissue disorder; DIF: direct immunofluorescence; ELISA: enzyme-linked immunosorbent assay; EM: erythema multiforme; FDR: fixed-drug reaction; FMF: familial Mediterranean fever; HIDS: hyperimmunoglobulin D syndrome; HIV: human immunodeficiency virus; HSV: herpes simplex virus; LE: lupus erythematosus; NOMID: neonatal-onset multisystem inflammatory disease; PFAPA: periodic fever, aphthous stomatitis, pharyngitis, and adenitis; RFT: renal function test)

Examination points to be considered: Site, number of lesions, size of lesions, types of lesions (erosions, bullae, aphthae, and ulcers), findings in surrounding mucosa, or other mucosal features apart from ulcers. Apart from mucosae labial commissures, lymph nodes, temporomandibular joint, cranial nerve examination should also be performed. ABCDE rule should be considered for solitary chronic ulcer especially in elderly males.

APPROACH FOR DIAGNOSIS

Approach has been outlined in **Flowchart 1**. First, we must observe if the ulcer is single or multiple and weather ulcer is chronic and recurrent. Then according to distinguished features as mentioned in **Tables 3 to 11** and history points and investigations we may arrive at final diagnosis. Though in real practice scenario sometimes it is really difficult to pinpoint to a diagnosis pertaining to unavailability of certain specific tests.

Number of lesions (Table 5):[1] Number of lesions can point toward etiology. Single ulcer is usually because of trauma, infective organisms, drug-induced fixed-drug reaction (FDR), major aphthous or malignancy. On the other hand, multiple oral ulcers are mainly seen in autoimmune and inflammatory disorders apart from minor and herpetiform RAS. Major and minor RAS have 1–10 ulcers compared to up to 100 in herpetiform RAS.

SITE OF LESIONS, TYPE OF LESIONS, AND CHANGES IN SURROUNDING MUCOSA

Distinguished feature of herpetiform aphthous ulcer is that it also affects nonkeratinized mucosa along with classically involving lateral or under surface of tongue **(Fig. 2)** which can be helpful in differentiating it from recurrent herpes simplex infection **(Fig. 3)** which predominantly involves keratinized mucosa like palate or gingiva along with lips. Type of lesions and changes in surrounding mucosa are fine examination points and their relevance are enumerated in **Tables 6 and 7** respectively. Significance of site is mentioned in **Tables 8 to 10**, where distinguished feature of individual diseases are discussed.

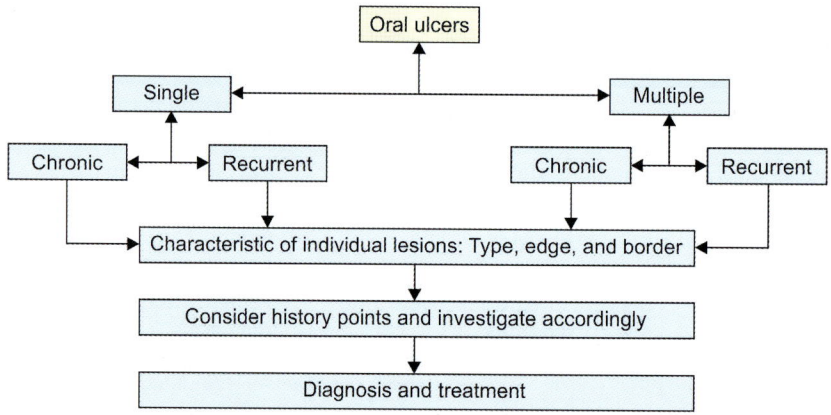

FLOWCHART 1: Diagnostic approach in cases of oral ulcers.

Table 5: Etiological possibilities according to number of lesions.

Single ulcer		Multiple ulcer	
Chronic	Recurrent	Chronic	Recurrent
Persistent traumatic ulcer	Occasionally aphthous ulcer	PV	Aphthous stomatitis
Necrotizing sialometaplasia (acute/chronic)	EM	BP	EM
SCC	FDR	MMP	Cyclic neutropenia
Eosinophilic ulcer	Sutton's disease (major aphthous)	LAD	Behçet's disease
CMV, TB, syphilis		LP	Herpes viral infection
Deep fungal		Chemotherapy/cytotoxic drugs	

(BP: bullous pemphigoid; CMV: cytomegalovirus; EM: erythema multiforme; FDR: fixed-drug reaction; LAD: linear immunoglobulin A dermatosis; LP: lichen planus; MMP: mucous membrane pemphigoid; PV: pemphigus vulgaris; SCC: squamous cell carcinoma; TB: tuberculosis)

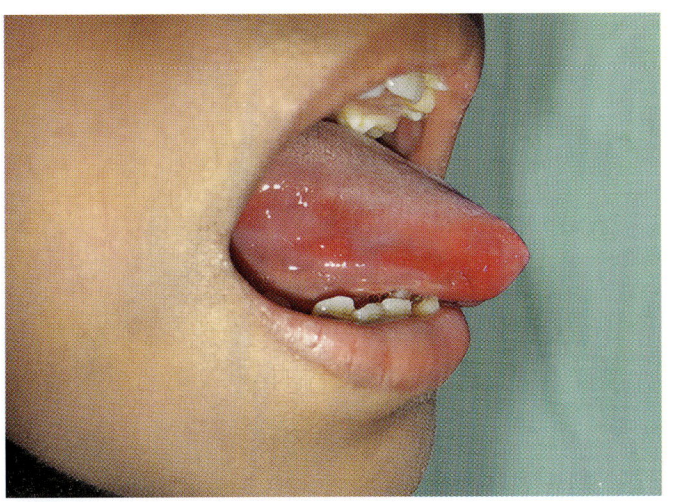

FIG. 2: Herpetiform recurrent aphthous ulcers involving characteristically lateral border of tongue.

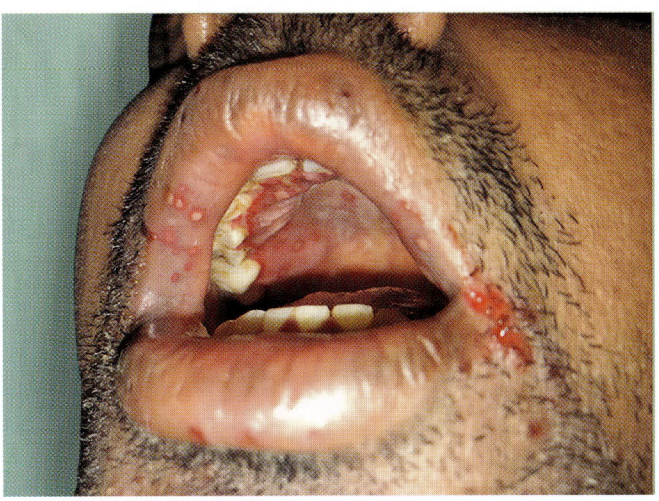

FIG. 3: Recurrent herpes simplex virus (HSV) lesions involving characteristically keratinized mucosa of palate and gingiva. Patient also had recurrent erythema multiforme.

Table 6: Type of lesions.[7,8]	
Erosions	Lichen planus, chronic erythema multiforme, pemphigus vulgaris (PV), cicatricial pemphigoid
Bullae	MMP, early stage of PV, cicatricial pemphigoid
Aphthae like ovoid ulcers	Aphthous ulcers, Behçet's syndrome, Sweet syndrome, ulcers associated with various systemic diseases like immune deficiency, celiac disease, Crohn's disease, autoinflammatory syndromes, etc.
Other type of ulcers	See **Table 8** of characteristic of solitary chronic ulcers
Desquamative gingivostomatitis	Pemphigoid group of disorders PV, lichen planus, LE GVHD, lichenoid drug reaction, chronic ulcerative stomatitis, contact dermatitis, lichenoid contact/foreign body gingivitis

(GVHD: graft-versus-host disease; LE: lupus erythematosus; MMP: mucous membrane pemphigoid)

Table 7: Changes in surrounding mucosa.[1,7,8,13]	
Surrounding red hallo **(Fig. 1)**	Aphthous ulcers and similar lesions associated with systemic disease, ulcers due to infective organisms
Minimal halo	Drug-induced agranulocytosis
Erythematous and glazed	Lichen planus (LP)
Reticular pattern **(Fig. 4)**	Lichen planus
Pigmentation	Lichen planus and nutritional deficiency, smoking associated malignant ulcer
Loss of papillae **(Fig. 5)**	Vitamin B12 deficiency, LP, benign migratory glossitis, centrally in median rhomboid glossitis
Scarring	LP, mucous membrane pemphigoid (MMP), major aphthous (Sutton's disease)
Mucosal pallor and petechiae, swollen gums	Leukemia, myelodysplastic syndrome
Cobblestone appearance (thickening and folding of mucosa), mucosal tags, cheilitis, and lip swellings	Crohn's disease
Swollen and inflamed papillae	Granulomatosis with polyangiitis
Strawberry gums	Wegener's granulomatosis

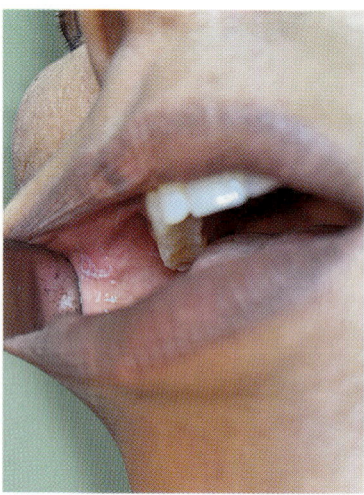

FIG. 4: Whitish reticular pattern over buccal mucosa in case of erosive lichen planus (LP).

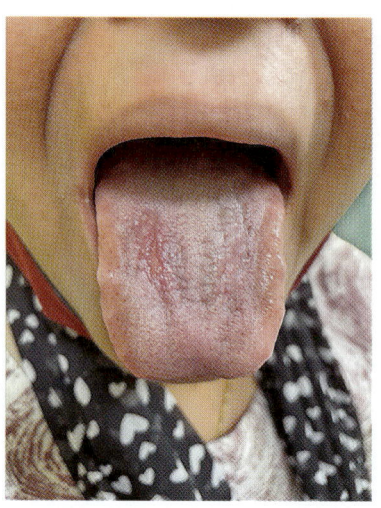

FIG. 5: Erosion involving dorsal surface of tongue with loss of papillae and scaring. Patient responded well to oral hydroxychloroquine.

Table 8: Characteristic of solitary chronic ulcers.[1,7]

Disease	Location of ulcer	Shape/border of ulcer/erosions	Distinguished features
Persistent traumatic ulcer	Tongue, lip, buccal mucosa	Regular/irregular edge	Rolled border of surrounding epithelium
Tuberculosis	Tongue, gingivae, floor of the mouth	Undermined border, ragged and indurated border	Occasionally painful
Syphilis	Lips, tongue, palate	Ragged rolled border	Clean, purple or brown base, cervical lymphadenopathy
Mucormycosis	Palate	Large and deep	Necrotic and verrucous, involvement of other organs
Blastomycosis	Any site	Painless, irregular rolled borders	Verrucous mucous hyperplasia
Necrotizing sialometaplasia	Palate, retromolar pad, lips	Crater like	Deep ulcer with yellow base
SCC	Lower lip, floor of the mouth, tongue	Crater like, rolled, indurated borders velvety base	Velvety base
Eosinophilic ulcer	Tongue, buccal mucosa	Punched out, rolled border	Slow healing, surrounding keratosis and erythema
CMV (rarely multiple)	Any	Large, minimally rolled border	Painful, necrotic, immunocompromised patients

(CMV: cytomegalovirus; SCC: squamous cell carcinoma)

Table 9: Characteristic of oral ulcers in vesiculobullous disease.[3-8]

Disease	Location	Shape/border of ulcer	Distinguished feature
Pemphigus vulgaris (Figs. 6 and 7)	Buccal mucosa, palate, gingivae, any part of mucosae	Map like, irregular borders	Positive Nikolsky sign, bullae ruptures easily, rarely desquamative gingivitis
Bullous pemphigoid	Gingivae	Vesicle	Desquamative gingivitis, early remission
MMP	Gingivae, buccal mucosa, palate	Nonspecific	Desquamative gingivitis (glazed sore gingiva), occasional blood blisters, blisters last longer, lesions may scar
LAD	Hard and soft palate, tonsillar pillars, buccal mucosa	Nonspecific, vesicles	Desquamative gingivitis/cheilitis, painful

(LAD: linear immunoglobulin A dermatosis; MMP: mucous membrane pemphigoid)

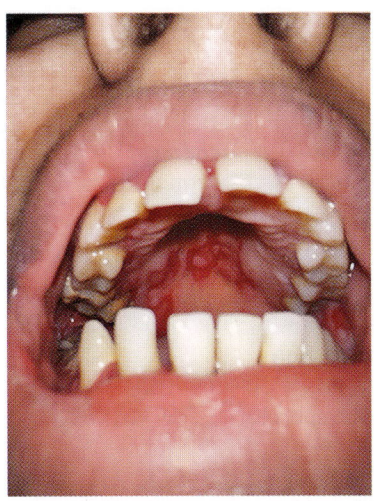

FIG. 6: Persistent map like ulcers of pemphigus vulgaris which were refractory to rituximab.

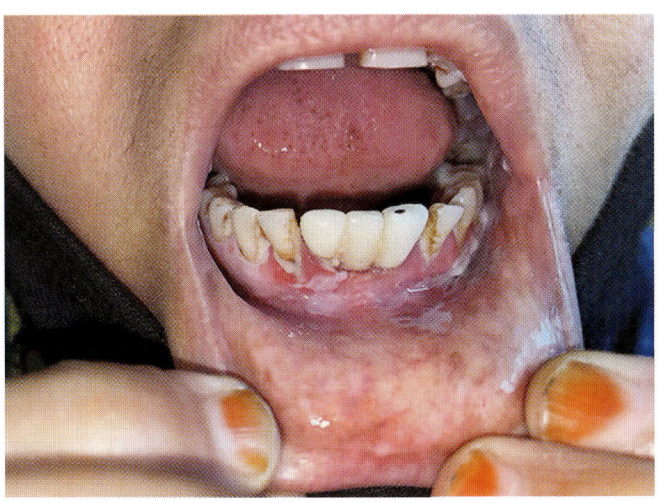

FIG. 7: Desquamative gingivitis in a case of pemphigus vulgaris.

Table 10: Distinguished features of LP and alike conditions.[7,8,10]						
	Oral LP	**Lichenoid drug reaction**	**LE**	**Chronic ulcerative stomatitis**	**Contact dermatitis**	**Lichenoid contact stomatitis/ foreign body gingivitis**
Age /sex	Middle aged F > M	–	F > M	Middle aged F > M	–	–
History points	Lesions at other site in skin and nail changes	Drugs (most common are NSAIDs, antihypertensives, antimalarials)	Associated symptoms **(Table 2)**	Rarely involves skin, ocular, and genital mucosa	History of contact with allergens, loss of taste, burning, numbness, itching	History of dental amalgam, teeth with crowns, cinnamon contact
Site and symmetry	Multifocal and roughly symmetrical	Single	Centrally on posterior aspect of hard palate, rarely other sites in SLE **(Fig. 8)**	Buccal mucosa, gingiva, tongue, symmetrical	Any site	In area of contact, unilateral lateral surface of tongue, buccal mucosa
Pain	+	+/–	–	++	+/–	
Appearance	Large irregular slit-like erosions with surrounding lace-like pattern and pigmentation	Same as LP	Irregular ulcers in SLE with white border in DLE **(Fig. 9)**	Superficial erosions	Presents as stomatitis/ cheilitis, geographic tongue, oral lichenoid reactions, burning mouth syndrome	Ulcers on contact side **(Fig. 10)**
H&E	Saw toothing, appearance of granular layer, interphase mucositis with lymphocytes	Parakeratosis, band-like infiltrate of lymphocytes, plasma cells and eosinophils, more apoptotic keratinocytes	Hyperkeratosis, basal cell vacuolization and perivascular lymphocytic infiltrate	Interphase mucositis with lymphocytes and plasma cells	Nonspecific spongiotic mucositis	Similar to LP

Continued

Continued

	Oral LP	Lichenoid drug reaction	LE	Chronic ulcerative stomatitis	Contact dermatitis	Lichenoid contact stomatitis/ foreign body gingivitis
DIF	Fibrinogen in shaggy pattern at BMZ, IgM staining of cytoid bodies	Similar as LP IIF may show string of pearls appearance of annular staining of basal cells	IgG, IgM, IgA, C3 deposition at BMZ in SLE	Staining of basal/parabasal cell nuclei (SES-ANA) with speckled pattern IgG, occasional IgA staining IIF (with epithelial substrate) findings similar as DIF	Negative	Similar to LP IIF: Negative
Treatment	Steroids, HCQ, immunomodulators and immuno-suppressives		HCQ, steroids and immunosuppres-sives, biologics	HCQ 200 mg/day, Dapsone Limited response to steroids	Elimination of contact allergen, cold compress, lignocaine, steroids	Elimination of contact allergen and symptomatic treatment

(BMZ: basement membrane zone; DIF: direct immunofluorescence; DLE: discoid lupus erythematosus; HCQ: hydroxychloroquine; IgM: immunoglobulin M; IIF: indirect immunofluorescence; LE: lupus erythematosus; LP: lichen planus; NSAIDs: nonsteroidal anti-inflammatory drugs; SES-ANA: stratified epithelial-specific antinuclear antibody; SLE: systemic lupus erythematosus)

Table 11: Distinguished feature of ulcers in inflammatory bowel disease.[7,8]

Disease	Location	Shape of ulcers/border	Distinguished feature
Crohn's disease (if localized to mouth it is termed as orofacial granulomatosis)	Buccal sulcus	Linear	Granulomatous masses at edges Aphthous like
		Superficial	Lip swelling, gingival swelling and/or facial nerve palsy (**Fig. 12**)
Ulcerative colitis		Superficial	Aphthous like
		Multiple pustules (pyostomatitis vegetans)	Cheilitis may be associated
		Solitary	Pyoderma gangrenosum-like

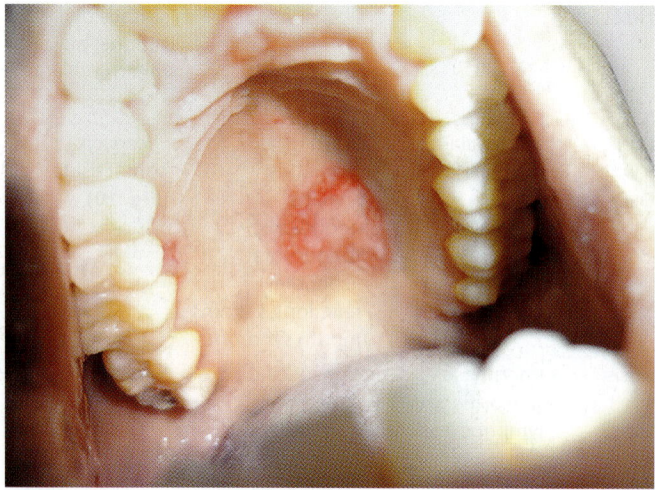

FIG. 8: Irregular linear ulceration on hard palate which were a presenting sign in a case of systemic lupus erythematosus with no other cutaneous symptoms at the time of presentation.

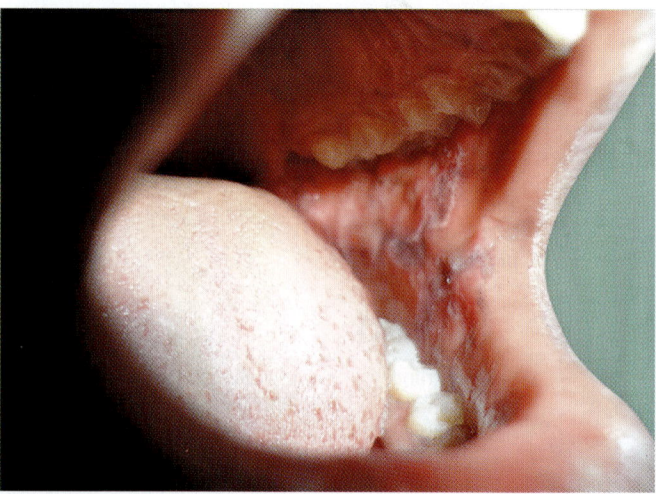

FIG. 9: Oral ulcerative lesions of discoid lupus erythematosus with characteristic white border.

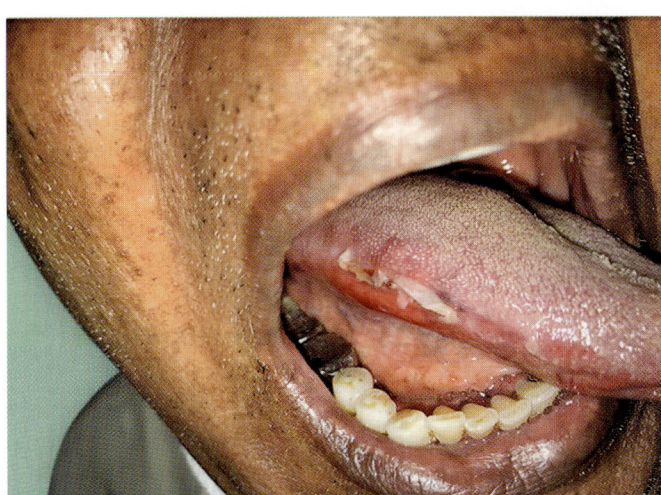

FIG. 10: Ulceration on the contact surface of tongue with metallic cap.

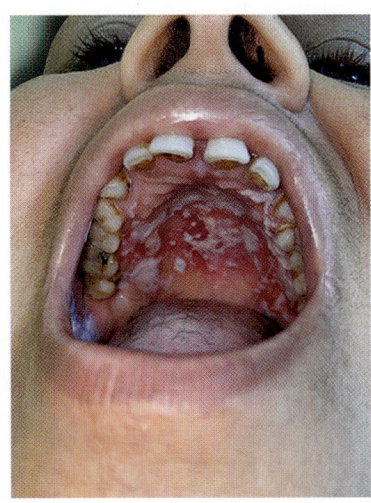

FIG. 11: Secondary candidiasis (whitish membrane) in a case of pemphigus vulgaris.

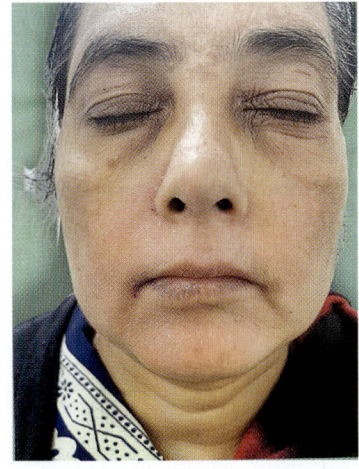

FIG. 12: Lip and surrounding skin erythema and mild scaling in a case of orofacial granulomatosis.

COMPARATIVE FEATURES OF INFECTIVE, APHTHOUS ULCERS, AND ULCERS OF SYSTEMIC DISEASES

Oral ulcers in viral infections are usually acute and associated with prodrome unlike aphthous ulcers. Aphthous like ulcers in systemic diseases are usually flat and large with associated symptoms as mentioned in **Table 4**.

Distinguished feature of oral ulcers individual diseases: Every disease has characteristic features and direct examinations of mucosa and cutaneous findings are always helpful in approaching a patient of oral ulcers. All characteristics of chronic and recurrent oral ulcers are compiled in **Tables 8 to 11**.

Collagen vascular disorders like dermatomyositis (DM) and mixed connective tissue disease (MCTD) might present with nonspecific erosions in oral mucosae. Herpes simplex virus (HSV) lesions are usually recurrent in nature but in setting of immunosuppression they can be chronic.

Presence of secondary candidiasis: Chronic oral ulceration might get complicated by secondary candidiasis. This is commonly observed with superficial erosions rather than deep ulcers **(Fig. 11)**. It appears as whitish membrane covering oral ulcers. Postcricoid web can be observed in cases of chronic mucocutaneous candidiasis (CMC).

Presence of periodontitis: Severe periodontitis might suggest immune defects. Probably that is why it is a feature of cyclic neutropenia along with ulcers.

Sensory disturbance can be seen in lymphoma and leukemia.

Motor function impairment: Facial nerve palsy in cases of orofacial granulomatosis.

INVESTIGATION

Baseline Investigations

Complete blood count (CBC): Nutritional deficiency can be identified. Anemia could reflect gastrointestinal (GI) disorders. Low white blood cell (WBC) count and anemia could be a pointer toward CTD. It might reflect cyclical neutropenia (if taken at proper time), it might help us to identify drug-induced neutropenia or pancytopenia as well as hematological disorders such as leukemia and myelodysplastic syndromes.

Inflammatory markers: Raised C-reactive protein (CRP) can be associated with inflammatory disorders and infections.

Erythrocyte sedimentation rate (ESR): It can be elevated in TB. Occasionally, it can be elevated in acute disease process associated with infections, rheumatological diseases, malignancy, and many other systemic and inflammatory diseases.

Additional Tests

Tzanck smear:[14] It is a useful test specially for acantholytic disorders (dyskeratotic cells and acantholytic cells) and herpes simplex (epithelial giant cells and cytopathic changes). It can also help in identifying secondary candidiasis. Presence of eosinophils might suggest BP. Other disorders may be associated with nonspecific changes may be seen and might not add in diagnosis.

Patch test: It can help to identify oral contact allergen and irritants.

Pathergy test: Positive pathergy test points toward Behçet's syndrome.

Antibody tests: Anti-desmoglein 3 (anti-Dsg3) antibodies can be obtained in suspected cases of pemphigus vulgaris. Autoantibodies in submucosal blisters can be obtained but these tests are not widely available in India. ANA and ANA profile can be ordered if LE is suspected. Autoantibodies like perinuclear antineutrophil cytoplasmic antibody (p-ANCA) and various antimicrobial antibodies can be ordered if history suggests toward IBD.[15] Antitissue transglutaminase 2 antibodies can be advised if gluten sensitive enteropathy is suspected.[16]

Histopathology and Direct Immunofluorescence

Histopathology in vesiculobullous disorders appears as same in mucosal lesions. Pemphigus vulgaris of oral cavity intraepithelial acantholysis and fishnet pattern on DIF. Submucosal blistering disorders can be differentiated by direct immunofluorescence (DIF). Histopathology and DIF findings in LP and alike conditions are described in **Table 10**.

Drug-induced ulcers:[17] FDR (basal cell vacuolization with lymphocytic infiltrate with occasional eosinophils, melanophage); cytotoxic drugs (nonspecific ulcers with marked inflammation).

TREATMENT[2,18]

General Treatment

- *Oral rinses*: Sterile water/saline solutions/chlorhexidine mouth wash.
- *Anesthetic agents*: Xylocaine and lignocaine solutions/gel.
- *Oral nonsteroidal anti-inflammatory drugs (NSAIDs)*: In cases with unbearable pain.
- *Nutritional deficiency corrections*: Iron, vitamin B12, Fa supplements.
- *Topical steroids*: Triamcinolone gel can be given in cases of noninfective ulcers. Other topical steroid available in oral formulation can also be used.
- Topical tacrolimus ointments can also be used.
- *Antifungal agents*: Clotrimazole lozenges or oral solutions in cases of secondary candidiasis. Oral fluconazole can also be given for same.

Specific Treatment

Aphthous and Aphthous-like Oral Ulcers in Systemic Diseases[2,18]

- If does not respond to general measures as stated above oral steroids, montelukast, antimicrobials (dapsone, clofazimine), anti-inflammatories (colchicine, pentoxifylline), immunomodulators (thalidomide, levamisole) or immunosuppressives (azathioprine) can be added.
- Other therapies like sucralfate, cimetidine, low energy laser, nicotine, interferon-α has also been tried.
- Cyclosporine has been shown to be effective for ocular lesions of Behçet's disease. Mycophenolate mofetil (MMF) has not been found effective in Behçet's.
- *Hydroxychloroquine (HCQ) and sulphapyridine* can be useful in ulcers associated with IBD. Treatment of IBD improves oral ulcers.
- *Biologics*: Adalimumab[19] has been tried in RAS.

Oral steroids (prednisolone)	25 mg/day
Dapsone	25 mg/day × 3 days → 50 mg/day × 3 days → 75 mg/day × 3 days → 100 mg/day (maintenance dose)
Clofazimine	100 mg/day × 6 months
Colchicine	0.5 mg/day × 7 days → increase by 1 mg/day → 1.5 mg/day (maintenance dose)
Pentoxifylline	400 mg tds /day × 3 months
Levamisole	150 mg 3 days a week × 6 months
Thalidomide	50–100 mg/day

Oral Ulcers in Vesiculobullous Disorders

Apart from general measures, intralesional steroids, oral steroids, intravenous Immunoglobulin (IVIG), and immunosuppressives are effective. Somehow in author's personal experience rituximab is not very much effective in oral lesions of pemphigus vulgaris. Dapsone and tetracycline might be effective.

Oral Erosive Lichen Planus[20]

Treatment response is poor and systemic treatment in form of oral steroids and other immunomodulators and immunosuppressive such as methotrexate, mycophenolate, minocycline, cyclosporine, HCQ, and acitretin can be tried.

In author's personal experience HCQ and oral acitretin are very effective in maintenance therapy.

Photochemotherapy, cryotherapy, CO_2, and neodymium-doped yttrium aluminum garnet (Nd-YAG) laser therapy have also been used.

PFAPA: Oral steroids, cimetidine, tonsillectomy, and adenoidectomy.

Chemotherapy-induced Mucositis and Oral Ulcers[21]

Treatment: Dental floss, oral rinses (sterile water/saline solutions >> chlorhexidine), xylocaine and lignocaine solutions, morphine gel, cryotherapy (contraindication in patients on oxaliplatin), granulocyte-macrophage colony-stimulating factor (GM-CSF) (limit extent and duration of disease), zinc, folic acid, laser therapy, drug-specific antidotes in cases of toxicity [example: leucovorin in case of methotrexate (MTX) toxicity].

For both prevention and treatment: Benzydamine, glutamine.

For prevention: Amifostine, IVIG, histamine gels, vitamin E, palifermin, zinc, and laser therapy.

REFERENCES

1. Mortazavi H, Safi Y, Baharvand M, Rahmani S. Diagnostic Features of Common Oral Ulcerative Lesions: An Updated Decision Tree. Int J Dent. 2016;2016:7278925.
2. Edgar NR, Saleh D, Miller RA. Recurrent Aphthous Stomatitis: A Review. J Clin Aesthet Dermatol. 2017;10(3):26-36.
3. Field EA, Allan RB. Review article: oral ulceration—aetiopathogenesis, clinical diagnosis and management in the gastrointestinal clinic. Aliment Pharmacol Ther. 2003;18:949-62.
4. Porter SR, Leao JC. Review article: oral ulcers and its relevance to systemic disorders. Aliment Pharmacol Ther. 2005;21:295-306.
5. Siu A, Landon K, Ramos DM. Differential diagnosis and management of oral ulcers. Seminars in Cutaneous Medicine and Surgery. 2015;34:171-7.
6. Tarakji B, Gazal G, Al-Maweri SA, Azzeghaiby SN, Alaizari N. Guideline for the Diagnosis and Treatment of Recurrent Aphthous Stomatitis for Dental Practitioners. J Int Oral Health. 2015;7(5):74-80.
7. Scully C. Dermatoses of the oral cavity and lips. In: Griffiths C, Barker J, Bleiker T, Chalmers R, Creamer D (Eds). Rook's Textbook of Dermatology, 9th edition. West Sussex, Willey Blackwell; 2016. pp. 110.1-110.94.
8. Allen CM, Camisa C. Oral disease. In: Bolognia JL, Jorizzo JL, Schaffer JV (Eds). Dermatology, 3rd edition. Philadelphia, PA: Elsevier; 2012. pp. 1149-70.
9. Nair A, Jose AS, Kaushik H, Poonja P, Kini R, Rao PK. Chronic Ulcer of Lateral Tongue—A Case Report. Austin J Dent. 2018;5(5):1119.
10. Müller S. Oral lichenoid lesions: distinguishing the benign from the deadly. Mod Pathol. 2017;30(s1):S54-S67.
11. Horwitz MS, Corey SJ, Grimes HL, Tidwell T. ELANE mutations in cyclic and severe congenital neutropenia: genetics and pathophysiology. Hematol Oncol Clin North Am. 2013;27(1):19-41, vii.
12. Slebioda Z, Szponar E, Kowalska A. Recurrent aphthous stomatitis: genetic aspects of etiology. Postepy Dermatol Alergol. 2013;30(2):96-102.
13. Chung JY, Ramos-Caro FA, Ford MJ, Mullins D. Recurrent scarring ulcers of the oral mucosa. Sutton disease (periadenitis mucosa necrotica recurrens). Arch Dermatol. 1997;133(9):1162-3, 1165-6.
14. Panwar H, Joshi D, Goel G, Asati D, Majumdar K, Kapoor N. Diagnostic Utility and Pitfalls of Tzanck Smear Cytology in Diagnosis of Various Cutaneous Lesions. J Cytol. 2017;34(4):179-82.
15. Mitsuyama K, Takedatsu H, Yamasaki H, Kuwaki, K, Yoshioka S, Yamauchi R. Antibody markers in the diagnosis of inflammatory bowel disease. World J Gastroenterol. 2016;22(3):1304-10.
16. Alaedini A, Green PH. Autoantibodies in celiac disease. Autoimmunity. 2008;41(1):19-26.
17. Jinbu Y, Demitsu T. Oral ulcerations due to drug medications. Jpn Dent Sci Rev. 2014;50:40-6.
18. Altenburg A, El-Haj N, Micheli C, Puttkammer M, Abdel-Naser MB, Zouboulis CC. The Treatment of Chronic Recurrent Oral Aphthous Ulcers. Dtsch Arztebl Int. 2014;111:665-73.
19. de Perosanz-Lobo D, Latour I, Ortega-Quijano D, Fernández-Guarino M, Torrelo A. Severe recurrent aphthous stomatitis treated with adalimumab: A case report in a teenage patient. Pediatr Dermatol. 2019;36(6):986-7.
20. Gupta S, Jawanda MK. Oral lichen planus: An update on etiology, pathogenesis, clinical presentation, diagnosis and management. Indian J Dermatol. 2015;60:222-9.
21. Naidu MUR, Ramana GV, Rani PU, Mohan IK, Suman A, Roy P. Chemotherapy-induced and/or Radiation Therapy–induced Oral Mucositis—Complicating the Treatment of Cancer. Neoplasia. 2004;6(5):423-31.

16

A Patient with Hyperkeratotic Lesions on Palm and/or Sole

Deblina Bhunia, Ravi Ranjan

INTRODUCTION

Hyperkeratotic lesions on palm and/or sole in a patient may be either the only skin finding or a part of generalized skin disease or some systemic disease/syndrome. The lesions may involve the whole palmoplantar surface or may be focal or punctate. It may be an early onset hereditary palmoplantar keratoderma (PPK) or an acquired disease. A detailed history, thorough clinical examination and sometimes histopathology or some laboratory investigations are required for definitive diagnosis and management of such cases.

CLASSIFICATION

Classification of palmoplantar hyperkeratotic lesions is based on their clinical features, pathological findings, and inheritance pattern. They are broadly divided into two groups: (1) hereditary and (2) acquired disease (**Tables 1 and 2** respectively). The hereditary PPKs are subdivided by its extent of involvement, i.e., diffuse, focal, striate, and punctate. Diffuse PPKs can be either nontransgradient (involving only the palmar and plantar sites) or transgradient (extending into the dorsal areas—**Fig. 1**). A number of PPKs

Table 1: Hereditary palmoplantar keratodermas (PPKs).		
Diffuse	*Focal/Striate*	*Punctate*
Nontransgradient: • Vorner, Unna–Thost PPK • Diffuse PPK with DSG1 mutation • Bart–Pumphrey syndrome • Howel–Evans syndrome • Naxos syndrome • KLICK (keratosis linearis with ichthyosis congenita and sclerosing keratoderma) *Transgradient*: • Nagashima PPK • Bothnian PPK • Greither syndrome • Mal de Maleda, Gamborg–Nielsen syndrome • Vohwinkel syndrome • Camisa syndrome/Loricrin keratoderma • Papillon-Lefèvre syndrome	• Focal (Brünauer–Fuhs–Siemens/Wachters) • Pachyonychia congenita • Howel–Evans syndrome • Richner–Hanhart syndrome • Carvajal syndrome • PPK and woolly hair • Focal palmoplantar and gingival keratosis	• Buschke–Fischer–Brauer (type 1 punctate PPK) • Spiny keratoderma (type 2 punctate PPK) • Marginal papular keratoderma/acrokeratoelastoidosis/focal acral hyperkeratosis (type 3 punctate PPK) • Punctate keratoses of the palmar creases • Porokeratosis punctata palmaris et plantaris (PPPP) • Cole disease • PLACK (peeling skin with leukonychia, acral punctate keratoses, cheilitis, and knuckle pads) syndrome

Continued

Continued

Diffuse	Focal/Striate	Punctate
• Haim–Munk syndrome • Huriez syndrome • Olmsted syndrome • Sybert syndrome • Clouston syndrome • Oculodentodigital dysplasia syndrome • Odonto-onycho-dermal dysplasia		

Table 2: Acquired palmoplantar keratodermas.

Diffuse	Focal/Striate	Punctate
Dermatoses: • Psoriasis • Chronic eczemas • Pityriasis rubra pilaris • Keratoderma blennorrhagica • Lichen planus *Infections*: • Dermatophytosis • Scabies • Human papillomavirus (HPV) • Syphilis • Tuberculosis • Leprosy *Drugs/chemicals*: Arsenic, lithium, verapamil, chemotherapeutic agent, halogenated herbicides *Systemic disease*: • Hypothyroidism • Myxedema • Chronic lymphedema • Circulatory disease • Lupus erythematosus • Dermatomyositis • Malnutrition *Malignancy*: • Acrokeratosis paraneoplastica (Bazex) • Tripe palm • Cutaneous T-cell lymphoma • Other visceral malignancy *Others*: • Keratoderma climactericum • Aquagenic • Idiopathic	• Frictional (callosities/corn) • *Neuropathic*: Diabetes, leprosy • *Infection*: Verruca, tuberculosis, chromoblastomycosis	Acrokeratoelastoides marginalis of hands

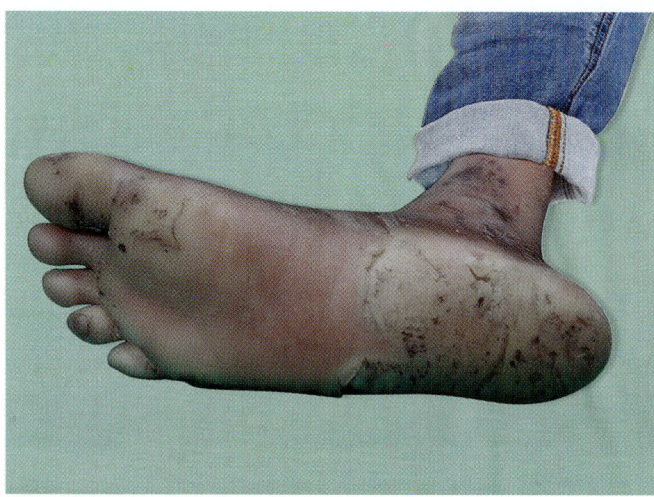

FIG. 1: Transgradient diffuse keratoderma affecting sole and extending over dorsum of foot.
Courtesy: Dr Nayan Patel.

may be mutilating, i.e., causing deformities or constriction bands leading to autoamputation of the digits. Some of the hereditary PPKs are associated with other systemic abnormalities or syndromes. Acquired palmoplantar keratotic lesions can also be diffuse, focal, or punctate. Although few cases of acquired PPK are idiopathic; several dermatosis, infections, malignancies, systemic diseases, and others can be associated with most of the acquired palmoplantar keratotic lesions.

APPROACH

History

Appearance of keratoderma during childhood with a positive family history or history of consanguineous marriage of the parents usually denotes hereditary PPK. Although a negative family history or late presentation does not exclude the possibility of hereditary disease and vice versa. For example, in childhood onset pityriasis rubra pilaris the presentation is earlier. A positive family history of keratoderma may be present in chronic arsenicosis in arsenic endemic regions. History of blistering may be present in few types of hereditary PPK. History of hyperhidrosis or hypohidrosis can be associated with some types of PPK. Hereditary PPK is persistence and also relative treatment resistant.

In acquired keratoderma, patient's residence, occupation, history of certain drug/chemical exposure, history of allergies/atopy, other medical conditions or history of previous/preexisting dermatosis should be pertained.

EXAMINATION

Cutaneous

Hereditary Palmoplantar Keratoderma
- *Type of keratotic lesions*: Diffuse, focal, striate, or punctate.
- *Distribution*: Symmetric or asymmetric.
- Transgradiens or nontransgradiens **(Table 1)**
- *Most involved site*: Palm or sole, pressure areas or others.
- Presence of scaling, inflammation, blistering, maceration **(Table 3)**
- Presence of mutilation, deformity, pseudoainhum **(Table 3)**
- *Presence of hyper-/hypohidrosis*:
  - *Hyperhidrosis*: Nagashima, Bothnian, Greither, Vohwinkel, Papillon–Lefèvre, Mal de Meleda, and Olmsted syndrome.
  - *Hypohidrosis*: Ectodermal dysplasias, and Olmsted syndrome.
- *Lesions on other sites in hereditary disease*:
  - *Extensors*: Nagashima, Greither, Sybert, Papillon–Lefèvre, and Haim–Munk syndrome.
  - *Periorificial*: Olmsted and Sybert syndrome.
  - *Flexures*: Greither and KLICK syndrome.
  - *Knuckle pads*: Bart-Pumphrey syndrome.
  - *Dorsum*: "Starfish-like" lesion in Vohwinkel syndrome, etc.

Changes on water exposure: White spongy appearance in Nagashima, Bothnian PPK after a short time water exposure.

Mucosal, Nail, and Hair Examination (Tables 3 and 4)

Wood's lamp examination: This might be helpful to diagnose punctate porokeratotic keratoderma where white fluorescence **(Figs. 4 and 5)** can be observed and mechanism of which has not been identified yet.

Other systemic examinations are ophthamological, auditory, dental, cardiovascular, neurological, and skeletal system **(Tables 3 to 5)**.

Acquired Diseases[6]

Differentiating features of palmoplantar psoriasis, chronic eczemas, dermatophytic keratoderma, and keratoderma climactericum are discussed in **Table 6**. Diffuse, yellowish/orangish, and waxy keratodermas are seen in pityriasis rubra pilaris **(Fig. 6)**, along with other cutaneous findings. In chronic arsenicosis, minute to large keratotic papules/

Table 3: Clinical features of hereditary diffuse palmoplantar keratoderma (PPK).[1-3]

Type	History	Cutaneous features	Mutilation	Mucosa, nail, hair	Other systemic
Vorner Unna–Thost syndrome	Acral blistering in infancy (Vorner)	Thick diffuse PPK	–	–	–
Diffuse PPK with DSG1 mutation		Thick diffuse PPK	–	Mild onycholysis with yellow discoloration of nails	–
Bart–Pumphrey syndrome		Diffuse, focal or punctate PPK, knuckle pads	–	Leukonychia	Sensorineural hearing loss
Howel–Evans syndrome (Figs. 2 and 3)		Focal or diffuse, yellowish callosity like PPK with fissuring	–	Oral leukoplakia	Chronic rhinitis, maxillary decalcification, alveolysis/tooth loss. Esophageal carcinoma in mid/late life
Naxos syndrome		Diffuse PPK	–	Woolly hair	Right ventricular cardiomyopathy
Nagashima	Hyperhidrosis, white spongy changes on water exposure	• Mild diffuse PPK with erythema; Lesion over knees, elbow, Achilles tendon area • Maceration, foul odor	–	–	–
Bothnian	Hyperhidrosis, white spongy changes on water exposure	Mild to thick diffuse hyperkeratosis	–	Curved nails, ragged cuticle	–
Huriez		Scleroatrophy, parchment-like skin on dorsum of hand and feet; increased chance of squamous cell carcinoma (SCC)	–	Nail dystrophy, hypoplasia	–
Greither	Transient blistering at infancy (epidermolytic type), hyperhidrosis	Thick diffuse PPK; Lesion over flexures, elbows, knees, Achilles tendon area	±	–	–
Sybert		• Lesions over elbow, knees • Periorbital and perioral erythema	±	–	–
Vohwinkel syndrome Camisa syndrome	Hyperhidrosis	Diffuse, severe, yellowish honeycomb-like PPK; "Starfish-like" lesions on dorsum. Mild ichthyosis in Camisa syndrome	+	Alopecia, nail dystrophy	• Deafness, myopathy, (spastic paraplegia possible), focal epilepsy • No deafness in Camisa syndrome
Olmsted syndrome	Hyper-/anhidrosis	• Periorificial/intertriginous hyperkeratotic plaques • Recurrent skin infection • Development of SCC and melanoma over keratoderma	+	Diffuse alopecia, onychodystrophy, oral leukokeratosis	Corneal dystrophy, delayed growth, bone deformities, deafness
Mal de Meleda syndrome [Gamborg–Nielsen (GN)/Norrbotten type]	• Hyperhidrosis • Onset in early infancy	• Diffuse, thick PPK; maceration, foul odor, bacterial superinfection; lesion on knee, elbow, wrist, ankles, dorsum of hands/feet and perioral areas • Knuckle pads in GN type	+	Subungual keratosis, koilonychia, dystrophy of great toe nail	Joint stiffness/contracture, corneal lesion, high arched palate

Continued

Continued

Type	History	Cutaneous features	Mutilation	Mucosa, nail, hair	Other systemic
Papillon–Lefèvre syndrome (PLS)	Hyperhidrosis	Psoriasiform plaques on knees, elbows, interphalangeal joints, pyogenic infections	+	–	Periodontitis, tooth loss
Haim–Munk	Hyperhidrosis	Similar to PLS	+	Atrophic nail changes	PLS with additional arachnodactyly, acro-osteolysis, pes planus, finger deformities
KLICK syndrome		Hyperkeratotic plaques, ichthyosis, and papules on the arm flexures and wrists with linear distribution	+	–	–

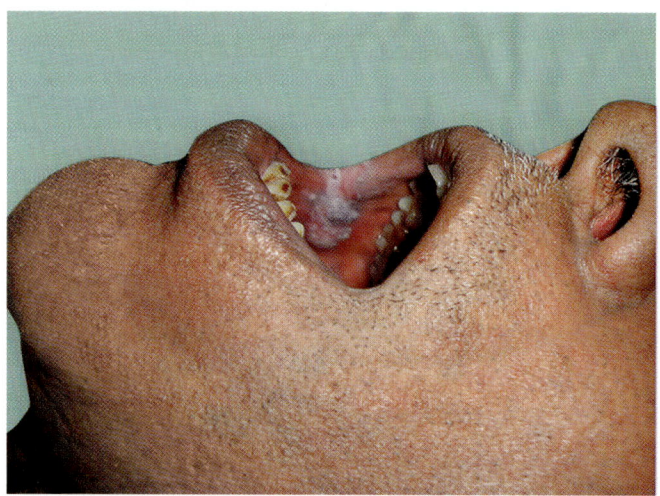

FIG. 2: Oral leukoplakia in a case of Howel–Evans syndrome.
Courtesy: Dr Nayan Patel.

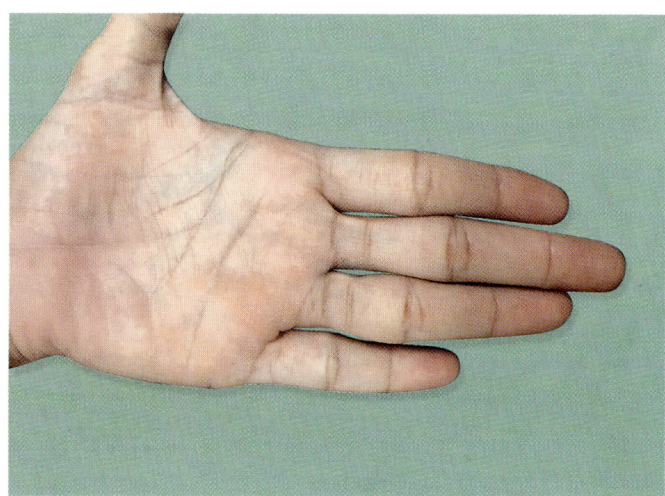

FIG. 4: Small, tiny punctate lesions coalescing to form plaque in punctate porokeratotic keratoderma.
Courtesy: Dr Jigna Padhiyar.

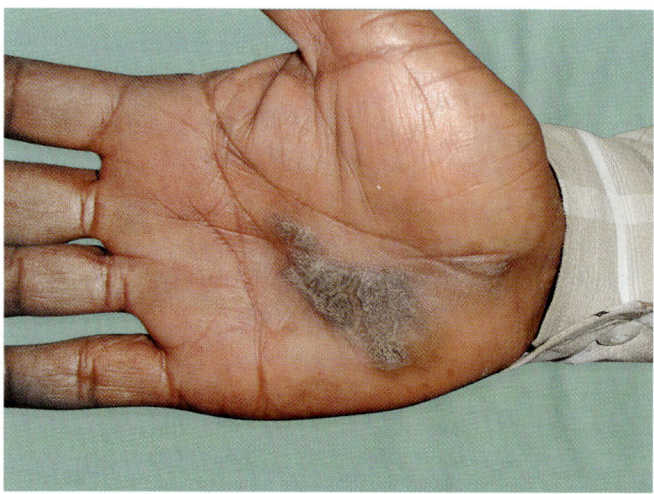

FIG. 3: Focal callosity like thickened keratoderma with fissures in Howel–Evans syndrome.
Courtesy: Dr Nayan Patel.

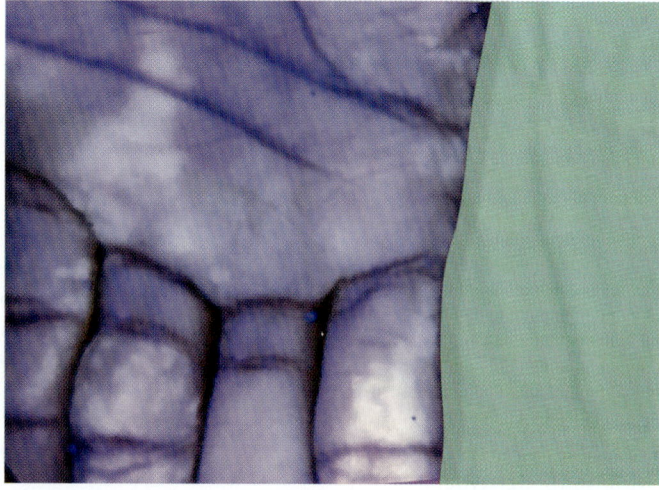

FIG. 5: Whitish fluorescence in punctate porokeratotic keratoderma on Wood's lamp examination.
Courtesy: Dr Jigna Padhiyar.

Table 4: Focal, striate, and punctate keratoderma.[1,2,4]

Type	Subtype	History	Cutaneous features	Other features
Focal	Focal PPK	Childhood onset, may be triggered by mechanical stimulation, painful	Focal PPK, plantar blistering	Follicular hyperkeratosis, minimal oral, or anogenital leukokeratosis
Striate	Type 1 Type 2 Type 3		Linear keratotic bands on the palms and flexor aspects of the fingers, island-like areas of hyperkeratosis over pressure points	Rarely hyperkeratosis over knee and elbow, foul odor
Punctate	Type 1	Numerous tiny punctate keratotic papules commonly appear during adolescence or early adulthood; gradually coalesce. Worsening on water exposure (1A)	Punctate lesions initially appear translucent, later become opaque and verrucous; plaques on pressure points. After removal of lesions, depression persists	
	Type 2	Onset at puberty	Tiny punctate keratotic lesions on palm and sole	
	Type 3	Lesions appear after adolescent	Small keratotic papules, sometimes umbilicated, appear on the margin of palm and sole	
	Punctate keratosis of palmar crease	African and American patients; age group of 15–40 years, can aggravate on friction	Punctate keratoses appear on the creases of palm and digits, less commonly sole	
	Porokeratosis punctata palmaris et plantaris (PPPP)	Lesions appear in adolescent or early adulthood	Punctate PPK; may later involve in other areas in disseminated type	
Focal palmoplantar keratoderma (PPK) with associate features	Pachyonychia congenita		Painful focal keratotic lesions, blistering on sole	Thickened nail plates, oral leukokeratosis, steatocystomas
	Richner–Hanhart syndrome		Painful plantar keratosis	Dendritic keratitis, corneal ulcers, intellectual disability
	Carvajal syndrome		Striate lesions on palms	Woolly hair, left ventricular cardiomyopathy
	PPK and woolly hair		Striate lesions on palms	Woolly hair, hypotrichosis, leukonychia
	Focal palmoplantar and gingival keratosis		Painful keratosis on soles, epidermolytic	Gingival leukokeratosis
Punctate PPK with associate features	Cole syndrome			Guttate hypopigmentation, calcinosis cutis
	PLACK syndrome			Peeling skin, leukonychia, cheilitis, knuckle pads
	Darier disease		Discrete, punctate keratotic papules on palm and sole; may coalesce	Dirty warty papules on seborrheic distribution, nail changes, cobblestoning on oral mucosa

Table 5: Hereditary palmoplantar keratoderma (PPK) with associated diseases.[5]		
Association	Disease	Clinical features
PPK with cardiomyopathy and woolly hair	Naxos syndrome	See **Table 3**
	Carvajal syndrome	See **Table 4**
	PPK with arrhythmogenic right ventricular cardiomyopathy	Right ventricular myocardial degeneration, mild striate PPK
PPK with deafness	Vohwinkel syndrome	See **Table 3**
	Bart–Pumphrey syndrome	See **Table 3**
	KID syndrome	Ichthyosiform erythroderma in infants, ichthyosis, alopecia, acrofacial verruciform hyperkeratosis, sensorineural deafness, keratitis, increased risk of bacterial infections, and squamous cell carcinoma
	PPK with hearing loss	Focal or diffuse PPK
	Ichthyosis hystrix with deafness	Verrucous or spinous hyperkeratosis
	Mitochondrial PPK with deafness	PPK predominantly on pressure areas, with sensorineural hearing loss
PPK with ectodermal dysplasia	Clouston syndrome	Diffuse PPK, nail dystrophy, hair abnormalities
	Naegeli–Franceschetti–Jadassohn syndrome	Diffuse PPK, nail dystrophy, anhidrosis, dental defects, reticulate hyperpigmentation
	Odontoonychodermal dysplasia	Diffuse PPK, hyperhidrosis, hypodontia, smooth tongue, hypotrichosis, nail dystrophy
	Schöpf–Schulz–Passarge syndrome	In addition to features of oculoonychodermal dysplasia, cystic eyelids, and skin cancers can occur
	Skin fragility syndrome	Systemic skin fragility, diffuse PPK with painful fissures, hypotrichosis or woolly hair, growth retardation
PPK with periodontitis	Papillon–Lefèvre syndrome	See **Table 3**
	Haim–Munk syndrome	See **Table 3**
PPK with predisposition to carcinogenicity	Howel–Evans syndrome	See **Table 3**
	Huriez syndrome	See **Table 3**
	Olmsted syndrome	See **Table 3**
	KID syndrome	Description above
	Cowden syndrome	Punctate PPK, intraoral mucosal papillomatosis, facial trichilemmoma, benign hamartomas in gastrointestinal tract, mammary gland, etc.; liver, breast, thyroid, uterine cancer

Table 6: Features of common causes of acquired palmoplantar keratoderma (PPK).[6-10]					
Type	Age of onset	History/symptoms	Clinical features	Dermoscopy	Histopathology
Palmoplantar psoriasis (**Fig. 7**)	20–60 years	Mild pruritus, pain if fissured, seasonal aggravation	Symmetric, well-defined plaques with scaling, erythema, fissuring. Involvement of instep of feet, knuckles and other extensors, coarse and irregular nail pitting	Regular vascular distribution pattern, white scale color	Confluent parakeratosis, hypogranulosis, regular acanthosis, neutrophil in stratum corneum and spinosum, suprapapillary thinning
Chronic eczema	Commonly middle age	Intense pruritus, history of exudation, history of exposure to chronic irritants and allergen	Ill-defined, asymmetrically distributed plaques	Yellow crust and scale, patchy scale and vascular pattern, dull-red background color, brownish orange globule	Intact granular layer, severe spongiosis with vesiculation, irregular acanthosis

Continued

Continued

Type	Age of onset	History/symptoms	Clinical features	Dermoscopy	Histopathology
Dermatophytosis	Adults	History of using occlusive shoes or excessive water exposure; pruritus ±	Diffuse hyperkeratosis with erythema and scaling. Onychomycosis may be associated. Symmetry ±	Whitish scale mostly localized to the creases	Hyperkeratosis, acanthosis, and sparse perivascular infiltrate in dermis; fungal filaments on periodic acid-Schiff (PAS) or methenamine silver stain
Keratoderma climactericum	Middle aged perimenopausal women; often associated with obesity and hypertension	First appears at plantar pressure points, extends to become confluent, later involves palm; rarely pruritic	Keratotic lesions on sole and palm; associated with erythema, fissuring, and pain	–	Compact orthokeratotic hyperkeratosis with hypergranulosis

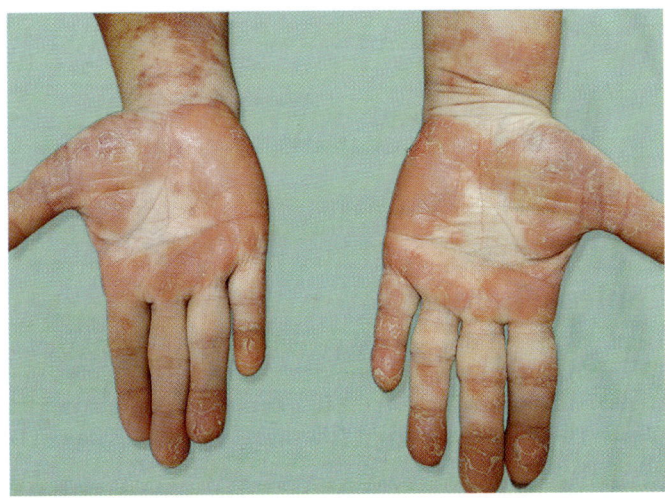

FIG. 6: Orange plaque involving palms in pityriasis rubra pilaris "PRP Sandal".
Courtesy: Dr Nayan Patel.

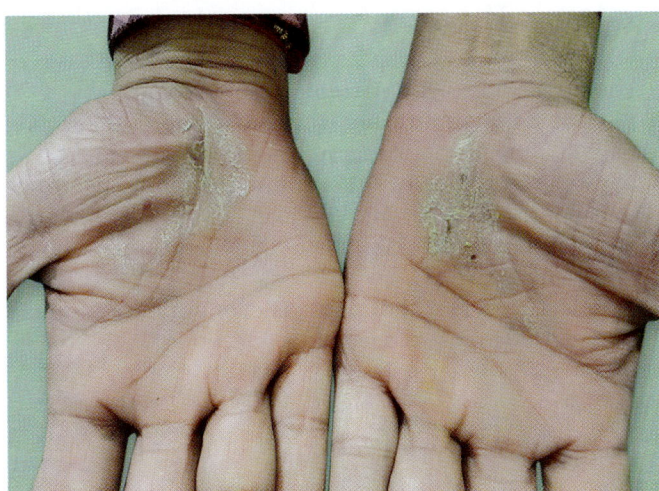

FIG. 7: Palmar psoriasis.
Courtesy: Dr Jigna Padhiyar.

nodules on palm and sole are distributed symmetrically with rain-drop pigmentation, diffuse hyperpigmentation, leukomelanosis, multiple Bowen's disease, squamous cell carcinoma, and basal cell carcinomas in the body. Keratoderma of acrokeratosis paraneoplastica of Bazex starts with psoriasiform lesions on fingers/toes, later becomes diffuse with violaceous color and other features like painful fissuring, paronychia, psoriasiform lesions on helices, and nasal bridge. Sezary syndrome can present with diffuse PPK and erythroderma. In Norwegian scabies, hyperkeratotic and/or crusted lesions appear with web space involvement, sometimes associated with erythroderma. In acquired aquagenic PPK, there is thickening and whitish, pebbly appearance of palm within 3 minutes of water exposure, which disappears on drying.

Other Cutaneous Examination

- Presence of hypoesthesia around the lesion and nerve thickening (leprosy)
- Other skin findings associated with the diseases

Systemic examination: To rule out systemic etiology of the PPK.

INVESTIGATIONS

Histopathology
Histopathological features of hereditary PPK are described in **Table 7**.

Acquired Diseases[6]
- Specific histological features are seen in specific dermatosis (e.g., psoriasis, dermatitis, etc.).
- In other acquired keratodermas, features are mostly nonspecific with marked hyperkeratosis with variable degree of parakeratosis, hypergranulosis, acanthosis, and perivascular inflammatory infiltrates.

Table 7: Histopathological features of hereditary palmoplantar keratoderma (PPK).[2]

Histopathological features	Disease
Epidermolytic hyperkeratosis	Vorner, Greither (epidermolytic variants), focal palmoplantar, and gingival keratosis
Orthohyperkeratosis, acanthosis, papillomatosis	Bothnia, Nagashima, Greither (nonepidermolytic variant), Mal de Meleda, Huriez, Howel–Evans, Papillon–Lefèvre, Vohwinkel syndrome
Orthohyperkeratosis with focal parakeratosis, acanthosis, and papillomatosis	KLICK, KID syndrome
Hyperkeratosis with focal parakeratosis and hypergranulosis with focal perinuclear vacuolization	Camisa syndrome/Loricrin keratoderma
Widening of intercellular spaces and partial dehiscence of keratinocytes	Striate PPK types 1 and 2, diffuse PPK due to DSG1 mutation, Carvajal syndrome
Keratinocytes with pale cytoplasm and eosinophilic inclusions	Pachyonychia congenita, Richner–Hanhart
Orthohyperkeratotic column overlaying depressed epidermis	Punctate PPK (Buschke–Fischer–Brauer type), punctate keratoses of the palmar creases
Parakeratotic column overlaying depressed epidermis without vacuolization or dyskeratosis	Spiny keratoderma
Focally parakeratotic column overlaying depressed epidermis with fragmentation and loss of elastic fibers	Acrokeratoelastoides
Parakeratotic column overlaying depressed epidermis with vacuolization and dyskeratosis	Porokeratosis

- *Dermoscopy*: Dermoscopic findings of palmoplantar psoriasis, eczema and dermatophytosis are discussed in **Table 6**.
- Skin scraping for fungal elements or scabies mite.
- *Investigations to rule out systemic diseases or malignancies in acquired diseases (as required)*: Routine blood examinations, thyroid profile, venereal disease research laboratory test (VDRL), antinuclear antibody (ANA), creatine phosphokinase (CPK), lactate dehydrogenase (LDH), chest radiography, ultrasonography of abdomen, CT scan, age and sex specific malignancy screening, etc.
- *In suspected chronic arsenicosis*: Arsenic estimation of hair, nail, and drinking water.
- Genetic analysis in hereditary PPK.

MANAGEMENT[2,11,12]

General Measures
- Proper footwear to avoid further trauma/friction
- Regular hand and foot bath followed by application of moisturizer
- Mechanical keratolysis when required

Topical Therapies

Lactic acid and urea-based cream/lotion, 50% propylene glycol in water under plastic occlusion several nights per week, and salicylic acid 4–6% in petrolatum (should not be given in larger areas to avoid salicylism), retinoids, vitamin D analogs, etc.

In palmoplantar psoriasis: Topical potent steroid, vitamin D analogs, coal tar, dithranol 1%, tazarotene, and soak psoralen plus ultraviolet A (PUVA) therapy are advised.

Systemic Therapy
- Systemic retinoids can be considered in severe cases of hereditary PPK, except in epidermolytic types.
- Retinoids, methotrexate can be considered in severe, debilitating palmoplantar psoriasis.
- Systemic steroids or other immunosuppressive drugs may be useful in chronic eczemas.
- In other acquired cases, the underlying diseases should be treated.
- Topical/Systemic antifungals and/or antibiotics should be advised in case of secondary infections.

REFERENCES

1. Dev T, Mahajan VK, Sethuraman G. Hereditary Palmoplantar Keratoderma: A Practical Approach to the Diagnosis. Indian Dermatol Online J. 2019;10(4):365-79.
2. Metze D, Oji V. Palmoplantar keratodermas. In: Bolognia JL, Schaffer JV, Cerroni L (Eds). Dermatology, 4th edition. Philadelphia (PA): Elsevier Health Sciences; 2018. pp. 924-43.
3. Rai R, Ramachandran B, Sundaram VS, Rajendren G, Srinivas CR. Naxos disease: a rare occurrence of cardiomyopathy with woolly hair and palmoplantar keratoderma. Indian J Dermatol Venereol Leprol. 2008;74(1):50-2.
4. Kim C, Fangman W. Keratosis follicularis (Darier-White disease), with an unusual palmoplantar keratoderma. Dermatol Online J. 2007;13(1):7.
5. Yoneda K, Kubo A, Nomura T, Ishida-Yamamoto A, Suga Y, Akiyama M, et al. Japanese guidelines for the management of palmoplantar keratoderma. J Dermatol. 2021;48:e353-e367.
6. Patel S, Zirwas M, English JC 3rd. Acquired palmoplantar keratoderma. Am J Clin Dermatol. 2007;8(1):1-11.
7. Çetinarslan T, Türel Ermertcan A, Temiz P. Dermoscopic clues of palmoplantar hyperkeratotic eczema and palmoplantar psoriasis: A prospective, comparative study of 90 patients. J Dermatol. 2020;47:1157-65.
8. Rao A, Khandpur S, Kalaivani M. A study of the histopathology of palmo-plantar psoriasis and hyperkeratotic palmo-plantar dermatitis. Indian J Dermatol Venereol Leprol. 2018;84(1):27-33.
9. Errichetti E, Stinco G. Dermoscopy in General Dermatology: A Practical Overview. Dermatol Ther (Heidelb). 2016;6(4):471-507.
10. Nigam PK, Saleh D. Tinea Pedis. In: StatPearls [Internet]. Treasure Island (FL): StatPearls Publishing; 2022.
11. Schiller S, Seebode C, Hennies HC, Giehl K, Emmert S. Palmoplantar keratoderma (PPK): acquired and genetic causes of a not so rare disease. J Dtsch Dermatol Ges. 2014;12(9):781-8.
12. Nair LV. Management of recalcitrant palmoplantar psoriasis. J Skin Sex Transm Dis. 2019;1:8-12.

17
A Case of Indurated Facial Plaque

Kiruthika Subburaj, Rahul Mahajan

INTRODUCTION

Indurated facial plaque is a very broad morphologic diagnosis that can encompass a wide variety of cutaneous diseases ranging from innocuous to sinister in prognosis. Many conditions look alike and hence cause diagnostic dilemmas requiring biopsy for histologic confirmation. But, even the histology may be less than conclusive in many patients, especially with granulomatous dermatitis. Hence, a dermatologist has to often rely on one's own clinical acumen and certain good clinical pointers to arrive at a diagnosis or a set of differential diagnoses with reasonable accuracy. Indurated facial plaques can be of varied etiologies ranging from infectious to neoplastic and can be of varied morphology and configuration. The classification based on etiology is listed in **Table 1**.

AGE AND SEX PREDILECTION

The prevalence of certain diseases in a particular age group, for example, basal cell carcinoma (BCC) in the elderly and actinic prurigo in children/adolescents aids in diagnosing the condition. The male to female ratio of cutaneous juvenile xanthogranuloma (JXG) is about 1.4:1 in children, while in adults no sex predilection exists. Children with multiple skin lesions and those who are younger than 2 years are at greater risk for ocular involvement.[1] Erythematous plaques in infancy can be of conditions like infantile hemangioma and in the elderly, it can be angiosarcoma (Wilson-Jones angiosarcoma) in whom it is often misdiagnosed as a hematoma. The age and sex predilection of common disorders have been listed in **Table 2**.

PRESENTING SYMPTOMS AND SIGNS

Most of the indurated lesions are painless and chronic in nature, which includes both infective and noninfective etiologies. Erythematous plaques are seen in erysipelas (Milian's ear sign—refer to **Table 2**), cellulitis (often tender), syphilis, leprosy, angiosarcoma, acute cutaneous lupus erythematosus (ACLE), Sweet syndrome, and

Table 1: Etiological causes of diseases manifesting as indurated facial plaque.

Etiology	

Infections	• *Bacterial*:
	  ○ Cellulitis
	  ○ Erysipelas
	  ○ Psychosis barbae
	  ○ Mycobacterial infection
	  ○ Leprosy
	• *Fungal*:
	  ○ Tinea faciei
	  ○ Sporotrichosis
	  ○ Mucormycosis
	  ○ Chromoblastomycosis
	  ○ Lobomycosis
	  ○ Conidiobolomycosis
	  ○ Aspergillosis
	• *Viral*:
	  ○ Giant molluscum contagiosum
	• *Others*:
	  ○ Syphilis
	  ○ Actinomycosis
	  ○ Leishmaniasis

Continued

Continued

Etiology	

Lymphocytic disorders	• *Benign*:
	  ○ Pseudolymphoma
	  ○ IgG4-related disease
	  ○ Jessner's lymphocytic infiltrate
	• *Malignant*:
	  ○ Folliculotropic mycosis fungoides
	  ○ Folliculocentric B-cell lymphoma
	  ○ Midline lethal lymphoma (NK T-cell lymphoma)
	• *Non-Hodgkin lymphoma neoplasm*:
	  ○ Langerhans cell histiocytosis
	  ○ Non-Langerhans cell histiocytosis—juvenile xanthogranuloma, necrobiotic xanthogranuloma

Disorders of keratinocytes	• *Benign*:
	  ○ Seborrheic keratosis
	  ○ Premalignant
	  ○ Keratoacanthoma
	  ○ Actinic keratosis
	• *Malignant*:
	  ○ Basal cell carcinoma
	  ○ Squamous cell carcinoma

Pilosebaceous unit disorder	• Morbihan's disease (solid facial edema) • Rhinophyma • Rosacea fulminans • Lupus miliaris disseminatus faciei
Deposition disorder	• Xanthoma • Scleromyxedema • Nodular amyloidosis • Colloid milium • Calcinosis

Granulomatous disorders	• *Noninfectious*:
	  ○ Sarcoidosis
	  ○ Foreign body granuloma
	  ○ Granuloma faciale
	  ○ Annular elastolytic giant cell granuloma
	• *Infectious*:
	  ○ Leprosy
	  ○ Tuberculosis
	  ○ Deep fungal infection

Panniculitis	• Lupus panniculitis • Morphea—en coup de sabre, Parry-Romberg syndrome

Continued

Continued

Etiology	
Vascular lesions	• Port-wine stain • Pyogenic granuloma • Infantile hemangioma • Angiolymphoid hyperplasia • Kimura disease • Arteriovenous malformation • Angiosarcoma
Pigmented disorders	• Congenital melanocytic nevi • Lentigo maligna melanoma

Adnexal tumors and genodermatoses	Epidermal cyst
	Lipoma
	• *Hair follicle tumors*:
	  ○ Trichoepithelioma
	  ○ Pilomatricoma
	  ○ Microcystic adnexal carcinoma
	  ○ Trichogenic adnexal tumor
	  ○ Apocrine gland tumors
	  ○ Syringocystadenoma papilliferum
	• *Nevi*:
	  ○ Nevus comedonicus
	  ○ Milia en plaque
	  ○ Becker's nevus
	  ○ Smooth muscle hamartoma
	  ○ Neurofibroma
	  ○ Fibrous cephalic plaque of tuberous sclerosis

Other inflammatory disorders	• Urticaria
	• Discoid lupus erythematosus
	• Subacute cutaneous lupus erythematosus
	• Seborrheic dermatitis
	• Facial psoriasis
	• Atopic eczema
	• Actinic lichen planus
	• Urticated plaques of chronic bullous disease of childhood, bullous pemphigoid
	• Porokeratosis
	• Sweet syndrome
	• Vasculitis
	• Granulomatosis with polyangiitis
	• Cryoglobulinemia
	• Levamisole vasculitis (cocaine)
	• *Environmental disorders*:
	  ○ Pernio
	  ○ Hydroa vacciniforme
	  ○ Actinic prurigo
	  ○ Chronic actinic dermatitis

Table 2: Cutaneous examination of facial plaque.

Disease	Age	Sex M:F	Symptoms	Morphology	Distribution
Erysipelas	Newborn and young children; 60 and 80 years of age	F > M	Sudden onset, areas of erythema, and edema enlarge with well-defined margins. High fever, and adenopathy, and lymphangitis	Bright red erythema with smooth surface limited from the environment by a steep, clearly marked heaped-up edge. Streaky protrusions are often caused by the spread of infection via the lymphatic vessels. The accumulation of exudative fluid in the papillary layer causes separation of the epidermis and the formation of blisters (erysipelas bullosum) and the severe course of erysipelas may lead to necrosis and gangrene (erysipelas gangraenosum)	• The erythematous change usually starts on the bridge of the nose, spreading symmetrically to the cheeks, often with massive eyelid edema. Very rarely the chin area and lower lip are affected • *Milian's ear sign:* Ear involvement in erysipelas; it is a feature distinguishing erysipelas from cellulitis because the pinna has no deeper dermis and subcutaneous tissue[9]
Cellulitis	Middle-aged and older adults	1:1	Swelling and pain and constitutional symptoms of generalized malaise, fatigue, and fever	Ill-defined erythematous swelling with warmth and tenderness, skin breaks, bullae, or areas of necrotic tissue may be present in severe cellulitis[10]	Usually unilateral
Sycosis barbae	20–40 years	Males. Nape of the neck in both sexes	Pus-filled lesions following shaving. Pain and itching	Erythematous papules or papulopustules with central hair with crusting without destruction of hair follicles. Lesions become hard and heal with hypertrophic scars. Lupoid sycosis: Deep folliculitis with the destruction of hair follicles and extensive scarring[11]	Beard, upper lip, below angles of the mouth, nape of the neck
Lupus vulgaris	All age groups	1:2–3	Chronic progressive plaques in a patient with active tuberculosis	Brownish-red soft macule or papule gradually progresses to a plaque with deep brown color. Expansion on one end with involution on the other end of the plaque. Morphological types: (1) plaque or planar form, (2) ulcerative or mutilant form, (3) vegetant form, (4) tumor-like form, and (5) papulonodular form[12,13]	90% head and neck. Usually starts on the nose, ear lobe, cheek, or scalp. The mucosa can be involved
Leprosy	All age groups		Single or multiple hypoesthetic or normoesthetic plaque	• Spectrum ranges from TT, BT, BB, BL, and LL • Hypoesthetic to normoesthetic plaques or nodules, dry scaly infiltrated in TT and BT to shiny nodules in BL and LL	• Facial plaques are predominantly seen in TT and BT. Indeterminate leprosy in children has a small to medium-sized hypopigmented patch with vague edges and some loss of sensation. Diffuse infiltration of face—leonine facies • Diffuse infiltration of ears present; madarosis[14]

Continued

CHAPTER 17 A Case of Indurated Facial Plaque

Continued

Disease	Age	Sex M:F	Symptoms	Morphology	Distribution
Actinomycosis ("lumpy jaw syndrome")	40–50 years	3:1	Slowly progressive painless indurated mass progresses into multiple discharging sinuses. At advanced stages, pain and trismus can occur	Multiple abscesses with draining sinus tracts on the skin surface or oral mucosa, sometimes expressing a typical thick yellow exudate with characteristic sulfur granules. Acute suppurative forms with rapid abscess formations are less common and are usually febrile and painful. Regional adenopathy is rare. Bone involvement is observed in approximately 10% of cases	Cervicofacial actinomycosis usually involves tissues surrounding the upper (maxillary expansion of the jaw) or lower mandible, including the mandible itself in approximately 50% of cases, cheek (15%), chin (15%), and submaxillary ramus and angle (10%)[15]
Syphilis	15–49 years	1.6:1	Extragenital primary syphilis and secondary syphilis. Painless chancre and annular or erythematous skin lesions on the face	• Great mimicker • Annular papules and plaques (nickels and dimes), corymbose plaques, necrotic ulcers (malignant syphilis), seborrheic dermatitis-like rash along the hairline (crown of Venus or corona veneris), split papules at the corners of the mouth[16]	Around mouth and nose, along the hairline
Mucormycosis			One-sided headache behind the eyes and lethargy are the earlier presentation. Nausea, fever, nasal congestion and rhinorrhea, epistaxis, nasal hypoesthesia, facial pain and numbness, history of black nasal discharge, and sinusitis. Common eye complaints are retro-orbital or periorbital pain, amaurosis, diplopia, and blurring of visions. CNS involvement presents with convulsions, dizziness, altered mental status, and gait. In widespread cases, respiratory involvement shows difficulty in breathing, cough, and hemoptysis. Vomiting and abdominal pain are common in gastrointestinal involvement	• Lesions are indurated plaques that are erythematous to purple. These become necrotic with an erythematous halo that can develop into an eschar. Other presentations include targetoid lesions, tender nodules, ulcers, purpuric lesions, and swollen and scaly plaques. In patients with surgical wound infections and burns it often appears as cellulitis and necrosis • Nasal and orbital cellulitis, redness and swelling of nasal bridge and skin of cheek in later stages, and eventually turn black due to necrosis are the common findings. Black eschar visible on nasal mucosa or palatine mucosa. Bleeding from the nose may be present in severe cases. An intraoral examination can show palatal ulceration. Some series of studies revealed proptosis as the most common orbital sign followed by ophthalmoplegia and visual loss. Other eye signs are conjunctival chemosis, nystagmus, and fixed pupil. Patients with cerebral involvement and vascular compromise may be in a coma or may show signs of a stroke. Neurological examination may reveal palsies of loss of second to seventh cranial nerves[17]	Periocular, perinasal
Conidiobolomycosis		10:1	Unilateral or bilateral nasal obstruction and painless centrofacial swelling	Swelling either in the ala or inferior turbinate of the nose along with swelling of the dorsum of the nose, cheek (nasolabial and nasofacial region), upper lip, or glabella. In the more advanced cases, the lesions can also affect the nasopharynx, oropharynx, palate, and laryngopharynx[18]	Ala or inferior turbinate and dorsum of nose or cheek

Continued

Continued

Disease	Age	Sex M:F	Symptoms	Morphology	Distribution
Aspergillosis			Invasive aspergillosis spreads beyond the confines of the sinuses and consists of AIA, CIA, and GIA. AIA occurs as a result of the invasion of the mucosa and blood vessels by fungal elements causing thrombosis, necrosis, and eschar formation. It has a fulminant course and is seen commonly in immunocompromised patients	• Primary aspergillosis, caused by direct inoculation of *Aspergillus* in damaged skin; secondary aspergillosis, involvement of skin by hematogenous dissemination; and contiguity aspergillosis, where aspergillosis of the PNS or neighboring cavity can spread contiguously to involve the skin. Contiguity aspergillosis usually presents as a necrotic, black, indurated plaque with eschar formation • Primary cutaneous aspergillosis may present as erythematous, indurated macules, papules, plaque, or hemorrhagic bullae, which may progress to necrotic ulcers that are covered by black eschar. Nodules and pustular lesions although rare might also occur[19,20]	Nasal ala, cheeks
Pseudolymphoma		1:3	Middle-aged females and elderly	Results from known or unknown stimuli, like insect bites, scabies, borreliosis, trauma, folliculitis, drugs, human immunodeficiency virus infection, herpes zoster, vaccination, tattoos, acupuncture, jewellery, and contact allergens like gold earrings	It usually manifests as an itchy solitary or multiple nodules or plaques with skin-colored or erythematous or brownish to the violaceous surface with a soft consistency[21]	Head, ear lobules, nose, and in children, the thorax
Jessner's lymphocytic infiltrate		1:1	30–50 years, few cases in children	Asymptomatic, which have been present for weeks to months. History may reveal the onset or exacerbation of the lesions following sun exposure. The lesions may have cleared spontaneously without sequelae and reoccurred at the original site or in previously unaffected areas. Few cases can have burning or pruritus	The lesions are well-demarcated, erythematous solitary, or numerous plaques or papules in sun-exposed areas and can appear annular or seen to be expanding peripherally. The surface of the lesions is nonscaly without evidence of follicular plugging or atrophy. The lesions are arranged in crescents of rings ranging from 2 mm to 2 cm in diameter	Malar area of the face and the upper back. However, lesions can be found in any area, including the forehead, neck, mastoid region, arms, legs, and trunk[22]

Continued

Continued

Disease	Age	Sex M:F	Symptoms	Morphology	Distribution
Fol-liculotropic mycosis fungoides	4.4:1	55–60 years	Itchy papules or plaques, swelling at the eyebrows with loss of hair, and diffuse infiltration of face	The initial lesions have an acneiform aspect or show follicular papules, erythematous plaques, cysts, and prurigo-like lesions. The heavy involvement of the hair follicle with follicular hyperplasia can result in the formation of tumor-like lesions even in the absence of a true tumor. Eyebrow involvement with alopecia is typical. With disease progression, there is the formation of bulky tumor masses and the face acquires a leonine appearance often associated with folliculotropism and blood involvement. Other rare presentations include lichen spinulosus-like lesions in association with hypopigmentation and alopecia, pseudotumors, lupus tumidus-like plaques, and rosacea-like lesions[23,24]	Preferentially on the face, neck, and upper trunk
LCH	1.2–1.4:1	Can occur at any age. Peak incidence 1–4 years	LCH can be completely asymptomatic. The most frequent presenting signs and symptoms include painful bone lesions and rash. Often nonspecific symptoms such as fever, poor appetite, weight loss, fatigue, irritability, and changes in behavior. Finally, more characteristic symptoms associated with the involvement of bones, skin, the pituitary gland, liver, spleen, the hematopoietic system, lungs, lymph nodes, the CNS, thymus, and the gastrointestinal tract, may appear	• Skin lesions are the second most common clinical manifestation of LCH (30–60%). Congenital cutaneous LCH in neonates is an uncommon Hashimoto–Pritzker disease characterized by self-regressive red–brown cutaneous nodules • Cutaneous presentations vary from crusted or scaly nodules and papules, blisters, vascular tumor-like lesions, scaling orange to red or purpuric macules (frequently in the seborrheic region), superficial ulcerations, nodules, and petechia • A maculopapular desquamative rash, which is located mainly within the scalp, retroauricular, inguinal or axillary area, can also appear in older children. Rare lesions include hemangioma-like lesion, a varicella-like eruption, or purpura. "Blueberry muffin baby syndrome" has also been described as a presentation of LCH in neonates. A seborrhea-like eruption on the scalp and lesions in the large body folds were also more frequent in the group with MS-LCH, with these lesions being more erosive and ulcerative compared to the skin-only group[25]	• The eruption may be extensive and involve the scalp, face, trunk, buttocks, and intertriginous area. The trunk is the most affected site • The involvement of the hands and feet suggests there is a self-regressive form, and necrosis might also be associated with a good prognosis • Lung involvement has been described in approximately 50% of patients with nail involvement

Continued

Continued

Disease	Age	Sex M:F	Symptoms	Morphology	Distribution
JXG	The first year of life. In 5–17% of cases, the skin lesions may appear soon after birth, adulthood: 20–30 years, rare in adults		Asymptomatic yellowish skin lesions	Well-defined nodules of different sizes and colors, usually yellow or red-brown, measuring up to 1 cm, single (60–82% of patients) or multiple, plaque-like lesions. Uncommon manifestations of JXG include the giant form with lesions up to 10 cm in size, the distorting face type called *Cyrano type* and lichenoid JXG. A solitary tumor located subcutaneously or deep in soft tissues may be another clinical presentation of JXG. Similar to multifocal cutaneous lesions they affect children in the first month of life[1,26]	Most typically are located on the head, neck, and upper trunk, but lesions may affect any site of the body, whereas mucosal lesions associated with JXG are hardly ever observed
NXG	17–85 years; peak in sixth decade		• The lesions may be associated with pruritus or a burning sensation • Involvement of the internal organs has been described: Heart, lungs, kidneys, intestines, ovaries, larynx, pharynx, skeletal muscles, and CNS	Firm, yellow nodules and plaques of <25 cm in diameter, starting with xanthelasma-like papules that progress to plaques. Central atrophy and ulceration can develop[5,27]	Periorbital lesions form the most characteristic sign. Other sites include elsewhere on the face, trunk, extremities, and within scars
SK	Middle age, >50 years	1:1	Usually asymptomatic and slow-growing; depending on the lesion location, there can be chronic inflammation, which leads to pain, pruritus, erythema, and bleeding around the site. There should be a concern, if there is sudden growth or emergence of multiple SK	Dull, waxy papules or plaques with verrucous surfaces result in their characteristic "stuck on" appearance. The color of SK can vary from light to dark brown, yellow, and gray, and they can present as an isolated lesion to tens or even hundreds of lesions[28]	These tumors can generally occur anywhere on the body, except for the palms, soles, and mucous membranes. The sign of Leser–Trelat refers to the sudden appearance of SK that is suggestive of internal malignancy, commonly associated with gastrointestinal or pulmonary carcinomas
AK	>40 years	M > F	Asymptomatic in most of the cases, although some patients refer to the experience of discomfort, such as burning, pain, bleeding, and pruritus	• Erythematous or reddish brown, scaly macules or papules or hyperkeratotic plaques. They are often better felt than seen. Clinically, different subtypes can be differentiated including keratotic, verrucous, pigmented, atrophic, and lichenoid forms, and cornu cutaneum • Transformation into SCC should be suspected if there is ulceration, increased mucosa thickness, lip texture changes, or loss of definition between the transition from labial commissure to adjacent skin[29]	Chronically sun-exposed areas such as the bald scalp, ears, face, forearms, and dorsum of the hands

Continued

Continued

Disease	Age	Sex M:F	Symptoms	Morphology	Distribution
BCC (Fig. 1)		40 and 79	Nonhealing nodule that bleeds occasionally	*Clinical types:* Superficial, nodular, micronodular, and infiltrative or morpheaform. Nodular BCC is the classic form, which most often presents as a pearly pink to white dome-shaped papule surrounded by a well-demarcated rolled border; prominent telangiectatic vessels may superficially traverse the lesion usually present on the face and ears. Superficial BCC presents as a scaly erythematous patch or plaque. The morpheaform type, also known as sclerosing, fibrosing, or infiltrative BCC, typically appears as an indurated, whitish, scar-like plaque with indistinct margins. Rare variants include cystic, micronodular, Basosquamous, Fibroepithelioma of Pinkus[30,31]	Above the tear line, periocular or perinasal. Superficial BCC presents usually on the trunk or extremities
SCC	9–14% for men and 4–9% for women		Asymptomatic nonhealing ulcer	Erythematous, pink, scaling plaque, papule, or nodule on sun-exposed skin that may have ulceration. Lesions can be crusted plaques or firm nodules, patchy, papulonodular, papillomatous, or exophytic[30,32]	Predominantly sun-exposed sites
Morbihan's disease	Third or fourth decades	F > M	Pain and itching and reported worsening of the edema after sun exposure	Nondepressive edema of the upper two-thirds of the face, with no tendency for spontaneous regression. The facial erythema is described as poorly defined or as discrete patches or isolated plaques. Its evolution is initially fluctuating but becomes permanent with time, leading to a disfigurement of facial contours. Eye involvement with rosacea is common, especially in the form of blepharitis and conjunctivitis[33]	The upper portion of the face, with accentuation in the periorbital region, forehead, glabella, nose, and cheeks
Sarcoidosis	Two-thirds of the cases are females	>40 years of age	Asymptomatic but may have itching, redness, persistent swelling, and unusual warmth at the site of inflammation	• Papules and plaques can be red, reddish-brown, violaceous, translucent, or hyperpigmented in color. Rare presentations include rare presentations follicular, verrucous, ichthyosiform, hypomelanotic, atrophic and ulcerative, psoriasiform, angiolupoid, and annular lesions[34,35] • Lupus pernio presents as chronic violaceous to telangiectatic (i.e., pinpoint, vascular-appearing) indurations, predominantly on the nose and cheeks causing disfigurement	Papular sarcoidosis is present on the face, especially around the eyelids and the folds, corners, and creases of the nose and lips
Granuloma faciale	Two-thirds of men	Third to fifth decades	Asymptomatic	Well-circumscribed smooth erythematous papules, nodules, or plaques with follicular accentuation on sun-exposed sites[36]	The majority of the lesions are confined to face with rare involvement of extra facial sites such as back, arms, chest, shoulders, and thighs

Continued

Continued

Disease	Age	Sex M:F	Symptoms	Morphology	Distribution
Lupus panniculitis (Fig. 2)	Female predilection	Third to the sixth decades	Tender or asymptomatic, asymmetry of the face, erythematous-indurated lesions, skin dimpling, depression, or scarring	Subcutaneous nodules, plaques with overlying normal skin, or from conditions ranging from erythematous to those of DLE (e.g., scaling, follicular plugging, dyspigmentation, telangiectasias, or atrophy, ulcers, skin hyperpigmentation, and atrophy)[37]	Predominantly on the face, upper arms, upper trunk, breasts, buttocks, and thighs
Morphea	F > M	Linear morphea is common in children	Asymptomatic plaque	• Linear morphea presents as single, unilateral binding down of skin in linear distribution; atrophic and slightly depressed, and skin is smooth, shiny, hard, and maybe pigmented • En coup de sabre (Fig. 3)—slowly progressive course and is generally limited to the hemiface. Lesions often start with contraction and stiffness of the affected area, forming a depressed groove on the parietal region and extending to the scalp, developing an area of linear alopecia. The groove may extend to the nasal region, upper lip, and, sometimes, to the gingiva. The ipsilateral tongue may be atrophic and the spacing and direction of teeth may be altered. The jaw may be involved and the bones of the skull may be affected. In case of deformity of the jaw, it may result in poor dental occlusion, poor teeth implantation, tooth root atrophy, and delayed appearance of teeth[38]	Linear morphea involves the extremities, face, or scalp
Infantile hemangioma (Fig. 4)	More common in females	At birth or in the first 2 months	Lesions develop in the first 2–4 weeks of life, but 20% of them can be present at birth. The lesion is at first a pale-white to the blue–gray macula, depending on its profoundness, or a papule with the same characteristics. They grow during a variable period until 6–9 months, after which they involute, following the characteristic evolution. Thus 50% regress by the age of 5 years and 90% regress by the age of 9	Superficial hemangiomas present as round or oval tumors, lobulated or with a fine surface, more often in the head-neck area, 1–25 cm in size. Deep hemangiomas come as soft, bluish masses, with or without telangiectasia. The common complications are ulceration, infection, and hemorrhage. Systemic complications come with Kasabach–Merritt syndrome, characterized by the association of cutaneous and visceral lesions of variable aspects and dimensions, and with extracutaneous manifestations, such as consumption coagulopathy	Chin hemangiomas are frequently associated with hemangiomas in the upper airway system. Eyelid or periocular hemangiomas express low visual acuity, amblyopia, or strabismus. Facial hemangiomas are associated with CNS malformations or ophthalmic vessel anomalies[39]

Continued

Continued

Disease	Age	Sex M:F	Symptoms	Morphology	Distribution
Angiosarcoma	At any age, more common in elderly	2:1	Asymptomatic Angiosarcomas have a poor prognosis compared to other soft tissue sarcomas, with a 5-year survival of 35%	• Initially appear as bruises or raised purplish papules but can further grow and look like ulcerated, fungating masses • The diagnosis of angiosarcomas can often be delayed due to misdiagnosis as a fungal infection, bacterial infection, Kaposi's sarcoma, melanoma, or ulcers since they have a wide range of appearance	Commonly occur in the head and neck, followed by the breasts and extremities[40]
LM melanoma	Elderly		Asymptomatic, although advanced tumors may produce pain, burning, itching, or bleeding	LM presents as an irregular brown macule or patch on chronically sun-damaged skin. Lesions are asymmetric, light-brown to black, with color variegation, and tend to have an ill-defined border. As lesions progress, skip areas occur with a patchy, noncontiguous pattern Due to its in situ nature, LM is typically smooth and nonpalpable. In invasive lesions, i.e., in LM melanoma a papular or dermal component may be felt	About 86% of LM occurs on the head/neck, predominantly on the cheeks[41]
Microcystic adnexal carcinoma	Middle-aged to elderly (44–64 years)	Equal distribution with a slight female predominance	Asymptomatic, locally aggressive and infiltrative tumor	Solitary, slow-growing 1–3-cm white-yellowish firm papule, plaque or cyst-like tumor, can have ulceration or paraesthesia, if there is a perineural invasion	Head and neck predominantly in the centrofacial area, including the upper and lower lips. Other sites include axilla, buttocks, and trunk[42,43]
DLE	Mid-adulthood occurs at a later age in men		Photosensitivity, erythematous or depigmented lesion over face, upper back, or sun-exposed sites	Acute cutaneous LE can manifest as a classical malar rash which presents as symmetrical erythematous plaques across the malar eminences and nasal bridge, with sparing of the nasolabial folds SCLE is characterized by a nonscarring photosensitive rash presenting as psoriasiform or annular lesions DLE presents as indurated discoid lesions with an overlying scale	• SCLE rash occurs on the face, V area of the neck, or extensor surfaces of the arms and upper back • DLE occurs most commonly on the face and scalp[44]
Sweets syndrome	Common in women	Classic type: Middle age	Fever, malaise, arthralgia, and headache	• Classical Sweet's syndrome: The abrupt onset of tender papulonodular skin lesions • Malignancy-associated Sweet's syndrome: Bullous or ulcerated and resemble pyoderma gangrenosum • Drug induced: Similar presentation with temporal association with the drug intake	Face, neck, and upper extremities with asymmetrical distribution[45]
Porokeratosis	Third and fourth decades	DSAP: 2:1	Asymptomatic or minimal pruritus	DSAP: Multiple superficial, mildly pigmented, annular, keratotic plaques with a central atrophic area, and a prominent peripheral ridge	DSAP—sun-exposed sites like nose, cheeks, and eyelids but paradoxically, the limbs are more affected than the face[46,47]

(AK: actinic keratosis; AIDS: acquired immunodeficiency disease syndrome; ACLE: acute cutaneous lupus erythematosus; AIA: acute invasive aspergillosis; BCC: basal cell carcinoma; BT: borderline tuberculoid; BB: borderline borderline; BL: borderline lepromatous; CIA: chronic invasive aspergillosis; CNS: central nervous system; DSAP: disseminated superficial actinic porokeratosis; DLE: discoid lupus erythematosus; GIA: granulomatous invasive aspergillosis; HIV: human immunodeficiency virus; JXG: juvenile xanthogranuloma; LCH: Langerhans cell histiocytosis; LL: lepromatous leprosy; MS: multisystem; NXG: necrobiotic xanthogranuloma; PNS: paranasal sinus; SCC: squamous cell carcinoma; SLE: systemic lupus erythematosus; SCLE: subacute cutaneous lupus erythematosus; SK: seborrheic keratosis; TT: tuberculoid leprosy)

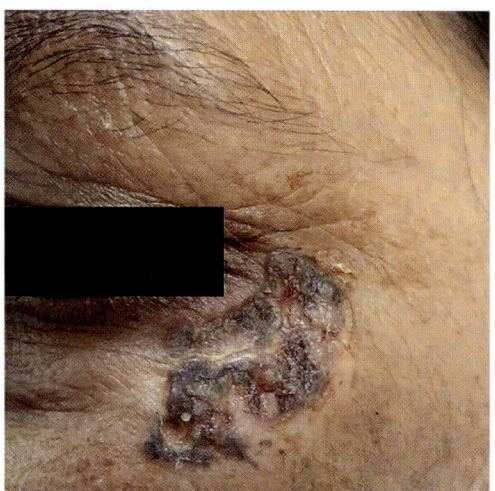

FIG. 1: Pigmented basal cell carcinoma—a well-defined hyperpigmented plaque with rolled-out borders and ulceration and crusting close to left lower eyelid.
Courtesy: Dr Adhyatm Bhandari, Department of Dermatology, PGIMER, Chandigarh, India.

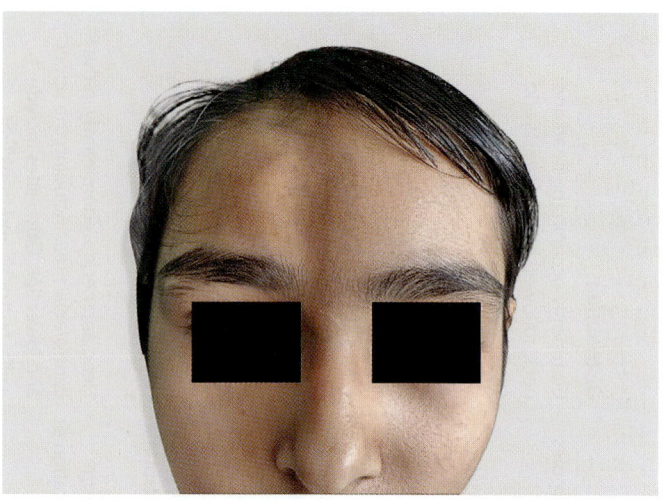

FIG. 3: En coup de sabre—well-defined depressed indurated plaque present on forehead extending up to the eyebrow.
Courtesy: Dr Adhyatm Bhandari, Department of Dermatology, PGIMER, Chandigarh, India.

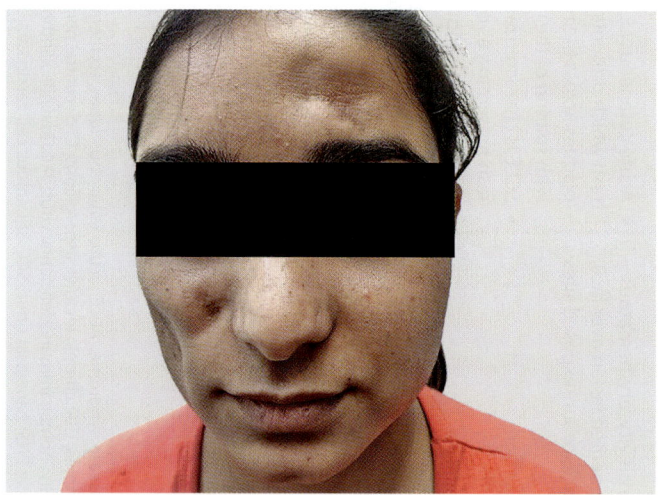

FIG. 2: Lupus panniculitis—multiple depressed atrophic lesions over the forehead and right cheek denoting the lipoatrophy occurring as a sequel of lupus panniculitis.
Courtesy: Dr Adhyatm Bhandari, Department of Dermatology, PGIMER, Chandigarh, India.

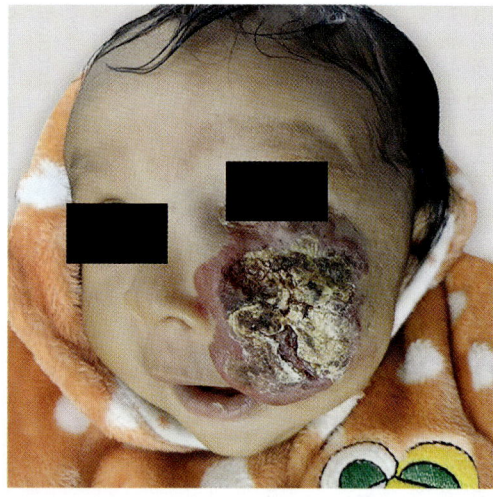

FIG. 4: Infantile hemangioma—well-defined erythematous infiltrated plaque with ulceration and crusting abutting the lower eyelid present on the cheek.
Courtesy: Dr Adhyatm Bhandari, Department of Dermatology, PGIMER, Chandigarh, India.

infantile hemangioma. Associated fever, malaise, and lymphadenopathy are seen in cellulitis, erysipelas, and Sweet syndrome. Ill-defined edematous subcutaneous plaques with minimal surface changes are seen in conidiobolomycosis (can have a nasal extension and fingers can be insinuated under the swelling), aspergillosis, folliculotropic mycosis fungoides (MF), Morbihan's disease, and lupus panniculitis. Ulcerative lesions are found in lupus vulgaris (nonulcerated plaques with apple jelly nodules upon diascopy), sporotrichosis, leishmaniasis, squamous cell carcinoma (SCC), and BCC. Necrotic plaques can be seen in mucormycosis. Itching can be present in tinea faciei, sycosis barbae, necrobiotic xanthogranuloma (NXG), sarcoidosis, Morbihan's disease, and actinic keratosis (AK).

ORIGIN AND PROGRESS

The onset of the disease is important as most of the infectious conditions like cellulitis, erysipelas are acute in onset as opposed to insidious onset in chronic infections like lupus vulgaris or deep fungal infections, or other noninfectious conditions. The presence of lesions since birth indicates birthmarks like a port-wine stain or congenital melanocytic nevus (CMN). The history of exacerbation during seasonal change can be useful in conditions like hydroa vacciniforme, atopic dermatitis, etc. Associated systemic symptoms like fever and sinusitis, epistaxis can be present in Sweet syndrome and granulomatosis with polyangiitis (GPA), respectively. Ulceration and bleeding in AK indicate malignant transformation. The plaques of borderline tuberculoid (BT) Hansen **(Fig. 5)** tend to become more erythematous and swollen during type 1 reaction along with other systemic symptoms and neuritis.

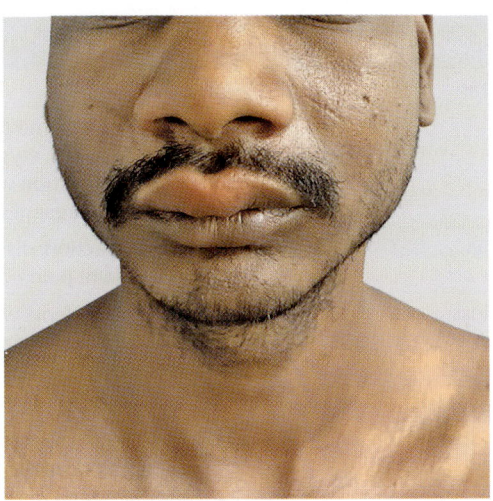

FIG. 5: Borderline tuberculoid Hansen—ill-defined skin-colored plaque with associated swelling of lower lip mimicking orofacial granulomatosis in a 27-year-old male patient.
Courtesy: Dr Adhyatm Bhandari, Department of Dermatology, PGIMER, Chandigarh, India.

SIGNIFICANT PAST/PRECEDING HISTORY

The history of travel or residing in regions endemic to leishmaniasis **(Fig. 6)** could help arrive at a diagnosis. Past history of medical illness like diabetes, human immunodeficiency virus (HIV) infection, or transplantation can be present in deep fungal infection, cutaneous tuberculosis (TB), or cutaneous malignancies. The risk factors for mucormycosis include diabetes mellitus, with or without ketoacidosis, hematological malignancies (HM), other malignancies, transplantation, prolonged neutropenia, corticosteroids, trauma, iron overload, illicit intravenous drug use, neonatal prematurity, malnourishment, and COVID-19 virus infection.[2] The preceding history of trauma or barrier disruption can be found in cellulitis, pseudolymphoma, or sporotrichosis. A sudden proliferation in preexisting nevus like CMN or nevus sebaceous can lead to the diagnosis of melanoma or syringocystadenoma papilliferum or BCC, respectively. The history of systemic symptoms should be thoroughly assessed as many of the facial lesions could be a manifestation of a part of underlying systemic disease.

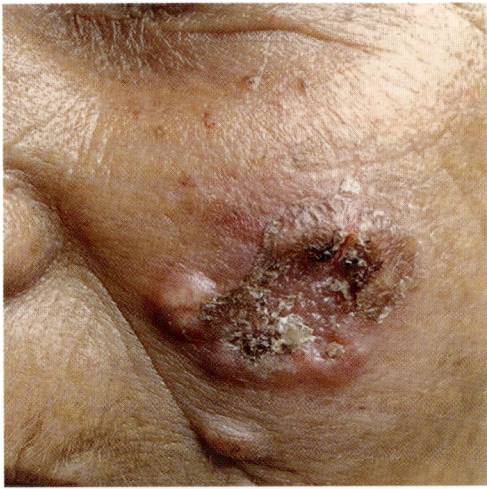

FIG. 6: Leishmaniasis—a well-defined erythematous indurated plaque with a central depression and crusting and raised borders (volcano sign) and a satellite papule present over the left cheek.
Courtesy: Dr Adhyatm Bhandari, Department of Dermatology, PGIMER, Chandigarh, India.

ASSOCIATED SYMPTOMS

Fever is a common symptom associated with facial indurated plaque. However, the pattern can provide a clue to diagnosis, for example, cutaneous TB with concurrent internal organ TB can have evening rise of temperature, downgrading leprosy with erythema nodosum leprosum (ENL), can have a high-grade fever, fever associated with night sweats, and weight loss can be seen in cutaneous B-cell lymphoma. The "red flags/warning signs" in mucormycosis are cranial nerve palsy, diplopia, sinus pain, proptosis, periorbital swelling, orbital apex syndrome, or a palatine ulcer.[3] Malignancy is associated with NXG, Sweet syndrome, and nodular amyloidosis. Other associated symptoms are listed in **Table 3**.

GENERAL EXAMINATION

The examination done by the clinician as the patient walks into the dermatology outpatient clinic can be helpful upon correlation with the cutaneous examination. PHACE syndrome (posterior fossa abnormalities, hemangiomas, arterial lesions, cardiac abnormalities, eye abnormalities)

Table 3: Systemic symptoms in facial plaques.	
Symptoms	**Disease**
Fever	Fever is present in multiple conditions whether infective or inflammatory or in lesions with secondary infection. Cellulitis, erysipelas, lupus vulgaris with concurrent internal organ TB, leprosy in reaction, deep fungal infection with fungal sepsis, SLE patients with ACLE, DLE, SCLE lesions, and Sweet syndrome can present with fever
Arthralgia	Leprosy in reaction, disseminated fungal infections, SLE with cutaneous lesions, psoriasis can have associated joint pain
Weight loss	HIV-infected patients with disseminated histoplasmosis, Kaposi sarcoma of the face, giant molluscum contagiosum in HIV can have significant weight loss. Malignancy-like lymphoma should be ruled out in the elderly
• Upper respiratory symptoms • Nasal obstruction • Nasal bleeding • Nasal deformity	• Aspergillosis, mucormycosis, conidiobolomycosis GPA, leprosy. More than 90% of patients with GPA have upper respiratory symptoms[4] • Leprosy (saddle nose deformity, facies leprosa), midline lethal lymphoma, GPA, deep fungal infections, lupus pernio, Cyrano nose deformity in infantile hemangioma of nose
• Lower respiratory symptoms • Breathlessness • Cough • Chest pain • Hemoptysis	• Cough and breathlessness are a manifestation of GPA due to pulmonary infiltrates pleural effusion and hemoptysis secondary to pulmonary hemorrhage.[4] Sarcoidosis can manifest with dry cough and dyspnea. In case of secondary deep fungal infections disseminated from the lungs, patients can have a cough, dyspnea, or hemoptysis. Histiocytosis like LCH or JXG or NXG can have lung involvement with respiratory symptoms • Interstitial lung disease can occur in dermatomyositis (DM)
• Gastrointestinal symptoms • Abdominal pain, diarrhea, constipation	Metastatic Crohn's disease can present with diffuse swelling of lips. Abdominal pain can be the presenting symptom in angiolipoma associated with tuberous sclerosis. Hereditary angioneurotic edema can manifest with facial swelling and abdominal pain
• Peripheral nervous system • Sensory loss • Motor weakness	Sensory loss and motor weakness are present in leprosy. Sensory loss can be found in sarcoidosis
Central nervous system	Seizures, psychosis, and central nervous system vasculitis can be associated with SLE. Port-wine stain can be associated with Sturge–Weber syndrome and manifest with seizures. Tuberous sclerosis with cortical tubers, subependymal giant cell astrocytoma can present with seizures and decreased intelligence
• Ophthalmic • Eye pain • Glaucoma • Blindness	Periorbital cellulitis, mucormycosis can extend into the eyeball causing pain, photophobia, and blindness. In 50–80% of cases of NXG eye involvement can be present with symptoms of diplopia, sclerosis, decreased visual acuity, exophthalmos, blepharoptosis, and decreased ocular motility.[5] En coup de sabre can present with glaucoma
Auditory	External ear destruction can occur in lupus vulgaris, chilblain LE; whereas infiltration is seen in leprosy, deposition disorders
• Renal • Hematuria • Proteinuria	Hematuria and proteinuria can be features of GPA or SLE. Renal amyloidosis can occur in leprosy or psoriasis
• Reproductive • Testicular pain	Epididymo-orchitis can occur in leprosy with type 2 reaction. Paraneoplastic DM has been reported with testicular cancer
• Vascular Raynaud's phenomenon • Acrocyanosis digital ulceration	The presence of Raynaud's phenomenon and vasculitis are associated with SLE and DM

(ACLE: acute cutaneous lupus erythematosus; DLE: discoid lupus erythematosus; GPA: granulomatosis with polyangiitis; HIV: human immunodeficiency virus; JXG: juvenile xanthogranuloma; LCH: Langerhans cell histiocytosis; LE: lupus erythematosus; NXG: necrobiotic xanthogranuloma; SLE: systemic lupus erythematosus; SCLE: subacute cutaneous lupus erythematosus; TB: tuberculosis)

CHAPTER 17 A Case of Indurated Facial Plaque

Table 4: General examination findings in patients with facial plaque.

Area of examination	Examination findings	Possible interpretation and associations
Scalp	Diffuse hair loss	SLE, DM, chronic telogen effluvium associated with chronic illness
	Lupus hair	SLE
	Cicatricial alopecia	Associated with ACLE, SCLE, DLE lesions on the face; en coup de sabre
	Erythematous scaly plaques	Psoriasis, seborrheic dermatitis
Eye	Conjunctival pallor	Anemia secondary to SLE
	Proptosis	Orbital involvement in GPA
	Red eye, scleritis, episcleritis	Leprosy
	Exophthalmos, blepharoptosis, decreased ocular motility	NXG; mucormycosis can present with necrosis of the eyeball
Eyebrow	Loss of eyebrow	Leprosy, folliculotropic MF
Nose	Nasal mass, nasal septum deviation, saddle nose deformity	Leprosy, GPA, lupus pernio, aspergillosis, syphilis
	Cyrano nose deformity	Infantile hemangioma
	Widening of the nasal root	Conidiobolomycosis
Oral cavity	Chronic recurrent ulcers	SLE
	Ulcer, induration, perforation GPA of the hard palate	Leprosy, syphilis, mucormycosis, squamous cell carcinoma, GPA
	Gingival hyperplasia (strawberry gingiva)	GPA
Nail	• Nail clubbing • Periungual telangiectasias SLE-associated vasculitis • Tortures capillaries with prominent subpapillary plexus on nail fold capillaroscopy	Chronic lung insufficiency in GPA, sarcoidosis
	Splinter hemorrhages	Psoriasis, SLE
	Brittleness, splitting, fissuring, pitting, onycholysis, elkonyxis, Beau's lines, onychomadesis, nail loss	Syphilis
	Longitudinal grooving, onycholysis, subungual hyperkeratosis, subungual pustules, purpuric striae of the nail bed, V-shaped notches, pterygium formation, elkonyxis and paronychial erythema, and swelling	LCH
Lymph node	Enlarged cervical lymph nodes	Infection, e.g., cellulitis, erysipelas, deep fungal infections, TB. Metastasis from SCC
	Generalized lymphadenopathy	Lymphoma, AIDS, histiocytosis

(ACLE: acute cutaneous lupus erythematosus; AIDS: acquired immunodeficiency disease syndrome; DLE: discoid lupus erythematosus; DM: dermatomyositis; GPA: granulomatosis with polyangiitis, HIV: human immunodeficiency virus; JXG: juvenile xanthogranuloma; LCH: Langerhans cell histiocytosis; MF: mycosis fungoides; NXG: necrobiotic xanthogranuloma; SLE: systemic lupus erythematosus; SCLE: subacute cutaneous lupus erythematosus; SCC: squamous cell carcinoma; TB: tuberculosis)

and lumbar syndrome are also disorders seen with infantile hemangiomas and are characterized by the association with several other anomalies in the upper or lower part of the body. The common findings in the general examination of the patient are listed in **Table 4**.

CUTANEOUS EXAMINATION

The site of presentation of the plaque can help in differentiation one condition from the other. Lesions with predominant distribution are listed as below:

- Nose[6]—lupus pernio, lymphocytoma cutis, rhinophyma, rosacea, SCC, BCC, granuloma faciale, AK, keratoacanthoma, Kaposi sarcoma, conidiobolomycosis
- Periorbital[7]—lupus miliaris disseminatus faciei (LMDF), sporotrichosis, histoplasmosis, JXG, NXG, angioedema, mucormycosis, aspergillosis, anthrax, rosacea, eccrine-derived tumors, SCC, BCC, sebaceous carcinoma, Merkel cell carcinoma, trichilemmal carcinoma
- Forehead—syphilis, SCC, folliculotropic MF, annular sarcoidosis, leprosy
- Jaw, chin, and perioral—rosacea, LMDF, sarcoidosis, trichoepithelioma

- Cheek—amyloidosis, lupus panniculitis, Jessner's lymphocytic infiltrate (JLI), lupus vulgaris, granuloma faciale, ACLE, BT Hansen, angiosarcoma

A significant part of the diagnosis depends on the color of the lesion, e.g., yellowish in JXG, sebaceous hyperplasia, juvenile colloid milium, sarcoidosis, seborrheic dermatitis, granulomatous rosacea, pityriasis rubra pilaris; skin-colored lesions are present predominantly in appendageal tumors.

Annular lesions[8] can be seen in leprosy, syphilis, lupus vulgaris, discoid lupus erythematosus (DLE), dermatophytosis, leishmaniasis, erythema multiforme, urticarial, JLI, psoriasis, lichen planus, porokeratosis, sarcoidosis, granuloma faciale, neonatal lupus, seborrheic dermatitis, Sweet syndrome, superficial BCC, and MF. The morphology and distribution of lesions are listed in **Table 2**.

Figure 7 shows plaque over lip and papules over the eyelid with the diagnosis of venous malformation.

Approach to facial plaque based on secondary skin changes is given in **Flowchart 1**.

DERMOSCOPY

The noninvasive analysis using dermoscopy has gained a unique importance because of the simplicity and ease of diagnosis without the need for histopathological evaluation. **Figure 9** shows the dermoscopic picture of porokeratosis. The dermoscopic findings of common facial plaques are listed in **Table 5**.

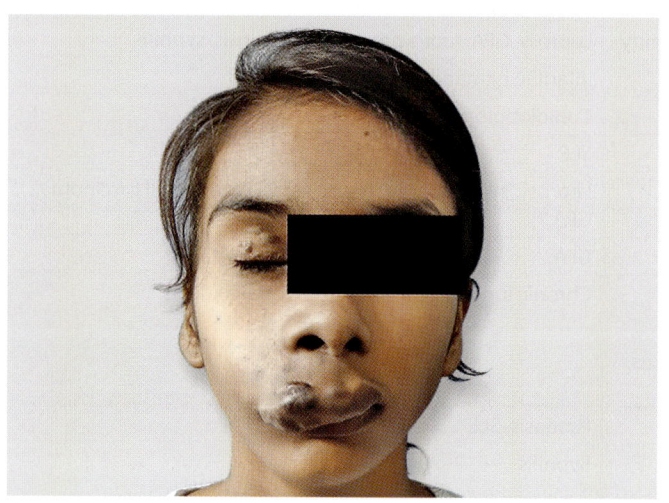

FIG. 7: Venous malformation—well-defined bluish to skin colored plaque over upper lip and papules over right eyelid.
Courtesy: Dr Neha Thakur, Department of Dermatology, PGIMER, Chandigarh, India.

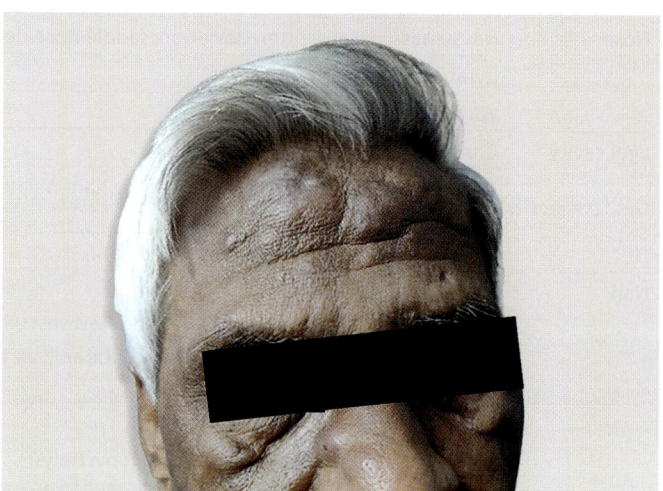

FIG. 8: Actinic reticuloid—well to ill-defined edematous skin colored plaques over forehead and cheeks with chronic actinic damage.
Courtesy: Dr Priyansh Gupta, Department of Dermatology, PGIMER, Chandigarh, India.

Secondary skin changes					
Atrophy	Telangiectasia	Ulceration/Erosion	Scaling	Keratin plug with a crateriform appearance	Edema
• DLE • Sarcoidosis • Leprosy • Lupus vulgaris • NXG • Lupus panniculitis • Infantile hemangioma • Leishmania recidivans cutis	• DLE • BCC • Lupus vulgaris • NXG • Rosacea	• Lupus vulgaris • NXG • Infantile hemangioma • Cellulitis • Mucormycosis • SCC • BCC • Sweet syndrome	• DLE • SCLE • Psoriasis • Leprosy • Lupus vulgaris • Seborrheic dermatitis	• KA • KA-like SCC	• DLE • SCLE • Sweet syndrome • Leprosy • Angiosarcoma • Tumid LE • Actinic reticuloid (Fig. 8)

(BCC: basal cell carcinoma; DLE: discoid lupus erythematosus; KA: keratoacanthoma; NXG: necrobiotic xanthogranuloma; SCC: squamous cell carcinoma; SCLE: subacute cutaneous lupus erythematosus)

FLOWCHART 1: Approach to facial plaque based on secondary skin changes.

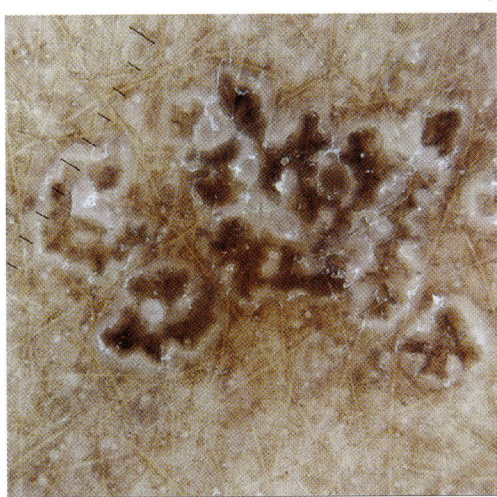

FIG. 9: On dermatoscopy, homogenous tan brown globules surrounded by white track-like structure in porokeratosis.
Courtesy: Dr Divya Joshi, Department of Dermatology, PGIMER, Chandigarh, India.

INVESTIGATIONS

Investigations should be focused on achieving the diagnosis and for planning further management of the patient. The diagnosis should be narrowed down by detailed history and examination as much as possible to avoid unwarranted investigations. Other than screening investigations, associated suspected systemic involvement should guide selection for further specialized investigations.

Following basic investigations should be ordered as screening:
- Complete blood count with differential leukocyte count
- Routine urine analysis
- Erythrocyte sedimentation rate (ESR)
- C-reactive protein levels (CRP)
- Liver function study
- Renal function study
- Skin biopsy for histopathological and direct immunofluorescence (DIF) study

Table 5: Dermoscopy of common facial plaques.	
Disease	**Dermoscopy findings**
Lupus vulgaris	• Yellowish-white globules, white structureless areas, white scales, telangiectasias (long linear, branching and short linear vessels). Pinkish-red background, white shiny streaks, white rosettes, and bluish hue. Facial lesion have increased frequency of follicular plugs, patulous follicles, and white rosettes. • Fine focused telangiectasias on a yellow to golden background correlate with the apple-jelly sign[48]
Granuloma faciale	Translucent white-gray background intermingled with orthogonal whitish streaks and elongated telangiectasias and amorphous yellowish or yellow-brown areas[49]
FMF	Perifollicular accentuation seen as a white halo around the follicle, comedo-like openings, white structureless areas, and dotted/fine linear vessels. Milky-white globules and black dots/broken hair, as well as keratotic cone-shaped spicules, in FMF and spiky MF, respectively[50]
JXG	The "setting sun" pattern is characterized by a yellow-orange central area, which may show areas of lighter yellow, correlating with the dermal xanthogranulomatous infiltrate, and an erythematous halo, which may occur at any stage of evolution. Linear telangiectasias have also been described. Other nonspecific characteristics found include discrete pigment network, whitish streaks indicating areas of fibrosis, and fine branched vessels[51]
SK	Fissures and ridges, hairpin vessels with white halo, comedo-like openings, and milia-like cysts. The histological counterparts are papillomatous epidermis, enlarged dermal capillaries, pseudohorn cysts, and intraepidermal cysts[52]
AK	• Grade 1 AKs are typified by red pseudonetwork pattern and discrete white scales; grade 2 corresponds to an erythematous background intermingled by white to yellow, keratotic, and enlarged follicular openings (strawberry pattern); and grade 3 AKs exhibit either enlarged follicular openings filled with keratotic plugs over a scaly and white-yellow-appearing background or marked hyperkeratosis seen as white-yellow structureless areas[53] • Dermatoscopy can be also helpful in differentiating grade 1 and 2 AKs from fully developed SCC. This is due to the fact that fully developed SCC often reveals vascular patterns as expression of tumoral neoangiogenesis. Effectively, vascular patterns including dotted or glomerular vessels, hairpin vessels, and linear irregular vessels occur at much higher frequency in SCC compared with AK. The development of initially dotted or glomerular vessels and later hairpin and linear vessels indicate progression toward a more aggressive invasive growth of SCC
BCC	• The most significant features in all types, were a scattered vascular pattern, featureless areas, atypical red vessels, arborizing vessels, comma vessels, background of white-red structureless areas, and telangiectasias. Hemorrhage-ulceration, hypopigmented areas, and blue-gray ovoid nests were all more likely to be observed in sBCCs, than in nBCCs. • Arborizing and atypical red vessels in addition to featureless areas were more frequent in nodular than in sBCCs. Telangiectasias, white-red structureless areas, red dots, and red globules were more common in nonpigmented than in pigmented BCCs. Arborizing vessels were described in pigmented lesions in comparison to nonpigmented[54]

Continued

Continued

Disease	Dermoscopy findings
SCC	Targetoid hair follicles, keratin/scales, blood spots, white circles, white structureless areas, hairpin vessels, linear-irregular vessels perivascular white halos, and ulceration[55]
Sarcoidosis	Linear vessels overlying the translucent orange ovoid structures[35]
CMN	Reticular pattern, globular pattern, reticular-globular pattern, homogeneous pattern, reticular-homogeneous pattern, globular-homogeneous pattern, cobblestone pattern, reticular patchy pattern. Atypical dots and globules, focal hypopigmentation, and perifollicular hypopigmentation are the most common dermoscopic features of CMN. The rarest dermoscopic feature is the blue-whitish veil[56]
Lentigo maligna melanoma	Polygons/rhomboids/zigzag pattern (angulated lines), annular-granular pattern, asymmetric pigmented follicular openings, circle within circle[57]
Bowen disease	Yellowish-white opaque scales and clusters of two types of roundish vascular pattern: small dotted vessels and glomerular or coiled vessels. Both patterns often appear within the same lesion and are distributed in small, densely packed clusters or groups. In pigmented Bowen disease, other dermoscopic features are represented by small brown globules, which are regularly packed or aligned in a patchy distribution, and by gray to brown homogeneous pigmentation. White circles are a specific feature of early SCC and AK. They are white structures within the hair follicle that might present a ring-like or targetoid appearance[55]
DLE	In nonscalp DLE, the most frequent features were follicular keratotic plugs, white perifollicular halo, white scale, speckled brown pigmentation, white structureless areas, and arborizing vessels[58]

(AK: actinic keratosis; BCC: basal cell carcinoma; CMN: congenital melanocytic nevus; DLE: discoid lupus erythematosus; FMF: folliculotropic mycosis fungoides; JXG: juvenile xanthogranuloma; MF: mycosis fungoides; nBCC: nodular basal cell carcinoma; SK: seborrheic keratosis; SCC: squamous cell carcinoma; sBCC: superficial basal cell carcinoma)

If primary cutaneous examination (plaque with scarring, necrosis, cutaneous ulceration) or associated systemic symptoms **(Table 4)** suggest infective etiology then Mantoux test, chest X-ray, urine for acid-fast bacilli, and retroviral status can be done. If there is a history of loss of sensation, fever with evanescent nodules, facial palsy then nerve conduction study, ultrasound of nerves, and nerve biopsy can be advised. In case of edematous indurated swelling associated with photosensitivity, scarring alopecia or malar rash, then antinuclear antibody (ANA), ANA immunoblot testing, and 24-hour urine protein could be ordered. Eosinophilia, elevated ESR and CRP and hypergammaglobulinemia, is markers of activity, usually seen in association with generalized, deep, and pansclerotic morphea. Elevated creatinine kinase and aldolase are seen in patients with new lesions.

Consumptive coagulopathy in Kasabach–Merritt phenomenon of infantile hemangioma is accompanied by thrombocytopenia, hypofibrinogenemia, low D-dimmers, and low coagulation factors.

Necrobiotic xanthogranuloma is associated with hematologic alterations, with the most common being monoclonal gammopathy of the immunoglobulin (Ig) G-kappa type (65%), followed by Ig G lambda (35%). Other reported associations comprise non-Hodgkin lymphoma, Waldenstrom's macroglobulinemia, amyloidosis, and myelodysplastic syndrome.

Details of positive findings in history and examination on presentation should clearly be mentioned in case paper of the patient to justify your rationally behind ordered investigations. Imaging studies like ultrasound, computed tomography, and magnetic resonance imaging can be done to assess the extent of the lesion.

BIOPSY TECHNIQUE

For conditions like cellulitis, erysipelas, or pseudofolliculitis where the diagnosis is predominantly clinical, no biopsy is required. However, in infective plaques, establishing a diagnosis becomes difficult without biopsy and culture/sensitivity or polymerase chain reaction (PCR) from the tissue sample. Biopsy should be taken preferably from the actively progressing edge of the lesion, e.g., in BCC, SCC, lupus vulgaris, leprosy, with adequate depth including epidermis, dermis, and subcutaneous tissue. DIF testing in biopsy sample is useful in lupus erythematosus. In a rapidly progressing necrotic plaque like mucormycosis, a fresh frozen biopsy to look for branching nonseptate hyphae. Histopathological examination plays a major role in establishing diagnosis in case of granulomatous dermatoses. Histologically six subtypes of granulomas found in granulomatous skin diseases—tuberculoid, sarcoidal, necrobiotic, suppurative, foreign body, and histoid type.[59] Granulomas are characterized by a focal collection of epithelioid cells or histiocytes, admixed with a variable number of lymphocytes, and multinucleated giant cells. Granulomatous reaction is a type IV hypersensitivity reaction evoked by poorly soluble reactive substances. Location of the granulomas around the neurovascular bundles and involvement of arrector pili muscle and adnexa in the background of proper clinical presentation cues to diagnose tuberculoid and BT leprosy. However, most of the borderline lepromatous (BL) and all lepromatous leprosy (LL) cases exhibit histiocytic granulomas and will be strongly positive for lepra bacilli in modified Ziehl–Neelsen stain. Tuberculoid granuloma has epithelioid histiocytes, giant cells, lymphocyte cuffing with or without caseous

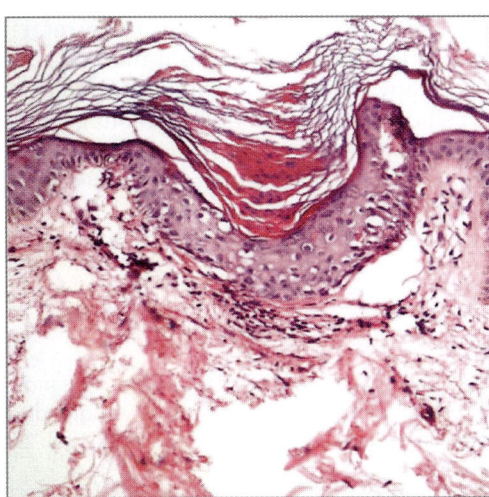

FIG. 10: Section shows a coronoid lamella with a packed parakeratotic column with underlying epidermis showing lack of granular layer. Adjacent epidermis appears essentially unremarkable. (Hematoxylin and eosin, 200×)
Courtesy: Dr Divya Aggarwal, Department of Histopathology, PGIMER, Chandigarh, India.

necrosis. Suppurative granuloma formation and giant cells are a very common inflammatory reaction against the chitinous wall of sporangium and spores in case of deep fungal infections. Microscopy of cutaneous leishmaniasis will reveal heavy plasma cell infiltration at subepithelial tissue and macrophages containing amastigote forms [Leishman-Donovan (LD)] bodies in case of early lesions. Sarcoidosis can have noncaseating epithelioid granuloma devoid of inflammatory cells and Langhans giant cells.[59] Histopathological features of porokeratosis have been described in **Figure 10**.

MANAGEMENT

Management of indurated facial plaque largely depends on etiology, the extent of systemic involvement and underlying factors. A broad approach in the management of the various types of indurated plaques on the face in concise has been described here. Readers are advised to refer to other resources for details.

Infections

Cellulitis, erysipelas—oral or intravenous antibiotics with both antistreptococcal and antistaphylococcal activity, such as flucloxacillin. Patients with severe or necrotizing infections should have an agent with activity against toxin production in group A streptococci, such as clindamycin or linezolid added.[60]

Lupus vulgaris—antituberculosis therapy according to extrapulmonary tuberculosis regimen.

Leprosy—World Health Organization (WHO) paucibacillary and multibacillary multidrug therapy according to the spectrum.

Syphilis—primary and secondary—injection Benzathine penicillin 2.4 MIU intramuscular single dose.

Tinea faciei—itraconazole 100 mg twice daily or terbinafine 250 mg daily along with topical antifungal.

Mucormycosis—extensive surgical debridement, antifungal therapy, correction of the underlying metabolic or impaired immunological status, and control of other concomitant infections intravenous liposomal amphotericin B, posaconazole.[2]

Aspergillosis—voriconazole, echinocandins. In cases of aspergillosis in burns or massive soft tissue wounds, surgical debridement is recommended, in addition to antifungal therapy.[61]

Leishmaniasis—local therapy—intralesional antimonials, cryotherapy, thermotherapy, lasers (carbon dioxide, argon, erbium glass, neodymium-doped yttrium aluminum garnet laser), topical paromomycin.[62]

Systemic therapy—meglumine antimoniate and sodium stibogluconate, ketoconazole, itraconazole and fluconazole, amphotericin B, Miltefosine, pentamidine isethionate, cyclosporine, imiquimod, and immunotherapy.

Conidiobolomycosis—saturated solution of potassium iodide (SSKI), ketoconazole (200–400 mg/day), itraconazole (200–400 mg/day), fluconazole (100–200 mg/day), miconazole, voriconazole, terbinafine, amphotericin B, clotrimazole, and hyperbaric oxygen.[62]

Jessner's lymphocytic infiltrate—topical and intralesional steroids, antimalarials, tacrolimus, thalidomide, etretinate, methotrexate, oral auranofin, and proquazone. Cosmetic camouflage, photoprotection, and excision of small lesions can eliminate or mask the appearance of the disease. Other less common treatment options include laser therapy, photodynamic therapy, and cryotherapy.[63]

Folliculotropic MF—for the treatment of early disease, topical medications are used, such as corticosteroids, bexarotene, and nitrogen mustard, as well as phototherapy or electron beam therapy. Other modifiers of the biological response, such as interferon-alpha, can be used for advanced disease. Polychemotherapy regimens are indicated in cases with lymph node and/or visceral involvement and for the cases refractory to topical treatment. Due to the deeper location of the infiltrate, folliculotropic MF are less responsive to treatments directed to the skin.[23]

Langerhans cell histiocytosis (LCH)—systemic therapy is indicated for all patients with multiple lesions within one single system (SS-m) and multisystem (MS)-LCH as well as for special localizations. A standard two-drug regimen with vinblastine and prednisone consisting of an initial intensive phase for 6–12 weeks, followed by maintenance therapy for a total treatment duration of at least 12 months, is recommended. Nonresponders, particularly those with progressive disease in a high-risk organ, are eligible for salvage therapy with cladribine, cytarabine, clofarabine, or combinations of those medications as well as bone marrow and/or solid organ transplantation.[25]

Morbihan's disease—isotretinoin, systemic antibiotics (tetracyclines, metronidazole), antihistamines (ketotifen), and systemic corticosteroids (prednisone, prednisolone), Clofazimine, and thalidomide.[33]

Sarcoidosis—strong-potency topical corticosteroids, systemic steroids, antimalarials, methotrexate, minocycline, thalidomide, tumor necrosis factor (TNF)-alfa inhibitors.[34]

Lupus panniculitis—antimalarials, steroids, thalidomide, dapsone, cyclosporine, intravenous Igs, and rituximab[37]).

Actinic keratosis—topical 5-fluorouracil (5-FU), diclofenac, imiquimod, and ingenol mebutate (IM), CO_2 laser, cryotherapy, curettage, and photodynamic therapy.[53]

Basal cell carcinoma and SCC—curettage and electrodesiccation, cryosurgery, surgical excision, and Mohs micrographic surgery, radiotherapy, topical and injectable therapy, and photodynamic therapy.[30]

REFERENCES

1. Pajaziti L, Hapçiu SR, Pajaziti A. Juvenile xanthogranuloma: A case report and review of the literature. BMC Res Notes. 2014;7(1):174.
2. Castrejón-Pérez AD, Welsh EC, Miranda I, Ocampo-Candiani J, Welsh O. Cutaneous mucormycosis. An Bras Dermatol. 2017;92(3):304-11.
3. Skiada A, Pavleas I, Drogari-Apiranthitou M. Epidemiology and diagnosis of mucormycosis: An update. J Fungi. 2020;6(4):265.
4. Hoffman GS, Kerr GS, Leavitt RY, Hallahan CW, Lebovics RS, Travis WD, et al. Wegener granulomatosis: an analysis of 158 patients. Ann Intern Med. 1992;116(6):488-98.
5. Geoloaica LG, Pătrașcu V, Ciurea RN. Necrobiotic xanthogranuloma: case report and literature review. Curr Health Sci J. 2021;47(1):126-31.
6. Sand M, Sand D, Thrandorf C, Paech V, Altmeyer P, Bechara FG. Cutaneous lesions of the nose. Head Face Med. 2010;6(1):7.
7. Chang P, Moreno-Coutiño G. Periocular dermatoses. Int J Womens Dermatol. 2017;3(4):206-18.
8. Narayanasetty NK, Pai VV, Athanikar SB. Annular lesions in dermatology. Indian J Dermatol. 2013;58(2):157.
9. Bonnetblanc JM, Bédane C. Erysipelas: recognition and management. Am J Clin Dermatol. 2003;4(3):157-63.
10. Brown BD, Watson KLH. (2021). Cellulitis. [online] In: StatPearls [Internet]. Treasure Island (FL): StatPearls Publishing. Available from https://www.ncbi.nlm.nih.gov/books/NBK549770/ [Last accessed November, 2022].
11. Sun KL, Chang JM. Special types of folliculitis which should be differentiated from acne. Dermatoendocrinol. 2017;9(1):e1356519.
12. Hjira N, Frikh R, Boudhas A, Baba N, Oukabli M, Boui M. Facial lupus vulgaris neglected for 50 years. J Dermatol Surg. 2018;22(1):33.
13. Can B. Disseminated lupus vulgaris: A case report. North Clin Istanb. 2014;1(1):53-6.
14. Bhandari J, Awais M, Robbins BA, Gupta V. (2021). Leprosy. [online] In: StatPearls [Internet]. Treasure Island (FL): StatPearls Publishing. Available from https://www.ncbi.nlm.nih.gov/books/NBK559307/ [Last accessed November, 2022].
15. Ferry T, Valour F, Karsenty J, Breton P, Gleizal A, Braun E, et al. Actinomycosis: Etiology, clinical features, diagnosis, treatment, and management. Infect Drug Resist. 2014;7:183-97.
16. Payne LC, Egan KM, Aziz N. Abrupt onset of ulcerative papules and nodules on the face and genitals. JAMA Dermatol. 2016;152(7):829.
17. Hernández JL, Buckley CJ. (2021). Mucormycosis. [online] In: StatPearls [Internet]. Treasure Island (FL): StatPearls Publishing. Available from https://www.ncbi.nlm.nih.gov/books/NBK544364/ [Last accessed November, 2022].
18. Das SK, Das C, Maity AB, Maiti PK, Hazra TK, Bandyopadhyay SN. Conidiobolomycosis: An unusual fungal disease—our experience. Indian J Otolaryngol Head Neck Surg. 2019;71(S3):1821-6.
19. Tahir C, Nggada H, Abubakar A, Garbati M, Yawe ET. Primary cutaneous aspergillosis in an immunocompetent patient. J Surg Tech Case Rep. 2011;3(2):94.
20. Liu X, Yang J, Ma W. Primary cutaneous aspergillosis caused by aspergillus fumigatus in an immunocompetent patient: A case report. Medicine (Baltimore). 2017;96(48):e8916.
21. Shetty S, Hegde U, Jagadish L, Shetty C. Pseudolymphoma versus lymphoma: An important diagnostic decision. J Oral Maxillofac Pathol. 2016;20(2):328.
22. Williams CT, Harrington DW. (2021). Jessner lymphocytic infiltration of the skin. [online] In: StatPearls [Internet]. Treasure Island (FL): StatPearls Publishing. Available from https://www.ncbi.nlm.nih.gov/books/NBK562281/ [Last accessed November, 2022].
23. Malveira MIB, Pascoal G, Gamonal SBL, Castañon MCMN. Folliculotropic mycosis fungoides: Challenging clinical, histopathological and immunohistochemical diagnosis. An Bras Dermatol. 2017;92(5 suppl 1):73-5.
24. Arun B, Coupland S, Parslew R. Cysts and erythematous plaques on the face and scalp. Clin Exp Dermatol. 2009;34(4):547-8.
25. Jezierska M, Stefanowicz J, Romanowicz G, Kosiak W, Lange M. Langerhans cell histiocytosis in children: a disease with many faces. Recent advances in pathogenesis, diagnostic examinations and treatment. Adv Dermatol Allergol. 2018;35(1):6-17.
26. Szczerkowska-Dobosz A, Kozicka D, Purzycka-Bogdan D, Biernat W, Stawczyk M, Nowicki R. Juvenile xanthogranuloma: A rare benign histiocytic disorder. Adv Dermatol Allergol. 2014;3:197-200.
27. Fasciani IA, Valente NYS, Luce MCA, Kakizaki P. Necrotic xanthogranuloma with disseminated annular lesions. An Bras Dermatol. 2020;95(1):117-9.
28. Greco MJ, Bhutta BS. (2021). Seborrheic keratosis. [online] In: StatPearls [Internet]. Treasure Island (FL): StatPearls Publishing. Available from https://www.ncbi.nlm.nih.gov/books/NBK545285/ [Last accessed November, 2022].
29. Reinehr CPH, Bakos RM. Actinic keratoses: Review of clinical, dermoscopic, and therapeutic aspects. An Bras Dermatol. 2019;94(6):637-57.
30. Halem M, Karimkhani C. Dermatology of the head and neck. Dent Clin North Am. 2012;56(4):771-90.
31. Dourmishev LA, Rusinova D, Botev I. Clinical variants, stages, and management of basal cell carcinoma. Indian Dermatol Online J. 2013;4(1):12.

32. Combalia A, Carrera C. Squamous cell carcinoma: An update on diagnosis and treatment. Dermatol Pract Concept. 2020;10(3):e2020066.
33. Cabral F, Lubbe LC, Nóbrega MM, Obadia DL, Souto R, Gripp AC. Morbihan disease: A therapeutic challenge. An Bras Dermatol. 2017;92(6):847-50.
34. Garg R, Aggarwal S, Kaur J, Kumar S. Isolated facial cutaneous sarcoidosis. J Nat Sci Biol Med. 2012;3(1):87.
35. Conforti C, Giuffrida R, de Barros MH, Resende FSS, Cerroni L, Zalaudek I. Dermoscopy of a single plaque on the face: An uncommon presentation of cutaneous sarcoidosis. Dermatol Pract Concept. 2018;8(3):174-6.
36. Oliveira CC, de Carvalho Ianhez PE, Marques SA, Marques MEA. Granuloma faciale: Clinical, morphological and immunohistochemical aspects in a series of 10 patients. An Bras Dermatol. 2016;91(6):803-7.
37. Zhao YK, Wang F, Chen WN, Xu R, Wang Z, Jiang YW, et al. Lupus panniculitis as an initial manifestation of systemic lupus erythematosus: A case report. Medicine (Baltimore). 2016;95(16):e3429.
38. Careta MF, Romiti R. Localized scleroderma: Clinical spectrum and therapeutic update. An Bras Dermatol. 2015;90(1):62-73.
39. Bota M, Popa G, Blag C, Tataru A. Infantile hemangioma: A brief review. Clujul Med. 2015;88(1):23.
40. Lara-Martinez H, Weinberg M, Baratam P, Horn J, Ward K, Styler M. Angiosarcoma of the face: A case study and literature review of local and metastatic angiosarcoma. Case Rep Oncol Med. 2021;2021:8823585.
41. Xiong M, Charifa A, Chen CSJ. (2020). Lentigo maligna melanoma. [online] In: StatPearls [Internet]. Treasure Island (FL): StatPearls Publishing. Available from https://www.ncbi.nlm.nih.gov/books/NBK482163/ [Last accessed November, 2022].
42. Kim DW, Lee G, Lam MB, Harris EJ, Lam AC, Thomas T, et al. Microcystic adnexal carcinoma of the face treated with definitive chemoradiation: A case report and review of the literature. Adv Radiat Oncol. 2020;5(2):301.
43. Gordon S, Fischer C, Martin A, Rosman IS, Council ML. Microcystic adnexal carcinoma: A review of the literature. Dermatol Surg. 2017;43(8):1012-6.
44. Blake SC, Daniel BS. Cutaneous lupus erythematosus: A review of the literature. Int J Womens Dermatol. 2019;5(5):320.
45. Mollaeian A, Roudsari H, Talebi E. Sweet's syndrome: A classical presentation of a rare disease. J Investig Med High Impact Case Rep. 2019;7:2324709619895164.
46. Hegde SK, Panchagavi A, Narayanasetty NK. Exclusive facial actinic porokeratosis. Indian Dermatol Online J. 2018;9(6):469.
47. Riad H, Mansour K, Sada HA, Shaika SA, Ansari HA, Mohannadi HA. Disseminated superficial actinic porokeratosis on the face treated with imiquimod 5% cream. Case Rep Dermatol. 2013;5(3):283.
48. Ankad BS, Adya KA, Gaikwad SS, Inamadar AC, Manjula R. Lupus vulgaris in darker skin: Dermoscopic and histopathologic incongruity. Indian Dermatol Online J. 2020;11(6):948.
49. Jardim MML, Uchiyama J, Kakizaki P, Valente NYS. Dermoscopy of granuloma faciale: A description of a new finding. An Bras Dermatol. 2018;93:587-9.
50. Geller S, Rishpon A, Myskowski PL. Dermoscopy in folliculotropic mycosis fungoides—a possible mimicker of follicle-based inflammatory and infectious disorders. J Am Acad Dermatol. 2019;81(3):e75-6.
51. de Oliveira TE, Tarlé RG, de Forville Mesquita LA. Dermoscopy in the diagnosis of juvenile xanthogranuloma. An Bras Dermatol. 2018;93(1):138-40.
52. Wollina U. Recent advances in managing and understanding seborrheic keratosis. F1000Res. 2019;8:F1000 Faculty Rev-1520.
53. Zalaudek I, Piana S, Moscarella E, Longo C, Zendri E, Castagnetti F, et al. Morphologic grading and treatment of facial actinic keratosis. Clin Dermatol. 2014;32(1):80-7.
54. Trigoni A, Lazaridou E, Apalla Z, Vakirlis E, Chrysomallis F, Varytimiadis D, et al. Dermoscopic features in the diagnosis of different types of basal cell carcinoma: A prospective analysis. Hippokratia. 2012;16(1):29.
55. Kato J, Horimoto K, Sato S, Minowa T, Uhara H. Dermoscopy of melanoma and non-melanoma skin cancers. Front Med (Lausanne). 2019;6:180.
56. Cengiz FP, Emiroglu N, Ozkaya DB, Su O, Onsun N. Dermoscopic features of small, medium, and large-sized congenital melanocytic nevi. Ann Dermatol. 2017;29(1):26.
57. Iznardo H, Garcia-Melendo C, Yélamos O. Lentigo maligna: Clinical presentation and appropriate management. Clin Cosmet Investig Dermatol. 2020;13:837-55.
58. Lallas A, Argenziano G, Apalla Z, Gourhant JY, Zaballos P, Di Lernia V, et al. Dermoscopic patterns of common facial inflammatory skin diseases. J Eur Acad Dermatol Venereol. 2014;28(5):609-14.
59. Günaştı S, Aksungur VL. Granulomatous disorders. Clin Dermatol. 2014;32(1):47-65.
60. Sullivan T, de Barra E. Diagnosis and management of cellulitis. Clin Med (Lond). 2018;18(2):160-3.
61. Patterson TF, Thompson GR, Denning DW, Fishman JA, Hadley S, Herbrecht R, et al. Practice guidelines for the diagnosis and management of aspergillosis: 2016 update by the Infectious Diseases Society of America. Clin Infect Dis. 2016;63(4):e1-60.
62. Garza-Tovar TF, Sacriste-Hernández MI, Juárez-Durán ER, Arenas R. An overview of the treatment of cutaneous leishmaniasis. Fac Rev. 2020;9:28.
63. Collie JS, Harper CD, Fillman EP. (2021). Juvenile xanthogranuloma. [online] In: StatPearls [Internet]. Treasure Island (FL): StatPearls Publishing. Available from https://www.ncbi.nlm.nih.gov/books/NBK526103/ [Last accessed November, 2022].

18

A Female with Chronic and Recurrent Vaginal Discharge

Neela M Patel, Khushbu R Modi

INTRODUCTION

"Vaginal discharge" (VD) or "leukorrhea" is the most common health issue for women with reproductive age group, and the term is used traditionally by patients for presenting any genital discomfort with the symptoms of VD, odor, pruritus, and/or discomfort. The complaint must be verified to differentiate physiological discharge from pathological discharge and to determine diagnosis and treatment by physical and laboratory examination. Untreated vaginitis can cause physical, social, and psychological complications.

In premenopausal women, the vagina is rich in glycogen which acts as a substrate for Doderlein's bacilli to glucose into lactic acid. This creates an acidic vaginal environment (pH 4–4.5) which helps in maintaining normal vaginal flora and inhibit growth of pathogenic organisms. The vagina and cervix are susceptible to various pathogens depending on the type of epithelium. *Candida* species and *Trichomonas vaginalis* (TV) can cause infection at squamous epithelium of vagina and ectocervix.

CHRONIC AND RECURRENT VAGINAL DISCHARGE

Chronic VD is defined as women having continuous symptoms despite conventional treatment. Recurrent VD is defined as a woman who is asymptomatic after treatment but subsequently there is recurrence of symptoms, usually three or more episodes within a year.[1]

If it remains untreated for a long period of time, complications like increased risk of sexually transmitted infection (STI) and human immunodeficiency virus (HIV) (associated subsequent infertility), adverse outcomes of pregnancy, miscarriage, preterm delivery, low-birth-weight infants and choriamnionitis can occur, in turn causing a burden on healthcare system.

Chronic and recurrent VD is very frustrating for women, impacting significantly on their self-esteem, sexual relationships, and making them feel ashamed.

There are different causes of chronic and recurrent discharge which are as given here:
- Physiological
- *Pathological*:
  - Infective **(Table 1)**
  - Noninfective **(Table 2)**
- Others **(Box 1)**

Identifying the source of VD is challenging, as it is a distressing and subjective symptom. Though there are multitude of causes for chronic and recurrent VD, majority of them are caused by infection, while less common causes include vaginal atrophy/atrophic vaginitis, cervicitis, foreign body, irritants and allergens, etc. Hence only infective etiology is elaborated in this chapter.

Physiological Vaginal Discharge

The most common cause of VD in reproductive age group is physiological,[2] which tends to change with the menstrual cycle. It increases during high estrogen states such as ovulation, the luteal phase, puberty, pregnancy, with estrogen-based therapies such as combined hormonal contraception as well as hormone replacement therapies and also increased during sexual arousal. Physiological discharge is clear with a stretchable consistency, nonoffensive at the time around ovulation, then may be thicker and slightly yellow during the luteal phase. pH of the physiological

Table 1: Infective causes.[3-6]

	Recurrent BV	Recurrent CVV	Recurrent TV
Definition	*Recurrent BV*: Defined as three or more episodes in 12 months	*Recurrent CVV*: Four or more symptomatic episodes occur in 1 year or at least three episodes unrelated to antibiotic therapy occur within 1 year	*Recurrent TV*: Infection due to reinfections from untreated sexual partners Persistent infection are concerning for treatment failure due to: • Nitroimidazole resistance • Insufficient long absorption • Lack of adherence • Inadequate treatment
Estimated recurrence rate	50%	5%	12.5–18.5%

Microorganisms responsible	*Gardnerella vaginalis, Alysicarpus vaginalis, Mobiluncus* species, *Bacteroides* species, *Prevotelle* species, *Clostridiales* species, *Leptotrichia, Sneathia* species, *Lactobacillus, Peptostreptococcus, Fusobacterium*	• Resistance of non-*Candida albicans* species to antifungal agents
		• *C. albicans*
		• Non-albicans *Candida* species
		  ○ *Candida tropicalis*
		  ○ *Candida krusei*
		  ○ *Candida parapsolis*
		  ○ *Candida glabrata*
			TV

(BV: bacterial vaginosis; CVV: candidal vulvovaginitis; TV: *Trichomonas vaginalis*)

Table 2: Noninfective causes.[7-9]

	Atrophic vulvovaginitis (genitourinary syndrome of menopause)	DIV	GVHD
Characteristics	Gradual thinning and drying of vaginal walls, mostly occurs in postmenopausal women with less estrogen levels	• It is a diagnosis of exclusion, chronic rare condition in which patient have discharge for more than a year with mean duration of symptoms of 15–31 months • It occurs in 8% women with low-estrogen levels, during breastfeeding or postmenopausal women • Probable etiopathologies are: ○ Bacterial overgrowth, immune-mediated reaction, toxin-induced reaction to *Staphylococcus aureus*	Uncommon cause of chronic vaginal discharge, usually occurs in 25–50% female having allogenic blood transfusion or transplant patients

(DIV: desquamative inflammatory vaginitis; GVHD: graft-versus-host disease)

discharge is between 3.8 and 4.5. Normal healthy discharge should not be associated with itching, redness, or odor. Sometime profuse physiological VD may produce vaginal irritation.

Pathological Vaginal Discharge

Pathological vaginal discharge can be further classified into (1) infective and (2) noninfective.

Chronic infective discharge can be of (1) vaginal origin or (2) cervical origin. Chronic and recurrent vaginal and cervical discharge are due to multiple reasons, most common ones are candidal vulvovaginitis (CVV), bacterial vaginosis (BV), TV, while less common causes are *Neisseria gonorrhea* and *Chlamydia trachomatis*.

Others

Apart from the above listed, there are multiple other causes of chronic and recurrent VD.

APPROACH IN A PATIENT OF CHRONIC AND RECURRENT VAGINAL DISCHARGE

Patients of VD should be evaluated initially by taking history, doing physical examination, microscopy, and cervical

Box 1: Other causes of vaginal discharge.

- *Foreign body* (causes—retained tampon, pessary or condom—mechanical irritation) is often associated with offensive, copious, purulent, sometime blood stained VD, intermittent bleeding, and/or troublesome odor due to inflammation and secondary infection[10]
- *Chemical* (causes—douches, latex condoms, deodorants—chemical irritation, contact dermatitis, or allergy)—soreness is pronounced than discharge[11]
- *Excretions* (causes—contamination with urine or feces—secondary vaginitis) lead to offensive discharge with pruritus[11]
- *Vaginal warts:* Skin/pink colored ranging from smooth flattened papules to verrucous, papilliform lesions. Patients with extensive vaginal warts can present with VD, pruritus, bleeding, burning, tenderness, and pain
- *Presence of granulation tissue or infection at surgical site* can cause VD or bleeding[12]
- *Neoplasia* (fibroid polyps or genital malignancy—necrotic or inflammatory changes associated with malignancy) in the upper or lower genital tract can result in Serosanguinous and often offensive VD, with more common complaint of spotting[12]
- *Disorders like pemphigus, drug reactions* can present with recurrent purulent or Serosanguinous discharge
- *Erosive vulvovaginitis:* The presence of multifocal rounded macular erythematous lesions with purulent discharge and tenderness

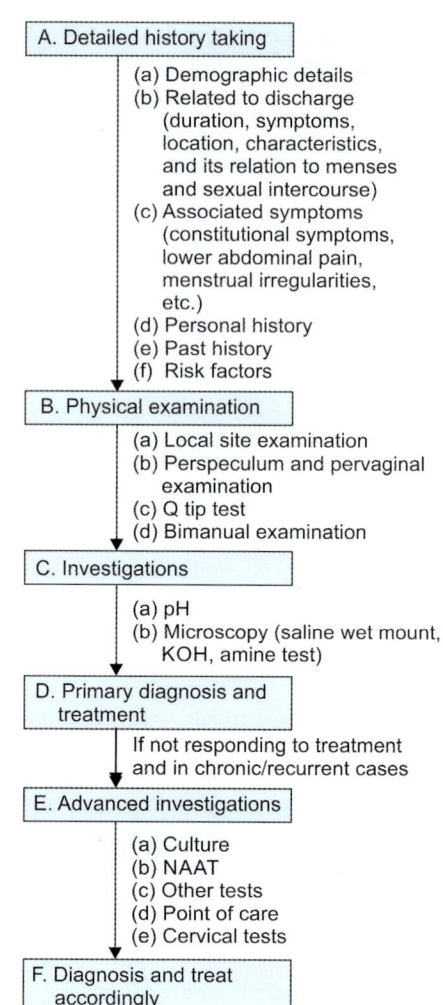

FLOWCHART 1: Basic approach in a patient of vaginal discharge.
(KOH: potassium hydroxide; NAAT: nucleic acid amplification test)

tests. Women whose initial evaluation confirms a diagnosis received targeted treatment and those who remain without a diagnosis or whose symptoms recur, go through a more detailed evaluation process.

Detailed History Taking

- *Demographic details*: Related to age, socioeconomic and marital status, education, occupation, etc., helps us in narrowing the diagnosis and easy management of the patients. Age gives us an idea about the etiology of discharge and differentiating physiological from pathological discharge. Early age of marriage and early age of sexual activity makes cervical epithelium more susceptible to ascending infections, in turn increasing the risk of STIs. The chances of recurrence, chronicity, and complications like pelvic inflammatory disease (PID), related to reproductive system are increased in lower socioeconomic status due to lower literacy rate, poor sanitation, nutrition and hygiene practices, ignorance, use of over the counter medications, etc. Similarly, in women with higher economic status the use of spermicides, fancy hygiene products, lubricants, douching, shaving practices, contraceptives, sprays, soaps, detergents increases the chances of chronicity, allergic and irritant dermatitis.
- *Characteristics of discharge* **(Tables 3 and 4)**: The symptoms and characteristics of discharge can vary from its classical presentation due to a variety of reasons. Specific history of relation to menses and sexual intercourse gives us a general idea about the etiology. Symptoms that develop soon after sexual exposure are suggestive of STI.
- *Associated symptoms* **(Table 5)**: Provides guide in approaching patient of discharge. Associated systemic symptoms like constitutional symptoms, pelvic pain or tenderness, and menstrual irregularities help in differentiating between vaginal and cervical infections. Dysuria and dyspareunia are suggestive of inflammatory disorders such as allergy, infection, or vulvovaginal atrophy.

Table 3: Symptoms of infective discharge.[3,4,6,13]

	Recurrent CVV	Recurrent BV	Recurrent TV
Symptoms	Pruritus, vaginal discharge, soreness, external dysuria, vulvar edema, and superficial dyspareunia	• Vaginal discharge • History of recurrence + • 50% cases are asymptomatic	• Vaginal discharge • Pruritus • Dyspareunia • Dysuria • 50–75% cases are asymptomatic
Relation with menses	Premenses	Postmenses	Postmenses
Relation with sexual intercourse	Aggravation of pruritus	Aggravation of fishy odor	–

(BV: bacterial vaginosis; CVV: candidal vulvovaginitis; TV: *Trichomonas vaginalis*)

Table 4: Symptoms of noninfective discharge.[7-9]

	Atrophic vulvovaginitis (genitourinary syndrome of menopause)	Desquamative inflammatory vaginitis	Graft-versus-host disease
Symptoms	Vaginal dryness, itching, irritation, dyspareunia, burning micturition	Symptoms like *Trichomonas vaginalis*, itching, burning, redness, dyspareunia, bleeds on touch	Itching, dryness, dyspareunia, burning with irritation, contact bleeding

Table 5: Associated symptoms.

Symptoms	Condition
Dysuria	• External dysuria (vulvovaginal irritation results in burning due to micturition): *Candida*, herpes • *Internal dysuria (felt inside the body)*: UTI, gonorrhea, chlamydia
Dyspareunia	Due to inflammatory reaction (*Candida, Trichomonas, Chlamydia trachomatis, Neisseria gonorrhea*)
Pruritus	• Intensely pruritic—*Candida* • Less pruritic—*Trichomonas* • Rarely pruritic—bacterial vaginosis • Allergic dermatoses • Persistent complaint of pruritus in a localized area is suggestive of neoplasia or malignancy
Lower abdominal pain, pelvic pain, pelvic tenderness, fever, tenesmus[14]	• Red flag signs of PID • Inflammatory causes of vaginitis or nonvaginal sources like vulvodynia and pelvic floor myofascial pain
Dysuria, menstrual irregularities, bleeding after intercourse[15]	Cervicitis, erosive causes of vaginitis or a uterine source
Burning, irritation, or other discomfort	Infective conditions like candidal vulvovaginitis and noninfective conditions like vulvodynia

(PID: pelvic inflammatory disease; UTI: urinary tract infection)

- *Personal history* (**Box 2**)
- *Past history*: Similar complaints and history of treatment taken for the same, symptoms in partner, history of urinary tract infection
- *Risk factors*: The risk factors to be kept in mind are risky sexual behavior, history of immunocompromised status, prolonged use of hormonal contraceptives, immunosuppressive drugs, and antibiotics as well as inadequate treatment.[16]

Physical Examination

The physical examination assesses (1) the degree of vulvovaginal inflammation, (2) characteristics of the VD, and (3) presence of lesions or foreign bodies.

- *Cutaneous examination of local sites*: Look for discharge, swelling, erythema, excoriation marks, pustules, papules, satellite lesions, genital ulcers, growth/wart, mass, etc., at following sites. Sites to be examined:

- Pubis, labia majora and minora, urethral meatus, vaginal opening, and perianal skin
- *Other sites*: Oral mucosa, lips, trunk, palms, and soles
- Abdomen can be examined for lymph node, guarding, tenderness, and abdominal mass
- *Perspeculum and pervaginal examination*: Done after taking patient's consent with patient in dorsal supine lithotomy position after explaining the procedure to the patient. It is performed to evaluate the vagina and cervix for:
  - VD, characteristics and signs of which can suggest the type of infection (**Tables 6 and 7**).
  - Foreign body, growth/warts, malignancy, necrotic/inflammatory changes, signs of allergic and irritant dermatitis

> **Box 2: Personal history.**
>
> - *Hygiene practices*: History of douching, shaving, use of hair removal creams, vaginal washes, etc., can cause mechanical, chemical, or allergic irritation leading to contact dermatitis
> - *Sexual history*:
>   - Different modes of sexual practices, number of partners, sex of the patient's partner, recent change in partner, complaints in partner, age of starting sexual activity, and sexual behavior have a role to play in aggravating the symptoms
>   - Penovaginal sex, vaginal sex after anal sex, females who have sex with females, and females who have sex with both females and males, are at increased risk of BV
>   - Sexual activity in extremes of age like early age and postmenopausal women increases chances of STI
> - *Medication history*:
>   - Antibiotics predispose to CVV by eliminating protective bacterial flora in the vagina, i.e., *Lactobacillus*, thus allowing overgrowth of *Candida*
>   - Use of OCP and barrier contraceptives including IUD's increases both physiological and pathological discharge
>   - Use of OTC's change the clinical presentation, altering diagnosis
>   - Use of lubricants and oils can cause allergic and irritant dermatitis
> - *Medical history*: Medical conditions can act as a risk factor for chronic/recurrent VD like:
>   - *Diabetes mellitus*: CVV
>   - *HIV*: Vaginal infections
>   - *Graft-versus-host disease*: Vaginal irritation, discharge, ulceration, and stenosis
>   - *Steven–Johnson syndrome/toxic epidermal necrolysis*: Vulvovaginal sequelae
>   - *Herpes simplex virus and Behçet syndrome*: Vulvovaginal ulcers
> - *Surgical history*: Recent transvaginal surgery, repair of perineal lacerations after childbirth, tubectomy, insertion of IUD, etc. Vaginal symptoms may be related to foreign body, bacterial infection, granulation tissue, or vaginal fistula. Vaginal fistula can develop after surgery like hysterectomy and can present with vaginal discharge
>
> (BV: bacterial vaginosis; CVV: candidal vulvovaginitis; HIV: human immunodeficiency virus; IUD: intrauterine device; OCP: oral contraceptive pills; OTC: over-the-counter; STI; sexually transmitted infection)

Table 6: Infective: Characteristics and signs of discharge (Fig. 1).

	Recurrent CVV	**Recurrent BV**	**Recurrent TV**
Amount	Scanty to moderate	Moderate to profuse	Profuse
Consistency	• Cheesy or curdy (cottage cheese like) • Watery to homogenous thick	Mucoid, thin	Thick, frothy
Color	White	Grayish white	Yellow greenish
Odor	No offensive smell	Fishy (worse at midcycle, after intercourse)	Foul smelling
Signs	*Cervix uteri*: Normal	Discharge coating the vagina	• Blisters developing in one-third cases • *Strawberry cervix*: Punctuate hemorrhagic lesions
Cutaneous examination of vulva	Erythema, edema or fissures, excoriation, satellite lesions	Normal, excoriation marks can be seen	Erythema, edema, or fissures

(BV: bacterial vaginosis; CVV: candidal vulvovaginitis; TV: *Trichomonas vaginalis*)

Erythematous, friable cervix (cervical inflammation), and mucopurulent discharge with a normal vagina and associated symptoms of cervicitis are suggestive of cervicitis rather than vaginitis.
- *Q tip test*: A cotton swab is applied with pressure at the labia or introitus, if patient complains of pain this is suggestive of candidiasis.[17]
- *Bimanual examination*: It is performed by inserting two fingers into vagina with the other hand over lower part of belly. It helps in assessing the pelvic/cervical motion tenderness in PID or in malignancy.

Symptoms can lead the approach, but alone cannot differentiate between the causes of discharge, office-based test, or laboratory testing must be used with the history and physical examination findings to make the diagnosis in patients of chronic and recurrent VD.

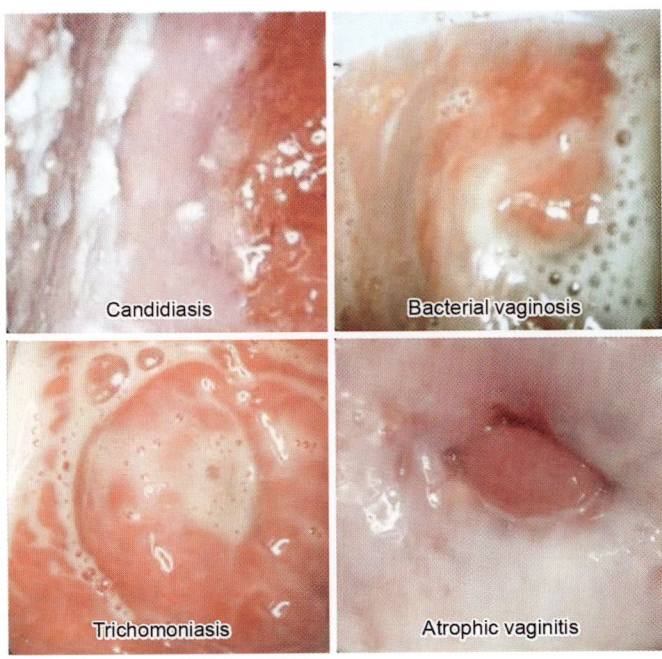

FIG. 1: Infective causes of vaginal discharge
Courtesy: Pillowtalk with Doc Mitch—Dr Michelle Dado; Philippines.

Investigations (Table 8)

Whenever required routine investigations like complete blood count, liver function tests, renal function tests, urine routine microscopy, random blood sugar and in cases of suspected STI's rapid plasma reagin (RPR), HIV, human papillomavirus (HPV), hepatitis B surface antigen (HBsAg), and Pap smear should be considered.

- *pH*: Vaginal pH checking is an outpatient department (OPD)-based procedure and is used for screening purpose, as it has high sensitivity and low specificity. pH strip is applied for few seconds to the middle one-third of vaginal side wall to avoid contamination by blood, semen, or cervical mucus in the posterior fornix. Alternatively, dry swab can be used instead of pH paper strip. For diagnosis of BV, trichomoniasis, or candidiasis, pH measurement is less useful at the extremes of age due to altered pH in these age groups. Vaginal pH may be altered by contamination with lubricating gels, semen, blood, douches, intravaginal medications, and amniotic fluid. ColorpHast pH test strips are commercially available paper strips. The FemExam TestCard pH and amine tests are also available as card tests that contains pH indicators as well as visual evaluation system for amines.[18]
- *Microscopy* **(Flowchart 2)**: Three samples of patient's VD were obtained with a cotton swab and evaluated under the microscope by saline mount, 10% potassium hydroxide (KOH), and amine test.[15,19]

Additional swab can be taken for gram staining of cervical discharge.
- *Saline wet mount*: Sample mixed with one to two drops of normal saline at room temperature on a glass slide, cover slips are then placed on the slides. Primary goal of the examination is to look for *Trichomonas*, clue cells, and increased no. of polymorphonuclear neutrophils (PMNs). Sample should be examined within 10–20 minutes to reduce the possibility related to loss of motility of *Trichomonas*.
- *10% KOH*: Identifying hyphae and budding yeast for diagnosis of candidiasis becomes easier with addition of 10% KOH, as it destroys cellular elements.

Table 7: Noninfective: Characteristics and signs of discharge.

	Atrophic vulvovaginitis (genitourinary syndrome of menopause)	Desquamative inflammatory vaginitis	Graft-versus-host disease
Amount	Scanty discharge	Profuse	–
Color	White	Yellow green	White
Signs	Normal/atrophy of vulva and vagina	• Purulent yellowish–green discharge, erythema, vaginal rash (petechial or ecchymotic) • Excoriation marks on vulva and vestibule in severe cases	Purulent discharge, vulvovaginal atrophy, vulval synechiae, vaginal stenosis

Table 8: Microscopic findings in infective vaginal discharge.

	CVV	BV	TV
pH test of the vaginal fluid/discharge from vaginal walls	4–4.5	>4.7	>4.5; Often exceeds 6
Sample collection (preferably from site)	Lateral vaginal wall	Posterior fornix	Posterior fornix
Microscopy First vaginal swab • Wet mount	Negative	*Clue cells:* >20% of the total epithelial cells (Normal vaginal cells; Clue cells: Vaginal cells with bacteria stuck to them; Vaginal cell, Nucleus, Bacteria)	*Trichomonas* (flagellates with pear-shaped morphology and whip-like processes) — 4 free flagelets anteriorly, Blepharoplast (mass or granules), Single nucleus, Cytostome, Vacuole with bacteria rarely RBC, Axostyle, 1 Flagellum attached by undulating membrane, 15 μm — *Trichomonas vaginalis*
• 10% KOH	Yeast cells and mycelia (Blastospores, Chlamydospore, Pseudohyphae — *Candida albicans*)	Negative	Negative
Whiff test	Negative	Positive	Negative
Second vaginal swab • Gram stain	–	*Nugent score:* Score > 7 indicates BV	–

(BV: bacterial vaginosis; CVV: candidal vulvovaginitis; KOH: potassium hydroxide; TV: *Trichomonas vaginalis*)

- *Amine test*: Smelling (whiffing) the slide immediately after applying KOH helps in detecting fishy (amine) odor of BV.
- *Gram stain*: Slide is prepared from discharge and gram stained and looked for gram-positive and-negative bacterial score for BV.

Nugent score.[20]

Bacterial morphology	0	1+	2+	3+	4+
Lactobacilli type (gram positive)	4	3	2	1	0
Gardnerella type (gram variable coccobacilli)	0	1	2	3	4
Mobiluncus type (gram negative)	0	1	2	3	4

Calculation of score:	Score:
0/oil immersion field: 0	0–3: Normal
<1/oil immersion field: 1+	4–6: Intermediate (test to be repeated later)
1–5/oil immersion field: 2+	
6–30/oil immersion field: 3+	7–10: Bacterial vaginosis
>30/oil immersion field: 4+	

Microscopy is negative/not available: If microscopy is negative but *Candida* is suspected and in strongly suspected cases of BV or trichomoniasis, additional testing by culture or nucleic acid amplification test (NAAT) is important.

If microscopy is not available, rapid antigen, NAAT, and polymerase chain reaction (PCR) are used for differentiating and confirming clinical diagnosis of CVV, BV, and TV.

Advanced Investigations for Chronic and Recurrent Vaginal Discharge

- *Culture*: Infective vaginal discharge **(Table 9)**. For recurrent TV and recurrent CVV, culture is gold standard. As BV represents a polymicrobial infection, culture is not used for the diagnosis. But, if microscopy is negative in recurrently symptomatic women with normal pH of discharge, then culture of discharge should be done.

  Microscopy requires adequate trained person and is subjective. Recently available test like PCR is objective in nature.
- *NAAT:* It should be conducted after 3 weeks of treatment completion because of possible detection of residual nucleic acid.[23]
  - *PCR*: To identify and amplify specific DNA fragments. Probes and primer are two types of single stranded, oligonucleotides used in various types of PCR. PCR primer method has proven to be the most accurate diagnostic method for TV, BV, and CVV.
  - *DNA probe*: This is an objective test developed to detect directly the presence of *Candida, Trichomonas,* and *Gardnerella*. DNA probe test is relatively insensitive to diagnose BV as *Gardnerella vaginitis* is present in vagina as normal flora also. Various kits are available commercially that detects *Gardnerella, Trichomonas,* and *Candida* at the same time. For example: The Affirm VPIII (45 minutes).[24]
- *Other tests*:
  - Elevated levels of interleukin (IL)-6, IL-8, ferritin, and granulocyte colony-stimulating factor are some of the secondary predictors that confirm the role of intrauterine infection.[25]
  - In recurrent and persistent VD drug sensitivity testing is indicated.
  - Male partner should also be investigated as in the form of culture from the prepuce, urine routine microscopy, semen culture, and blood sugar.
- *Point of care test*:[18]
  - Proline iminopeptidase (PIP) activity test card (proline aminopeptidase test card)
  - Trimethylamine and high pH
  - *BV blue test*: It detects elevated levels of sialidase in vaginal fluid, which is produced by pathogens that cause BV. It is an office-based objective test that provides result in <1 minute.[26]
  - *Trichomonas* rapid test[27]
  - *Vulvovaginal candidiasis (VVC)*: Savvy check vaginal yeast assay[28]

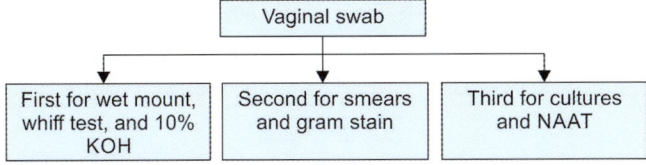

FLOWCHART 2: Vaginal swabs for investigations.
(KOH: potassium hydroxide; NAAT: nucleic acid amplification test)

Advantages of point of care test: Less than 30 minutes result, require minimal training, can be done at any peripheral

Table 9: Culture: Infective vaginal discharge.			
	CVV[21]	**BV**	**TV**[22]
Culture	• SDA • Nickerson's or Microstix-*Candida* • Chromogenic agar *Advantages of chromogenic agar*: It helps in differentiation of different *Candida* species and identification of polyfungal populations *Disadvantage of chromogenic agar*: Costly	BV not cultured as they are normal commensals	Vaginal swab culture *Culture media*: • Inoculate inPouch at bedside/ Amies transport medium • Kupferberg • Diamonds TV medium

(BV: bacterial vaginosis; CVV: candidal vulvovaginitis; SDA: sabourad's dextrose agar; TV: *Trichomonas vaginalis*)

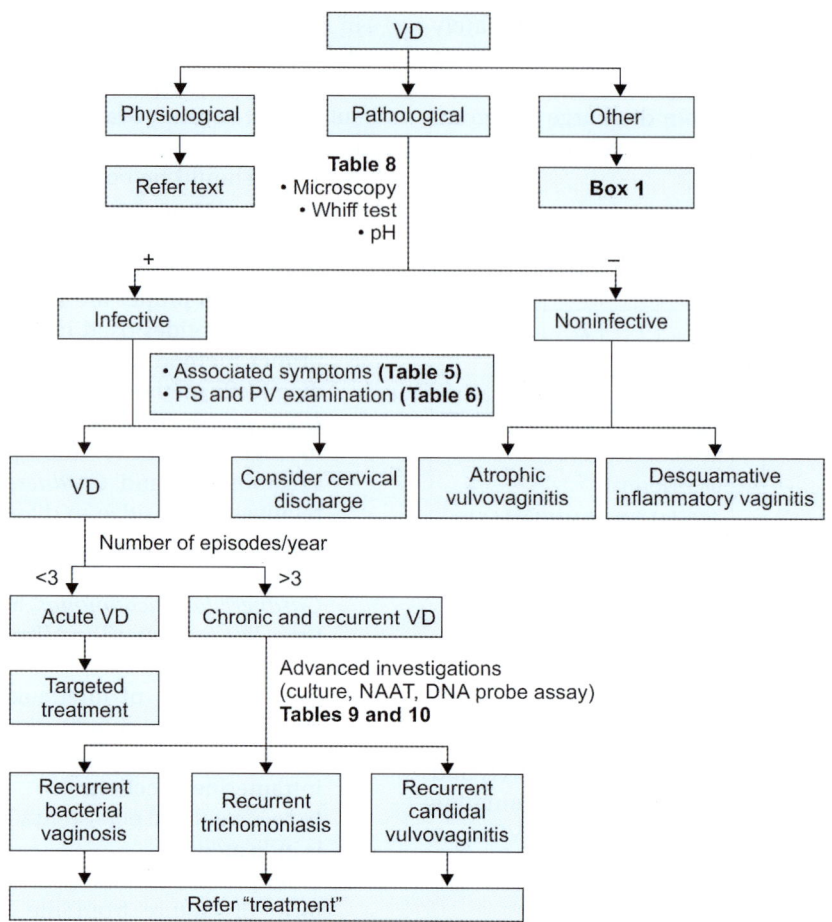

FLOWCHART 3: A practical approach in a female with chronic and recurrent vaginal discharge (VD).

Table 10: Characteristics of detection assays: Sensitivity%/specificity%.[23]				
Organism	*Microscopy (wet mount)*	*Culture*	*Antigen detection*	*DNA probe assay*
Candidiasis	35–45%/99%	67%/66%	61–81%/97%	80%/98%
Trichomoniasis	38–82%/100%	98%/100%	86%/100%	88–91%/100%
Bacterial vaginosis	81%/94%	89%/93%	93%/93%	94%/81%

clinic, whole blood-based procedure (no centrifuge/rotator), ingredients can be kept at room temperature, battery dependent

- *Cervical test*: An additional swab taken in suspected cases of cervicitis/cervical discharge is for culture and NAAT.

Diagnostic Criteria

The diagnostic criteria for infective and noninfective vaginitis are given in **Table 11**.

Treatment

Patients with symptoms and history of chronic and recurrent VD: (1) if not responding to empirical treatment, (2) have a risk for STI's, or (3) have symptoms indicative of upper genital tract infection should be investigate thoroughly and treat accordingly.

- *Infective conditions*: As basic management of VD is very well known, we comprise the treatment protocol for chronic and recurrent VD.
- *BV*:[26] For women who have recurrence, different recommended treatment regimens can be considered.
  ○ Retreatment with the same recommended regimen is an acceptable approach for treating persistent or recurrent BV after the first occurrence.
  ○ For women with multiple recurrences after completion of a recommended regimen, either 0.75% metronidazole gel or 750 mg metronidazole vaginal suppository twice weekly for >3 months.

Table 11: Diagnostic criteria.	
	Diagnostic criteria
CVV[29]	• Major criteria (≥5) • Discharge, dyspareunia, positive vaginal swab (at present or past), previous response to antifungal medication, exacerbation with antibiotics, cyclicity, swelling, soreness

BV[30,31]	• *Amsel's criteria:*
	  ○ Thin, white, homogenous discharge
	  ○ Clue cells on microscopy of wet mount
	  ○ pH of vaginal fluid >4.5
	  ○ Release of a fishy odor on adding 10% KOH
	(At least three of the four criteria are present for the diagnosis to be confirmed)
	In *Hay/Isoncriteria* gram-stained vaginal smear is evaluated as follows:
	• *Grade 0*: No bacteria present
	• *Grade 1 (normal)*: Lactobacillus morphotypes predominates
	• *Grade 2 (intermediate)*: Mixed flora with some Lactobacilli present, but *Gardnerella* or *Mobiluncus* morphotypes also present
	• *Grade 3 (bacterial vaginosis)*: Predominantly *Gardnerella* and/or *Mobiluncus* morphotypes. Few or absent Lactobacilli
	• Grade 4 gram-positive cocci predominate

Desquamative inflammatory vaginitis[32]	• At least one symptom (vaginal discharge, dysparunia, pruritus, pain, irritation, or burning) • Evidence of vulvovaginal inflammation • Vaginal pH > 6 • Leukorrhea ± parabasal cells on microscopy
Atrophic vulvovaginitis[24]	• pH > 4.6 • VMI—to assess the relative proportion of parabasal, intermediate, and superficial vaginal epithelial cell types. <5% superficial cells in postmenopausal women points would be suggestive of atrophic vulvovaginitis

(BV: bacterial vaginosis; CVV: candidal vulvovaginitis; KOH: potassium hydroxide; VMI: vaginal maturation index)

- ○ *Other treatment options are*:
  - Oral nitroimidazole (metronidazole or tinidazole 500 mg two times/day for 7 days), followed by intravaginal boric acid 600 mg daily for 21 days, and suppressive 0.75% metronidazole gel twice weekly for 4–6 months.
  - Monthly oral metronidazole 2 g administered with fluconazole 150 mg—as suppressive therapy; this regimen reduced the BV incidence and promoted colonization with normal vaginal microbiota.
  - A dendrimer-based microbicide 1% vaginal gel (astodrimer)—favorable results in prolonging the time to BV recurrence.
  - Lactobacillus crispatus CTV-05 (Lactin-05)-vaginal application for four consecutive days for week 1 then followed by twice daily dose for week 10 - decrease incidence of BV recurrence.
- *Vulvovaginal candidiasis*[28]

Treatment for Candida albicans:
- Most episodes of recurrent VVC caused by *C. albicans* respond well to basic first-line oral or topical azole therapy.

- To maintain clinical and mycological control, a longer duration of initial therapy is needed. Few other options are:
  - ○ *Induction therapy*: Topical azole therapy for 7–14 days or a 100 mg, 150 mg, or 200 mg oral dose of fluconazole every third day for a total of three doses (days 1, 4, and 7)
  - ○ *Maintenance therapy*: Oral fluconazole (i.e., a 100 mg, 150 mg, or 200 mg dose) weekly for 6 months. If this regimen is not feasible, use topical treatments intermittently.

Treatment for non-albicans Candida:
- The optimal treatment of non-albicans *Candida* VVC remains unknown.
- *Options available*:
  - ○ A longer duration of therapy (7–14 days) with a non-fluconazole azole regimen (oral or topical)
  - ○ 600 mg of boric acid in a gelatin capsule administered vaginally once daily for 3 weeks.
- *TV:*[27]
  - ○ *For recurrent infection*:
    - If re-exposed to an untreated partner and/or If treatment failure occurs-metronidazole 500 mg 2 times/day for 7 days.

- If no re-exposure—metronidazole or tinidazole 2 g once daily for 7 days.
  ○ For persistent infection: (Drug resistance should be evaluated)
    - Treatment for infections demonstrating in vitro resistance-metronidazole or tinidazole 2 g daily for 7 days.
    - If a patient has treatment failure after the 7-day regimen of high-dose oral metronidazole or tinidazole, two additional treatment options are:
      ▪ High-dose oral tinidazole 2 g daily plus intravaginal tinidazole 500 mg two times/day for 14 days
      ▪ High-dose oral tinidazole (1 g three times/day) plus intravaginal paromomycin (4 g of 6.25% intravaginal paromomycin cream at night) for 14 days
  ○ Intravaginal boric acid might be effective but has not been systemically evaluated.

Treatment in pregnancy:
- *BV and TV*: Oral therapy has not been reported to be superior to topical therapy for treating symptomatic BV and TV in effecting cure or preventing adverse outcomes of pregnancy. Pregnant women can be treated with any of the recommended regimens for nonpregnant women, in addition to the alternative regimens of oral clindamycin and clindamycin ovules.
- *VVC*: Topical azole therapy for 7 days.

Treatment in people living with HIV and immunocompromised patients: Same basic treatment regimen has to be followed.
- *Noninfective conditions*:
  ○ *Desquamated inflammatory vaginitis*:[33]
    - Clindamycin 2% vaginal cream, 5 g every night for 3 weeks followed by twice weekly for 2 months.
    - Clindamycin 200 mg vaginal pessary, once every night for 2 weeks followed by twice weekly for 2 months.
    - Hydrocortisone 300–500 mg vaginal pessary, once a night for 3 weeks followed by twice weekly for 2 months.
    - Clobetasol propionate is an ultrapotent steroid that can be used in refractory cases for few weeks to avoid remission before switching to mild potency steroids.
    - Women at risk of developing candidiasis (25%) with prolonged clindamycin can be given fluconazole 150 mg weekly suppressive therapy.
  ○ *Atrophic vaginitis:*[34]
    - First-line treatment: Vaginal moisturizer, lubricants, and probiotics
    - Second-line treatment: Localized hormone replacement therapy
      ▪ Vaginal cream—estradiol-17b
      ▪ Vaginal tablets—estradiol hemihydrate
      ▪ Vaginal capsules—estradiol-17b softgel capsules
    - Third-line treatment: Systemic hormone replacement therapy ospemifene [selective estrogen receptor modulator (SERM)] 60 mg daily

Prevention for Recurrence

These are some hygiene modifications for prevention. Like, wear 100% cotton underpants, and avoid overly tight clothing, sprays, and bubble baths. Keep the vagina clean by washing with a gentle, mild soap, and warm water from the outside. Always wipe from front to back and avoid jet sprays of toilet seats to prevent bacteria from getting into the vagina and causing an infection.

Treatment of every episode of infection with full course of treatment must be done with partner treatment when required.

FUTURE ASPECTS

- *CVV:*[35] A new virulence factor candidalysin secreted by candidal hyphae which is a cytolytic peptide toxin. It triggers protective immune response in form of host cell activation, neutrophil recruitment, type 17 immunity that will help to prevent recurrence. This immune response will also open horizon about targeting new strategies for vaccination. Few are under trial, like NDV-3A (antigen Als-3). Several other antigens to target are virosomal Sap2, Beta-glucan-CRM-conjugate/MF59, HyR-1.
- *BV:*[36] An updated conceptual model on the pathogenesis of BV that centers on the roles of virulent strains of *Gardnerella vaginalis*, as well as *Prevotella bivia* and *Atopobium vaginae* that forms a biofilm which is responsible for the continuance and high-recurrence rates of BV. Absence of inflammation in BV leads to considerable overgrowth of gram-negative and positive anaerobes. Lack of inflammation in BV may be due to majority of vaginal bacteria originates from gut microbiota which leads to immune tolerance acquired through evolution and presence of short-chain fatty acids which modulates the immune response.
- *TV:*[37] Vaccination against *Trichomonads* species infection is already in use for systemic infections in infants. Immune response to *T. vaginalis* infection is heterogenous. Some immunogenic epitopes for *T. vaginalis* are 115 kDa alpha actin protein, 100 kDa protein, and heat shock protein.

TAKE HOME MESSAGE

"Our knowledge of leukorrhea is unsatisfactory and incomplete. The majority of physicians neither appreciate the gross aspects of the condition, nor

discover the locality from which discharges arise, practically none of us possesses an adequate knowledge of the bacteria involved and most clinicians admit that their curative efforts yield poor results."
—**Arthur H Curtis**

This comprehensive approach for diagnosis and management in chronic and recurrent VD patients will result in symptom improvement and reduction in recurrence in majority of cases.

REFERENCES

1. Sim M, Logan S, Goh LH. Vaginal discharge: Evaluation and management in primary care. Singapore Med J. 2020;61(6):297-301.
2. Fernandopulle RC. An overview on approach to diagnosis and management of vaginal discharge in gynaecological practice. Sri Lanka J Obstet Gyn. 2012;34:73-8.
3. Faught BM, Reyes S. Characterization and treatment of recurrent bacterial vaginosis. J Womens Health (Larchmt). 2019;28(9):1218-26.
4. Sobel JD, Faro S, Force RW, Foxman B, Ledger WJ, Nyirjesy PR, et al. Vulvovaginal candidiasis: Epidemiologic, diagnostic, and therapeutic considerations. Am J Obstet Gynecol. 1998;178(2):203-11.
5. Sheary B, Dayan L. Recurrent vulvovaginal candidiasis. Aust Fam Physician. 2005;34(3):147-50.
6. Seña AC, Bachmann LH, Hobbs MM. Persistent and recurrent Trichomonas vaginalis infections: Epidemiology, treatment and management considerations. Expert Rev Anti Infect Ther. 2014;12(6):673-85.
7. Goje O. (2019). Three difficult-to-diagnose forms of chronic vaginitis. [online] Available from https://consultqd.clevelandclinic.org/three-difficult-to-diagnose-forms-of-chronic-vaginitis/ [Last accessed November, 2022].
8. Mayo Clinic. (2022). Vaginal atrophy. [online] Available from https://www.mayoclinic.org/diseases-conditions/vaginal-atrophy/symptoms-causes/syc-20352288?p=1 [Last accessed November, 2022].
9. Reichman O, Sobel J. Desquamative inflammatory vaginitis. Best Pract Res Clin Obstet Gynaecol. 2014;28(7):1042-50.
10. Paradise JE, Willis ED. Probability of vaginal foreign body in girls with genital complaints. Am J Dis Child. 1985;139(5):472-6.
11. Konar H. DC Dutta's Textbook of Gynecology, 7th edition. New Delhi: Jaypee Brothers Medical Publishers; 2016.
12. Sobel JD. (2022). Vaginal discharge (vaginitis): Initial evaluation. [online] Available from https://www.uptodate.com/contents/approach-to-females-with-symptoms-of-vaginitis [Last accessed November, 2022].
13. Paladine HL, Desai UA. Vaginitis: Diagnosis and treatment. Am Fam Physician. 2018;97(5):321-9.
14. Hakakha MM, Davis J, Korst LM, Silverman NS. Leukorrhea and bacterial vaginosis as in office predictors of cervical infection in high-risk women. Obstet Gynecol. 2002;100(4):808-12.
15. Sardana K, Sinha S, Rani S. Compendium of Dermatology for Examinations, 1st edition. New Delhi: CBS Publisher and Distributors; 2020.
16. Lema VM. Recurrent vulvo-vaginal candidiasis: Diagnostic and management challenges in a developing country context. Obstet Gynecol Int J. 2017;7(5):00260.
17. Kelly KG. Tests on vaginal discharge. In: Walker HK, Hall WD, Hurst JW (Eds). Clinical Methods: The History, Physical, and Laboratory Examinations, 3rd edition. Boston: Butterworths; 1990. Also available https://www.ncbi.nlm.nih.gov/books/NBK288 [Last accessed November, 2022].
18. Workowski KA, Bolan GA; Centers for Disease Control and Prevention. Sexually transmitted diseases treatment guidelines, 2015. MMWR Recomm Rep. 2015;64(RR-03):1-137.
19. Miller JM, Binnicker MJ, Campbell S, Carroll KC, Chapin KC, Gilligan PH, et al. A guide to utilization of the microbiology laboratory for diagnosis of infectious diseases: 2018 Update by the Infectious Diseases Society of America and the American Society for Microbiology. Clin Infect Dis. 2018;67(6):e1-e94.
20. Nugent RP, Krohn MA, Hillier SL. Reliability of diagnosing bacterial vaginosis is improved by a standardized method of gram stain interpretation. J Clin Microbiol. 1991;29(2):297-301.
21. Melville C, Nandwani R. Comparative study of clinical management strategies for vaginal discharge in family planning and genitourinary medicine setting. J Fam Plann Reprod Health Care. 2005;31:26-30.
22. Garber GE. The laboratory diagnosis of Trichomonas vaginalis. Can J Infect Dis Med Microbiol. 2005;16(1):35-8.
23. Aetna. (2022). Diagnosis of vaginitis. [internet] Hartford, last accessed and updated November 2022, available from https://www.aetna.com/cpb/medical/data/600_699/0643.html
24. Hess R, Austin RM, Dillon S, Chang CCH, Ness RB. Vaginal maturation index self-sample collection in mid-life women: acceptability and correlation with physician-collected samples. Menopause. 2008;15(4 Pt 1):726-9.
25. Leitich H. Controversies in diagnosis of preterm labour. BJOG. 2005;112(Suppl 1):61-3.
26. Centers for Disease Control and Prevention. (2021). Sexually transmitted infections treatment guidelines, 2021 for bacterial vaginosis. [online] Available from https://www.cdc.gov/std/treatment-guidelines/bv.htm [Last accessed November, 2022].
27. Centers for Disease Control and Prevention. (2021). Sexually transmitted infections treatment guidelines, 2021 for trichomoniasis. [online] Available from https://www.cdc.gov/std/treatment-guidelines/trichomoniasis.htm [Last accessed November, 2022].
28. Centers for Disease Control and Prevention. (2021). Sexually transmitted infections treatment guidelines, 2021 for vulvovaginal candidiasis (VVC). [online] Available from https://www.cdc.gov/std/treatment-guidelines/candidiasis.htm [Last accessed November, 2022].
29. Hainer BL, Gibson MV. Vaginitis. Am Fam Physician. 2011;83(7):807-15.
30. Amsel R, Totten PA, Spiegel CA, Chen KC, Eschenbach D, Holmes KK. Nonspecific vaginitis. Diagnostic criteria and microbial and epidemiologic associations. Am J Med. 1983;74(1):14-22.
31. Ison CS, Hay PE. Validation of a simplified grading of gram stained vaginal smears for use in genitourinary medicine clinics. Sex Transm Infect. 2002;78(6):413-5.

32. Stockdale CK. Clinical spectrum of desquamative inflammatory vaginitis. Curr Infect Dis Rep. 2010;12(6):479-83.
33. Sobel JD, Reichman O, Misra D, Yoo W. Prognosis and treatment of desquamative inflammatory vaginitis. Obstet Gynecol. 2011;117(4):850-5.
34. Bachmann GA, Nevadunsky NS. Diagnosis and treatment of atrophic vaginitis. Am Fam Physician. 2000;61(10):3090-6.
35. Cassone A. Vulvovaginal *Candida albicans* infections: pathogenesis, immunity and vaccine prospects. BJOG. 2015;122(6):785-94.
36. Muzny CA, Taylor CM, Swords WE, Tamhane A, Chattopadhyay D, Cerca N. An updated conceptual model on the pathogenesis of bacterial vaginosis. 2019;220(9):1399-405.
37. Sehgal R, Goyal K, Sehgal A. Trichomoniasis and lactoferrin: Future prospects. Infect Dis Obstet Gynecol. 2012;2012:536037.

19

A Female Patient with Vulvar Pruritus

Neela M Patel, Khushbu R Modi

INTRODUCTION

Pruritus is defined as an unpleasant sensation of the skin that provokes the urge to scratch. It is a characteristic feature of many skin diseases and an alarming sign of some systemic diseases. Pruritus manifest as acute or chronic condition and can be localized or generalized. Considering its intractable and incapacitating nature, pruritus is diagnostic and therapeutic challenge.

Pruritus vulvae or simply quoted as itching of the female external genitalia, is a common complaint for which women of all age groups can present to dermatologists. In addition to itching, there is a sensation of irritation, chafing, pain or burning, and women commonly self-treat with increased washing and over-the-counter (OTC) hygiene or medicinal products.

The true prevalence of vulvar pruritus may be difficult to assess as it is commonly unregistered. Prevalence varies according to the age group. Atopic dermatitis and irritant contact dermatitis have been reported to the most common cause of vulvar symptoms in prepubertal girls.[1] Approximately 81.4% patients with vulvar itch were found to have at least one positive contact allergen on patch testing.[1] Considering the postmenopausal women age group, the prevalence is approximately 50% according to Indian studies.[2] Despite its high prevalence, it can be challenging to reach an accurate diagnosis.

Complications of pruritus vulvae include severe discomfort and irritability, painful and uncomfortable sexual intercourse, secondary bacterial and fungal infections, social awkwardness and emotional stress, and psychological trauma. So, to prevent all these complications thorough history taking, examination, and investigations are crucial to provide effective treatment.

APPROACH TO A PATIENT WITH VULVAR PRURITUS

Approach to a female patient of vulvar pruritus should be directed toward establishing diagnosis, finding possible etiology, and if any systemic involvement and individualizing treatment.

The causes of pruritus vulvae are countless in number, just like the causes of pruritus. Thus, most common conditions causing vulvar pruritus are discussed in this chapter **(Table 1)**.

HISTORY TAKING

- *Demographic characteristics* **(Table 2)**: Give an idea of pruritic dermatomes which are common in the respective age groups.
- *Symptoms* **(Table 3)**:
  - *Duration of symptoms*: If pruritus vulvae persists for <6 weeks, it is considered to be acute in nature, as seen in infection and contact irritant dermatitis and if it persists for >6 weeks, it is considered chronic in nature as seen in chronic inflammatory dermatoses, malignancy, and secondary causes.[4]
  - *Onset of pruritus*: Pruritus occurred before skin lesions (e.g., neoplastic, secondary causes, and prodrome to herpes flare)/after skin lesion (e.g., chronic inflammatory dermatoses and infectious cause)
  - *Location of pruritus*: Localized as seen in infections and neoplastic conditions or generalized as seen with other causes like scabies, lichen planus (LP), etc.

Table 1: Differential diagnoses of pruritus vulvae (conditions causing vulvar pruritus are classified into four categories).

Chronic inflammatory dermatoses	Infections	Neoplastic	Secondary causes
• Lichen sclerosus atrophicus (LSA) • Lichen planus (LP) • Lichen simplex chronicus (LSC) • Psoriasis • Dermatitis (atrophic vulvitis, seborrheic dermatitis, irritant dermatitis, allergic dermatitis) • *Other inflammatory etiology*: seborrheic dermatitis, plasma cell vulvitis and Fox–Fordyce disease	• *Fungi*: Vulvovaginal candidiasis (VVC), tinea cruris. • *Virus*: Genital warts, herpes progenitalis • *Protozoa*: Trichomoniasis • *Parasites*: Enterobius vermicularis (pin worm) infestation • *Arthropod*: Scabies, pubic lice • *Bacterial*: Folliculitis, bacterial vaginosis and β-hemolytic streptococcal infection	• *Benign*: Syringomas and hidradenoma papilliferum • *Premalignant*: Vulvar intraepithelial neoplasia (VIN), extra mammary Paget's disease, Bowen's disease • *Malignant*: Squamous cell carcinoma	• *Systemic*: Diabetes mellitus, hepatic and renal diseases, urinary tract infection (UTI) • Drug reaction • *Local*: Tight clothing, intimate hygiene, shaving, incontinence • *Psychological*: Vulvodynia • *Hormonal*: Atrophic vulvovaginitis, pregnancy

Table 2: Frequent pruritic dermatoses during different age groups.[3]

Prepubertal	Reproductive age	Postmenopausal
• *Chronic inflammatory dermatoses*: 　○ Lichen sclerosus atrophicans 　○ Atopic dermatitis 　○ Psoriasis • *Infections*: 　○ Beta hemolytic streptococcal vulvovaginitis • *Others*: 　○ Irritant contact dermatitis 　○ Napkin dermatitis	• *Chronic inflammatory dermatoses*: 　○ Lichen simplex 　○ Psoriasis 　○ Atopic dermatitis 　○ Lichen sclerosus (less frequent than in other age groups) • *Infections*: 　○ Vulvovaginal candidiasis 　○ Bacterial vaginosis 　○ Trichomonas vaginitis 　○ Herpes progenitalis • *Secondary causes*: 　○ Allergic contact dermatitis 　○ Irritant contact dermatitis • *Neoplasia*: Rare	• *Chronic inflammatory dermatoses*: 　○ Psoriasis 　○ Lichen sclerosus 　○ Lichen simplex chronicus • *Neoplasia*: 　○ Vulvar intraepithelial neoplasia 　○ Squamous cell carcinoma of vulva 　○ Extramammary Paget's disease 　○ Bowen's disease • *Secondary causes*: 　○ Irritant contact dermatitis 　○ Atrophic vulvovaginitis 　○ Allergic contact dermatitis (less frequent) • *Infections*: Uncommon

Table 3: Symptoms of vulvar dermatoses.

Name of condition	Chronic inflammatory dermatoses	Infections	Neoplastic	Secondary causes
Symptoms	• Severe itching • Burning • Pain	Pruritus associated with discharge	Asymptomatic or can present with persistent/intermittent and localized pruritus	• Pruritus, dryness, and burning micturition • Recurrent UTI
Associated symptoms	• Dyspareunia • Dysuria • Vulvar soreness	• Dyspareunia • Dysuria	• SCC can be associated with bleeding or pain • Pruritus of VIN is refractory to anti-inflammatory treatment	Pain, dyspareunia, dysuria
Risk factors	• History of atopy • Use of irritants • Family history of similar lesions • Sacral spinal compression, postherpetic neuralgia, diabetic neuropathy associated with LSC • Autoimmune conditions	• Young age • Lower socioeconomic status • Increased number and recent changes in sexual partners • Prostitution • Drug use	• Immunocompromised individuals • HPV infection • Increasing age • Precancerous lesions	• Uncontrolled DM • Psychiatric illness • Systemic illness

(DM: diabetes mellitus; HPV: human papillomavirus; LSC: lichen simplex chronicus; SCC: squamous cell carcinoma; UTI: urinary tract infection; VIN: vulvar intraepithelial neoplasia)

- ○ *Nature of pruritus*: Intermittent/continuous/nocturnal
- ○ *Severity of symptoms*: Severity of itching can be assessed by variety of scales like
    - *Monodimensional:* Visual analog scale, numerical rating scale, verbal rating scale
    - *Multidimensional:* Itch severity scale, pruritus grading system[5]
- ○ *Aggravating factors*: Heat, sweat, stress, menstruation, etc.
- ○ *Associated symptoms*: Discharge, burning, irritation, dyspareunia, pain, bleeding from lesions, dysuria, vulvar soreness, dryness, constipation.
- ○ Relieved on taking antihistaminics or not
- ○ Any systemic complaints/constitutional symptoms at present
- *Personal history*: Smoking, recurrent urinary tract infections, urine or stool continence, any systemic illness, use of systemic drugs, immunosuppressants, OTC drugs, and topical application.
- *Family history*: Similar complaints in partner, diabetes mellitus, hypertension, hypothyroidism, atopy/allergies, hepatic and renal diseases, and neoplasia.
- Detailed gynecological, obstetric history, and sexual history
- *Past history*: History of similar complaints and treatment for the same in past. History of sexually transmitted diseases in past, history of fistulas, or surgery done over vulvae.
- Impact on social, psychological, and sexual life

PHYSICAL EXAMINATION (TABLE 4)

Local site examination of vulva, vagina, and surrounding skin gives us a clue about diagnosis and helps in differentiating other vulvar dermatomes. General examination helps us in evaluating systemic involvement.

- *Examination of local site*: Refer **Table 4**
- *General/complete skin examination*: A full examination of anogenital region, flexural areas, mucosal sites, lips, trunk, palms, and soles. Lymph nodes should be palpated along with abdomen to look for any mass, tenderness, or lymphadenopathy.
- *Vulvoscopy and colposcopy*

Table 4: Examination of genitals (Figs. 1 to 8).		
Condition	**Examination**	**Differential diagnosis**
a. Chronic inflammatory dermatoses		
Lichen sclerosus	• Atrophy, erosions, fissures and bruising • Figure-of-eight shaped porcelain white plaque around vulva and anus • Loss of genital architecture with subsequent effacement of labia minora and clitoris • Parchment like or cigarette paper skin • Vestibular involvement is rare and vaginal lesions do not occur, as LS spare mucosal involvement • <5% risk of developing squamous cell carcinoma (SCC)[6]	• Lichen simplex chronicus • Lichen planus • Vitiligo
Lichen planus	Three types of vulvar lichen planus have been described: Erosive, classical, and hypertrophic • Erosive LP is characterized by erosions involving the introitus, clitoris and clitoral hood, labia minora and majora. A lacy white edge to the erosions. Healing erosions may appear as a glazed erythema. Vaginal involvement is very common and presents with vaginal erythema, contact bleeding, erosions, and scarring with synechiae. In rare cases, vaginal lesions may be the only manifestation • The classical type presents with small purple, polygonal papules, with sometimes a reticulate lace pattern • Hyperkeratotic lichen planus presents as single or multiple white-hyperkeratotic papules and plaques	• Lichen sclerosus • Autoimmune blistering diseases
Lichen simplex chronicus	• Skin is thickened, lichenified and often hyperpigmented due to chronic rubbing and scratching • Thickened plaques with exaggerated skin markings over the hair bearing labia majora and sparing mucosal vulvar skin and labia minora	• Lichen sclerosus • Contact dermatitis

Continued

Continued

Condition	Examination	Differential diagnosis
Psoriasis	- Well demarcated symmetric, smooth red plaques without scaling in the vulvar and perianal region - Vaginal mucosa is spared	- Contact dermatitis - Candidiasis - Intertrigo - Hailey–Hailey disease - Lichen simplex chronicus
Dermatitis (atrophic vulvitis, seborrheic dermatitis, contact dermatitis)	In acute cases, erythematous and scaly or nonscaly plaques that may ooze, drain, or crust with warm, tender skin. Lichenified plaques with rugosity and dyspigmentation are seen in chronic cases	Lichen simplex chronicus
Plasma cell vulvitis	Few well-defined shallow ulcers, with a clean, red-orange base	
Fox–Fordyce disease	Small dome-shaped papules +/- involvement of axillae, intensely itchy and often presenting as lichenification	
b. Infections		
Fungal		
Vulvovaginal candidiasis	Curdy, white, adherent discharge associated with vulvovaginal redness Satellite lesions on inner thigh	- Bacterial vaginosis - Trichomoniasis
Dermatophytic infection	Erythematous hyperpigmented patch with progressing borders	- Candidial intertrigo - Erythrasma
Viral		
Genital warts	Solitary or in clusters, corrugated or cauliflower like	Condyloma lata
Herpes progenitalis	Grouped fluid-filled vesicles, erosions and ulcer	Insect bite
Parasitic		
Trichomoniasis	Green yellow frothy discharge on erythematous vaginal wall, erythema extends up to cervix	- Vulvovaginal candidiasis - Bacterial vaginosis
Pinworm infestation	Excoriation marks and eczematized lesions over vulva and perianal area	
Protozoal		
Scabies	- Scabetic nodules over vulva - Burrows alongside of fingers and front of wrists	- Atopic dermatitis - Contact dermatitis - Insect bite
Pubic lice	Nits in pubic hair	
Folliculitis	Few discrete/multiple pustules seen in hair bearing areas	
Bacterial vaginosis	Moderate to profuse, mucoid/thin, grayish-white discharge associated with fishy odor	- Vulvovaginal candidiasis - Trichomoniasis
Beta hemolytic streptococcal infection	- *Acute*: There is a sudden onset of an erythematous swollen painful vulva and vagina with a thin mucoid discharge - *Subacute*: Pruritic erythematous patches and plaques in the vulvar and perianal region	
c. Neoplasia		
Benign		
Syringoma	Multiple or solitary, localized or generalized, small, skin-colored to yellowish papules up to 1–5 mm in diameter	- Fox–Fordyce disease - Lichen simplex chronicus - Condyloma acuminata
Hidradenoma papilliferum	The lesions are firm and freely movable. Ulceration and pain may develop if the lesion connects with the epithelial surface	- Syringocystadenoma papilliferum - Adenocarcinoma - Intraductal carcinoma

Continued

Continued

Condition	Examination	Differential diagnosis
Premalignant		
VIN	Skin colored or white or red papules, plaques, nodules, erosions	• Squamous cell carcinoma • Basal cell carcinoma • Paget's disease • Melanoma
Extramammary Paget's disease	• Florid, eczematous lichenified lesions associated with erythema and excoriation marks • Well demarcated with slightly raised edges and surrounding erythema	• Sqaumous cell carcinoma • Lichen simplex chronicus • Bowen's disease
Bowen's disease	Erythematous to violaceous, minimally indurated, nontender plaque	• Extramammary Paget's disease • Squamous cell carcinoma
SCC	Vulvar lump or mass, which may present ulcerated, leukoplakic, fleshy, or warty	• VIN • Bowen's disease • Extramammary Paget's disease
d. *Secondary causes*		
Vulvodynia	Excoriation marks that is out of proportion to lesion or without lesion	Diagnosis of exclusion
Atrophic vulvovaginitis	• Pale, dry, thin vaginal epithelium that is smooth and shiny with loss of most rugosity • Vulva—atrophic • Vagina—pale	Lichen sclerosus atrophicus

(LP: lichen planus; LS: lichen sclerosus; VIN: vulvar intraepithelial neoplasia)

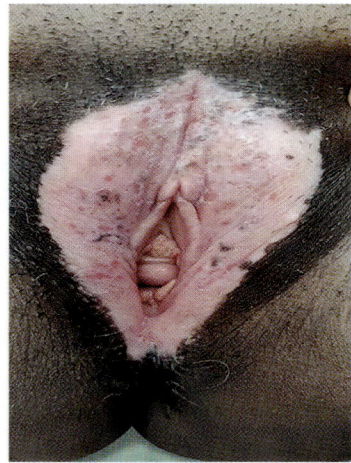

FIG. 1: Lichen sclerosus et atrophicus.

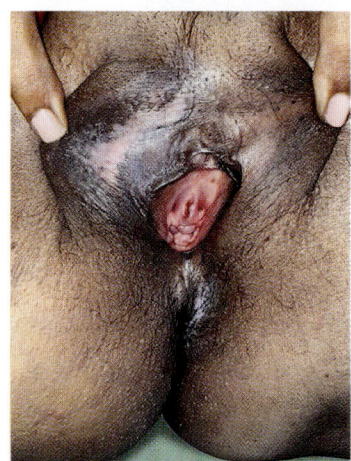

FIG. 2: Lichen simplex chronicus.

Vulvoscopy (Table 5): Done especially for chronic inflammatory dermatomes and neoplastic conditions.

Vulvoscopy is a noninvasive, rapid, and efficient diagnostic method that has been established as an essential part of the clinical examination for more detailed assessment of vulvar lesions. It helps in (1) improving the diagnostic accuracy, (2) deciding the site of biopsy, and (3) helps in early identification of precancerous lesions.

Colposcopy: It is an office-based procedure is used to find out cancerous cells or abnormal cells in cervix, vagina, and vulva, guides in deciding site of biopsy and immunohistochemistry. After inserting speculum to open up vagina in proper position, cervix-vagina-vulva will be lightly wiped with a 3–5% acetic acid, which washes away mucus and allows us to see whitish abnormal cells.

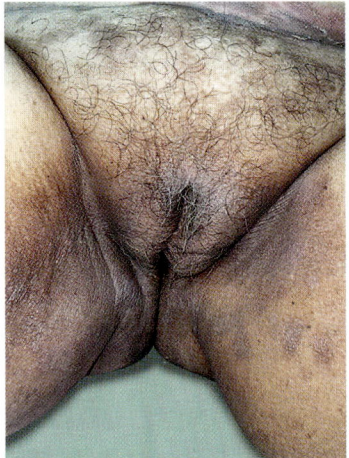

FIG. 3: Vulvar psoriasis.

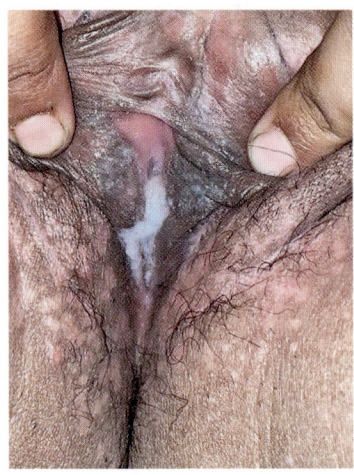

FIG. 6: Vaginal discharge.

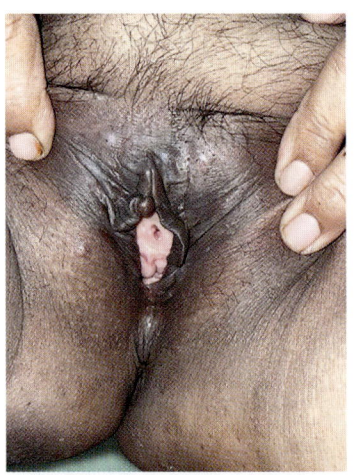

FIG. 4: Scabetic nodules.

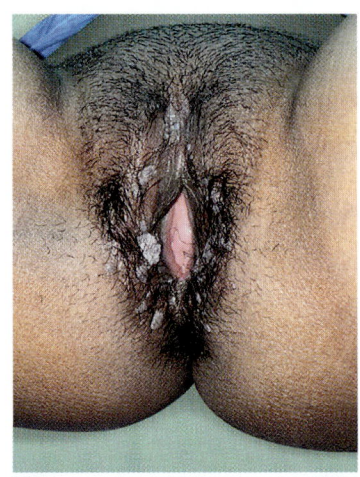

FIG. 7: Bowen's disease.

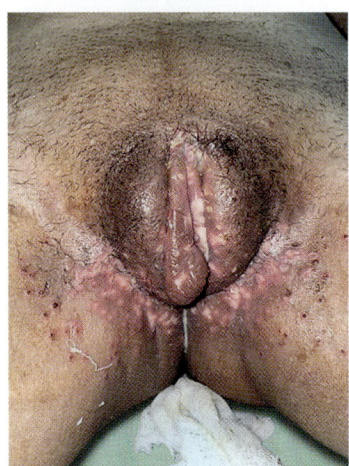

FIG. 5: Herpes progenitalis.

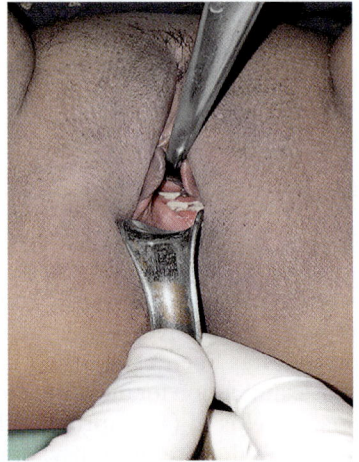

FIG. 8: Vulvovaginal candidiasis.

Table 5: Evaluation of vulvoscopy findings.	
Condition	**Vulvoscopy findings**
Chronic inflammatory dermatoses	
Lichen sclerosus[7]	• Patchy, structureless areas, whitish to white-yellowish to pink-whitish in color over a diffuse whitish background • Gray-blue dots, usually with a characteristic peppered arrangement, corresponding to dermal melanophages • Comedo-like openings and scales were observed
Lichen simplex chronicus[8]	Regularly distributed dotted vessels corresponding to dilated vessels in elongated dermal papillae
Lichen planus[9]	The dermoscopic hallmark of active lichen planus is Wickham striae, which are intersecting crossing white lines forming a network
Psoriasis[10]	Regular red dots arranged in glomerulus pattern and white scales on erythematous background
Atrophic vulvovaginitis[7]	White structureless areas indicate hyperkeratosis and epidermal atrophy; telangiectasia and dotted vessels represent atrophic epidermis with dilated blood vessels
Neoplasia	
Vulvar intraepithelial neoplasia (VIN)[11]	Papillomatous hyperkeratotic scales with an erythematous center and whitish peripheral borders
Extramammary Paget's disease[12]	White small round clods with white structureless areas ("cloud-like structureless areas") and thick branching white lines with intermingled white clods ("lava lake structures")
Bowen's disease[13]	Glomerular and dot vessels grouped in clusters (glomerular vessels are tortuous capillaries often distributed in clusters, usually larger than dotted vessels) and surrounded by a white halo (sign of keratinization) and surface scales

Vulvar Q-tip examination: It is commonly used objective diagnostic tool for vulvodynia. Patient is asked to rate her pain using a 0-10 scale while touching vulva and vestibule in a clockwise direction.[14]

INVESTIGATIONS

Following investigations can be done to reach definitive diagnosis and deciding a line of treatment. Investigations can be done according to the clinical diagnosis, as ordering all the investigations in all patients can increase physical and mental burden. Other than screening investigations, further specialized investigations can be done wherever required.

Screening Tests

- *Routine blood investigations*: Complete blood count, liver function tests, kidney function tests, and blood sugar
- *Urine analysis*: Urine routine microscopy and urine culture sensitivity
- *Other investigations*: vulvar and perianal swab, X-ray, antinuclear antibody (ANA) titer, serum immunoglobulin E (IgE) whenever required.

Special Investigations (Table 6)

- *pH and microscopy*: To rule out infectious causes (for details refer to Chapter 18 of this book, a female with

Table 6: Special investigation.	
pH and microscopy	Infections, atrophic vulvitis
Patch test	Allergic contact dermatitis, atopic dermatitis
Biopsy	Chronic inflammatory dermatoses and neoplasia
Immunohistochemistry (IHC)	Neoplasia

chronic and recurrent vaginal discharge), vaginal secretions are tested using pH paper. If pH is <4.5 then candidal cause, and if pH >4.5 then bacterial or trichomonal cause may be the probable etiology for discharge and pruritus. A cotton swab is used to make slide for wet mount (to see mobile trichomonads or clue cells), KOH preparation (yeast and epithelial cells), Gram stain (gram-negative and positive cocci-bacilli)

- *Patch test*:
  ○ Patch testing is recommended to rule out allergic contact dermatitis and may be helpful to distinguish between atopic and allergic contact dermatitis.
  ○ Four main groups of allergens are generally responsible: (1) metals (e.g., nickel, cobalt, and chromium); (2) medications (e.g., hydroxyzine, an ethylenediamine-derived antihistamine, or oral medications that contain propylene glycol); (3) plant and herbal products, fragrances, and flavorings (e.g., citrus, wine, beer, cinnamon, cola, curry,

Table 7: Chronic inflammatory dermatoses.[6]	
Pathologic correlates	*Clinical condition*
Spongiotic pattern	Atopic, allergic, irritant dermatitis
Acanthotic pattern	Psoriasis, lichen simplex chronicus, primary (idiopathic), secondary (superimposed on lichen sclerosus atrophicus, lichen planus or other vulvar disease)
Lichenoid pattern	Lichen sclerosus atrophicus, lichen planus
Dermal homogenization/sclerosis pattern	Lichen sclerosus
Vesiculobullous pattern	Pemphigoid (cicatricial type), linear immunoglobulin A (IgA) disease
Acantholytic pattern	Hailey–Hailey disease, Darier's disease
Granulomatous pattern	Crohn's disease, Melkersson–Rosenthal syndrome
Vasculopathic pattern	Aphthous ulcers, Behçet's disease, plasma cell vulvitis

Table 8: Neoplastic conditions.	
Pathologic correlates	*Clinical condition*
Single-to-double layered epithelial cells with pale eosinophilic cytoplasm. Epithelial cells, forming nests, cords or tubules, with a typical comma-like tail. Within the tubular lumen, periodic acid-Schiff (PAS)-positive eosinophilic material exists	Syringoma[17]
Dermal tumor with cells in papillary folds, tubules, and cystically dilated spaces. The lumen was lined by columnar cells with oval staining nucleus located near base and faintly eosinophilic cytoplasm	Hidradenitis papilliferum[18]
Parakeratosis, dyskeratosis, nuclear pleomorphism, hyperchromatism, and increased mitoses	Vulvar intraepithelial neoplasia (VIN)[19]
Abundant round cells with pale cytoplasm are most evident in the basal layers of the epithelium	Extramammary Paget's disease[20]
Hyperkeratosis, parakeratosis, dyskeratosis, abnormal mitoses, and the presence of proliferating atypical cells that do not evade the dermis with a typical round-to-oval giant Bowen cells, windblown appearance	Bowen's disease[21]
Nests of squamous epithelial cells arising from the epidermis and extending into the dermis. The malignant cells are often large with abundant eosinophilic cytoplasm and nucleus. Keratin pearls are present	Squamous cell carcinoma[22]

vanilla, or other flavorings); and (4) preservatives (e.g., formaldehyde in aspartame).[15] In addition to standard series of allergens, the patient's own topical medications, popular remedies, or other suspected products should also be tested.
  ○ Fragrances, medications, and preservatives are most frequently responsible allergens for vulvar dermatitis.
  ○ Contact allergy induced by topical corticosteroid application is an important cause of vulvar dermatitis that should not be missed.
- *Biopsy*: Biopsy is not routinely performed in patients with vulvar dermatitis. However, a biopsy may be necessary if the diagnosis cannot be made on clinical grounds or there is a suspicion of neoplasia and refractory chronic inflammatory dermatoses. Following are the biopsy findings of various chronic inflammatory dermatoses and neoplastic conditions causing vulvar pruritus **(Tables 7 and 8)**.

Neoplastic conditions: Indications for vulvar biopsy to exclude vulvar intraepithelial neoplasia (VIN):[16]
- Raised moist or eroded lesions
- Discrete lumps
- White, erythematous, or pigmented
- Pain
- Warty lesion
- Multifocal
- Persistent lesions
- *Immunohistochemistry*:
  ○ *VIN*:[23] Increased MIB-1 staining, p16 extensively positive in classic VIN, p53 overexpression in differentiated/simplex VIN.
  ○ *Extramammary Paget's disease*:[24] Paget cells usually stain for markers of eccrine and apocrine derivation including low molecular weight cytokeratins (CK), periodic acid-Schiff (PAS), gross cystic disease fluid protein (GCDFP-15), and carcinoembryonic antigen (CEA). S100 staining is negative.
    The main histological differential diagnoses to exclude in the vulva are superficial spreading malignant melanoma (PAS negative, S100 positive, cytokeratin negative, and CEA negative) and anogenital intraepithelial neoplasia (S100 negative, PAS negative).
  ○ *SCC*:[22] Typically stain strong for high molecular weight keratins AE1/AE3, CEA, and CD44.

MANAGEMENT

Management largely depends on etiology, associated conditions, and possible precipitating factors. Readers are advised to refer other resources for details.

General Measures (Table 9)

- *Behavior modification*: Gentle skin care should be encouraged. Soaking in warm water, without additives, relieves vulvar discomfort, and pruritus. Patients should

Table 9: Preventive measures.[6]	
Do's	Don'ts
• Use soap substitute • Shower • Gently dab vulvar area • Dry with soft towel or hair dryer on a cool setting held away from skin • Wear loose fitting silk or cotton underwear • Sleep without underwear • Wear white or light colors of underwear	• Wash in plain water. Use small amount or emollient moth water, to avoid dry skin • Bath: Add bath emollient if bathing • Avoid sponges or flannels to wash but use emollients and apply with hand • Avoid fabric conditioner, biological washing powder, soaps, shower gel, scrubs, bubble bath, deodorants, baby wipes, and douches • Avoid colored toilet paper, panty liners and dark colored underwear, dark textile dyes may cause allergies

be reassured that skin issues are not the result of a lack of cleanliness and that excessive washing can worsen dermatitis.
- The patient's personal care practices should be reviewed at each visit to ensure ongoing good practices are being followed. Known or suspected allergens and irritants in the environment should be eliminated.
- Appropriate treatment of partner in cases of sexually transmitted diseases.

Treatment for Chronic Inflammatory Dermatomes
Topical Treatment
- Nonallergic emollients (white petroleum jelly, propylene glycol).
- *Astringent soaks*: Vulvar sores can be soothed by soaking in a bath with aluminum acetate solution.
- *Antibiotics (mupirocin 2% cream, fusidic acid 1% cream)*: To prevent secondary infection
- Cooling agents like calamine can be used.
- Moisture is sealed into the skin with the application of a nonallergenic emollient and a topical corticosteroid ointment ("soak and seal").

If patient is having mild symptoms:
- *Low- to medium-potency topical corticosteroid ointment*: Hydrocortisone 1% or 2.5%, desonide 0.05% or triamcinolone 0.1%.
- Topical corticosteroid can be used one or more times daily, for 2–4 weeks, although a clear benefit has not been demonstrated with more than once daily application.
- Therapy is continued for indefinitely period necessary to control pruritus with a goal of <14 days per month.

If patient is having moderate-to-severe symptoms:
- Start with medium-to high-potency corticosteroids such as clobetasol propionate 0.05% cream, betamethasone dipropionate 0.05% ointment at night daily for 30 days and then re-evaluate and switch over to low to medium-potency steroids according to response. Potent topical steroids can be used for up to 12 weeks on the vulva without adverse effects.
- Topical calcineurin inhibitors such as tacrolimus 0.03% ointment and pimecrolimus 1% cream is a good option for postmenopausal females.
- Local anesthetic and other antipruritic agents such as benzocaine, lignocaine, and pramoxine

Systemic Treatment
- *Antihistaminics*: Sedative antihistaminics such as diphenhydramine 25–50 mg or hydroxyzine 12.5–25 mg and nonsedative antihistaminics such as levocetirizine 5-10 mg, desloratadine 5 mg, fexofenadine 120–180 mg can be given to break itch-scratch cycle.
- Oral antibiotics
- *Oral immunosuppressants*: Systemic corticosteroids, azathioprine, cyclosporine, methotrexate, and mycophenolate mofetil are required for refractory generalized chronic inflammatory dermatomes.
- Phototherapy is also an option to treat various inflammatory condition such as atopic dermatitis, psoriasis, and lichen sclerosus.

Treatment for Infections
For treatment of vaginal discharge refer to CDC guidelines July 2021.[25-27]

Treatment for Neoplasia
In this group for treatment multidisciplinary approach is needed. For excision and further follow-up oncologist referral is mandatory.

Treatment of Secondary Causes
Treatment of primary cause, management of systemic illness and withdrawal of irritants is the first-line management.

Atrophic Vulvovaginitis
- *Nonhormonal treatments*: Current OTC treatments include nonhormonal vaginal moisturizers and lubricants for dyspareunia.
- *Hormonal treatments*:
  - *Local*: Vaginal moisturizers, lubricants, probiotics, and vaginal cream (estradiol 17β)
  - *Systemic*: Ospemifene 60 mg daily [selective estrogen receptor modulator (SERM)]

Vulvodynia
- Psychiatry refer for psychosexual counseling
- *Topical treatment*: Lignocaine 5% ointment can be applied to maximum points of tenderness.
- *Systemic treatment*:
  - *Antidepressants*: Doxepin (10–25 mg up to 75 mg), amitriptyline (25 mg up to 100 mg), gabapentin.
  - *Selective serotonin reuptake inhibitor (SSRI)*: Fluoxetine, paroxetine, sertraline, fluvoxamine, mirtazapine, and citalopram used for patients with intractable pruritus resistant to routine therapy.

TAKE HOME MESSAGE

Comprehensive history taking and examination can help narrow down differential diagnoses. To diagnose some conditions, clinical examination is sufficient enough and their preliminary management includes avoidance of irritant substances and antihistaminics. Invasive investigational procedures are required to confirm diagnoses of chronic inflammatory dermatomes and mainstay treatment for this group includes immunosuppressants. Treatment resistant or suspicious malignant lesions require multidimensional approach for diagnosis and treatment.

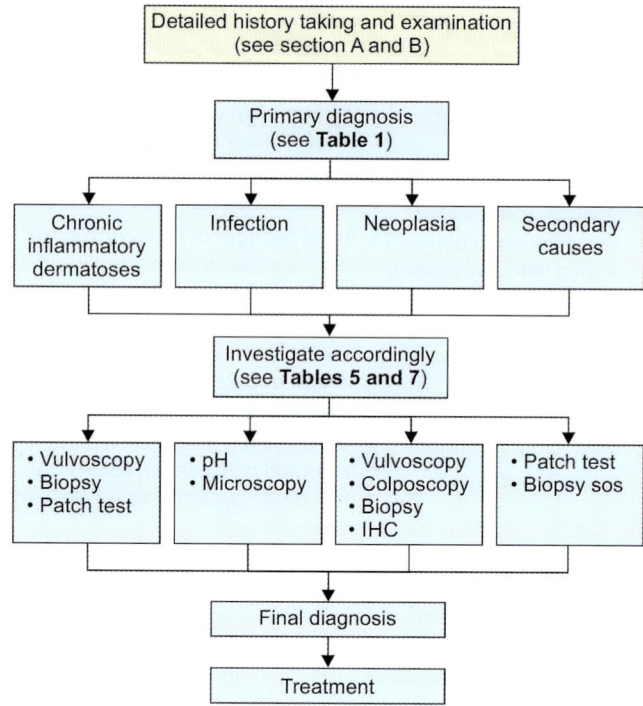

FLOWCHART 1: Approach in a female patient with vulvar pruritus. (IHC: immunohistochemistry)

REFERENCES

1. Raef HS, Elmariah SB. Vulvar Pruritus: A Review of Clinical Associations, Pathophysiology and Therapeutic Management Front Med (Lausanne). 2021;8:649402.
2. Kaur J, Kalsy J. Study of pruritus vulvae in geriatric age group in tertiary hospital. Indian J Sex Transm Dis AIDS. 2017;38(1):15-21.
3. Lambert J. Pruritus in female patients. BioMed Res Int. 2014;2014:1-6.
4. Wölber L, Prieske K, Mendling W, Schmalfeldt B, Tietz H, Jaeger A. Vulvar Pruritus—Causes, Diagnosis and Therapeutic Approach, Dtsch Arztebl Int. 2020;116(8):126-33.
5. Pereira MP, Ständer S. Assessment of severity and burden of pruritus. Allergol Int. 2017;66(1):3-7.
6. Gopal G, Hadoura E, Mahmood T. Pruritus vulvae. Obstet Gynaecol Reprod Med. 2016;26(4):95-100.
7. Borghi A, Corazza M, Minghetti S, Bianchini E, Virgili A. Dermoscopic Features of Vulvar Lichen Sclerosus in the Setting of a Prospective Cohort of Patients: New Observations. Dermatology. 2016;232(1):71-7.
8. Errichetti E, Ankad B, Neema S, Sadek A, Hossam D, Jha AK, Kaliyadan F, Puravoor J, Khare S, Lallas A. Papulosquamous disorders. Errichetti E, Lallas A (Eds). Dermoscopy in General Dermatology for Skin of Color. New York: CRC Press, Taylor and Francis Group; 2021. pp.1-23.
9. Lallas A, Kyrgidis A, Tzellos T, Apalla Z, Karakyriou E, Karatolias A, et al. Accuracy of dermoscopic criteria for the diagnosis of psoriasis, dermatitis, lichen planus and pityriasis rosea. Br J Dermatol. 2012;166(6):1198-205.
10. Ankad B, Madarkar M. Red dots caught red handed: Dermoscopy of genital psoriasis. Clin Dermatol Rev. 2017;1(1):25.
11. Barisani A, Dika E, Fanti P, De Iaco P, Tosti G, Patrizi A, et al. Dermoscopic findings of vulvar intraepithelial neoplasia: a series of four cases. Br J Dermatol. 2016;176(1):227-30.
12. Ngan V. (2020). Extramammary Paget disease of skin. [online]. Available from https://dermnetnz.org/topics/extramammary-paget-disease [Last accessed December, 2022].
13. Bhat Y, Bashir S, Wani R, Hassan I. Dermoscopy of Bowen's Disease. Indian J Dermatopathol Diagn Dermatol. 2019;6(1):60-1.
14. Kelly KG. Tests on Vaginal Discharge. Walker HK, Hall WD, Hurst JW (Eds). Clinical Methods: The History, Physical, and Laboratory Examinations, 3rd edition. Boston: Butterworths; 1990.
15. Johnson NR, Scheinman PL. (2021). Vulvar dermatitis. [online]. Available from https://www.uptodate.com/contents/vulvar-dermatitis [Last accessed December, 2022].
16. Bansal J, Datta S. Pruritus vulvae. Obstet Gynaecol Reprod Med. 2019;29(6):170-4.
17. Nibhoria S, Tiwana KK, Yadav A. Vulvar syringoma: a rare case report. J Clin Diagn Res. 2014;8(8):FD06.
18. Kambil S, Bhat R, D'Souza D. Hidradenoma papilliferum of the vulva. Indian Dermatol Online J. 2014;5(4):523.
19. Ayala M, Fatehi M. (2021). Vulvar Intraepithelial Neoplasia. [online]. Available from https://www.statpearls.com/articlelibrary/viewarticle/31278/ [Last accessed December, 2022].

20. Yadav S, Gahalaut P, Soodan HS, Mishra N, Rastogi MK. Extramammary Paget's disease of vulva: A rare entity. Indian J Sex Transm Dis AIDS. 2017;38(1):76-7.
21. Mishra J, Pandia A, Padhy A, Mahapatra M, Mohapatra J, Nayak B, et al. Bowen's disease of vulva: A rare case of vulvar premalignant disorder. Clin Cancer Investig J. 2020;9(5):210.
22. Wilkinson EJ, Rush DS. The histopathology of vulvar neoplasia. Glob Libr Women's Med. 2017;doi 10.3843/GLOWM.10256.
23. Santos M, Montagut C, Mellado B, García A, Ramón y Cajal S, Cardesa A, et al. Immunohistochemical staining for p16 and p53 in premalignant and malignant epithelial lesions of the vulva. Int J Gynecol Pathol. 2004;23(3):206-14.
24. McDaniel B, Brown F, Crane JS. (2021). Extramammary Paget Disease. [online]. Available from https://www.statpearls.com/articlelibrary/viewarticle/26522/ [Last accessed December, 2022].
25. Centers for Disease Control and Prevention. (2021). Sexually transmitted infections treatment guidelines, 2021 for bacterial vaginosis. [online]. Available from https://www.cdc.gov/std/treatment-guidelines/STI-Guidelines-2021.pdf [Last accessed December, 2022].
26. Centers for Disease Control and Prevention. (2021). Sexually transmitted infections treatment guidelines, 2021 for vulvovaginal candidiasis. [online]. Available from https://www.cdc.gov/std/treatment-guidelines/candidiasis.htm [Last accessed December, 2022].
27. Centers for Disease Control and Prevention. (2021). Sexually transmitted infections treatment guidelines, 2021 for trichomoniasis. [online]. Available from https://www.cdc.gov/std/treatment-guidelines/trichomoniasis.htm [Last accessed December, 2022].

Part 4: Pediatric Dermatology

20
A Child with Genital Lesions

Kalgi Baxi Majmundar, Ashish Jagati

INTRODUCTION

The skin of the perineum includes the perianal, groin folds, and the external genitalia. Dermatoses of the perineum, especially in the pediatric population, trigger considerable apprehension in parents and caretakers, as the perineum and genitals are considered as "sensitive" and lesions in this region are invariably linked to the suspicion of child sexual abuse, more so in the female patients. As dermatologists, a thorough knowledge and competent approach is essential, because common dermatological conditions, which are easily recognizable on other parts of the body, pose a diagnostic challenge in the perineal region, owing to their unique, specific morphological appearance in this area. This can be attributed to an alteration of the flexural microenvironment due to heat, moisture, and friction.

This chapter focuses on the classification of anogenital dermatoses occurring in the pediatric population, as well as approach to their diagnosis, evaluation, and management.

CLASSIFICATION
Infectious
- *Staphylococcal*: Folliculitis, impetigo, staphylococcal scalded skin syndrome
- *Streptococcal*: Folliculitis, vulvovaginitis, streptococcal perianal dermatitis, recurrent toxin-mediated perianal erythema, impetigo, and toxic shock syndrome
- *Gram-negative enteric bacteria*: *Enterococcus*, *Escherichia coli* abscess, pyoderma, and pruritus
- *Shigella* and *Salmonella*
- *Yersinia enterocolitica*, *Streptococcus viridans*, *Haemophilus influenzae*—pediatric vulvovaginitis (hemorrhagic type)
- *Treponema pallidum*: Primary chancre
- *Haemophilus ducreyi*: Chancroid
- *Viral infections*: Molluscum contagiosum, condyloma acuminata, herpes genitalis, herpes zoster involving the sacral dermatoses, hand, foot, and mouth disease, Lipschutz ulcers, and HIV
- *Fungal infections*: Dermatophytosis and candidiasis
- *Parasitic and helminthic infections*: Scabies, enterobius vermicularis (pinworm) infection—pruritus ani with or without dermatitis
- *Rare*: Chancriform pyoderma

Noninfectious
Inflammatory dermatosis:

A. *Predominant morphological presentation with papules, plaques, and scaling*:
Broadly encompassing the entity called as "diaper dermatitis":
- Allergic and irritant contact dermatitis
- Napkin (flexural) psoriasis
- Infantile seborrheic dermatitis
- Perianal pseudoverrucous papules and nodules (PPPN)

Other inflammatory dermatoses:
- Atopic dermatitis
- Lichen sclerosus et atrophicus (LSeA) and balanitis xerotica obliterans
- Lichen planus
- Lichen nitidus
- Kawasaki's disease

B. *Vesiculobullous, erosive, and ulcerative lesions*:
- *Severe forms of irritant contact dermatitis*: Jacquet's erosive dermatitis, granuloma gluteale infantum
- *Immunobullous diseases*: Linear immunoglobulin A (IgA) bullous dermatosis, bullous pemphigoid
- Darier disease and Hailey–Hailey disease

Rarely, mucous membrane pemphigoid, pemphigus vulgaris
- *Erythema multiforme*, Steven–Johnson syndrome, toxic epidermal necrolysis, and bullous fixed drug reaction
- *Aphthous ulcers*: Minor or herpetiform aphthae, recurrent aphthosis associated with pediatric Behçet's disease
- Erosive LSeA
- Systemic lupus erythematosus (sometimes may be associated with idiopathic genital ulcers)
- Vasculitis
- *Rare*: Cutaneous Crohn's disease

Nevoid entities and vascular malformations (VMs):
- *Pigmentary nevi*: Congenital and acquired melanocytes nevi
- Epidermal nevi
- Infantile and congenital (RICH, PICH, and NICH): Hemangiomas
- Arteriovenous malformations
- Lymphangioma circumscriptum

Developmental and anatomical:
- Ambiguous genitalia
- Cloacal opening
- Infantile perineal pyramidal protrusion
- Hymenal tags
- Median raphe cyst
- *Physiological entities*: Pearly penile papules and vulvar vestibular papillomatosis, and Fordyce spots

Neoplastic conditions:
- Langerhans cell histiocytosis
- Melanoma
- Granular cell tumor
- Syringoma
- Juvenile xanthogranuloma

Miscellaneous:
- *Nutritional*: Acrodermatitis enteropathica
- Hidradenitis suppurativa
  Flowcharts 1 to 3 outlining an arbitrary approach to pediatric genital dermatosis are depicted below.

PRACTICAL CONSIDERATIONS WHILE EXAMINING LESIONS INVOLVING THE ANOGENITAL LESIONS

A complete examination of anogenital dermatosis involves inspection and palpation of both the cutaneous and mucosal surfaces, internal examination as well as the other mucosae, and lymph nodes. The dermatological examination should focus on the following attributes:
- *Number or lesions*: Single or multiple, grouped or discrete
- Chronic/relapsing/recurrent
- Bilateral/unilateral, symmetrical
- Extent, with sparing or involvement of folds
- Presence of similar lesions over other parts/mucosae
- Presence of satellites
- *Demarcation*: Sharp or ill-defined
- Presence of lichenification

Moreover, as a dermatologist, one should also focus on ruling out pediatric sexual abuse.

The following signs are suggestive of child sexual abuse, based on the World Health Organization (WHO) guidelines.[1]
- Acute abrasions, lacerations, or bruising of the labia, perihymenal tissues, penis, and scrotum or perineum
- Hymenal notch/cleft extending through >50% of the width of the hymenal rim
- Scarring or fresh laceration of the posterior fourchette not involving the hymen (but unintentional trauma must be ruled out)
- Condyloma in children over the age of 2 years
- Significant anal dilatation or scarring

In this chapter, we have arbitrarily classified the genital lesions morphologically and outlined an approach likewise for diagnosis and therapy.

ARBITRARY MORPHOLOGICAL CLASSIFICATION OF PEDIATRIC GENITAL DERMATOSES

1. Papular, papulopustular, and papulonodular lesions
2. *Papulosquamous lesions*: Presenting as papules and plaques with scaling
3. Vesiculobullous and erosive lesions
4. Genital ulcers
5. Urethral or vaginal discharge

PAPULAR, PAPULOPUSTULAR, AND PAPULONODULAR LESIONS (TABLE 1)

Lesions may be folliculocentric, perifollicular or nonfollicular papules, pustules, or nodules. Infective folliculitis is the most common cause of pustular and papulopustular lesions in the genital area.

Other Rarer Causes of Genital Papular, Papulopustular and Papulonodular Lesions

- *Lichen nitidus*: Asymptomatic or mildly pruritic, pinpoint, flat-topped brownish to skin colored, grouped papular lesions
- *Eosinophilic folliculitis*: Sterile pustular and papulopustular, pruritic lesions
- *Lichen scrofulosorum*: Type of tuberculid, closely grouped skin colored to erythematous, multiple perifollicular or follicular papules with central necrosis, present over acral areas

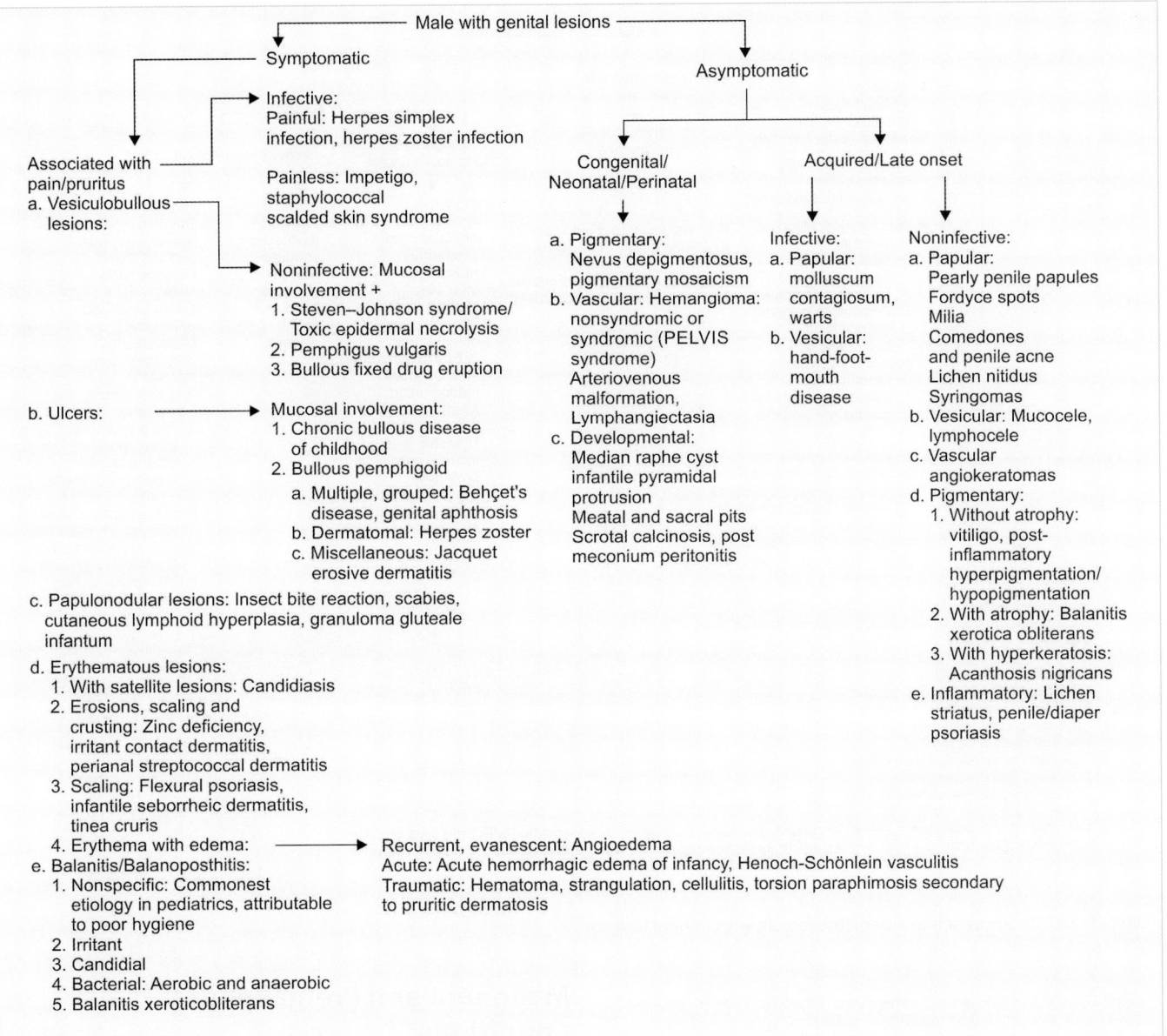

FLOWCHART 1: Approach to a pediatric male with genital lesions.

- *Xanthoma disseminatum*: Multiple rounds to oval, yellow-orange or brown papules, nodules, and plaques. Rare cases of vulvar intraepithelial neoplasia, squamous cell carcinoma of vulva, and primary B-cell lymphoma have been reported.
- *Verruciform xanthomas*:[2] Asymptomatic, pale or hyperkeratotic lesions with a pebbled surface and verrucous appearance.
- *Hidradenitis suppurativa*:[3,4] Painful abscesses, sinuses and scarring can uncommonly be seen in children and adolescents. Like in adults, axilla and groin regions are most commonly involved in children also. Pediatric patients with HS should be examined for any associated endocrine comorbidities (premature adrenarche or diabetes). Mild cases may be treated with topical clindamycin or topical 15–20% azelaic acid with or without systemic treatments. Systemic therapeutic options include antibiotics (clindamycin, rifampicin, moxifloxacin, and metronidazole used alone or in combination), oral prednisolone (0.5–1 mg/kg), and oral isotretinoin (0.7–1 mg/kg body weight/day). Other systemic modalities include antiandrogens (finasteride) and immunosuppressants [such as tumor necrosis factor (TNF-α) blockers]. Surgery may be needed for treating scars and sinuses.

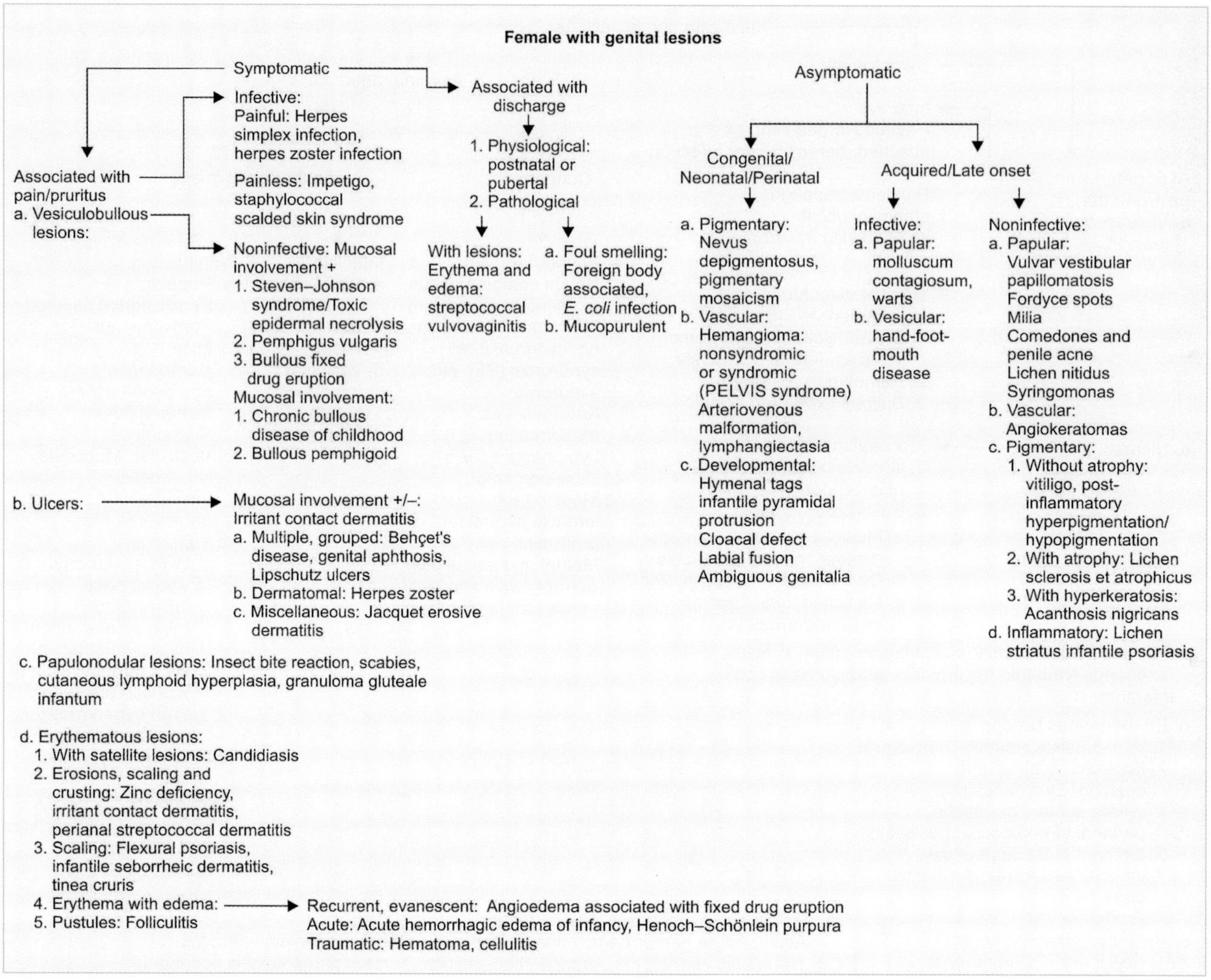

Female with genital lesions
Symptomatic
Asymptomatic
Associated with pain/pruritus
a. Vesiculobullous lesions:
Infective:
Painful: Herpes simplex infection, herpes zoster infection
Painless: Impetigo, staphylococcal scalded skin syndrome
Noninfective: Mucosal involvement +
1. Steven–Johnson syndrome/Toxic epidermal necrolysis
2. Pemphigus vulgaris
3. Bullous fixed drug eruption
Mucosal involvement:
1. Chronic bullous disease of childhood
2. Bullous pemphigoid
b. Ulcers:
Mucosal involvement +/–:
Irritant contact dermatitis
a. Multiple, grouped: Behçet's disease, genital aphthosis, Lipschutz ulcers
b. Dermatomal: Herpes zoster
c. Miscellaneous: Jacquet erosive dermatitis
c. Papulonodular lesions: Insect bite reaction, scabies, cutaneous lymphoid hyperplasia, granuloma gluteale infantum
d. Erythematous lesions:
1. With satellite lesions: Candidiasis
2. Erosions, scaling and crusting: Zinc deficiency, irritant contact dermatitis, perianal streptococcal dermatitis
3. Scaling: Flexural psoriasis, infantile seborrheic dermatitis, tinea cruris
4. Erythema with edema:
5. Pustules: Folliculitis
Recurrent, evanescent: Angioedema associated with fixed drug eruption
Acute: Acute hemorrhagic edema of infancy, Henoch–Schönlein purpura
Traumatic: Hematoma, cellulitis
Associated with discharge
1. Physiological: postnatal or pubertal
2. Pathological
With lesions: Erythema and edema: streptococcal vulvovaginitis
a. Foul smelling: Foreign body associated, E. coli infection
b. Mucopurulent
Congenital/ Neonatal/Perinatal
a. Pigmentary: Nevus depigmentosus, pigmentary mosaicism
b. Vascular: Hemangioma: nonsyndromic or syndromic (PELVIS syndrome) Arteriovenous malformation, lymphangiectasia
c. Developmental: Hymenal tags infantile pyramidal protrusion Cloacal defect Labial fusion Ambiguous genitalia
Acquired/Late onset
Infective:
a. Papular: molluscum contagiosum, warts
b. Vesicular: hand-foot-mouth disease
Noninfective:
a. Papular: Vulvar vestibular papillomatosis Fordyce spots Milia Comedones and penile acne Lichen nitidus Syringomonas
b. Vascular: Angiokeratomas
c. Pigmentary:
1. Without atrophy: vitiligo, post-inflammatory hyperpigmentation/ hypopigmentation
2. With atrophy: Lichen sclerosis et atrophicus
3. With hyperkeratosis: Acanthosis nigricans
d. Inflammatory: Lichen striatus infantile psoriasis

FLOWCHART 2: Approach to a pediatric female with genital lesions.

Pediatric genital dermatoses and genital involvement as a part of generalized dermatological conditions
a. Inflammatory dermatoses:
– Presenting with papules, plaques:
Psoriasis vulgaris: Vulval and penile lesions
Lichen planus: Erosive, papular, reticulate
Atopic dermatitis
Darier disease
– Presenting with erythema and scaling:
Recurrent toxin mediated perianal erythema (RTPE)
Kawasaki disease
Toxic shock syndrome
Convalescent phase
b. Neoplastic: Langerhans cell histiocytosis
c. Infections:
– Sexually transmitted infections: Congenital syphilis, condyloma lata, herpes genitalis (in victims of pediatric sexual abuse)
– Non STI: TB: Tuberculous chancre, Lymphadenopathy, sinus, cold abscess Neiserria meningitidis

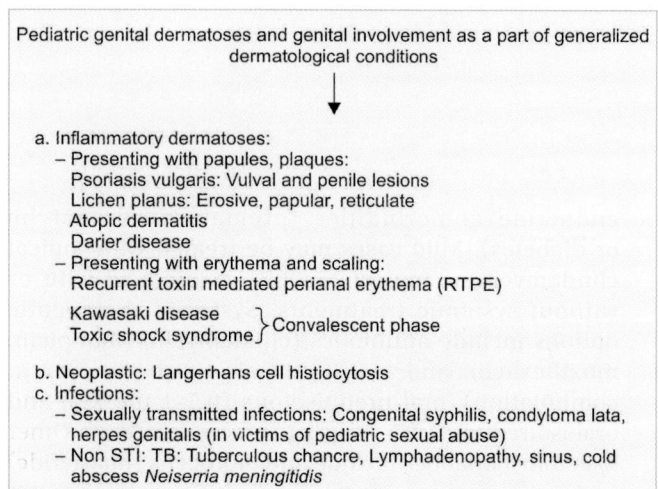

FLOWCHART 3: Approach to a pediatric patient with perineal involvement as a part of generalized dermatosis.

(STI: sexually transmitted infection; TB: tuberculosis)

Malignant and Premalignant Conditions[5-7]

- *Rhabdomyosarcoma*: Firm painless swelling over penis, perineum, or vagina

Involvement of genitalia in these dermatoses is extremely rare.

PAPULOSQUAMOUS DERMATOSES (TABLE 2)

The most commonly encountered entity in this group falls under the broad classification of "diaper dermatitis".

A history of diaper usage, use of various soaps, antiseptics, and topical applications in the area is important for consideration of differentials. Involvement of key extragenital sites serves as a diagnostic marker for many conditions.

CHAPTER 20 A Child with Genital Lesions

Table 1: Papular, papulopustular, and papulonodular lesions.

Dermatological condition	Mucocutaneous lesions of perineal region	Extraperineal involvement	Extracutaneous features if any	Salient distinguishing features	Differential diagnosis	Investigations	Management
Scabies History points: • Family history of pruritus, similar lesions • Nocturnal aggravation of pruritus	Extremely pruritic papules associated with the burrows (so-called as the "larval papules", burrows and nodules)	Burrows and pruritic papules over interdigital areas, axillae, neck, and periumbilical area (circle of Hebra) In infants and neonates, lesions occur over the head and neck	• Poststreptococcal glomerulonephritis may occur as a complication • Secondary impetigo	The flexural crease between the buttock and upper thigh is one of the hallmark sites	• Papular urticaria • Atopic dermatitis • Lichen planus • Infantile acropustulosis • Cutaneous mastocytosis	• Direct microscopy of burrow scraping (KOH mount) • Dermoscopy of the burrow showing "jet with contrail" or "delta sign"	• First-line therapy for infants >2 months of age is topical permethrin 5% cream to be applied overnight over the entire body, to patient and close contacts • ≤2 months of age: precipitate sulfur ointment in (2–10%) in petrolatum base Crotamiton (10%) • Other topical antiscabetic agents for children >5 years include: topical benzyl benzoate, sulfur (10–25%) • For infants and children >15 kg, oral ivermectin 200 µg/kg is considered safe for therapy
Molluscum contagiosum History points: History of similar lesions in close contacts, siblings	Dome-shaped pearly white papules with or without central umbilication BOTE sign— "Beginning of The End" Sign. It is regarded as a sign of impending resolution	Similar lesions over other parts of body	Giant genital molluscs and extensive mollusca: look for HIV and immunocompromised status	Asymptomatic, pearly, umbilicated appearance	• Milia • Verruca plana • Lichen nitidus	• Giemsa staining reveals molluscum bodies • Dermoscopy shows radial, punctiform or crown-like vessel pattern	• In immunocompetent pediatric patients spontaneous resolution is the rule • Extraction of the molluscum body with a curette may be done • Ranitidine: 5 mg/kg dose over 8 weeks has been reported to show response

Continued

Continued

Dermatological condition	Mucocutaneous lesions of perineal region	Extraperineal involvement	Extracutaneous features if any	Salient distinguishing features	Differential diagnosis	Investigations	Management
• Genital warts History: History of warts in caretaker or siblings, history of sexual abuse, where relevant • Mode of transmission: >3 years, sexual abuse should be ruled out Nonsexual transmission via autoinoculation (HPV2), Hand-genital contact from affected children or adults has been described <3 years—vertical transmission during vaginal delivery	Cauliflower-like flat or pedunculated growths, more over the perianal region	Verruca vulgaris or verruca plana over other body sites	In cases of perinatal transmission, especially of HPV6 and -11, recurrent respiratory papillomatosis is a rare complication involving the upper respiratory tract and is usually detected between 1 and 3 years of age, presenting with hoarseness and respiratory problems	Typical morphology	• Molluscum • Verrucous herpes simplex infection in immunocompromised patient • Perianal pseudoverrucous papules and nodules • Condyloma lata	—	• "Wait and watch (75% spontaneous remission within 3 years) • 5% imiquimod cream • Cryotherapy for large (persisting) anogenital warts: CO_2 laser, pulsed-dye laser, surgical removal
Condyloma lata	See **Table 4A** (syphilis)						
Perianal pseudoverrucous papules and nodules	See text (chronic irritant diaper dermatitis: Complications)						
Granuloma gluteale infantum	See text (chronic irritant diaper dermatitis: Complications)	May or may not be involved					
Gram-positive: Staphylococcus aureus—most common	Painful, tender, papules, pustules and suppurative nodules, with or without purulent discharge		Furunculosis and abscess more likely to develop	MRSA and panton valentine leukocidin factor producing variants are associated with larger, more erythematous, painful lesions, with a positive family history		Generally, a clinical diagnosis; swab culture and sensitivity for suspected MRSA cases	• Topical mupirocin 1% cream or ointment, topical fusidic acid 2% cream • Oral amoxicillin, cefixime in weight appropriate dosage

Continued

Continued

Dermatological condition	Mucocutaneous lesions of perineal region	Extraperineal involvement	Extracutaneous features if any	Salient distinguishing features	Differential diagnosis	Investigations	Management
Gram-negative folliculitis Hot tub folliculitis—Pseudomonas species History of exposure to hot bath, shared bath tubs, contaminated swimming pool	Papular, vesiculopustular, urticarial pruritic eruption	Buttocks, proximal extremities, trunk An associated otitis externa may coexist	With or without associated fever and malaise	Pleomorphic lesions with history of exposure to hot bath tubs/contaminated tub toys, swimming pool		Generally, a clinical diagnosis Gram stain may identify presence of multiple gram-negative rods	Simple cases subside spontaneously within 2 weeks: • Topical mupirocin, with or without systemic cephalosporins (cephalexin, cefixime, cefadroxil)
Herpes simplex folliculitis	Presents similarly as bacterial folliculitis; however, tendency to form papulovesicles and grouped distribution is clinically suggestive of herpetic folliculitis	May be associated with herpes genitalis		Papulovesicles, tendency to grouping		A Tzanck smear from the papulovesicular lesion may show presence of multinucleated giant cells	Acyclovir in the dose of 10–15 mg/kg in 3–4 divided doses
Molluscum contagiosum folliculitis	Very rare Follicular, pruritic nonumbilicated papular lesions	Over head and neck region, extensive umbilicated and nonumbilicated erythematous papules and nodules have been reported		Extensive lesions have been associated with immunocompromised status		Giemsa stain may identify presence of molluscum bodies Histopathology is suggestive of molluscum bodies in the follicular epithelium	Cryotherapy
Malessezia folliculitis History of travel to tropical climate, immunosuppression±	Small, monomorphic, erythematous, pruritic papules Majority of cases are pubertal or postpubertal, and perineal lesions have generally not been described	Extragenital sites are more commonly involved; chest back, upper arms, neck and face	Associated seborrheic dermatitis and pityriasis versicolor may be present In neonates, it presents as neonatal acne	—	—	Direct microscopy of potassium hydroxide-based wet mount shows presence of Malessezia yeasts	Various azole antifungal creams or lotions: twice daily for 2 weeks
Candidial folliculitis	Follicular pustular, pruritic lesions, often seen as satellite lesions surrounding the plaques of candidiasis	Extragenital sites, including other flexures may be involving		Prolonged corticosteroid or antibiotic therapy		Gram stain shows presence of gram-positive yeast and pseudohyphae	Topical azole antifungals, clotrimazole, miconazole, are generally sufficient

Table 2: Papulosquamous dermatoses.

Dermatological condition	Mucocutaneous feature	Extragenital involvement	Salient differentiating feature	Differential diagnosis	Investigations, if any	Management
Candidiasis Perineal (candidosis of infancy or candidal diaper dermatitis) (Fig. 1)	Pruritic, red, glazed plaques with a scalloped margin, with peripheral, superficial, rapidly exfoliating pustule (Fig. 5). Satellite pustular lesions considered almost diagnostic of the condition	Similar lesions may be present over other flexures, especially the neck in infants	Satellite pustules, rapidly exfoliating "fragile" pustules surrounding the typical glazed plaques	Infantile seborrheic dermatitis Infantile flexural psoriasis Langerhans cell histiocytosis Acrodermatitis enteropathica	Presence of yeasts with pseudohyphae on Gram-stained preparation of contents of the pustules	Topical antifungals—clotrimazole 1% cream, miconazole 1% cream may generally suffice
Dermatophytosis (Fig. 2)	Erythematous scaly plaques with central clearing and peripheral scaling	Tinea corporis, Faciei, manuum, pedis, and onychomycosis may or may not coexist	Typical pruritic annular scaly plaques with central clearing	Erythema annulare centrifugum, granuloma annulare (however occurrence of these dermatoses in genital area is extremely rare)	Observation of hyphae under KOH mount	Itraconazole 5 mg/kg oral suspension, fluconazole (50 mg/mL solution available for pediatric use) Terbinafine is approved for use in age-group >4 years Topical antifungals (clotrimazole 1% cream, miconazole 1% cream) Duration of therapy is variable.[8]
Perianal infectious dermatitis (perianal streptococcal dermatitis/perianal cellulitis)	Most commonly encountered in the age-group of 6–10 months Sharply demarcated, intensely erythematous and edematous, painful perianal erythema with or without overlying mucopurulent exudate, superficial erosions and fissuring	Acral desquamation, following resolution after therapy, has been noted, and is exotoxin mediated	Sharply demarcated erythema, pain and edema over the perianal region Cellulitis-like appearance with variable exudate	Candidial intertrigo Infantile seborrheic dermatitis Congenital syphilis Desquamation phase resembles Kawasaki's disease Staphylococcal-scalded skin syndrome	Generally, not required Local and throat swab shows presence of group A beta-hemolytic Streptococcus	Topical—mupirocin 1% cream or ointment, fusidic acid 2% cream Systemic—amoxicillin, cefixime in weight appropriate dosage Bland emollients for local application in the desquamation phase
Recurrent toxin-mediated perianal erythema (Fig. 3)	Recurrent episodes of asymptomatic perianal erythema, followed by rapid desquamation	Acral areas may show similar desquamation	Recurrent asymptomatic episodes, conspicuously lacks any systemic symptoms	Kawasaki disease	Positive throat swab for Streptococcus; local swab—negative as it is an exotoxin-mediated disease	Amoxicillin in weight-based dosage
Allergic contact dermatitis	Erythema, papules, plaques, scaling, and papulovesicular lesions involving the whole of the diaper area including the folds		Involvement of folds and convexities History: Use of diapers, sanitary wiping tissues, inadvertent application of topicals, even emollients	Irritant contact dermatitis Atopic dermatitis Psoriasis Seborrheic dermatitis	—	Identification of the inciting agent and avoidance of the same Short course of low-potency topical corticosteroid

Continued

Dermatological condition	Mucocutaneous feature	Extragenital involvement	Salient differentiating feature	Differential diagnosis	Investigations, if any	Management
Irritant contact dermatitis (inflammation occurring secondary to contact with fecal and urinary irritants or scrubbing of diapers with a high pH detergent, in an occlusive microenvironment) (Fig. 4)	Erythema, papules, small plaques, scaling involving the areas in contact with the diaper, the convexities of the skin, including buttocks, inner sides of the thighs, mons pubis, and genitalia (labia, scrotum), sparing the folds		Sparing of folds with involvement of convexities Erosive lesions may concur	Same as allergic contact dermatitis	—	• Maintenance of proper hygiene, frequent diaper change, use of pH-buffered wipes • Use of disposable diapers to prevent hyperhydration of the perineal skin • Bland emollient
Infantile seborrheic dermatitis	Salmon-colored, well-demarcated plaques with yellowish greasy scales involving the diaper area, scalp, face, and other flexures Pruritus is minimal or absent as compared to contact eczema or atopic dermatitis	Well-demarcated, dry looking bilaterally symmetrical, flexural plaques Involvement of scalp (cradle cap) and other flexures	Pruritus is minimal or absent as compared to contact eczema or atopic dermatitis	Same as allergic contact dermatitis		• Generally benign and self-resolving • Low-potent topical corticosteroids (1% hydrocortisone cream) or topical calcineurin inhibitors for short time
Infantile atopic dermatitis History: Suggestive of atopy and presence of other atopic stigmata aid in the diagnosis	Diaper area is generally spared in atopic dermatitis. However, occasionally, it may involve the genitocrural and perianal regions, presenting as eczematous, erythematous rash, more pronounced over the convex surfaces	Involvement of the extensor aspects of the limbs, and cheek	Intense pruritus	Same as allergic contact dermatitis		Emollients and topical corticosteroids (low potency)
Infantile psoriasis Predilection in infants <2 years History of sore throat may be present	Sharply demarcated, erythematous, glazed looking plaques with scaling, involving the groin and perianal folds	• Other flexures, periumbilical region, scalp, retroauricular region and external auditory canals • Infantile psoriasis often develops secondary to perianal streptococcal dermatitis, probably as a Koebner's phenomenon or poststreptococcal pharyngitis	Lack of pruritus	Same as allergic contact dermatitis		Topical low- to mid-potent corticosteroids and emollients

Continued

Continued

Dermatological condition	Mucocutaneous feature	Extragenital involvement	Salient differentiating feature	Differential diagnosis	Investigations, if any	Management
Acrodermatitis enteropathica[9] History of diarrhea and failure to thrive	Presents in infancy as erythematous, desquamative, and erosive plaques involving the periorificial areas	Periorificial and acral involvement Alopecia Cheilitis, stomatitis		Same as allergic contact dermatitis Congenital syphilis	—	Supplementing with elemental zinc in a dosage of 3 mg/kg/day is required Among many available formulations, zinc sulfate is the preferred oral formulation and zinc chloride is preferred for parenteral supplementation
Langerhans cell histiocytosis[10]	Crusted or scaly papules and papulovesicles over the inguinal fold and other parts of body are the most common presentation of skin LCH	• The cutaneous presentation is variable and pleomorphic, with vesiculopustular, erosive, ulcerative, purpuric, and even vascular tumor-like lesions affecting the scalp, retroauricular areas and other flexures • Nail involvement can occur in the form of longitudinal grooving, onycholysis, subungual hyperkeratosis, subungual pustules, purpuric striae of the nail bed, V-shaped notches, pterygium formation, and end elkonyxis (oval depression in the nail plate) • Paronychial erythema and swelling as well as nailfold destruction have also been reported	Extracutaneous involvement of musculoskeletal and central nervous system Failure to thrive	Same as allergic contact dermatitis Jacquet erosive dermatitis Candidiasis	Imaging remains the gold standard for diagnosis and staging Presence of punched out lytic lesions of the bones-hallmark	Patients with LCH limited to the skin may be observed. If the skin lesions do not spontaneously resolve, a variety of methods may be used, including topical steroids, oral methotrexate or thalidomide, topical nitrogen mustard, or psoralens with UV light. A single bone lesion involving the frontal, parietal, occipital bones, and any other bones may be treated by curettage only or curettage with a local injection of methylprednisolone. Other skull lesions (mastoid, temporal, or orbital) should be treated with chemotherapy or radiotherapy or both

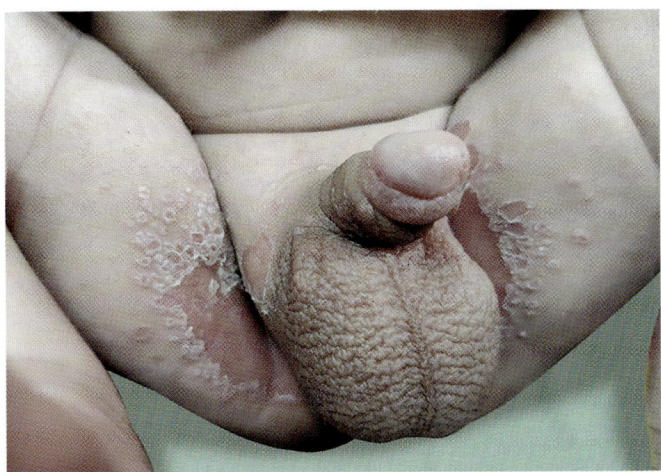

FIG. 1: Well-defined, bilaterally symmetrical plaques with an eroded surface, with multiple, grouped, peripheral arranged satellite lesions and marginal, whitish scales over groin fold, suggestive of candidal intertrigo.

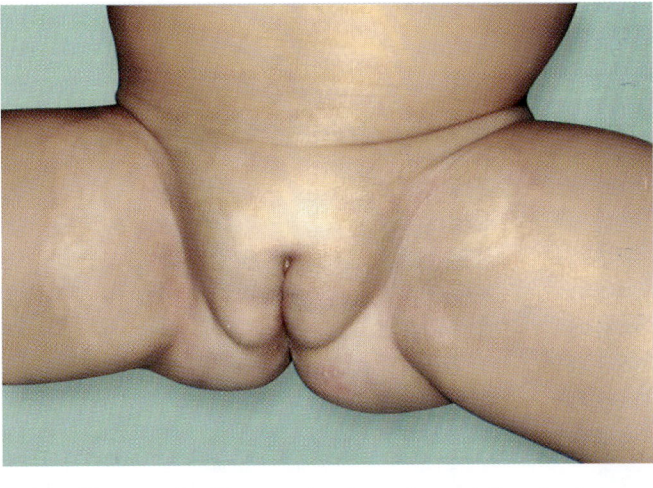

FIG. 2: Tinea cruris with secondary hypopigmentation due to topical steroid application.

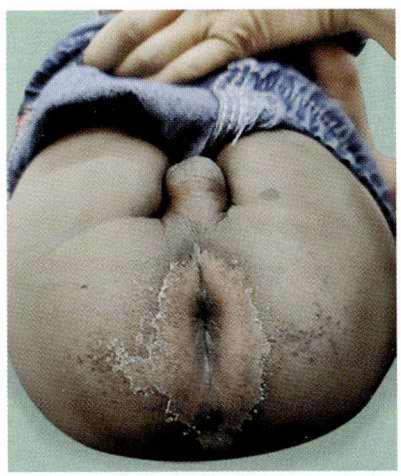

FIG. 3: Recurrent toxin-mediated perianal erythema: dry, brownish-red plaques with peripheral exfoliation over the intergluteal cleft, extending to the perianal area.

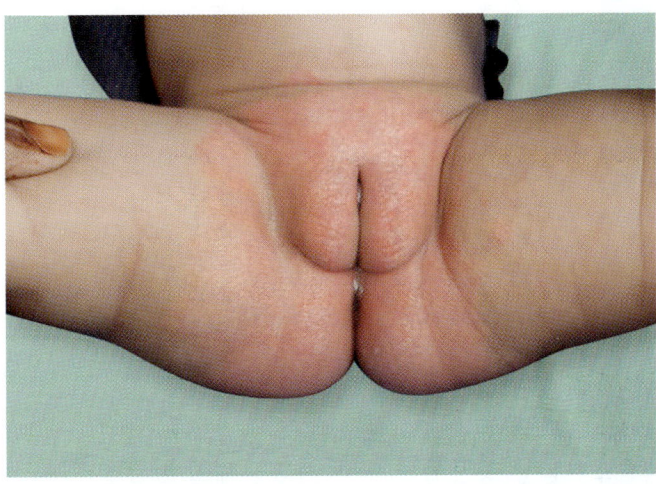

FIG. 4: Irritant contact dermatitis due to diaper wear in a patient with diarrhea. Involvement of convexities is characteristic.

Chronic Irritant Diaper Dermatitis: Complications

Chronic irritant contact dermatitis predisposes to occurrence of a spectrum of cutaneous manifestations of diaper dermatitis, encompassing the following three entities:
1. Granuloma gluteale infantum
2. Jacquet erosive dermatitis
3. Perianal pseudoverrucous papules and nodules

The predisposing factors are the same as irritant contact dermatitis, albeit of a chronic nature. Like chronic urinary and fecal incontinence due to spinal dysraphism, surgical anastomosis of the gut and stomas, and fistulas.

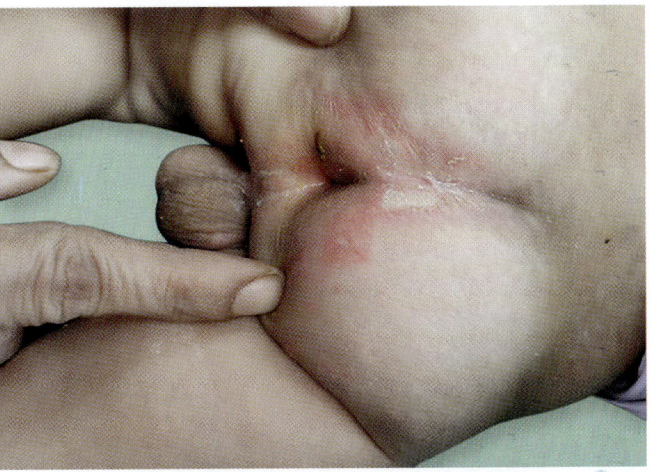

FIG. 5: Jacquet erosive dermatitis: severe irritant contact dermatitis of the diaper area with superficial erosions with a yellowish base.

Table 3: Vesiculobullous and erosive lesions.

Dermatological condition	Mucocutaneous lesions of perineal region/mucosal involvement	Extraperineal involvement	Differential diagnosis	Investigation	Management
Bullous impetigo (Fig. 6)	• Small vesicles that coalesce to form pus-filled bullae with surrounding erythema • Resolve with erythema surrounded by a collarette of scale and heal without scarring	Around mouth and nose, other parts of the body may also have discrete lesions	• Bullous FDE • Paederus dermatitis • Vulvar pemphigoid (childhood localized bullous pemphigoid)	• None • Local culture from fluid of an intact bullae may be positive	• Mupirocin 2% cream or ointment Retapamulin 1% ointment • Fusidic acid • Oral antibiotics for larger bullae—cephalexin, clindamycin augmentin
Staphylococcal scalded skin syndrome	• Generalized erythema and skin tenderness, followed by development of flaccid, large bullae • Extensive denudation leaving behind large raw areas, rapidly covered by thin crusting, accentuated over flexures • Nikolsky sign: positive	• Preceded by fever, irritability, and malaise • Characteristic perioral and perinasal radial fissuring and crusting • Conspicuous sparing of mucosa	• Steven–Johnson syndrome and toxic epidermal necrolysis • TEN-like lupus erythematosus	• Blood culture • Swab culture form perinasal, nasopharynx, perianal, and periurethral regions	• Require hospitalization and parenteral antibiotic drug therapy. • Supportive treatment for skin barrier recovery
Herpes simplex (Fig. 7)	Multiple grouped vesicles and erosions with polycyclic margins over an erythematous base, associated with burning and pain	• Presence of herpes-associated erythema multiforme • Herpes simplex virus may secondarily complicate atopic dermatitis and diaper dermatitis; generalized involvement (Kaposi's varicelliform eruption) can occur as a complication	• Insect bite reaction • Hand–foot–mouth disease • Lipshutz ulcers	• Tzanck smear • HSV, DNA, PCR from blister fluid	See **Table 4A** (pediatric STI)

Varicella	Frequently affects the genitals, manifesting as mucosal erosions and vesicles along with a blood-stained penile or vaginal discharge can be associated with pruritus. The lesions may be localized below napkin, especially when there is associated napkin dermatitis, without evident blistering elsewhere on the body. (Harper)	Pleomorphic rash with multiple umbilicated vesicles in different stages of evolution	• Kaposi's varicelliform eruption
			• Erythema multiforme (generalized rash)
			• For genital lesions:
			  ○ Genital herpes
			  ○ Lipshutz ulcers
			  ○ Genital aphthosis
				Tzanck smear	• *For uncomplicated cases,* acyclovir (20 mg/kg/dose in four divided doses over 5 days)
					• *For patients with CNS/lung involvement:* Injectable acyclovir 10 mg/kg in three divided doses over 7–10 days.

Continued

Continued

Dermatological condition	Mucocutaneous lesions of perineal region/mucosal involvement	Extraperineal involvement	Differential diagnosis	Investigation	Management
Herpes zoster	Sacral herpes zoster may present with unilateral genital erosions	Usually, dermatomal involvement	• Zosteriform HSV • Insect bite reaction	• Clinical diagnosis is the mainstay • Tzanck smear	Acyclovir 20 mg/kg/dose in four divided doses for 5–7 days
Hand–foot–mouth disease (Fig. 8)		• Vesicles surrounded by a thin halo of erythema, eventually rupturing and forming superficial ulcers with a gray-yellow base and erythematous rim • Involvement of buttocks and genitalia • Usually, nonpruritic and not painful • Macular, papular, or vesicular exanthem over dorsum of the hand, feet, buttocks, legs, and arms	Herpes simplex infection	Usually clinical diagnosis	Most patients recover within a few weeks without any residual sequelae. The acute illness usually lasts 10–14 days, and the infection rarely recurs or persists
Pemphigus vulgaris (childhood—<12 years, juvenile between 12 and 18 years)	Mucosal involvement common (oral>genital)	• Flaccid blister • Persistent painful erosion and crust	• Sexual abuse • Bullous FDR • Bullous lichen sclerosis • Erosive lichen planus	• *Histopathology*: Intraepidermal blister (acantholysis) • Dermal plasma-histiocytic infiltrate with eosinophils • *DIF*: Intercellular space deposition of IgG (Fishnet or chicken wire appearance)	• Systemic corticosteroid • Rituximab (moderate-to-severe refractory disease) • *Other*: Dapsone, MMF, azathioprine
Paraneoplastic autoimmune multiorgan syndrome (paraneoplastic pemphigus)	Mucosal involvement can be first manifestation (oral > genital)	Polymorphous cutaneous eruptions over body	• BP • EM • Lichen planus • Graft vs. host disease	• *Histopathology*: Suprabasal acantholysis with interface/lichenoid infiltrate associate necrotic keratinocyte • *DIF*: Intercellular and basement membrane deposition of IgG and C3	• Management of underlying associated neoplasm • Palliative immunosuppression with systemic corticosteroids, mycophenolate mofetil, rituximab, intravenous Ig plasmapheresis
Childhood bullous pemphigoid (infantile BP: First year of life, childhood BP: Peak around the age of 8 years)	Mucosal involvement common with childhood form	• Tense bullae with urticarial plaques over body • *Infantile form*: Predominantly involve palmoplantar region, genital lesions rare • *Childhood form*: Mainly involve face and external genitalia	CBDC Epidermolysis bullosa acquisita	• *Histopathology*: *Early lesion*—dermal edema, perivascular lymph histiocytic infiltrate with eosinophils and eosinophilic spongiosis • *Blisters*: Subepidermal blister with inflammatory cells including eosinophils (rarely the blisters can be cell-poor) • *DIF*: Linear deposition of IgG or C3 at the basement membrane zone	• Resolve spontaneously • Mild or localized—topical steroids • *Severe forms*: Systemic oral corticosteroids

Continued

Continued

Dermatological condition	Mucocutaneous lesions of perineal region/mucosal involvement	Extraperineal involvement	Differential diagnosis	Investigation	Management
Chronic bullous disease of the childhood	Can involve mucosa	• Tense, polymorphic bullae arranged in an annular configuration, often (string of pearls or ring of jewels) • *Site:* Lower extremities and genitals, occasionally face and upper arms	• Bullous impetigo • Dermatitis herpetiformis • Bullous pemphigoid • Erythema multiforme	• *Histopathology:* Subepidermal blister with neutrophilic predominant infiltrate • *DIF:* Linear IgA deposition along dermal–epidermal junction	Dapsone with or without systemic steroids
Bullous systemic lupus erythematosus	Can involve mucosa	• Noncicatricial bullous eruption • Mainly sun-exposed areas but can involve sun-protected area also	• Acquired epidermolysis bullosa • Dermatitis herpetiformis bullous	• *Histopathology:* Subepidermal blister filled with fibrin, lymphomononuclear cells and neutrophils • Thickening of the basement membrane with mild perivascular lymphoplasmacytic infiltrate in dermis • *DIF:* Linear IgG, IgA, and C3 deposition in the basement membrane zone and granular IgM	Dapsone, prednisone, azathioprine, cyclophosphamide or methotrexate
Epidermolysis bullosa (EB)	Genitourinary tract involvement in EB coincides with the severity of the EB subtype	Blistering, erosion, or ulceration over trauma-prone site	Immunobullous disorders Traumatic (suckling, friction blister)	• *Histopathology:* Usually not recommended • *Depending on subtype:* Intraepidermal to subepidermal cleavage (EB simplex—epidermolytic, junctional EB—lucidolytic, dystrophic EB—dermolytic) • *Immunofluorescence antigen mapping (IFM) is preferred*	Comprehensive multidisciplinary and multimodal approach
Bullous fixed drug eruption	Predilection sites: oral–genital mucosa, perineal area, trunk	Well-demarcated oval, erythematous patches, with overlying hemorrhagic bullae, associated with burning and itching	• Acute graft versus host disease • Stevens–Johnson syndrome or toxic epidermal necrolysis • Subacute cutaneous lupus erythematosus	• *Histopathology: Epidermis—*Dyskeratotic keratinocytes, parakeratosis vacuolar interface changes, lymphocytic exocytosis • *Dermis:* Eosinophils and plasma cells in dermis	• Withdrawal of the offending drug • Localized lesion topical corticosteroids • Generalized involvement may require short course of systemic corticosteroids

Continued

Continued

Dermatological condition	Mucocutaneous lesions of perineal region/mucosal involvement	Extraperineal involvement	Differential diagnosis	Investigation	Management
Erythema multiforme	• Oral mucosa (most common) • Oculogenital • Painful	Typical or atypical target lesions	• Urticaria • Erythema nodosum • Bullous pemphigoid • Dermatitis herpetiformis	*Histopathology:* *Epidermal—* • Apoptotic individual keratinocytes (earliest histological change) • Hydropic degeneration of basal keratinocytes • Intercellular edema • Intraepidermal/subepidermal blister • Epidermal necrosis without large sheets of epidermal necrosis *Dermal:* Moderate/dense perivascular lymphocytic infiltrate in the papillary dermis and along the dermoepidermal junction (DEJ) Superficial dermal edema *DIF:* Granular C3 and IgM at basement membrane and in vessels	• Management is multifaceted, with treatment of probable or proven causative agent
Bullous lichen planus	• Upper and lower extremities • Mucosae	Development of bullae over or near preexisting lesions	Lichen planus pemphigoides	*DIF:* • Fibrillar band of fibrin along dermoepidermal junction • Civatte bodies highlighted with IgM, IgA, and C3	• Topical potent corticosteroids • Systemic corticosteroids including oral mini pulse therapy • Dapsone has also been proved to be efficacious, especially in pediatric BLP

(DIF: direct immunofluorescence; FDR: fixed-drug reaction; HSV: herpes simplex virus; PCR: polymerase chain reaction; STI: sexually transmitted infection)

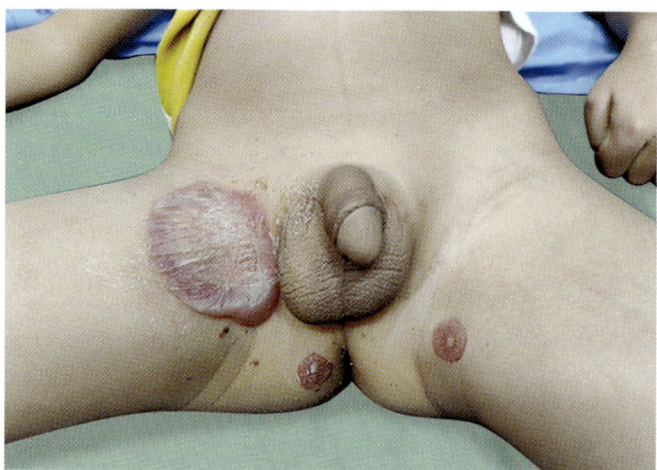

FIG. 6: Bullous impetigo: A large, flaccid bulla with sanguinopurulent fluid over the groin fold, two, circular erosions with a dry, hemorrhagic base and scaly margins over the lower aspect of perineal region.

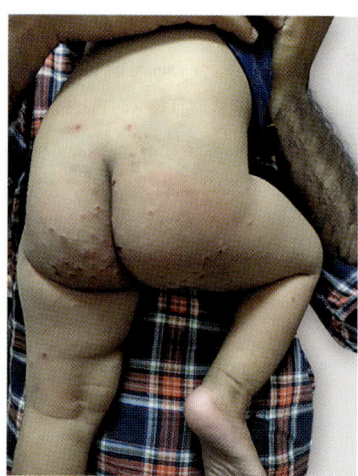

FIG. 8: Hand–foot–mouth disease: anogenital lesions—typical erythematous papulovesicles and small plaques with central erosions covered with hemorrhagic crusting present over the buttocks.

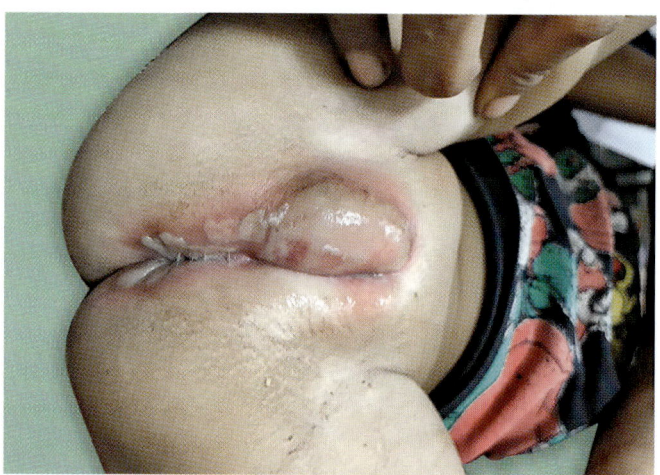

FIG. 7: Herpes genitalis in a sexual abuse victim.

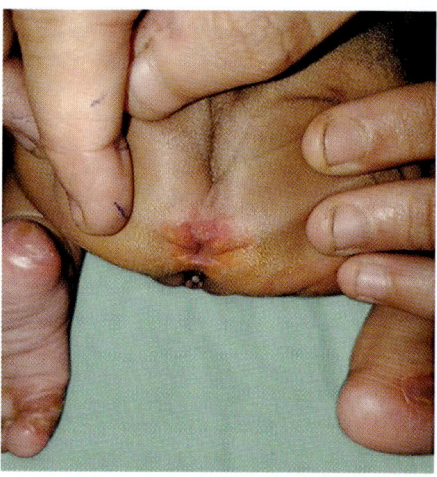

FIG. 9: Congenital syphilis: Erosive perianal dermatitis; patient's and maternal rapid plasma regain test in serial dilution strongly positive.

Granuloma Gluteale Infantum[11]

Contributory etiopathogenetic factors:
- Topical mid to high potent, fluorinated corticosteroids
- Foreign materials such as talc and starch
- Use of reusable diapers
- Candidiasis (Questionable role)
- Increased absorption of topical corticosteroids through inflamed skin of the diaper area can induce alterations in dermal collagen, which is responsible for some of the unique clinical features of granuloma gluteale infantum

Clinical features: An asymptomatic, reddish brown to purplish, firm, deep-seated papules and papulonodules with central erosion and ulceration, distributed over the convexities, with sparing of folds. Similar lesions can also occur in peristomal areas (e.g., in patients with Hirschsprung's disease).

The course is chronic and protracted with slow healing after removal of aggravating factors.

Management:
- Removal and subsequent avoidance of inciting and precipitating agents forms the cornerstone of therapy.
- *Local skin care*: Prevention of secondary bacterial infection, bland topical preparations with zinc oxide and petroleum jelly for restoration of skin barrier
- Low-potent topical corticosteroids (short contact) and topical calcineurin inhibitors (age >3 months) to minimize morbidity[12]

Jacquet Erosive Dermatitis

Clinical features: Also known historically as dermatitis syphiloides posterosiva, Jacquet erosive dermatitis is a severe variant of irritant diaper dermatitis, characterized by *papuloerosive lesions, sharp cut, punched out or crateriform ulcers* in the diaper area. Reddish purple umbilicated papules, which slowly evolve into ulcerative lesions that heal with atrophy and hypopigmentation, are classically described **(Fig. 5)**.

The clinical course is again chronic and protracted with variable response to various topical therapies.[13]

Management: On the lines of granuloma gluteale infantum. Use of oral antibiotics may be required in some cases. The response shows a high inter-individual variability and often a combination of multiple topical antimicrobials, antifungal, and barrier repair agents, after removal of inciting agent, results in a slow and complete remission.

Perianal Pseudoverrucous Papules and Nodules[14]

Considered as a unique type of chronic irritant dermatitis, PPPN is characterized by a hyperplastic response of the skin to chronic area. This reaction has been given various names: chronic papillomatous dermatitis, granulomas, hyperkeratosis, hyperplasia, pseudoepitheliomatous hyperplasia, and reactive acanthosis.

Age-group: Although any age-group is affected, generally infants rather than neonates.

Clinical features: Variously sized, shiny, moist-looking dome-shaped papules (≤10 mm) with a friable surface and small verrucous papules and small nodules over the convexities of groin and buttocks and also perianal area. Secondary infection is very common.

Management: Avoidance of precipitating factors, prevention of secondary infections by repeated swab cultures of perianal and peristomal sites. Topical application of potato protease inhibitors has been promoted as a novel approach in preventing protease-induced perianal dermatitis.[15]

VESICULOBULLOUS AND EROSIVE LESIONS

Table 3 represent various vesiculobullous and erosive lesions.

ULCERATIVE AND EROSIVE GENITAL DERMATOSIS (TABLES 4A AND B)

Genital ulcers can be a part of sexually transmitted infections or noninfective. For the purposes of simplicity in description, they are described separately in **Tables 4A and B**, with their specific clinical features and management guidelines.

URETHRAL OR VAGINAL DISCHARGE (TABLES 5A AND B)

For the purposes of simplicity of description, sexually and nonsexually transmitted causes are described separately in **Tables 5A and B**.

NEVOID CONDITIONS (TABLE 6)

The congenital nevi in skin represent developmental abnormalities caused by genetic mosaicism. They result from a proliferation of benign melanocytes in the dermis, epidermis, or both. They are believed to be the migratory paths of individual clones of genetically identical cells.[25] Congenital nevi are often present at birth while occasionally few nevi which may not be present at birth develop during the first 2 years of life. These are referred to as congenital nevus tardive.[26,27]

Genital nevi in children often concern the parents more frequently than nevi in any other body area.[28] While there are many studies on large congenital nevi, the exact prevalence of genital nevi in the pediatric population has not been studied in detail as most of these studies exclude genital area.[29]

DEVELOPMENTAL ANOMALIES OF GENITALIA

Table 7 represents the common developmental and anatomical abnormalities of genitalia.

VASCULAR LESIONS

Vascular lesions are divided into two groups by the International Society for the Study of Vascular Anomalies (ISSVA) classification: Vascular tumors (infantile hemangiomas being the most common) and VMs.

Vascular tumors are either present at birth, e.g., the congenital hemangiomas [rapidly involuting congenital hemangioma (RICH), partially involuting congenital hemangiomas (PICH), noninvoluting congenital hemangioma (NICH)], Kaposiform hemangioendothelioma (KHE), and multifocal lymphangioendotheliomatosis or are undetectable/minimally apparent at birth and appear in early life (infantile hemangiomas).[44] Any midline segmental vascular lesions involving lower back, buttocks, or perineum such as LUMBAR syndrome (Lower body hemangioma, Ulceration, Urogenital defects, Myelopathy, Bony deformities, Anorectal anomalies, Renal anomalies) should be considered for ultrasonography of the lower spine, abdomen, and pelvis.[45] Rarely, Blue Rubber Bleb Nevus Syndrome can present with hemangiomas over glans penis and vulva.[46]

Table 4A: Sexually acquired genital ulcerative disease.

Disease	Prepubertal mode of transmission	Vertical transmission	Clinical signs—perineal region	Clinical clues for diagnosis—extragenital region	Recommended evaluation	Management
Syphilis	Sexual transmission is most likely	+ Primary syphilis in a child > 4 months and secondary syphilis in a child >2 years is most probably an acquired infection	a. Syphilitic chancre: Chance begins as an erythematous macule —> papule —> ulcer Painless, well-defined and a rubbery base; associated with regional nontender adenopathy; in children, chancres are said to be smaller than in adults and less likely to be recognized. b. Secondary syphilis: Condyloma lata: flat-topped, moist papules over intertriginous areas, angle of mouth, external genitalia c. Congenital syphilis: Early congenital syphilis can present as multiple erythematous, eroded papules and/or erosions surrounding the periorificial and diaper areas **(Fig. 9)**	• Papular or papulosquamous rash in adult distribution, including palms and soles, with or without constitutional symptoms • Mucous patches have also been described • *Congenital syphilis:* About 60% of infants born with congenital syphilis are asymptomatic at birth Symptoms develop within the first 2 months of life • Vesiculobullous or a macular copper-color rash on the palms and soles and papular lesions around the nose and mouth and in the diaper area, as well as petechial lesions. • Other features include rhinitis, bone abnormalities, chorioretinitis, lymphadenopathy, hepatosplenomegaly, and nephrotic syndrome. Late congenital syphilis, which presents after 2 years of age, may have a variety of skeletal and dental defects, interstitial keratitis, and eighth nerve deafness (Hutchinson's triad)	• Direct dark-field examination or fluorescent antibody test or other specific test of skin lesions, lymph nodes or body fluids • Serum quantitative nontreponemal and treponemal serological investigations • IgM serology is highly recommended • Complete blood count and differential and platelet count • Cerebrospinal fluid analysis for VDRL, cell count and protein • Other tests as clinically indicated (long bone radiographs, chest radiograph, liver function tests, cranial ultrasound, ophthalmological examination)	Children with acquired syphilis: Benzathine benzylpenicillin, 50,000 IE/kg/IM (maximal dose: 2.4 million IE/dose) Ceftriaxone (children up to 12 years: 30–80 mg/kg/d, older children: 1–2 g/d IV, both in one dose for 10 days) is also an alternative, and there is no evidence in the literature that it is less efficient than penicillin.[31] In a recent meta-analysis, it was concluded that ceftriaxone was a good alternative to penicillin in penicillin-allergic people

Continued

Continued

Disease	Prepubertal mode of transmission	Vertical transmission	Clinical signs—perineal region	Clinical clues for diagnosis—extragenital region	Recommended evaluation	Management
Herpes simplex virus infection	Autoinoculation and child sexual abuse should be considered	About 75% of children with neonatal herpes are born to mothers who are not known to have herpes genitalis	• Genital HSV lesions are rare in pediatric patients • Vesicular or ulcerative, painful lesions involving the skin and mucosae, with or without regional lymphadenopathy • An acute napkin rash with ulcers over vulva has also been reported. • Rare complications: Sacral myeloradiculitis, neurogenic bladder postgenital HSV, though these are more commonly encountered in adolescents.	Generalized erosions and vesicles with involvement of other mucosae (oral, anal, nasal, conjunctival) in case of disseminated HSV infection	NAAT, HSV2 type specific serology HSV PCR for neonatal herpes with CNS involvement and dissemination	• Uncomplicated genital HSV infection—no need to treat. • Primary infection with severe symptoms is treated orally with 500 mg valaciclovir twice a day for 5 days. • For very severe symptoms, including neonatal infection, intravenous treatment with aciclovir is mandatory (10 mg/kg/dose three times daily for 5–10 days). • Neonatal herpes is always treated with aciclovir intravenously. The recommended regimen for infants treated for known or suspected neonatal herpes is aciclovir 20 mg/kg bodyweight intravenously every 8 hours for 21 days for disseminated and CNS disease or 14 days for disease limited to the skin and mucous membranes

(CNS: central nervous system; HSV: herpes simplex virus; PCR: polymerase chain reaction)

Table 4B: Nonsexually acquired genital ulcers.		
	Clinical features	*Management*

Lipschutz ulcers (Fig. 10)	• Painful, acute, necrotic genital ulceration in a sexually inactive young female; after exclusion of other infectious and noninfectious causes of orogenital ulceration
	• *Morphology*: The ulcers are deep, with red borders and a necrotic center covered by gray exudate or gray–black eschar, presenting in a kissing pattern. They primarily affect the medial aspect of the labia minora and vestibule, with variable size. Intense reactionary edema and erythema are evident
	• *Diagnostic criteria*:
	Suggested by Fahri et al.
	  ○ *Major criteria*:
	    – Age <20 years
	    – Ulcer with sudden onset and acute evolution
	    – First and unique episode
	    – No sexual contact in the 3 months prior to complaint
	    – Absence of immunodeficiency
	  ○ *Minor criteria*:
	    – One or more ulcers with necrotic or fibrinous core, with a well-delimited, painful, and symmetrical pattern
	For diagnosis, all major and minor criteria should be fulfilled
	• *Constitutional symptoms*: Infectious mononucleosis-like prodromal symptoms
	Etiology of Lipschutz ulcers is controversial. Onset has been reported with an exacerbated immune response to viral diseases, such as Epstein–Barr virus, cytomegalovirus, influenza virus, paratyphoid fever, toxoplasmosis, mycoplasma pneumoniae, and mumps. However, these associations are not uniformly confirmed.[16,17]
		No specific treatment is effective; pain management is central to the management of Lipschutz ulcers. Oral anti-inflammatory agents, analgesics and in severe cases, short course of oral corticosteroids (prednisolone 0.5–1 mg/day) may be required. Avoidance of soaps, disinfectants is advisable. For cases with associated flu-like symptoms and/or elevated inflammatory parameters, broad-spectrum antibiotics, amoxycillin should be given
		As painful as the lesions are, the natural course is generally benign, and spontaneous resolution by 2–3 weeks is the rule.[18]

Behçet's disease and recurrent genital aphthosis	Criteria for pediatric Behçet's disease: 1. Recurrent oral aphthosis: At least three attacks/year 2. Genital ulceration or aphthosis healing: Typically with scarring 3. Skin involvement: Necrotic folliculitis, acneiform lesions, and erythema nodosum 4. *Ocular involvement*: Anterior uveitis, posterior uveitis, and retinal vasculitis 5. *Neurological signs*: With the exception of isolated headaches 6. *Vascular signs*: Venous thrombosis, arterial thrombosis, and arterial aneurysm Three or more criteria are needed for diagnosis. Genital ulcers are less common than in adults; however, they are still the second most common finding in pediatric Behçet's, after oral aphthosis. They morphologically resemble oral ulcers, but are deeper, irregular shaped, with erythematous borders and often heal with scarring (as contrary to oral ulcers of Behçet's)[19]	For initial treatment of orogenital aphthae, topical corticosteroids such as triamcinolone gel are recommended. For severe cases with multisystemic involvement, the therapeutic armamentarium consists of systemic corticosteroids, colchicine, cyclosporine (contraindicated in neurological symptoms), azathioprine

Continued

Continued

	Clinical features	**Management**
Lichen sclerosus et atrophicus (LSeA) **(Fig. 11)**	Mean age of onset—5 years LSeA is characterized by porcelain white flat-topped papules, small plaques and atrophic patches (classically forming a "figure of 8" involving the labia minora, clitoral hood, and the perianal region) as the initial lesions, with secondary erosions and fissuring. Vulvar purpura is a hallmark manifestation Females are more commonly affected than males. The main presenting complaints include pruritus and significant vulvodynia. Secondary constipation is common, and may persist long after treatment of LSeA symptoms. Vulvar LSeA is a strong mimic of child sexual abuse Males present with involvement of glans penis as balanitis xerotica obliterans leading to acquired phimosis Extragenital lesions are common. Involvement of oral mucosa concurrently, in the form of porcelain white papules, sometimes mimicking vitiligo has been noted Associations with other autoimmune conditions such as vitiligo, alopecia areata, autoimmune thyroiditis, and celiac disease have been reported *Complications*: Chronic inflammation and a relapsing and remitting course can lead to scarring and distortion of vulvar architecture. Symptoms may persist up to adolescence Development of squamous cell carcinoma and vulvar melanoma over chronic LSeA has been reported, albeit rarely[20]	The European Academy of Dermatology and Venereology recommends the following management protocol for prepubertal LSeA[9] *Initial therapy*: Ultrapotent topical corticosteroids—clobetasol propionate 0.05% ointment, once or twice daily application, for the first 3 months, with possible reduction in application frequency after the first month. Depending on the patient, TCS may only need to be used once or twice a month, up to two to three times a week *Proactive maintenance*: Mometasone furoate 0.1% ointment twice weekly application for maintenance The first follow-up should be at 3 months and if the diseases remain uncomplicated, follow-up visits can be done at 6 months. Moisturizers and silk underwear were also recommended, as decreasing friction was associated with fewer symptoms. Topical calcineurin inhibitors are effective maintenance agents Use of moisturizers and silk underwear is recommended
Stevens–Johnson syndrome (SJS)/toxic epidermal necrolysis (TEN) and MIRM (mycoplasma-induced rash and mucositis)	Pediatric retrospective studies identify a drug as the cause of SJS and TEN in 72–90% of the reported cases. Antibiotics, anticonvulsants, and nonsteroidal anti-inflammatory drugs are implicated in the majority of pediatric cases. MIRM, triggered by mycoplasma pneumoniae, initially was considered SJS TEN in the past; however, the disease processes are distinctly different in both Incidence of genitourinary involvement in SJS TEN has been described to be around 50–60% in few studies. Meatal involvement is common, more often described in boys than girls. Clinical involvement of genitalia ranges from mild meatal erythema, discharge, erosions over the labia/glans penis, hemorrhagic crusting, acute scrotal swelling, presence of targetoid lesions and purpuric macules on the genitalia Severity of mucosal involvement in MIRM is at par with SJS/TEN; however, overall course and prognosis are favorable Sequelae include meatal stenosis and urethral stricture, labial adhesions, vaginal synechiae, hematocolpos, and hydrocolpos	General management of SJS/TEN, with specific importance to local wound care to prevent long-term sequelae. The decision to follow supportive care vs. active immunosuppression therapy is challenging as the reports of various studies on the usage of corticosteroids, IVIG, TNF-α inhibitors are controversial. A risk–benefit assessment is essential before starting therapy. Identification and withdrawal of the offending drug are the focus of management plan Although antibiotics are used to treat MP respiratory infections, the effect of antibiotics on the skin and mucous membrane changes of MIRM is dubious, with a recurrence rate of 20%. There is evidence of rapid response with use of cyclosporine 3 mg/kg in few case reports of MIRM[21] However, there is no available consensus on prophylactic genitourinary interventions such as catheterization to prevent meatal stenosis[22]
Pyoderma gangrenosum	Genital PG is very rare, and often presents as an isolated, refractory genital ulcer. Common site of predilection in children includes head and neck, genital, perianal and peristomal regions; as opposed to adults, where lower extremities are preferentially involved Classical ulcerative PG is characterized by a painful, deep, necrotic ulcer with violaceous margins, which heals with cribriform scarring	Local wound care, along with systemic corticosteroids and calcineurin inhibitors, has reported to be effective in pediatric PG Current evidence is in the favor of use of TNF-α inhibitors, especially infliximab, in pediatric IBD-associated PG[23]

(IVIG: intravenous immunoglobulin; MP: *Mycoplasma pneumoniae*; PG: pyoderma gangrenosum; TCS: topical corticosteroids; TNF: tumor necrosis factor)

Table 5A: Urethral and/or vaginal discharge.

Disease	Prepubertal mode of transmission	Vertical transmission	Clinical signs—perineal region	Clinical clues for diagnosis—extragenital region	Recommended evaluation	Management
Neisseria gonorrhoeae	Sexual contact most likely Pediatric gonorrhea is rare, but when diagnosed, it is almost always due to child sexual abuse	Ophthalmic gonorrhea (ophthalmia neonatorum) There is no data available as to the cut-off age-group for vertical transmission	Neonates: No anogenital manifestations; Older children: Females more commonly affected than males Females: Vulvovaginitis: presents with a profuse purulent yellowish, white to cream discharge, with staining of undergarments; with associated dysuria and vulval erythema Sometimes, the discharge may be scanty, simulating a benign condition Males: Present with scant or profuse urethral discharge, rarely associated with penile edema, epididymitis, and testicular pain Rectal involvement in both males and females may be asymptomatic or present with rectal discharge and pain	Neonates: Severe conjunctivitis with copious blood-stained purulent discharge, chemosis, lid edema can lead to corneal ulcers and blindness, if untreated Disseminated gonococcal infection is rare, arthritis is the most common manifestation Older children: Females: Lower abdominal pain in cases with ascending pelvic infections including salpingitis, perihepatitis (Fitz–Hugh–Curtis syndrome) proctitis Disseminated gonococcal infection Presentation of DGI is usually with dermatitis, arthropathy or both. Skin involvement is seen in about 50–70% of patients with DGI. The skin lesions are usually multiple, erythematous, maculopapular, vesicular, hemorrhagic, pustular, or necrotic lesions. They often progress from papules to pustular, hemorrhagic or necrotic lesions, and the presence of lesions in different stages of evolution is typical of DGI. The lesions are usually on the extremities and number from one to 40, and range in size from 1 to 20 mm Pharyngeal infections with N. gonorrhoeae are frequently asymptomatic.	Gram stains—inadequate for evaluating prepubertal children for gonorrhea and should not be used to diagnose or exclude gonorrhea. NAAT can be used to test for N. gonorrhoeae from vaginal and urine specimens from girls and urine for boys	Uncomplicated gonococcal cervicitis, urethritis, vulvovaginitis, and proctitis <45 kg: Ceftriaxone 25–50 mg/kg body weight IV or IM in a single dose, not to exceed 250 mg IM >45 kg: Injection ceftriaxone 500 mg as a single intramuscular dose Evidence of DGI + <45 kg: Injection ceftriaxone 50 mg/kg body weight (maximum dose: 2 g) IM or IV in a single dose daily every 24 hours for 7 days >45 kg: Ceftriaxone 1 g IM or IV in a single dose daily every 24 hours for 7 days

Continued

Continued

Disease	Prepubertal mode of transmission	Vertical transmission	Clinical signs—perineal region	Clinical clues for diagnosis—extragenital region	Recommended evaluation	Management
Chlamydia trachomatis	Sexual transmission most likely	There is no data available on age at which vertical transmission can be ruled out. However, perinatally transmitted C. trachomatis infection of the nasopharynx, urogenital tract, and rectum can persist for 2–3 years	Generally subclinical or asymptomatic	Inclusion conjunctivitis, chlamydial pneumonia in neonates and infants	NAAT—confirmatory	For infants and children, who weigh <45 kg: Erythromycin base or ethylsuccinate 50 mg/kg body weight/day orally divided into 4 doses daily for 14 days Data are limited regarding the effectiveness and optimal dose of azithromycin for treating chlamydial infection among infants and children weighing <45 kg. For children weighing ≥45 kg but aged <8 years: Azithromycin 1 g orally in a single dose For children aged ≥8 years: Azithromycin 1 g orally in a single dose or Doxycycline 100 mg orally 2 times/day for 7 days
Bacterial vaginosis	Both sexual and nonsexual transmission possible in prepubertal girls Very low prevalence in asymptomatic prepubertal girls Slightly more often in sexually abused prepubertal girls with a discharge	There is no data available on age at which vertical transmission can be ruled out	Vulvovaginitis, a thin, homogeneous gray-white to yellow discharge or a typical odor	—	*Postpubertal*: Amsel's criteria, Nugent score *Prepubertal*: any mention of clue cells, mixed anaerobes	"Wait and watch (spontaneous recovery) Metronidazole 30 mg/kg/day in 3 doses orally for 7 days Amoxicillin 50 mg/kg/day in 4 doses for 7 days (alternative)

Continued

Continued

Disease	Prepubertal mode of transmission	Vertical transmission	Clinical signs—perineal region	Clinical clues for diagnosis—extragenital region	Recommended evaluation	Management
Trichomonas vaginalis	Child sexual abuse should be considered Nonsexual transmission should be excluded because of inadequate hygiene Role of fomite transmission: The organism of TV can survive for several hours on wet towels and clothing which have been used by infected women	No evidence to establish the age at which vertical transmission can be excluded TV in a girl <2 months of age could be the result of a perinatal infection	*Females*: Transient vulvovaginitis in prepubertal age-group is the most common symptom. In adults, persistent infection with ascending involvement of cervix has also been described. *In males*: transient urethritis, with or without epididymitis, can occur; however, trichomoniasis is rare in males; as the TV requires estrogen to establish infection	—	Wet mount—very high sensitivity Culture NAAT	In prepubertal age-group, self-resolving, treatment is usually not necessary, due to lower concentration of estrogen If treatment is necessary, metronidazole 30 mg/kg/day in three doses given orally for 7 days is the first choice For children >12 years, the metronidazole dose is 500 mg orally twice daily for 5–7 days (first choice) or metronidazole 2 g or all

(DGI: disseminated gonococcal infection; NAAT: nucleic acid amplification test; IM: intramuscular; IV: intravenous)

Table 5B: Nonsexually transmitted causes of vaginal discharge.		
D/D of vulvovaginitis	**Salient clinical features and causative agent**	**Management**
Nonspecific vulvovaginitis Mild discharge, dysuria, pruritus, mucosal erythema	No identifiable bacterial pathogen on repeated cultures; most common	Hygiene and avoidance of irritants, if any Topical estrogen or topical steroid in severe inflammation
Non-STI bacterial vulvovaginitis	Culture positive; commonly isolated pathogens include: • Group A β-hemolytic streptococci: Painful, blood tinged, or mucopurulent discharge • *Staphylococcus aureus* • *H. influenzae, Neisseria meningitidis,* • *E. coli* • *Shigella, Yersinia enterocolitica*—hemorrhagic vulvovaginitis	Cephalosporins (cefixime and cefadroxil) or fluoroquinolone-based empiric oral antibiotic therapy based on the weight
Vaginal foreign body: Foul smelling vaginal discharge, less commonly associated with vaginal bleeding Recurrent symptoms	Common foreign body encountered—toilet paper	Flushing out of the foreign body using a pediatric feeding tube under topical or local anesthesia
Enterobius vermicularis	Although many patients with pinworm infestation are asymptomatic, it may commonly present with genital/vulval and perianal itching, with or without eczematous dermatitis.	• For confirmation of diagnosis, a clear tape can be applied to the perianal area and be observed under the microscope for presence of ova[24] • Management is symptomatic, along with systemic antihelminthic therapy (albendazole 200–400 mg as a single dose)
Candidial vulvovaginitis	Generally, it is unusual in prepubertal age-group, as vulvovaginal candidiasis manifests under estrogenic influence. However, in the neonates, up to 2 months of age, vulvovaginal candidiasis may occur under the influence of maternal estrogens. VVC presents as pruritic, bright red erythema with overlying curdy white discharge	Topical clotrimazole vaginal gel

(D/D: differential diagnosis; STI: sexually transmitted infection; VVC: vulvovaginal candidiasis)

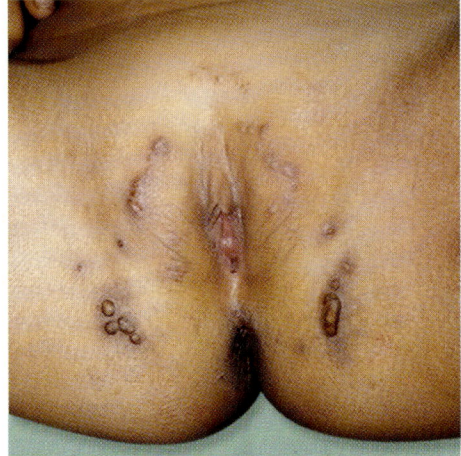

FIG. 10: Lipschutz ulcers in a 4-year-old girl.

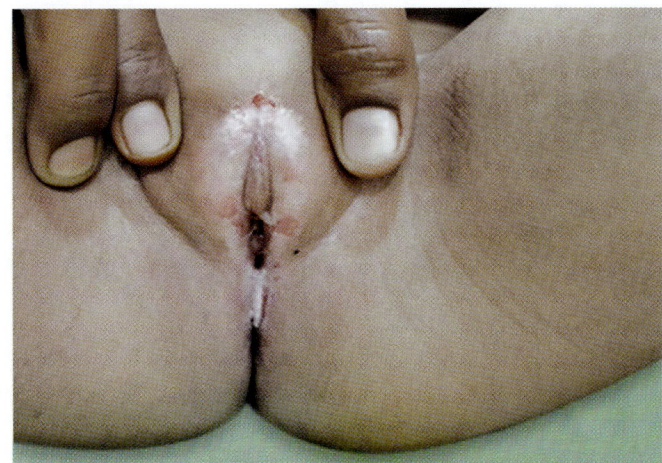

FIG. 11: Lichen sclerosus et atrophicus: Depigmented atrophic plaques over the mucosal aspect of vulva with superficial erythematous erosions.

Table 6: Nevoid lesions over perineal region.

	Clinical appearance	Extraperineal mucocutaneous features	Syndromic association/complications	Differential diagnosis	Management
Congenital melanocytic nevi	Genital nevi clinically present as macules or papules with color ranging from tan to dark brown. The genital nevi may be present at birth or develop early in life and may enlarge as the child grows	• Similar lesions on other parts of the body • In patients with giant CMN, neurocutaneous melanosis may be associated	• Neurocutaneous melanosis • Transformation to malignant melanoma	• Mucosal melanotic macule • Lentiginosis	• Gradual and symmetrical enlargement in size, changes in color or texture of genital nevi should not be an indication for biopsy • Indications for a biopsy: unusually rapid rate of growth of lesion, any firm new elevation, and asymmetry in border, color, or texture of lesion[28]
Mucosal melanotic macules	One or more brown to black macules with irregular borders and mottled pigmentation	—	Multiple genital melanotic macules can be a feature of Bannayan–Riley–Ruvalcaba syndrome and type 2 segmental Cowden disease (PTEN nevus)[30]	• Lentigines • Melanocytic nevi	—
Nevus depigmentosus or nevus achromicus	Hypopigmented macule or patch, since birth, with serrated margins	—	Associations have been reported with tuberous sclerosis, neurofibromatosis	• Vitiligo • Nevus anemicus	—
Epidermal nevi	• Present as patches, plaques, or nodules that are distributed on most of the body, including genitals. Usually, they are asymptomatic clinically except inflammatory linear verrucous epidermal nevus (ILVEN) • Though uncommon, lesions of verrucous epidermal nevus have been described in the perianal area and penis	Can occur anywhere on the body	*Pruritus is the chief complaint associated with ILVEN* Some reports of limb reduction defects with ILVEN suggests that ILVEN represents a limited form of congenital hemidysplasia with ipsilateral limb defect (CHILD) nevus, and more appropriately can be named, PEN, and PENCIL, respectively indicating psoriasiform epidermal nevus (PEN) with or without congenital ipsilateral limb defects (PENCIL)[31] Syndromes that can be associated with epidermal nevus include: • Proteus syndrome[32,33] Type 2 segmental Cowden disease (PTEN nevus)—Cowden syndrome is a multisystemic disorder characterized by the appearance of multiple hamartomas and tumors, including breast cancer, endometrial cancer, thyroid cancer, and colon cancer, trichilemmomas, oral papillomas, mucocutaneous neuromas, acral keratosis, *genital lentiginosis,* malformations, and vascular tumors and lipomas[34,35] • CHILD syndrome[34,36]	• Nevoid psoriasis, linear • Darier disease, warts[37] for ILVEN	Treatment of ILVEN includes topical corticosteroids with or without occlusion and intralesional steroids. Topical retinoids and Vitamin D analogs. Physical modalities such as cryotherapy, photodynamic therapy, and carbon dioxide laser therapy have been tried successfully. Surgical excision is associated with high chances of recurrence and requires deep dermal excision[38]

Continued

	Clinical appearance	Extraperineal mucocutaneous features	Syndromic association/complications	Differential diagnosis	Management
Nevus comedonicus	Hamartomatous malformation of the pilosebaceous apparatus, characterized by closely grouped dilated follicular openings with horny plugs mimicking comedones. Genital involvement has very rarely been reported on perineal region and labium majora[39,40]	It is most frequently located on the face or trunk	Noncutaneous developmental abnormalities include skeletal malformation (absent fifth finger, trichilemmal cysts, rudimentary toe, scoliosis), eccrine spiradenoma and hidradenoma, bilateral follicular basal cell nevus, Alagille syndrome, CNS abnormalities (brain dysgenesis, microcephaly, Sturge–Weber syndrome), multiple basal cell carcinoma, ipsilateral polysyndactyly and bilateral oligodontia, ipsilateral cataract, and trichilemmal cysts[41]	Familial dyskeratotic comedones	—
Nevus sebaceous	Clinically presents as a flat, smooth-surfaced, solitary plaque, few cases have been reported over genitals[42,43]	Occurs mainly on the face and scalp			Though most do not need any active treatment, therapeutic options available include cryotherapy, electrocautery, topical retinoids, and surgical excision

Table 7: Developmental/anatomical defect.[34,36,52,54-62]	
Developmental/anatomical defect	**Clinical presentation**
Ambiguous genitalia	*History*: • Family history of similar complaint/ambiguous genitalia, unexplained neonatal death, genital abnormality, and abnormal pubertal development • Consanguineous marriage in parents • History of any drug intake during pregnancy • History of maternal virilization or hormonal disorder *Clinical finding*: • Apparent males with nonpalpable testes in a full-term infant • Hypospadias associated with separation of the scrotal sacs • Undescended testis with hypospadias • Apparent female with clitoral hypertrophy • Foreshortened vulva with single opening • Inguinal hernia containing a gonad
Cloacal defect **(Fig. 13)**	• Single perineal orifice usually posterior to the clitoris and the urethra is inside the hymen or the absent anterior hymen • Diminutive and foreshortened labia minora and a clitoral hood • *Urethra distal to the hymen rules out cloaca*
Labial adhesion	Partially or entirely agglutinated labia minora
Bladder exstrophy	Fleshy mass prolapsing out of suprapubic area with continuous urine leakage
Hymenal defect **(Fig. 14)**	A transparent yellowish bulging mass seen at the introitus suggests imperforate hymen. Absence of hymeneal tissue extending to the base in the posterior half of the hymen suggests trauma and may (signify) be a sign of sexual abuse.
Epispadias	*Male*: Split dorsal urethra with dorsal chordee and ventral foreskin hood *Female*: Nonbulbar urethra, incomplete development of labia, bifid clitoris, and flat mons pubis
Hypospadias	*Male*: Ventrally incomplete prepuce with glandular groove and dorsal hood of foreskin *Female*: Shortening of the urethra and ectopia of the external urethral opening
Smegma pearl **(Fig. 15)**	Physiological collection of smegma in the subpreputial space of young uncircumcised boys *Differentials*: 1. *Preputial Epstein pearls*: Accumulation of keratinized epithelial cells 2. *Preputial cysts*: Collection of dead skin under the glans and presents as a nodular swelling 3. Penile median raphe cyst **(Fig. 16)**

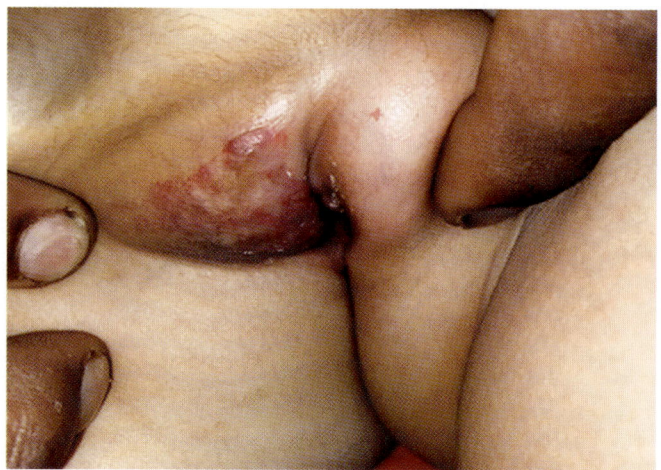

FIG. 12: Infantile hemangioma over the right labium majora.

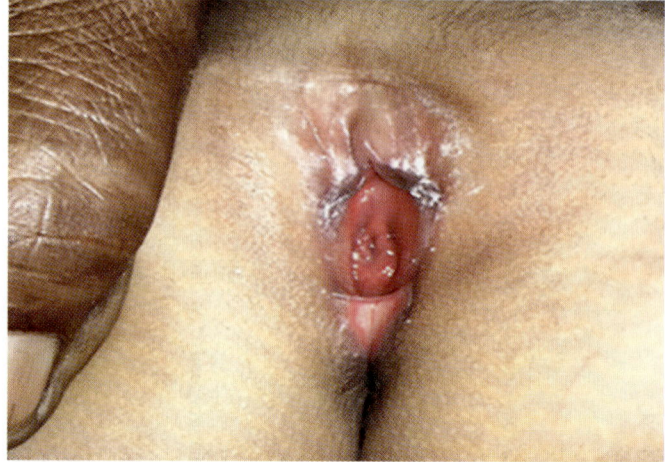

FIG. 13: Cloacal defect.

CHAPTER 20 A Child with Genital Lesions

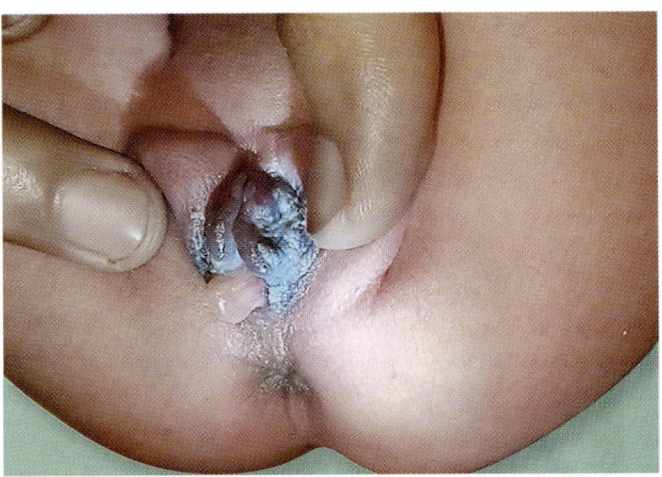

FIG. 14: Hymenal tag: tongue-like projection.

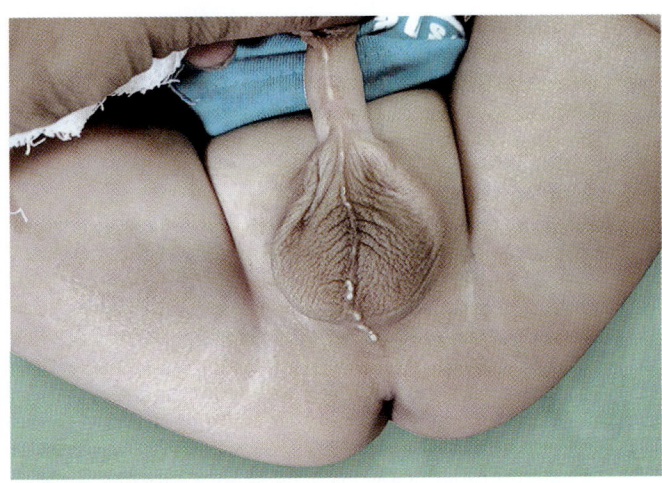

FIG. 16: Median raphe cyst.

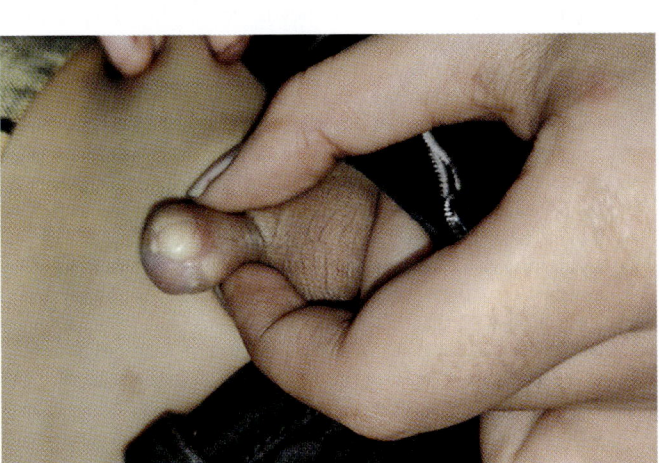

FIG. 15: Smegma pearl: milky white colored papule.

Infantile hemangiomas **(Fig. 12)** rarely need a treatment, but in children with giant lesions, ulcerating lesions or lesions interfering with urination/defecation active treatment modalities should be considered.[47]

Vascular malformations are a result of inborn errors in vascular embryogenesis. They are usually present at the time of birth or may sometimes present later. They develop gradually with age, with peak growth occurring at the time of puberty.[48] VMs can be classified based on the predominantly affected vessel (arterial, venous, lymphatic, capillary, or combination) or according to the type of flow: slow flow VM (capillary, venous, lymphatic, and complex combined) or fast-flow VMs (arterial malformation, arteriovenous fistula, arteriovenous malformation, and complex-combined VMs).[49]

Early detection of vascular anomalies is important, as this may affect childbirth decisions. Also, early awareness of vascular lesions and associated syndromic features can help in further evaluation and management strategies.[50]

Syndromes associated with VMs involving lower body:
- Klippel–Trenaunay syndrome (CM, VM, and/or LM, soft tissue hypertrophy and/or skeletal anomalies), RASA-1 AVM-CM (AVMs with multiple cutaneous CMs)[51]
- Parkes–Weber syndrome (CM, VM with arteriovenous fistula)[52,53]
- CLOVES (congenital lipomatous overgrowth, VMs, epidermal nevus, and spinal/skeletal scoliosis)[52]

ACKNOWLEDGMENTS

For **Figures 7 and 8**, We are thankful to the Department of Dermatology, GCS Hospital, for image contribution. We can acknowledge SCL General Hospital also.

REFERENCES

1. Adams JA, Farst KJ, Kellogg ND. Interpretation of medical findings in suspected child sexual abuse: An update for 2018. J Pediatr Adolesc Gynecol. 2018;31(3):225-31.
2. Guo Y, Dang Y, Toyohara JP, Geng S. Successful treatment of verruciform xanthoma with imiquimod. J Am Acad Dermatol. 2013;69(4):e184-6.
3. Vaiopoulos AG, Nikolakis G, Zouboulis CC. Hidradenitis suppurativa in paediatric patients: a retrospective monocentric study in Germany and review of the literature. J Euro Acad Dermatol Venereol. 2020;34(9):2140-6.
4. Patil S, Apurwa A, Nadkarni N, Agarwal S, Chaudhari P, Gautam M. Hidradenitis suppurativa: inside and out. Indian J Dermatol. 2018;63(2):91.

5. Otis CN, Fischer RA, Johnson N, Kelleher JF, Powell JL. Histiocytosis X of the vulva: a case report and review of the literature. Obstet Gynecol. 1990;75(3 Pt 2):555-8.
6. Agrons GA, Wagner BJ, Lonergan GJ, Dickey GE, Kaufman MS. From the archives of the AFIP. Genitourinary rhabdomyosarcoma in children: radiologic-pathologic correlation. Radiographics. 1997;17(4):919-37.
7. Paller A, Mancini AJ, Hurwitz A, Paller S, Mancini A. Histiocytosis and malignant skin diseases. Hurwitz Clin Pediat Dermatol. 2011;245-54.
8. Kaul S, Yadav S, Dogra S. Treatment of Dermatophytosis in Elderly, Children, and Pregnant Women. Indian Dermatol Online J. 2017;8(5):310-8.
9. Jagadeesan S, Kaliyadan F. (2020). Acrodermatitis enteropathica. StatPearls [Internet]. [online] Available from https://www.ncbi.nlm.nih.gov/books/NBK441835/#:~:text=Acrodermatitis%20enteropathica%20is%20a%20rare,biochemical%20pathways%20of%20the%20body. [Last accessed December, 2022]
10. Jezierska M, Stefanowicz J, Romanowicz G, Kosiak W, Lange M. Langerhans cell histiocytosis in children - a disease with many faces. Recent advances in pathogenesis, diagnostic examinations and treatment. Postepy Dermatol Alergol. 2018;35(1):6-17.
11. Ramos Pinheiro R, Matos-Pires E, Baptista J, Lencastre A. Granuloma Glutaeale Infantum: A Re-emerging Complication of Diaper Dermatitis. Pediatrics. 2018;141(2):e20162064.
12. Luger T, Boguniewicz M, Carr W, Cork M, Deleuran M, Eichenfield L, et al. Pimecrolimus in atopic dermatitis: consensus on safety and the need to allow use in infants. Pediatr Allergy Immunol. 2015;26(4):306-15.
13. Guerriero C, Paradisi A, Capizzi R, Silveri SL. Jacquet papuloerosive dermatitis. Pediatr Dermatol. 2009;60(3):AB145.
14. Dandale A, Dhurat R, Ghate S. Perianal pseudoverrucous papules and nodules. Indian J Sex Transm Dis AIDS. 2013;34(1):44-6.
15. Ruseler-van Embden JG, van Lieshout LM, Smits SA, van Kessel I, Laman JD. Potato tuber proteins efficiently inhibit human faecal proteolytic activity: Implications for treatment of perianal dermatitis. Eur J Clin Invest. 2004;34:303-11.
16. Farhi D, Wendling J, Molinari E, Raynal J, Carcelain G, Morand P, et al. Non-sexually related acute genital ulcers in 13 pubertal girls: a clinical and microbiological study. Arch Dermatol. 2009;145(01):38-45.
17. Pereira DAG, Teixeira EPP, Lopes ACM, Sarmento RJP, Lopes APC. Lipschütz ulcer: An unusual diagnosis that should not be neglected. Rev Bras Ginecol Obstet. 2021;43(5):414-6.
18. Sadoghi B, Stary G, Wolf P, Komericki P. Ulcus vulvae acutum Lipschütz: a systematic literature review and a diagnostic and therapeutic algorithm. J Eur Acad Dermatol Venereol. 2020;34(7):1432-9.
19. Yıldız M, Köker O, Adrovic A, Şahin S, Barut K, Kasapçopur Ö. Pediatric Behçet's disease - clinical aspects and current concepts. Eur J Rheumatol. 2019;7(Suppl 1):1-10.
20. Dinh H, Purcell SM, Chung C, Zaenglein AL. Pediatric Lichen Sclerosus: A Review of the Literature and Management Recommendations. J Clin Aesthet Dermatol. 2016;9(9):49-54.
21. Ramien M, Goldman JL. Pediatric SJS-TEN: Where are we now? F1000Res. 2020;9:F1000 Faculty Rev-982.
22. Van Batavia JP, Chu DI, Long CJ, Jen M, Canning DA, Weiss DA. Genitourinary involvement and management in children with Stevens–Johnson syndrome and toxic epidermal necrolysis. J Pediatr Urol. 2017;13(5):490.e1-490.e7.
23. Katherine V, Rebecca W, Simon RS Steven MS. Treatment of Pyoderma Gangrenosum in Pediatric Inflammatory Bowel Disease. JPGN Rep. 2020;1(2):e008.
24. Fischer OG. Genital Disease in Children. In: Hoeger P, Kinsler V, Yan A (Eds). Harpers' Textbook of Pediatric Dermatology, 4th edition. Hoboken, New Jersey, United States: Wiley-Blackwell Publishing; 2020. pp. 2159-94.
25. Kumar A, Kashyap S. Giant congenital melanocytic nevus. Int J Health Sci Res. 2016;6(6):444-6.
26. Farabi B, Akay BN, Goldust M, Wollina U, Atak MF, Rao B. Congenital melanocytic naevi: An up-to-date overview. Australas J Dermatol. 2022. Online ahead of print.
27. Clemmensen OJ, Kroon S. The histology of "congenital features" in early acquired melanocytic nevi. J Am Acad Dermatol. 1988;19(4):742-6.
28. Hunt RD, Orlow SJ, Schaffer JV. Genital melanocytic nevi in children: Experience in a pediatric dermatology practice. J Am Acad Dermatol. 2014;70(3):429-34.
29. Oliveria SA, Satagopan JM, Geller AC, Dusza SW, Weinstock MA, Berwick M, et al. Study of nevi in children (SONIC): baseline findings and predictors of nevus count. Am J Epidemiol. 2009;169:41-53.
30. Schaffer JV, Bolognia JL, Levy ML, Dellavalle RP, Corona R. Benign pigmented skin lesions other than melanocytic nevi (moles). [online] Available from https://www.uptodate.com/contents/benign-pigmented-skin-lesions-other-than-melanocytic-nevi-moles#:~:text=Benign%20pigmented%20skin%20lesions%20and,)%2C%20will%20be%20discussed%20below. [Last accessed December, 2022]
31. Dyopadhyay D, Abanti S. Genital/Perigenital Inflammatory Linear Verrucous Epidermal Nevus: A Case Series. Indian J Dermatol. 2015;60:593.
32. Lindhurst MJ, Sapp JC, Teer JK, Johnston JJ, Finn EM, Peters K, et al. A mosaic activating mutation in AKT1 associated with the Proteus syndrome. N Engl J Med. 2011;365:611-9.
33. Garcias-Ladaria J, Rosón MC, Pascual-López M. Epidermal nevi and related syndromes—part 1: keratinocytic nevi. Actas Dermo-Sifiliográficas (English Edition). 2018;109(8):677-86.
34. Murugesan A, Palaniappan Y, Kalaimani T. An Unusual Cause of Urinary Pseudoincontinence: Two Rare Cases of Labial Fusion in Adolescent and Postmenopausal Women. JSAFOG. 2020;12(3):197.
35. Gantner S, Rütten A, Requena L, Gassenmaier G, Landthaler M, Hafner C. CHILD syndrome with mild skin lesions: histopathologic clues for the diagnosis. J Cutan Pathol. 2014;41(10):787-90.
36. Anand S, Lotfollahzadeh S. Bladder Exstrophy. [Updated 2021 Oct 9]. In: StatPearls [Internet]. Treasure Island (FL): StatPearls Publishing; 2021. [online] Available from https://www.ncbi.nlm.nih.gov/books/NBK563156/. [Last accessed December, 2022]
37. Narang T, Kanwar AJ. Verrucous epidermal naevus on penis. Indian J Dermatol. 2006;51(3):222-3.
38. Gianfaldoni S, Tchernev G, Gianfaldoni R, Wollina U, Lotti T. A case of "inflammatory linear verrucous epidermal nevus" (ILVEN) treated with CO_2 laser ablation. Open Access Maced J Med Sci. 2017;5(4):454.
39. Ferrari B, Taliercio V, Restrepo P, Luna P, Abad ME, Larralde M. Nevus comedonicus: a case series. Pediatr Dermatol. 2015;32(2):216-9.
40. González-Martínez R, Marín-Bertolín S, Martínez-Escribano J, Amorrortu-Velayos J. Nevus comedonicus: report of a case with genital involvement. Cutis. 1996;58(6):418-9.

41. Cockerell CJ, Larsen F. Benign epidermal tumors and proliferations. In: Bolognia JL, Joseph LJ, Rapini RP (Edits). Dermatology, 2nd edition. India: Mosby; 2009. pp. 1661-80.
42. Feito J, Cebrián-Muiños C, Alonso-Morrondo EJ, García-Mesa Y, García-Piqueras J, Cobo R, et al. Hyperplastic sensory corpuscles in nevus sebaceus of labia minora pudendi. A case report. J Cutan Pathol. 2018;45(10):777-81.
43. Mandal RK, Das A, Chakrabarti I, Agarwal P. Nevoid sebaceous hyperplasia mistaken as nevus sebaceous: Report of four cases. Indian J Dermatol Venereol Leprol. 2017;83(2):213-6.
44. Wildgruber M, Sadick M, Müller-Wille R, Wohlgemuth WA. Vascular tumors in infants and adolescents. Insights Imaging. 2019;10(1):1-4.
45. Yu X, Zhang J, Wu Z, Liu M, Chen R, Gu Y, et al. LUMBAR syndrome: A case manifesting as cutaneous infantile hemangiomas of the lower extremity, perineum and gluteal region, and a review of published work. J Dermatol. 2017;44(7):808-12.
46. Having K, Bullock S. Blue Rubber Bleb Nevus Syndrome. J Diagnost Med Sonograph. 2008;24(6):365-8.
47. Léauté-Labrèze C, Hoeger P, Mazereeuw-Hautier J, Guibaud L, Baselga E, Posiunas G, et al. A randomized, controlled trial of oral propranolol in infantile hemangioma. N Engl J Med. 2015;372:735-46.
48. Del Pozo J, Gómez-Tellado M, López-Gutiérrez JC. Vascular malformations in childhood. Actas Dermo-Sifiliográficas (English Edition). 2012;103(8):661-78.
49. Samadi K, Salazar GM. Role of imaging in the diagnosis of vascular malformations vascular malformations. Cardiovasc Diagn Ther. 2019;9(Suppl 1):S143-51.
50. Blei F, Bittman ME. Congenital vascular anomalies: current perspectives on diagnosis, classification, and management. J Vasc Diag Intervent. 2016;4:23-37.
51. Clemens RK, Pfammatter T, Meier TO, Alomari AI, Amann-Vesti BR. Combined and complex vascular malformations. Vasa. 2015;44(2):92-105.
52. Burleigh A, Lam JM. A mobile yellow nodule under the foreskin of a toddler. Paediatr Child Health. 2017;22(8):459-60.
53. Ghosh SK. Combined Vascular Malformation. Vascular Malformations. Singapore: Springer; 2021. pp. 93-104.
54. Committee on Genetics Section on Endocrinology AS. Evaluation of the newborn with developmental anomalies of the external genitalia. Pediatrics. 2000;106(1; Part 1):138-42.
55. Halleran DR, Wood RJ. Cloacal Malformations. [Updated 2021 Aug 12]. In: StatPearls [Internet]. Treasure Island (FL): StatPearls Publishing; 2021. [online]Available from https://www.ncbi.nlm.nih.gov/books/NBK539730/. [Last accessed December, 2022]
56. Wróblewska-Seniuk K, Jarząbek-Bielecka G, Kędzia W. Gynecological Problems in Newborns and Infants. J Clin Med. 2021;10(5):1071.
57. Frimberger D. Diagnosis and management of epispadias. Semin Pediatr Surg. 2011;20(2):85-90.
58. Donaire AE, Mendez MD. (2022). Hypospadias. [online] Available from https://www.ncbi.nlm.nih.gov/books/NBK482122/. [Last accessed December, 2022]
59. Patil NA, Patil SB, Kundargi VS, Biradar AN. Female urethral anomalies in pediatric age group: Uncovered. J Surg Tech Case Rep. 2015;7(1):14-6.
60. Sonthalia S, Jha AK. Smegma pearl. Indian Dermatol Online J. 2017;8(6):520.
61. Faridi MM, Sharma A. Managing pearly prepuce: Active communication and masterly inaction. Indian J Child Health. 2017;4(1):107-9.
62. Alphones S, Phansalkar M, Manoharan P. Median raphe cyst of the penis: A startling diagnosis for the unaccustomed clinician. Urol Ann. 2019;11(3):314-6.

Approach to a Child with Erythroderma

Jeta Y Buch, Halak J Vasavada

INTRODUCTION

Von Hebra first described erythroderma (exfoliative dermatitis) in 1868, which refers to inflammation of skin manifesting as erythema and scaling involving >90% body surface area (BSA).[1]

The incidence of erythroderma in children is 0.11% in Indian population.[2,3]

In adults, erythroderma may be due to drugs or exacerbation of preexisting dermatosis whereas in children, the condition, although a rare entity, represents a common morphological phenotype encompassing a broad spectrum of underlying ailments ranging from transient and benign skin diseases to potentially fatal systemic disorders. Particularly in newborn and infants with extensive epidermal barrier disruption, failure to thrive, associated severe infections, neurologic, hemodynamic, and metabolic complications, the condition often warrants a rapid comprehensive differential diagnostic workup and a timely symptomatic or causal therapeutic intervention by a multidisciplinary panel.[4]

PATHOGENESIS

The exact pathogenesis of erythroderma is still a matter of debate. Data suggests a high and persistent expression of adhesion molecules [vascular cell adhesion molecule 1 (VCAM-1), intercellular adhesion molecule 1 (ICAM-1), E-selectin, P-selectin] which stimulates dermal inflammation in endothelium of erythroderma patients and increased production of inflammatory cytokines.[4] The complex interaction of cytokines and cellular adhesion molecules including interleukin 1, 2, and 8, ICAM-1 and tumor necrosis factor (TNF) leads to elevated epidermal turnover rate resulting in increased mitotic rates. The number of germinative cells increases while the transit time of the keratinocytes through the epidermis is shortened leading to significant loss of nucleic acid, amino acid, soluble protein via scales.[5-7] In addition to the basic changes, the mechanism underlying erythroderma of various etiologies is specific.

CLASSIFICATION[8]

Childhood erythroderma can be classified according to duration of illness, age of onset, etiology, and morphology.
- *Based on duration of illness*:
  - Acute (few days)
  - Chronic
- *Based on age of onset*:[9]
  - *Congenital:*
    - Infections
    - Ichthyosis
    - Primary immunodeficiency syndrome (PIDS) (rarely symptomatic at birth due to protective effect of maternal immunity)
    - Metabolic
    - Diffuse cutaneous mastocytosis[10]
    - Psoriasis (rare)[11,12]
    - Pityriasis rubra pilaris (PRP) (rare)[13]
  - *Neonatal (<1 month):*
    - Infections
    - Ichthyosis
    - PIDS
    - Metabolic
    - Drugs
    - Transient neonatal disorders
    - Diffuse cutaneous mastocytosis
    - Seborrheic dermatitis (rare)
    - Atopic dermatitis (rare)
    - Psoriasis (rare)

- Infantile (1 month–1 year):
  - Atopic dermatitis
  - Seborrheic dermatitis
  - Psoriasis, PRP
  - Ichthyosis
  - Immunodeficiency
  - Metabolic/nutritional
  - Cystic fibrosis (CF)
  - Drugs
- Late childhood/adolescent:
  - Atopic dermatitis
  - Seborrheic dermatitis
  - Psoriasis, PRP
  - Lichen planus
  - Drugs
  - Nutritional
  - Cutaneous T-cell lymphoma
  - Idiopathic

- Based on morphology:[9]
  - *Erythematous macules coalescing to papule, pustules/vesicles*:
    - Stevens–Johnson syndrome (SJS)
    - Congenital cutaneous candidiasis (CCC)
    - Neonatal herpes
    - Drug induced
  - *Bulla*:
    - Bullous ichthyosis
    - Bullous mastocytosis
    - Toxic epidermal necrolysis (TEN)
    - Staphylococcal scalded skin syndrome (SSSS)
    - Pemphigus foliaceus
    - Congenital syphilis (rare)
  - *Eczematous*:
    - Atopic dermatitis
    - Seborrheic dermatitis
    - Ichthyosis (some)
    - Scabies
    - Metabolic disorders—acrodermatitis enteropathica, biotinidase deficiency, holocarboxylase synthetase deficiency
    - PIDS
    - Cutaneous T-cell lymphoma
  - *Papulosquamous*:
    - Psoriasis
    - PRP

- Based on etiology:[14-20]
  - *Transient neonatal dermatoses*:
    - Miliaria
    - Erythema toxicum neonatorum **(Fig. 1)**
  - *Infections*:
    - SSSS
    - Scarlet fever
    - Toxic shock syndrome (TSS)
    - Congenital and neonatal candidiasis
    - Congenital and neonatal herpes simplex (rare)

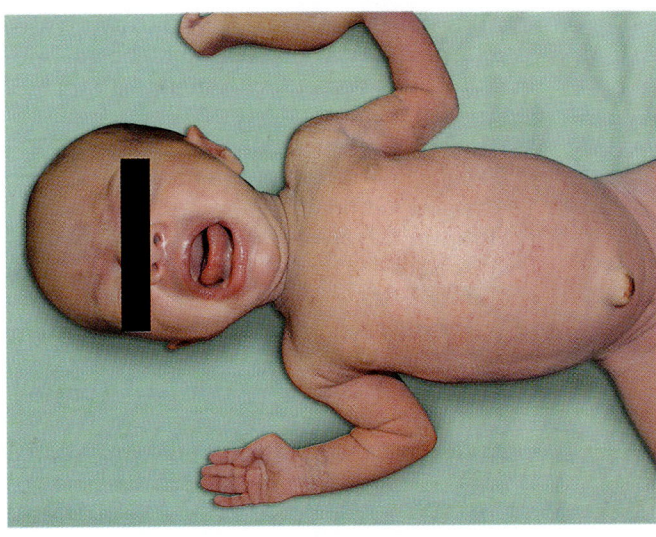

FIG. 1: Erythema toxicum neonatorum.

    - Congenital syphilis (rare)
  - *Infestations*:
    - Norwegian scabies
  - *Drugs*:[21-24]
    - Antiepileptic—valproic acid, carbamazepine, phenobarbitone, phenytoin, lamotrigine, levetiracetam
    - Antibiotics—macrolides, cephalosporins, trimethoprim/sulfamethoxazole, sulfonamides, cloxacillin, amoxicillin, penicillin, fluoroquinolones, vancomycin, tobramycin
    - Analgesics—ibuprofen, paracetamol (acetaminophen), nimesulide
    - Allopurinol
    - Nevirapine
    - Boric acid
    - Topical tar
    - Thioacetazone
    - Captopril
    - Cimetidine
    - Minocycline
    - Dapsone
    - Griseofulvin
    - Clindamycin
    - Fluoxetine
    - Antitubercular drugs
    - Oxymetazoline nasal spray
    - Ayurvedic and homeopathic medicines
  - *Ichthyosis*:[25]
    - Nonsyndromic:
      - X-linked recessive ichthyosis
      - Autosomal recessive—harlequin ichthyosis, lamellar ichthyosis **(Fig. 2)**, congenital ichthyosiform erythroderma (CIE), peeling skin syndrome

- Autosomal dominant—lamellar ichthyosis, ichthyosis hystrix **(Figs. 3A and B)**, epidermolytic ichthyosis, erythrokeratoderma variabilis
- Syndromic:
  - X-linked recessive ichthyosis
  - X-linked dominant—Conradi-Hunermann-Happle syndrome
  - Autosomal recessive with prominent neurologic signs—Sjögren-Larsson syndrome (SLS)
  - Autosomal recessive with hair abnormalities—Netherton syndrome, trichothiodystrophy (TTD)
  - Autosomal recessive with fatal course—Gaucher's disease
  - Autosomal recessive with other associated signs—keratitis-ichthyosis-deafness (KID) syndrome, neutral lipid storage disease (NLSD) with ichthyosis, severe dermatitis, multiple allergies, metabolic wasting (SAM) syndrome, ichthyosis prematurity syndrome
  - *Immunodeficiency*:
    - Combined defect—severe combined immunodeficiency (SCID), Omenn's syndrome
    - Wiskott-Aldrich syndrome, hyperimmunoglobulin E syndrome (HIES)
    - Complement defect—hemophagocytic lymphohistiocytosis (HLH)
    - T-cell defect—DiGeorge syndrome
    - Antibody deficiency—hypogammaglobulinemia
    - Graft-versus-host disease (GVHD)
    - Immune dysregulation, polyendocrinopathy, enteropathy, X linked (IPEX) syndrome
  - *Metabolic*:
    - Acrodermatitis enteropathica
    - Multiple carboxylase deficiency
    - Essential fatty acid deficiency
    - Organic academia—propionic academia, methylmalonic academia, glutaric academia
    - Urea cycle defects—ornithine transcarbamylase (OTC) deficiency, citrullinemia, carbamoyl phosphate synthetase (CPS) deficiency
    - Aminoacidopathy—maple syrup urine disease (MSUD)
    - CF
    - Renal failure
  - *Nutritional*:
    - Acquired zinc deficiency
    - Kwashiorkor
  - *Malignancies*:
    - Diffuse cutaneous mastocytosis
    - Cutaneous T-cell lymphoma

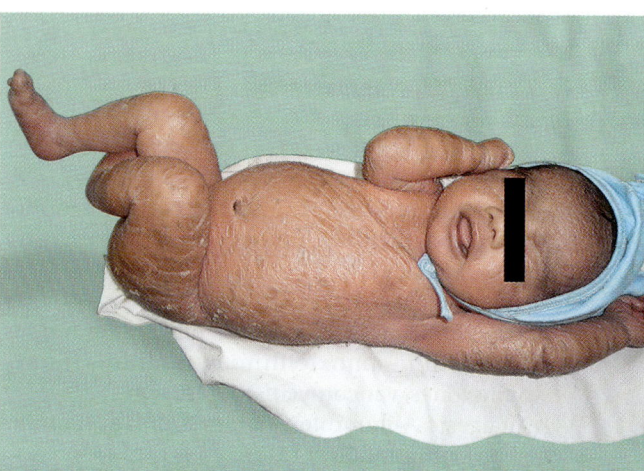

FIG. 2: Lamellar ichthyosis.

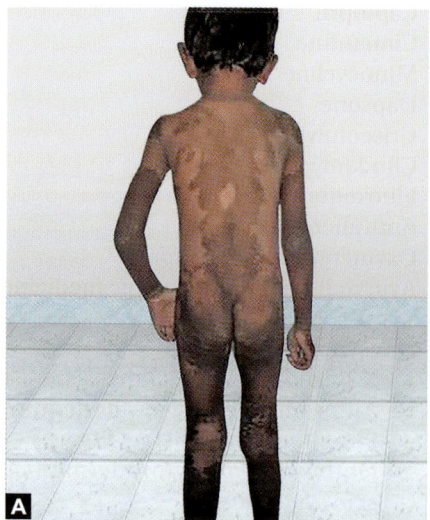
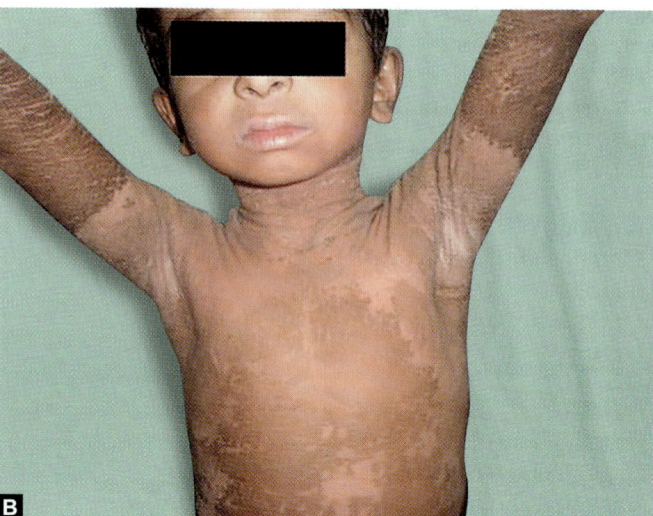

FIGS. 3A AND B: Ichthyosis hystrix.

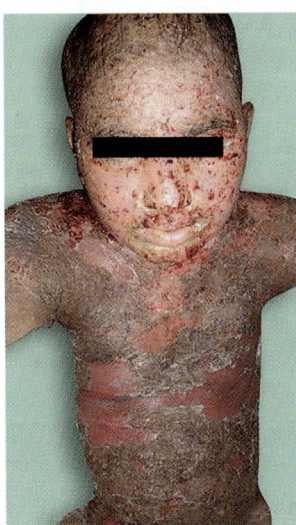

FIG. 4: Pemphigus foliaceus.

- Idiopathic
- Ectodermal dysplasia [ankyloblepharon-ectodermal defects-cleft lip/palate (AEC syndrome)]
- *Autoimmune*:
  - Kawasaki disease
  - Dermatomyositis
  - Pemphigus foliaceus **(Fig. 4)**
  - Sarcoidosis

APPROACH

Pediatric erythroderma is definitely a diagnostic challenge for pediatric dermatologists. A thorough history, clinical examination and investigative workup forms the cornerstone of appropriate therapeutic intervention.

HISTORY[14-20,26]

History of erythroderma is given in **Table 1**.

EXAMINATION

General Examination[14-20,26]

General **(Table 2)** and systemic examinations **(Table 3)** in childhood erythroderma are of vital importance as they give a clue to possible underlying etiology.

Table 3 depicts important findings on systemic examination in childhood erythroderma.

Mucocutaneous Examination[14-20,26]

Hair

- Alopecia/hypotrichosis in Omenn's syndrome
- Graft-versus-host reaction (GvHR)

- Netherton's syndrome
- IPEX syndrome
- SAM syndrome
- Acrodermatitis enteropathica
- Acquired zinc deficiency
- Biotin metabolism disorders
- Citrullinemia
- TTD (brittle hair); dark and light bands in malnutrition
- Erosive dermatitis in AEC syndrome
- Pemphigus foliaceus

Skin Examination

- *Type of scale:*
  - Hystrix (porcupine spine) like—hystrix-like ichthyosis with deafness (HID) syndrome, ichthyosis hystrix
  - Double edged—Netherton syndrome
  - Large plate like—Lamellar ichthyosis
  - Fine white on body and plate like on extensor—CIE
  - Fine scale—peeling skin syndrome
- *Distribution*:
  - Extensor—KID syndrome
  - Flexor—TTD
  - Blaschko's line—Conradi-Hunermann-Happle syndrome
  - Ipsilateral—CHILD (congenital hemidysplasia with ichthyosiform erythroderma and limb defects)
  - Sparing of diaper area and axilla—atopic dermatitis
- *Associated features/specific features*:
  - Periorificial dermatitis—metabolic and nutritional
  - Target lesions—TEN
  - Darrier's sign—mastocytosis
  - Cold abscess—HIES
  - Absence of sweating—ectodermal dysplasia
  - Aquagenic palmoplantar wrinkling, white marks when skin gets dry—CF
  - Nikosky sign—SSSS, TEN
  - Palmoplantar thickening—PRP, AEC syndrome, CF, SAM syndrome
  - Skip areas—PRP
  - Swirled pattern of erythroderma—Conradi-Hunermann-Happle syndrome
  - Well-defined erythematous scaly plague with involvement of diaper area—psoriasis
  - Keratotic follicular papules—PRP

Nails

- Paronychia, dystrophy—chronic cutaneous candidiasis
- Dystrophy—SAM syndrome, AEC syndrome
- Clubbing—CF

Mucosa

- Recurrent thrush in pelvic inflammatory disease (PID)
- Cleft palate in HIES
- Cleft lip/palate in ectodermal dysplasia
- Strawberry tongue in Kawasaki disease

Table 1: History of erythroderma.	
Consanguineous marriage and pedigree chart, previous child with same disease, similar complaint in other family member	• Ichthyosis (common) • IEM (rare) • PIDS (rare)
Failure to thrive	Malnutrition, Netherton syndrome, cystic fibrosis, IEM (rare), PID (rare), SAM syndrome (rare), Gaucher disease (rare)
Infection (recurrent, severe, fulminant, complicated, persistent infections, unusual sites), diarrhea, autoimmune disease, or hematological malignancy in family members, family history of PID	PID (Rule out (r/o) HIV)
Lethargy, poor feeding, vomiting, chronic hiccups, difficult to control seizures, acute deterioration after a period of normalcy, poor response to treatment to a supposedly acquired illness	IEM
Atopy	Atopic dermatitis, Netherton syndrome, Wiskott–Aldrich syndrome, SAM syndrome, HIES
Diarrhea	Omenn syndrome, GVHD, Netherton syndrome
Collodion baby	Lamellar ichthyosis, Non-BIE, trichothiodystrophy, NLSD, Conradi–Hunermann disease, Sjogren–Larsson syndrome, Gaucher's disease
Maternal history of still birth, nonimmune hydrops in fetus	Gaucher's disease
Family history of linear epidermal nevus	BIE
Family history of similar complaint	Atopy, psoriasis, PRP, BIE, Netherton's syndrome, PID, IEM
Persistent cough, breathing difficulty, cystic frothy, oily, foul smelling stool difficult to clean, floating of stool in water even after flushing, poor weight gain even after adequate food intake, recurrent abdominal pain, and rectum coming out which has to be pushed manually, salty taste on kissing the baby	Cystic fibrosis
Blisters	SSSS, mastocytosis, BIE
History of maternal vaginal candidiasis, prolonged rupture of membranes, administration of antibiotics (+/-)	Congenital cutaneous candidiasis
Preceding purulent infection	SSSS
Concomitant maternal infection	TSS
Irritability, diarrhea, poor appetite, weight loss, periorificial dermatitis	Acrodermatitis enteropathica
Hypogeusia, anosmia	Acquired zinc deficiency
Blood transfusion, diarrhea	GVHD
Nausea, vomiting, diarrhea, abdominal pain	Diffuse cutaneous mastocytosis

(BIE: bullous ichthyosiform erythroderma; GVHD: graft-versus-host disease; HIV: human immunodeficiency virus; HIES: hyperimmunoglobulin E syndrome; IEM: inborn errors of metabolism; NLSD: neutral lipid storage disease; PRP: pityriasis rubra pilaris; PID: pelvic inflammatory disease; PIDS: primary immunodeficiency syndrome; SSSS: staphylococcal scalded skin syndrome; SAM: severe dermatitis, multiple allergies, metabolic wasting; TSS: toxic shock syndrome)

INVESTIGATIONS[14-20,26,27]

Skin Biopsy

Skin biopsy is essential as in adults to take specimens from two to three different sites simultaneously to establish the underlying cause of erythroderma. Histopathology of childhood erythroderma showed histology of dermatitis or psoriasiform changes **(Table 4)**.

Routine Investigations

- *Complete blood count*:
    - Anemia—CF, malnutrition, Gaucher disease, diffuse cutaneous mastocytosis with systemic involvement
    - Leukocytosis—SSSS, TSS
    - Neutropenia—can be found in neutrophil defects
    - Eosinophil count—markedly increased in Omenn syndrome and Netherton syndrome. Mildly increased in atopic dermatitis and associated syndromes.
    - Thrombocytopenia—Wiskott-Aldrich syndrome, Gaucher disease, diffuse cutaneous mastocytosis with systemic involvement
- Liver function test—Chanarin–Dorfman syndrome, Gaucher's disease, Inborn errors of metabolism
- Elevated blood urea and serum creatinine—TEN
- Serum electrolytes—hypernatremic dehydration
Screening tests when an IEM is suspected **(Tables 5 and 6 and Flowchart 1)**.

Table 2: General examination.

Assessment	Examination findings	Possible etiology
Growth assessment	• Unexplained weight loss and wasting • Failure to thrive • Developmental delay and short stature • Wasting • Growth retardation	• Antibody deficiency, any chronic inflammatory state • Malnutrition, Netherton syndrome, IEM, PIDS, cystic fibrosis, SAM syndrome, Gaucher's disease • NLSD, trichothiodystrophy • Essential fatty acid deficiency • Acquired zinc deficiency
Facies: • Coarse facies • Dysmorphic facies	• Prominent forehead, broad nasal bridge, deep set eyes, broad outer canthal distance • Periorbital fullness, narrow upslanted palpebral fissure, prominent nose with large tip and hypoplastic nares, small mouth, everted upper lip, hypoplastic ears	• Hyper IgE syndrome • DiGeorge syndrome
Shock	–	TEN, TSS, diffuse cutaneous mastocytosis
Lymphoid tissue	• Absence of lymph nodes and tonsils • Lymphadenopathy • Asplenia • Hepatosplenomegaly	• SCID • Omenn's syndrome, GVHD, atopic dermatitis, DRESS, diffuse cutaneous mastocytosis, IPEX syndrome • Chronic GVHD • Omenn's syndrome, GVHD, NLSD, DRESS, diffuse cutaneous mastocytosis, Gaucher's disease, IPEX syndrome

(DRESS: drug reaction with eosinophilia and systemic symptoms; IPEX: immune dysregulation, polyendocrinopathy, enteropathy, X linked; Ig: immunoglobulin; IEM: inborn errors of metabolism; NLSD: neutral lipid storage disease; PIDS: primary immunodeficiency syndrome; SCID: severe combined immunodeficiency; SAM: severe dermatitis, multiple allergies, metabolic wasting; TEN: toxic epidermal necrolysis; TSS: toxic shock syndrome)

Table 3: Systemic examination.

Examination	Examination findings	Possible etiology
CNS	• Spasticity and mental retardation • Hypotonia, ataxia, and seizures • Seizures, abnormal muscle tone, athetosis	• Trichothiodystrophy, SLS, DiGeorge syndrome • Biotinidase deficiency • Holocarboxylase synthase deficiency
CVS	• Tachycardia	• Diffuse cutaneous mastocytosis
Respiratory	• Productive cough with mucoid or purulent sputum, wheeze or crackles, hyperresonant lungs • Hyperventilation, laryngeal stridor, apnea	• Cystic fibrosis • Biotinidase deficiency
Eye	• Ankyloblepharon • Ectropion • Cataract • Keratitis • Sectorial cataracts • Perifoveal glistening dots • Optic nerve atrophy, keratoconjunctivitis • Oculomotor apraxia	• AEC syndrome • Collodion baby • NLSD • KID syndrome • Conradi–Hunermann–Happle syndrome • SLS • Biotinidase deficiency • Gaucher's disease
ENT	• Scarred tympanic membranes or chronic perforation due to recurrent otitis media • Sensorineural hearing loss	• Hypogammaglobulinemia • KID syndrome, NLSD, biotinidase deficiency, hyper IgE syndrome
Musculoskeletal	• Myopathy • Congenital hemidysplasia and limb defects	• NLSD • CHILD syndrome
Genital	Hypogonadism	Zinc deficiency

(AEC: ankyloblepharon-ectodermal defects-cleft lip/palate; CHILD: congenital hemidysplasia with ichthyosiform erythroderma and limb defects; CNS: central nervous system; CVS: cardiovascular system; Ig: immunoglobulin; KID: keratitis–ichthyosis–deafness; NLSD: neutral lipid storage disease; SLS: Sjögren–Larsson syndrome)

Table 4: Histopathological findings in erythroderma of various etiologies.

Histopathological changes	Psoriasiform	Ichthyosiform	Lipid vacuoles	Eczematous	Basal layer pigmentation and mast cell deposition around blood vessels and throughout dermis	Necrosis of epidermal keratinocytes
Disease	Psoriasis, Netherton syndrome	Ichthyosis	NLSD	Atopic dermatitis, Seborrheic dermatitis	Mastocytosis	TEN

(NLSD: neutral lipid storage disease; TEN: toxic epidermal necrolysis)

Table 5: Screening tests when an inborn error of metabolism is suspected.[28]

Blood	• Complete blood count (neutropenia and thrombocytopenia seen in propionic academia and methylmalonic academia) • SGPT/SGOT, PT, and APTT • Creatinine • Uric acid • Calcium • Electrolytes • Arterial blood gas, anion gap $(Na^+ + K^+) - [Cl^- + HCO_3^-]$ • Ammonia (normal values in newborn: 90–150 mg/dL or 64–107 mmol/L) • Arterial blood lactate (normal values of lactate: 0.5–1.6 mmol/L) • Glucose
Urine	• Odor (burnt sugar in maple syrup urine disease, sweaty feet in organic acidemias, musty or mousy odor in phenylketonuria) • Ketones • Reducing substances by Benedict's reagent and glucose oxidase

(APTT: activated partial thromboplastin time; PT: prothrombin time; SGPT: serum glutamic pyruvic transaminase; SGOT: serum glutamic oxaloacetic transaminase)

Table 6: Categorization of common inborn errors of metabolisms causing erythroderma based on simple metabolic screening tests.[28]

Disorder	Acidosis	Ketosis	Ammonia	Lactate	Glucose
MSUD	N	++	N	N	N/↓
Organic acidemias	+	++	N/↑	N/↑	↓↓
Urea cycle disorders	N	N	↑↑	N	N

(MSUD: maple syrup urine disease)

Special Investigations

Once a differential diagnosis with the help of history, physical examination, and basic investigations as detailed above is made, specific investigations need to be performed in a targeted manner based on presumptive diagnosis.
- Muscle enzymes, serum lipid profile, peripheral blood smear for Jordan's anomaly in Chanarin-Dorfman syndrome
- Serum Vitamin D levels for undiagnosed and untreated rickets due to ichthyosis or treatment with retinoids
- Serum immunoglobulin (Ig)E—atopic dermatitis, Wiskott-Aldrich syndrome, Omenn syndrome, Netherton's syndrome, DiGeorge syndrome, GVHD, SAM syndrome, IPEX syndrome[29]
- Swabs from skin, eyes, nose, and umbilicus—SSSS, TSS, CCC
- Culture of urine, blood, and cerebrospinal fluid (CSF)—candidiasis
  ○ KOH mount—candidiasis
  ○ Tzanck smear—pemphigus foliaceus, herpes simplex virus (HSV) infection
  ○ Wet mount—sarcoptes mite
  ○ High-vaginal swab from mother—*Staphylococcus aureus* or CCC
  ○ Trichoscopy—trichorrhexis invaginata or bamboo hair in Netherton syndrome, hair shafts with nonhomogeneous structure of grains of sand with slightly wavy appearance in TTD,[30] pili torti in citrullinemia,[31] spindle-shaped intermittent hair shaft constrictions with fracturing at different lengths in acrodermatitis enteropathica.[32]

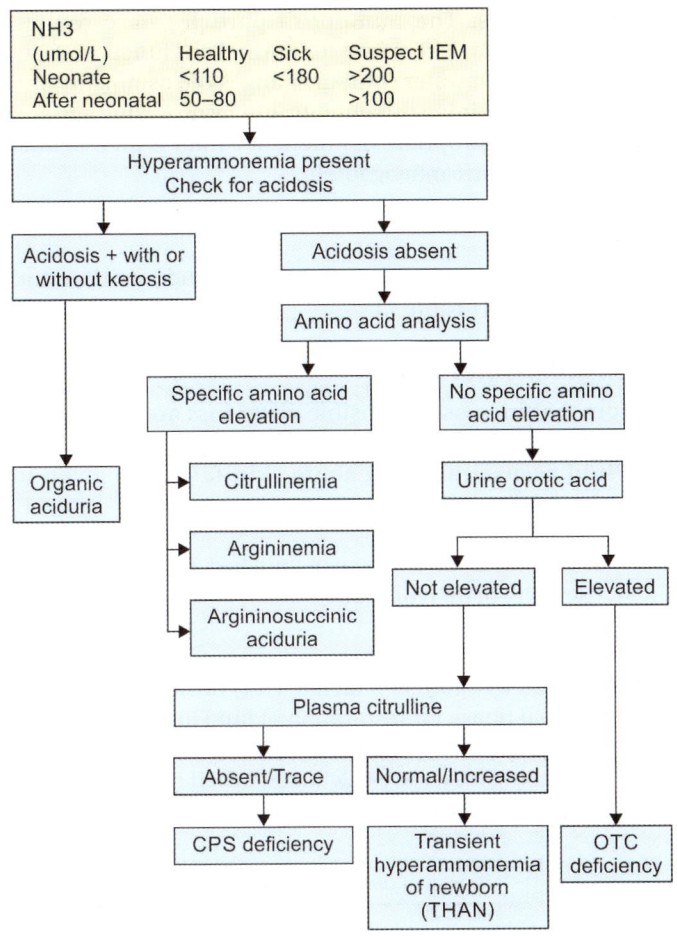

FLOWCHART 1: Algorithmic approach to diagnose an inborn errors of metabolism (IEM) presenting as erythroderma.[28]
(CPS: carbamoyl phosphate synthetase; OTC: ornithine transcarbamylase)

- Light microscopy/polarized microscopy—band-like pattern in Netherton syndrome;[33] trichoschisis on light microscopy and alternate dark and light bands: tiger tail pattern on polarized microscopy in TTD;[30] pseudomonilethrix nodal swelling, atypical trichorrhexis nodosa with stretch fractures and kinking, irregular pattern of alternate dark and light bands, variation in hair shaft diameter with a spindle appearance, cortex thinning in acrodermatitis enteropathica.[32]
- Complement level—Leiner's disease
- T- and B-lymphocytes count, antibodies level—immunodeficiency syndromes
- Oxygen saturation—SJS/TEN
- Serum zinc levels in mother and infant, zinc levels in maternal milk, serum albumin, serum alkaline phosphatase—acrodermatitis enteropathica
- Sweat chloride levels, sputum/cough swab, mutation analysis for *CFTR* gene (in cases with intermittent sweat chloride test results)—CF
- Acid beta-glucocerebrosidase enzyme assay in blood leucocytes, bone marrow biopsy for Gaucher's cells, chitotriosidase assay (up to 1,000 fold) to assess disease status—Gaucher's disease
- Blood for fatty acid levels (triene: tetraene ratio >0.4)—essential fatty acid deficiency
- Genetic analysis for *SPINK5*—Netherton syndrome
- Genetic analysis for *GBA*—Gaucher's disease
- X-ray chest-absent thymic shadow—SCID
- X-ray spine and pelvis—Gaucher's disease
- DEXA (dual energy X-ray absorptiometry) scan—Gaucher's disease
- Magnetic resonance imaging (MRI) spine and femur neck (optional)—Gaucher's disease
- Pulmonary (optional)
  - Pulmonary function tests ⎤ Gaucher's
  - Computed tomography chest ⎦ disease
- Two dimensional (2D) echo (if indicated)—Gaucher's disease
- Ultrasound (USG) abdomen in Gaucher's disease, Chanarin–Dorfman syndrome
- Histamine and its metabolite levels, tryptase in serum or urine—mastocytosis
- HLA-B17—positive in congenital psoriasis
- Audiometry—KID syndrome
- Fetal USG/2D echo—conotruncal defects in DiGeorge syndrome
- Organic acids by gas chromatography mass spectrometry (GC-MS) of urine for diagnosis of organic acidemias, biotinidase deficiency.
- Plasma amino acids by high performance liquid chromatography (HPLC)—required for diagnosis of organic acidemias and aminoacidopathies.
- Carnitine and acylcarnitine profile by tandem MS for diagnosis of organic acidemias, aminoacidopathies, and urea cycle defects.
- Lactate/pyruvate ratio in cases with elevated lactate.
- Urinary orotic acid in cases of hyperammonemia to classify urea cycle defect.
- Enzyme assay—biotinidase assay in serum or plasma in suspected biotinidase deficiency (metabolic ketolactic acidosis, hyperammonemia, and urinary excretion of 3-hydroxyisolvalerate)
- Neuroimaging—MRI may provide helpful pointers toward underlying etiology. Examples of neuroimaging findings in IEMs include:
  - MSUD—brainstem and cerebellar edema
  - Propionic and methylmalonic academia—basal ganglia signal change
  - Glutaric aciduria—frontotemporal atrophy, subdural hematoma
  - Biotinidase deficiency—cerebral atrophy, ventriculomegaly, widened extra cerebral spaces, subdural effusions, basal ganglion calcifications, T2 and fluid-attenuated inversion-recovery (FLAIR) hyperintensities in bilateral hippocampi and parahippocampal gyri[34]

- Magnetic resonance spectroscopy—may be helpful in selected disorders, e.g., leucine peak in MSUD
- Electroencephalography (EEG)—some EEG abnormalities may be suggestive of particular IEM, e.g., comb-like rhythm in MSUD, burst suppression in holocarboxylase synthase deficiency.
- Mutation analysis by next-generation sequencing (NGS) when available. Confirmed etiological diagnosis is essential for providing prenatal diagnosis and should be done even in cases of expected poor outcome or after death. In cases where there is no sample for DNA analysis, whole exome sequencing (WES) should be done in one or both the parents to identify carrier status for an autosomal recessive disorder in both of them or a heterozygous mutation for an X-linked disorder in mother. WES has an added advantage as it can also identify other genetic disorder with a presentation similar to IEM even when the clinician has not suspected it.
- CSF analysis of glucose, lactate, and amino acids.

Note: In a very sick neonate/child, metabolic investigations may not be always possible and most of the IEMs have a 25–50% risk of recurrence in subsequent pregnancy. In the absence of confirmed diagnosis, genetic counseling, and prenatal diagnosis is not possible. In such situations, blood, urine, CSF/tissue biopsy samples must be stored (metabolic autopsy) for diagnostic purposes.[28]

MANAGEMENT

Irrespective of the cause, erythroderma especially during the neonatal and infantile period is a dermatological emergency. Erythrodermic children are threatened by thermoregulatory disturbances, fluid and electrolyte imbalance, and infections due to barrier dysfunction. Hence, careful monitoring of fluid, electrolytes, and maintenance of oral and parenteral intake is mandatory.[18]

General Measures and Management of Complications

Fluid and Electrolyte Balance: The Rationale

Maintenance of fluid and electrolyte balance constitutes an important part of management of hospitalized children. Composition of body fluids is given in **Flowchart 2**.[35]
- Total body water at 26 weeks gestation is 80% which reduces to 60% of total body weight at around 1 year of age.
- Total maintenance of body fluid in various compartments occurs by colloid osmotic pressure, membrane permeability, and hydrostatic pressure.
- The extracellular fluid (ECF) consists of Na, Cl, and HCO_3.
- The intracellular fluid on the other hand is made up of phospholipid, creatinine kinase, and adenosine triphosphate. The number of particles here remain constant and it is required for normal cell function.
- Any change in water content changes the osmolality and hence maintaining this equilibrium by providing age and condition appropriate maintenance fluid is an essential part of pediatric management.

Fluid Losses[36]

The two categories of ongoing fluid loss include sensible and insensible losses **(Table 7)**.

Insensible Water Loss

Factors that increase insensible water loss are outlined in **Table 8**.

Fluid resuscitation in acute skin failure is given in **Flowchart 3**.[35]
- *Restoration of fluid loss*:
  - Depends upon the type of fluid lost
  - Severity of dehydration
  - Underlying disease
  - Age of the patient

Isotonic fluid like Ringer's lactate (RL) or normal saline is used in initial phase for restoration of fluid loss.
- *Replacement of ongoing losses*:
  - On going losses are calculated based on the extent of skin conditions.

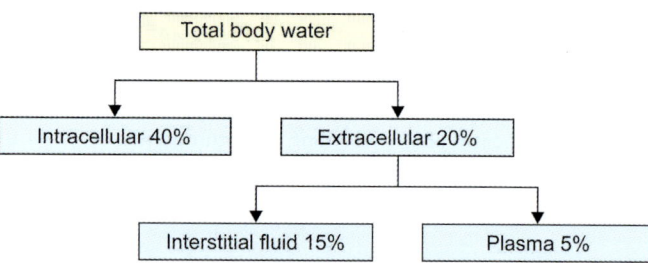

FLOWCHART 2: Composition of body fluids.

Table 7: Fluid losses.	
Sensible water losses	Seen and measured, e.g., urine, stool, gastric aspirate
Insensible water losses	Cannot be seen and measured, e.g., perspiration and respiration (skin and RS)
(RS: respiratory system)	

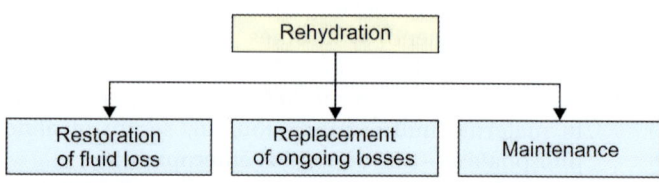

FLOWCHART 3: Fluid resuscitation in acute skin failure.

Table 8: Insensible fluid loss in erythroderma.	
Increased IWL	Tachypnea, fever, crying, skin loss, prematurity
Loss occurring through scales/erosions in blister fluid in TEN[33]	• 120–150 mmol/L Na$^+$ • 100 mmol/L Cl$^-$ • 5–10 mmol/L K$^+$ • 40 g/L protein
Normal TEWL[36,37]	400 mL/day
Increased TEWL[36]	• Two to fivefold higher in erythroderma patients than normal subjects • Loss is more in acute erythroderma than in chronic • In psoriasis, the TEWL is 10–20 times more than normal
Other factors affecting TEWL	• Humidity • Temperature • Time of year (season variation) • Moisture content of the skin (hydration level)

(IWL: insensible water loss; TEWL: transepidermal water loss; TEN: toxic epidermal necrolysis)

Table 9: Calculation of maintenance fluid.	
Weight	Fluid requirement
<10 kg	100 mL/kg
10–20 kg	1,000 + 50 mL/kg for every kg >10
>20 kg	1,500 + 20 mL/kg for every kg >20

- ○ Risk of fluid and electrolyte disturbance is higher in children because:
  - Increased metabolic rate → increased caloric expenditure
  - Relatively higher BSA → increased water loss from skin
  - Increased respiratory rate
  - Immaturity of renal system
- *Maintenance fluid:*[35]
  - ○ Calculation of maintenance fluid is done according to Holliday and Segar formula **(Table 9)**.
  - ○ Maintenance fluid should contain:
    - 30 mEq/L—Na and Cl
    - 5 mEq/L
    - 5 % dextrose

Traditionally, isolyte P is used as a maintenance fluid in pediatric patients. However, the recent concept is to use less hypotonic fluid, i.e., 0.45% dextrose saline (DNS) with added potassium chloride (KCl) as a maintenance fluid.

Based on the above concepts of fluid resuscitation, following is the plan for fluid administration for rehydration **(Table 10)**.

HYPERNATREMIC DEHYDRATION IN OTHER SKIN CONDITIONS[35]

In conditions characterized by ichthyosis and scaling, since children do not drink water on their own in response

Table 10: Plan for fluid administration for rehydration.	
Phase	Fluid and electrolytes
Initial phase (first 24 hours)	2 mL/kg/% BSA of RL + maintenance fluid by Holliday and Segar formula
Next 24 hours	0.25 mL/kg/% BSA 5% albumin in NS + D5W to maintain urine output 1 mL/kg/h
Maintenance phase (EWL + MF)	[(% BSA + 35) × BSA × 24]/2 + [1,500 × BSA (m^2)] of D5W ½ NS with potassium supplements (40 mEq/L at a rate of 3 mEq/kg/24 hours) (Gradually IV fluids are converted to oral fluids over next few days)

(BSA: body surface area; D5W: dextrose in water; IV: intravenous; NS: normal saline; RL: Ringer's lactate)

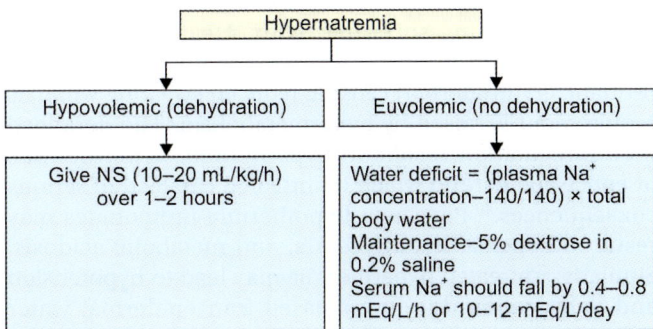

FLOWCHART 4: Fluid and electrolyte therapy in other conditions.

to hypernatremia → associated thirst → hypernatremic dehydration **(Flowchart 4)**.

Monitor a patient during fluid resuscitation **(Table 11)**.[38]

Thermoregulation: The Rationale

Maintenance of temperature is striking a balance between minimizing heat loss and the mechanisms of heat

Table 11: Noninvasive guide to fluid resuscitation.			
Vitals	**Physical signs**	**Laboratory investigations**	**Fluid losses**
• Temperature • Heart rate • Respiratory rate • Blood pressure • SpO$_2$	• Sensorium • Body weight • Peripheral circulation • Urine output	• Hematocrit • BUN and serum creatinine • Serum electrolytes • Urea electrolytes and osmolality • Blood gases and pH	• Urine • Stool • Gastric
(BUN: blood urea nitrogen)			

production. In older children and adults, heat production and conservation occurs via shivering, peripheral vasoconstriction, and diminished sweating. However, newborns have a distinct physiologic response. Apart from vasoconstriction, these factors have a limited role to play in newborns. Sympathetic stimulation of skeletal muscle is minimal and shivering (perceived as change in behavior and increased movement) plays little role in response to cold. Instead, the newborn largely accelerates heat production by nonshivering thermogenesis or direct heat production through metabolism of adipose tissue. In addition, in newborn especially the premature newborn, heat loss is a major factor. Heat loss occurs through four different mechanisms (1) conduction, (2) convection, (3) radiation, and (4) evaporation.[39] Also, newborns in comparison to adults are more susceptible to heat loss due to larger BSA to body mass ratio, rapid transepidermal water loss through a thinner and under keratinized epidermis, diminished amount of subcutaneous fat and greater body water content.

In erythroderma, heat conservation is impaired as the ability of affected skin to vasoconstrict fully in response to cold is decreased. In addition, because of increase blood flow and temperature, the cutaneous cold receptors are not activated thereby abolishing shivering reflex. Heat elimination is impaired due to occlusion of sweat gland (especially in psoriatic erythroderma) causing reduced sweating while its requirement is raised by hypermetabolism. The deranged thermoregulation results in hypothermia, hyperthermia, or concealed pyrexia which if untreated can lead to serious consequences.[40] Persistent hypothermia in neonates may result in hypoxia, hypoglycemia, and metabolic acidosis. Similarly, untreated hyperthermia may lead to hypotension and dehydration due to increased transepidermal water loss, seizures and apnea (due to high core temperature), and hypernatremia.

Recommendation[36]

Hypothermia is defined as rectal temperature <35.5°C or 95.5°F or axillary temperature <35°C or 95°F. In presence of hypothermia, always screen for *blood glucose* and screen for *infections*.

Prevention of Hypothermia[40]

Preventions of hypothermia are as follows:
- Appropriate clothing, skin-to-skin contact [kangaroo mother care (KMC)]
- Change wet clothing
- Windows closed, fans off
- Continue breastfeeding

Management of Hypothermia[40]

- *Mild hypothermia*:
  ○ Remove cold clothes
  ○ KMC, skin-to-skin contact
  ○ Keep room draught free, continue breastfeeding
  ○ Hot water bottles—placed away from baby
  ○ Monitor temperature and capillary refill time (CRT), apnea, and hypoglycemia.
- *Moderate-to-severe hypothermia*:
  ○ Rapid rewarming up to 34°C
  ○ Remove cold clothes
  ○ Radiant warmer/incubator
  ○ Monitor temperature, oxygen saturation with pulse oximeter, CRT, and blood sugar
  ○ Heating lamp/hot water bags/*angeethi*
  ○ KMC stabilization and transport to higher center

Supportive Management

Supportive management of hypothermia are as follows:
- Prompt detection and treatment of hypoxia, hypoperfusion, and hypoglycemia.
- Dextrose infusion 6–8 mg/kg/min
- RL or normal saline (NS) 20 mL/kg over 5 minutes
- Monitor axillary temperature every 30 minutes

Hyperthermia is defined as temperature >37.5°C (**Box 1**).

Always Remember

- In young infants, due to underdeveloped thermo-regulation mechanisms, the body temperature is affected by the environmental temperature.
- Hence, temperature of the room should be maintained at 31–32°C.

Box 1: Management of hyperthermia.
- Undress the baby partly/fully
- Monitor hydration, weight, urine output, and renal function
- Give frequent feeds
- Correct dehydration
- Tepid sponging, if temperature >39°C

NUTRITION: THE RATIONALE

Protein and iron are the principal nutrients lost through skin. Disturbed protein metabolism is due to protein loss through skin and gastrointestinal tract (GIT), due to malabsorption, decreased synthesis, increased catabolism, and decreased intake of protein.[41] In severe scaling, the cumulative effect of these factors results in negative nitrogen balance—hypoalbuminemia (decreased serum protein, reversal of albumin globulin ratio), edema, and loss of muscle mass.[42,43]

The severity of hypoproteinemia varies depending on the primary etiology, chronicity of illness, and inter individual differences. The amount of protein lost in psoriasis is significantly greater than (25–30%) in other conditions (10–15%), due to high-cell turnover which may be further exacerbated by intense dermal inflammation compared to other conditions where only inflammation plays a role.[42]

In addition to protein loss through scale, there is impaired utilization and absorption of iron and vitamin B12. Relative folate deficiency arises due to increased cellular turnover. All these factors contribute to anemia.[41]

Caloric requirement is also increased in erythrodermic children to meet the demands of hypermetabolic state and requirements of normal growth and development.

Recommendation

To replenish the losses, child's diet should be high in protein 3–4 g/kg body weight per day.[38]

In TEN, protein requirement—3 g/kg + 1 g/% BSA.[35] Supplementation with protein-rich diet, i.e., eggs, fish, milk, legumes or commercially available protein powders is required till scaling ceases clinically.[38]

Ferrous sulfate or fumarate to be given in a dose of 4 mg (elemental iron)/kg to combat anemia.

Formulae to meet the caloric requirements in TEN are given in **Box 2**.[35]

To replace the calories in a sick child, F75 and F100 preparations are used **(Table 12 and Boxes 3 and 4)**.[44]

Sample requirement calculation in a 10 kg child.
For example: A 10 kg child
- Protein required—2 g/kg
- Calorie required—100 kcal/kg
- 10 kg required—20 g protein and 1,000 kcal
- 12 hourly feed → so every 2 hourly feed = 1,000/12 = 80 mL/feed
- Start with F-75 = 100 mL

Box 2: Formulae to meet the caloric requirements in toxic epidermal necrolysis.
Sutherland formula:
- 60 kcal/kg + 35 kcal/% BSA as enteral feeding in equal amount of fluid

For example, 600 + 35 × 0.5 = 600 + 15.5 = 615.5 = 600 kcal

Modified Harris–Benedict formula:
- 0–12 months—2,100 kcal/m^2 + 1,000 kcal/m^2 TBSA involved:
  - 1–11 years—1,800 kcal/m^2 + 1,300 kcal/m^2
  - 12 years or older—1,500 kcal/m^2 + 1,500 kcal/m^2

(BSA: body surface area; TBSA: total body surface area) |

Table 12: Composition of WHO recommended F-75 and F-100 diets.

Amount per 100 mL		
Constituents	F75	F100
Energy (calories)	75	100
Protein (g)	0.9	2.9
Lactose (g)	1.3	3.0
Potassium (mmol)	3.6	5.9
Sodium (mmol)	0.6	1.9
Magnesium (mmol)	0.43	0.73
Zinc (mg)	2.0	2.3
Copper (mg)	0.25	0.25
Osmolality (mOsmol/L)	333	419

Box 3: Recipe for F-75.
Recipe for F75
- *Fresh cow's milk*: 30 mL (1/3 cup)
- *Sugar*: 6 g (1 tablespoon)
- *Puffed rice/cereal flour*: 3 g (1 tablespoon)
- *Vegetable oil*: 2.5 g (1/2+ tablespoon)
- *Water to make*: 100 mL
- Gives 75 kcal, 0.9 g protein, and 1 g lactose

Kept at room temperature for 6 hours and in fridge for 24 hours. |

Box 4: Recipe for F-100.
Recipe for F100
- *Fresh milk*: 75 g (1/2 cup)
- *Sugar*: 2.5 g (1/2 tablespoon)
- *Cereal flour/puffed rice*: 7 g (2 tablespoons)
- *Vegetable oil*: 2 g (1/2 tablespoon)
- *Water to make*: 100 mL

- 1 g lactogen is 4.89 kcal
- 3 scoops of lactogen—75 kcal
- Formula—100 mL milk—75 kcal + 1 tablespoon sugar—20 kcal + 1/2 tablespoon oil—5 kcal—100 m/100 kcal

SPECIFIC MEASURES

Ichthyosis

Congenital ichthyosis does not have a cure, has a major impact on quality of life (QoL), and therefore, requires lifelong treatment. Treatment includes a combination of different symptomatic therapeutic modalities ranging from skin care with frequent bathing, daily topical emollients, and environmental humidification to systemic treatment using retinoids.

Bathing

Parents/caregiver should be explained about the importance of intensive bath therapy in severe ichthyosis. Bathing cleanses, hydrates the skin, loosens the scales which facilitates mechanical removal, and clears the residual medicaments. Most patients prefer bathing over showers as it helps in scale removal. Children including newborns should be bathed in lukewarm water (27–30°C) once or twice daily for 30–60 minutes in absence of nondermatologic contraindications.[45] An ideal cleansing agent is a low pH, hypoallergenic, and fragrance-free agent. Parents should be advised to use syndets or lipid-free cleansers.[46] In resource-rich settings, pretreatment with temperature controlled steam bath or steam shower (for 5–15 min) is advisable to loosen the scales and hydrate the skin.

Bath Additives

The indication for use of bath additive depends on the requirement—lipid replacement or keratolysis. Moisturizing additives like oil is not ideal as it is messy, occlusive, not keratolytic, requires effort in cleaning the bathtub and associated with risk of slipping. On the other hand, saltwater baths (normal saline 0.9%) promotes hydration and keratolysis. However, children with erythrodermic ichthyosis, Netherton syndrome, those with extensive erosions may experience burning and irritation. In most other forms of ichthyosis, salt additives work well and can be used daily in a concentration not exceeding 3–4% (0.45 kg/3.79 L) in children.[45]

Keratolytic agents like sodium hydrogen carbonate (commercially available as baking soda) found to be most effective causes loosening of keratosis through increased activity of serine proteases. The treatment is generally recommended for patients ≥1 year of age. For infants and toddlers, the concentration should be 3 g/L. For adults, 6 g/L is required for adequate keratolysis. Other keratolytic products that can be tried, if sodium hydrogen carbonate is not helpful include wheat starch, rice starch, and corn starch.[45]

In congenital ichthyosis with recurrent and overt skin infections like KID syndrome or Netherton syndrome (including newborn), antiseptics such as diluted bleach baths (0.005%) (most commonly used), chlorhexidine (dilution 5/1,000 – 5/10,000) or potassium permanganate (1/10,000) should be used.[45] The bleach solution is to be prepared by adding 1 tablespoon of household bleaching powder to 1 L of water, and this should be diluted to a bucket of water (20 L).[46] The antiseptic bath should be used two or three times a week and the frequency can be reduced as the condition improves and continued as a maintenance treatment, to prolong the remission period. Iodine-based antiseptic baths are not recommended as they carry risk of thyroid dysfunction.[47]

Mechanical Keratolysis

After bathing or immediately after pretreatment in a steam bath, moderate scrubbing using sponges/loofah, soft wash cloth, microfiber household towels, or pumice stone is more effective in loosening the scales than topical keratolytics. The treatment frequency depends on the severity of ichthyosis (between once a day and once a week). The duration of treatment lasts for 60–90 minutes, if whole body is affected.[46] However, scrubbing is not recommended in Netherton syndrome and epidermolytic ichthyosis.

Emollients

The choice of emollient depends on the preference of the patient/caregiver. Ideally the emollient of choice should be dispensed in disposable sachets or pump dispenser. If the emollient is in a pot or jar, a disposable spoon or spatula and a dish should be used for decanting to avoid contamination. Emollients should be applied immediately after bathing and soft pat drying (soak and smear approach) in long smooth downward sweeping strokes in the direction of hair.[45] Do not rub in as it may cause itching thus preventing the emollient from forming a protective barrier. Bland emollients like petrolatum jelly, extra virgin coconut oil, and sunflower oil are considered safe and also possess antimicrobial properties.[48,49] Emollients must be applied thinly six to eight times a day in congenital ichthyosis [in neonatal intensive care unit (NICU)] and two or three times a day in newborn, infants, and children immediately after bathing.

Keratolytics

Keratolytic agents include urea (>20%) salicylic acid (>2%), propylene glycol (>20%), alpha hydroxyl acids (5–12%) with urea being most commonly used in clinical practice.

Systemic Retinoids

Systemic retinoids have proven to be a boon for patients with severe congenital ichthyosis including harlequin ichthyosis.[50]

Dose

- Isotretinoin (1 mg/kg/day) and acitretin (0.5 mg/kg/day) are the drug of choice. However, when recommended, acitretin is preferred over isotretinoin. The drug should be started on a low dose and then gradually escalated with careful monitoring of side effects.[50]
- Dose should be lowered and "retinoid holidays" may be considered during warm, humid months.

Storage
Retinoids are light sensitive and hence should be stored at room temperature.[14]

Mode of Administration
- Isotretinoin is a fatty liquid inside a hard gelatin shell (Box 5).
- Acitretin is a yellow–green crystalline lyophilized powder available in 10 and 25 mg gelatin coated capsules.

Acitretin can be compounded by:
- Extracting the powder, weighing and administering the appropriate dose.
- In a small aliquot of milk[51] OR
- Capsule is twist opened, extracted powder is dissolved in 1 mL bland/pleasantly flavored oil such as olive, rapeseed, or soy, in an amber.
- Colored dispenser. The desired dose is administered within 5–6 minutes.
- (To prevent degradation) using a syringe for dose titration.[52]

Caution[53]
- While on acitretin, patients should avoid getting pregnant 4 weeks before, during, and 3 years after discontinuation.
- Acitretin should be changed to isotretinoin before puberty, if at risk of pregnancy.
- Women on isotretinoin should take two effective birth control methods 1 month before and 1 month after starting isotretinoin.

Side Effects
Side effects of retinoids are dose (>1 mg/kg/day) and duration (4–6 years) dependent. Skeletal toxicities observed in children include premature epiphyseal closure, calcifications of tendons and ligaments, osteophytes or "bone spurs," DISH (diffuse idiopathic skeletal hyperostosis), and potential alterations in bone density and growth. Monitoring for these toxicities should include comprehensive personal and family history for risk factors of skeletal toxicity, annual growth assessment [height, weight, body mass index (BMI), growth curve], regular inquiry about musculoskeletal symptoms, about diet, and imaging of symptomatic areas.[54] BAD (British Association of Dermatology) guidelines does not recommend routine radiographic assessment as it exposes the children to unnecessary radiation.[53] However, some authors[48] recommend pretreatment X-rays for bone age and thereafter monitoring at yearly intervals in children on long-term therapy.

The choice of treatment however, depends on several factors:[48,54]
- Age of patient:
  - Keratolytic agents:
    - All keratolytics must be avoided in the newborn period and infants as chance of systemic absorption is high. Use of urea is contraindicated in those under 1 year except once daily application over palms and soles. Salicylic acid is contraindicated in children under 2 years but can be applied over stubborn areas in older children.
    - In older children, for hyperkeratotic skin, the concentration of urea can be increased from 20 to 40% to be applied once or twice daily and then tapered according to response.
  - Systemic retinoids:
    - No minimum age exists for using systemic retinoids.
    - In the neonatal period, in collodion baby, membrane shed in few weeks and therefore, oral retinoids are not usually necessary. In harlequin ichthyosis, in mild cases, systemic retinoids are not required. In severe cases of harlequin ichthyosis, systemic retinoids are recommended.
- Type of ichthyosis:
  - Systemic retinoids have been proven to be effective in CIE, epidermolytic ichthyosis, erythrokeratodermia variabilis, harlequin ichthyosis, KID syndrome, lamellar ichthyosis, NLSD with ichthyosis, ichthyosis with confetti, recessive X-linked ichthyosis, and SLS.
  - Systemic retinoids have not been tried or have proven to be ineffective CHILD syndrome, CHIME

Box 5: Tips for administering retinoid to child.

Keep out of direct sunlight, use immediately after removing from packaging
- Always wear disposable gloves while handling isotretinoin
- It is best to swallow the whole capsule with fatty food (whole milk, ice cream, pudding, peanut butter, whipped cream) to facilitate absorption OR
- Puncture the capsule with a sharp knife or nail clippers or cut with scissors and add to food (to be given within 1 hour) OR
- Freeze the capsule in bite sized, soft centered chocolate and chew chocolate and capsule OR
- Capsule is softened by placing in a small cup, adding warm water or milk for 2–3 minutes, and then drinking the milk/water with the softened capsule

Through feeding tube:
- The contents of the capsule are squeezed in 5–10 mL of warm milk or tube feed. The mixture is then pulled through into oral syringe and administered through feeding tube. The tube is then flushed with minimum 30 mL of milk or tube feed OR
- Puncture or cut open the capsule, draw the contents into an oral syringe, add 1–5 mL of soybean, or safflower oil into the same syringe, mix the contents in the syringe, administer the mixture through the feeding tube, flush the feeding tube well with 30 mL of milk or tube feed

Source: St Jude Children's Research Hospital. (2022). Isotretinoin. [online] Available from https://stjude.org/treatment/patient-resources/caregiver-resources/medicines/a-z-list-of-medicines/isotretinoin.html [Last accessed November, 2022].[49]

(Coloboma, Heart defects, Ichthyosiform dermatosis, Mental retardation, and Ear) syndrome, Conradi–Hunermann–Happle syndrome, peeling skin disease, Refsum syndrome, and TTD.
- In disorders with increased skin fragility like peeling skin syndrome or with atopic diathesis like Netherton syndrome, systemic retinoids may exacerbate the condition and hence should be used with caution.
- In CHILD syndrome caused by deficiency of cholesterol and toxic accumulation of steroid precursors, targeted topical therapy using combination of topical cholesterol with a topical statin should be used.
- *Severity of ichthyosis*:
  - Emollients, topical keratolytic agents, topical retinoids such as adapalene/tazarotene should be used in mild disease and when the risk of giving systemic therapy outweigh the benefits.
  - Systemic retinoids should be reserved for following cases after thorough discussion of the expected outcome and the adverse effects to the child and caregivers.
- Inadequate response to topical therapy
- Moderate to severe phenotype
- Functional impairment
- Distribution and presence/absence of inflammation and erosions
  - Emollients containing urea and keratolytic agents should be avoided on face and flexures, inflamed, eroded skin, and areas of fissuring.
- *Morphology*:
  - Topical retinoids are useful in reducing scale, improving digital contractures, and reversing ectropion.
  - Systemic retinoids are effective in removing scales, improving hypohidrosis, ectropion and eclabion, hearing and shortening the time spent in skin care.

VITAMIN D SUPPLEMENTATION

Rickets has been previously reported in ichthyosis due to:
1. Alterations in epidermal cholesterol metabolism possibly involving vitamin D receptors leading to defective synthesis of vitamin D in diseased epidermis and excessive loss of calcium through skin.
2. Increased keratinocyte proliferation leading to poor or no penetration of skin by sunlight
3. Dark skinned individuals with ichthyosis have poor penetration of sun rays
4. Associated vitamin D dependent rickets
5. Children with ichthyosis loose water through skin easily leading to dehydration and constipation which can interfere with food intake
6. Limited sun exposure to prevent sunburn and sunstroke
7. Preference to stay indoors because of social embarrassment
8. Use of systemic retinoids which reduced calcium absorption from gut

To prevent the development of rickets: Oral vitamin D 600,000 IU once weekly for 8 weeks then 2,000 IU once a day needs to be supplemented.

RECENT ADVANCES

Once daily oral liarozole, a retinoic acid metabolism-blocking agent, may be used in moderate to severe lamellar ichthyosis as an alternative to systemic retinoid therapy.[55]

Topical 10% N-acetyl cysteine in combination with 5% urea may be beneficial not only for correcting cutaneous lesions but also ectropion thus avoiding surgical procedure in lamellar ichthyosis.[56]

PRIMARY IMMUNODEFICIENCY[57]

Treatment of PID should be tailored to counteract the immune defect and prevent complications **(Table 13)**.

Table 13: Treatment of primary immunodeficiency syndrome (PID).

Disease	Treatment
Severe combined immunodeficiency	Immunoglobulin (Ig) replacement, hematopoietic stem cell transplantation
Combined immunodeficiency	Ig replacement, hematopoietic stem cell transplantation
Wiskott–Aldrich syndrome	Ig replacement, hematopoietic stem cell transplantation, splenectomy, immunomodulation as required
DiGeorge syndrome	• Thymus transplantation • Supplementation with vitamin D or calcium and with parathyroid hormone • Surgical repair for cleft palate and other heart defects
Hyper IgE syndrome[58]	• Hematopoietic stem cell transplantation • Antimicrobial treatment • Immunomodulation, if needed • Multidisciplinary care
Agammaglobulinemia	Ig replacement, antimicrobial treatment, and prophylaxis
Familial hemophagocytic lymphohistiocytosis	Hematopoietic stem cell transplantation, antimicrobial treatment, chemotherapy, and immunomodulation as needed
IPEX syndrome	Hematopoietic stem cell transplantation, antimicrobial treatment, chemotherapy, and immunomodulation as needed

(Ig: immunoglobulin; IPEX: immune dysregulation, polyendocrinopathy, enteropathy, X linked)

Early treatment and prevention of infections by reducing pathogen exposure, aggressive use of antimicrobials, and early institution of immunoglobulin therapy is essential in all forms of PID.

INBORN ERRORS OF METABOLISM[28]

The aim of treatment includes:
- Removal of toxic metabolite by reducing substrate availability (by stopping feeds).
- Enhance excretion of toxic metabolite.
- Provide adequate calories to prevent endogenous catabolism and aggravation of encephalopathy.
- Institute cofactor therapy
- Supportive therapy

For all sick neonates, discontinue all feeds. Provide adequate calories by intravenous (IV) 10% glucose and lipids. If hyperglycemia occurs, consider insulin. After stabilization, add small amounts of protein orally no later than 24–48 hours (0.5 g/kg/day) and gradually increased to 1 g/kg/day.

The biochemical abnormalities need urgent intervention. To decrease ammonia levels, sodium benzoate, sodium phenylbutyrate/phenylacetate, L-arginine, and L-carnitine are best given by IV route (IV preparation not available in India). For rapid removal of ammonia, dialysis should be initiated. Although hemodialysis is more effective and fast, peritoneal dialysis is widely available and feasible.

For suspected organic academia, sodium bicarbonate is initiated as per NICU protocol. In addition, carnitine, biotin, B12 [vitamin B12 responsive methylmalonic acidemia (MMA)], and thiamine (thiamine responsive MSUD) are supplemented.

For intractable seizures, 100 mg IV pyridoxine is administered. If seizures persist, folinic acid 5 mg/kg/day orally or IV in three divided doses is initiated daily for 3 days.

Sodium valproate is best avoided in patients with IEM for treating seizures. For long-term therapy, special diets including protein restriction and exclusion of amino acids specific to particular disorder are now made available in India.

CYSTIC FIBROSIS[59]

To reduce the progression of disease, following measures should be taken:
- *Optimize lung function by*:
  ○ Drinking more water
  ○ Taking appropriate amount of salt
  ○ Regular chest physiotherapy
  ○ Inhalation with hypertonic saline, salbutamol, budecort/foracort, tobamist, and DNase
- *Nutritional therapy*:
  ○ Pancreatic enzyme supplements—available in capsule/spherule form to be given before meals.
  ○ Fat soluble vitamins A, D, and E.
  ○ Salt, water, and potassium—syrup Potklor has a bitter taste so mix with sugar/water.
  ○ Inhalational antibiotics according to culture sensitivity report.
- *Suppression of inflammation*:
  ○ Steroids/high-dose ibuprofen
- Identifying and managing complications, e.g., intestinal obstruction, CF-related diabetes, CF liver disease, and respiratory failure.

MISCELLANEOUS[8]

Specific treatment for erythroderma with an underlying etiological diagnosis is as outlined in **Table 14**.

GENETIC EVALUATION[60]

Due to the genetic nature of certain diseases like ichthyosis, PIDs, IEMs, acrodermatitis enteropathica, Gaucher's disease, etc., genetic testing for the individual affected by these conditions and their family members becomes very important to provide comprehensive care.

Table 14: Treatment of miscellaneous conditions.

Disease	Treatment
• Bacterial infection • Herpes simplex • Candidiasis • Scabies	• Antibiotics • Antiviral • Antifungal • Scabicidal
• Dermatomyositis • Psoriasis • Pemphigus foliaceus sarcoidosis	Immunosuppressant, biologics
• Atopic dermatitis • Drug-induced erythroderma	Short course of systemic steroids
Biotinidase deficiency[34]	Oral biotin 5–20 mg/day
Holocarboxylase synthase deficiency[34]	Oral biotin 10–40 mg/day
Gaucher's disease	ERT with imiglucerase (type 1 and 3)
Acrodermatitis enteropathica	Zinc-rich food and replacement therapy
SJS/TEN	Short course of systemic steroids or IVIg or cyclosporine
Mastocytosis	Avoidance of triggers, H1 antagonist for cutaneous symptoms, H2 antagonist for systemic symptoms
Kawasaki disease	IVIg + Aspirin

(ERT: enzyme replacement therapy; IVIg: intravenous immunoglobulin; SJS: Stevens–Johnson syndrome; TEN: toxic epidermal necrolysis)

Molecular genetic testing is now preferred for characterization of exact genetic etiology. Sanger sequencing of that gene alone might be done, if clinical diagnosis suggests the possibility of involvement of a specific gene that has only a small number of exons. But for conditions that are genetically heterogeneous or with overlapping phenotypes or with large genes, an NGS-based focused exome sequencing panel can be used as the first-tier test. If no significant variants are found, WES and/or whole-genome sequencing can be done further.

Following an accurate diagnosis of the affected individual, appropriate genetic counseling can be provided to the patient and the family about the nature of the disorder, natural course and prognosis, available management options, and the surveillance/monitoring plan. Many of the genetic disorders have associated systemic/multiorgan involvement, as mentioned above, and therefore, require multidisciplinary management.

Based on the identified genetic etiology and the pattern of inheritance, the risk of recurrence in subsequent pregnancies in the family can be ascertained. Carrier testing of other family members is also possible. Prenatal diagnosis can be offered as an option for at-risk pregnancies through targeted mutation analysis after identifying the pathogenic variant(s) in the affected proband and/or carrier parents, to prevent the recurrence of severe genetic disorders in the family.

REFERENCES

1. Austad SS, Athalye L. (2021). Exfoliative dermatitis. [online] In: StatPearls [Internet]. Treasure Island (FL): StatPearls Publishing. Available from https://www.ncbi.nlm.nih.gov/books/NBK554568/ [Last accessed November, 2022].
2. Sarkar R, Sharma RC, Koranne RV, Sardana K. Erythroderma in children: A clinico-etiological study. J Dermatol. 1999;26:507-11.
3. Kalsy J, Puri K. Erythroderma in children: Clinico-etiological study from Punjab. Indian J Paediatr Dermatol. 2013;14:9-12.
4. Ott H. Guidance for assessment of erythroderma in neonates and infants for the pediatric immunologist. Pediatr Allergy Immunol. 2019;30(3):259-68.
5. Sigurdsson V, de Vries IJ, Toonstra J, Bihari IC, Thepen T, Bruijnzeel-Koomen CA, et al. Expression of VCAM-1, ICAM-1, E-selectin, and P-selectin on endothelium in situ in patients with erythroderma, mycosis fungoides and atopic dermatitis. J Cutan Pathol. 2000;27(9):436-40.
6. Okoduwa C, Lambert WC, Schwartz RA, Kubeyinje E, Eitokpah A, Sinha S, et al. Erythroderma: Review of a potentially life-threatening dermatosis. Indian J Dermatol. 2009;54(1):1-6.
7. Sehgal VN, Srivastava G, Sardana K. Erythroderma/exfoliative dermatitis: A synopsis. Int J Dermatol. 2004;43:39-47.
8. Swarnkar B, Sarkar R. Neonatal and infantile erythroderma revisited. Indian J Paediatr Dermatol. 2020;21:15-21.
9. Fraitag S, Bodemer C. Neonatal erythroderma. Curr Opin Pediatr. 2010;22:438-44.
10. Oranje AP, Soekanto W, Sukardi A, Vuzevski VD, van der Willigen A, Afiani HM. Diffuse cutaneous mastocytosis mimicking staphylococcal scalded-skin syndrome: Report of three cases. Pediatr Dermatol. 1991;8(2):147-51.
11. Henriksen L, Zachariae H. Pustular psoriasis and arthritis in congenital psoriasiform erythroderma. Dermatologica. 1972;144:12-18.
12. Salleras M, Sanchez-Regana M, Umbert P. Congenital erythrodermic psoriasis: Case report and literature review. Pediatr Dermatol. 1995;12:231-4.
13. Champion RH, Burton JL, Ebling FJG, Griffiths WAD, Leigh IM, Marks R. Disorders of keratinization. In: Champion RH, Burton JL, Ebling FJG (Eds). Rook/Wilkinson/Ebling Textbook of Dermatology, 5th edition. Oxford: Blackwell Scientific Publishers; 1992. pp. 1325-90.
14. Hoeger PH, Harper JI. Neonatal erythroderma: Differential diagnosis and management of the "red baby". Arch Dis Child. 1998;79:186-91.
15. Sarkar R. Neonatal and infantile erythroderma: "The red baby". Indian J Dermatol. 2006;51:178-82.
16. Sarkar R, Garg VK. Erythroderma in children. Indian J Dermatol Venereol Leprol. 2010;76:341-7.
17. Sehgal VN, Srivastava G. Erythroderma/generalized exfoliative dermatitis in pediatric practice: An overview. Int J Dermatol. 2006;45:831-9.
18. Dhar S, Banerjee R, Malakar R. Neonatal erythroderma: Diagnostic and therapeutic challenges. Indian J Dermatol. 2012;57:475-8.
19. Kotrulja L, Murat-Susić S, Husar K. Differential diagnosis of neonatal and infantile erythroderma. Acta Dermatovenerol Croat. 2007;15:178-90.
20. Ott H, Hütten M, Baron JM, Merk HF, Fölster-Holst R. Neonatal and infantile erythrodermas. J Der Dtsch Dermatol Ges. 2008;25:6 Suppl 12:1070-86.
21. McPherson T, Exton LS, Biswas S, Creamer D, Dziewulski P, Newell L, et al. British Association of Dermatologists' guidelines for the management of Stevens-Johnson syndrome/toxic epidermal necrolysis in children and young people, 2018. Br J Dermatol. 2019;181(1):37-54.
22. Liotti L, Caimmi S, Bottau P, Bernardini R, Cardinale F, Saretta F, et al. Clinical features, outcomes and treatment in children with drug induced Stevens-Johnson syndrome and toxic epidermal necrolysis. Acta Biomed. 2019;90(3-S):52-60.
23. Das S, Ramamoorthy R. Stevens-Johnson syndrome and toxic epidermal necrolysis in children. Indian J Paediatr Dermatol. 2018;19:9-14.
24. Mori F, Caffarelli C, Caimmi S, Bottau P, Liotti L, Franceschini F, et al. Drug reaction with eosinophilia and systemic symptoms (DRESS) in children. Acta Biomed. 2019;90(3-S):66-79.
25. Oji V, Tadini G, Akiyama M, Bardon CB, Bodemer C, Bourrat E, et al. Revised nomenclature and classification of inherited ichthyoses: Results of the First Ichthyosis Consensus Conference in Sorèze 2009. J Am Acad Dermatol. 2010;63(4):607-41.
26. Sarkar R, Garg S, Garg VK. Neonatal erythroderma (red baby). Indian J Paediatr Dermatol. 2013;14:47-53.

27. Sharma S, Kumar P, Agarwal R, Kabra M, Deorari AK, Paul VK. Approach to inborn errors of metabolism presenting in the neonate. Indian J Pediatr. 2008;75(3):271-6.
28. Puri RD, Phadke SR. Inborn errors of metabolism presenting in the newborn period: Representative phenotypes and diagnostic approach. In: Ranganath P (Ed). Genetics Update for the Next Generation Clinician. India: Indian Academy of Medical Genetics; 2017. pp. 57-69.
29. Schaffer JV, Paller AS. Primary immunodeficiencies. In: Bolognia JL, Jorizzo JL, Schaffer JV (Eds). Dermatology, 3rd edition. India: Reed Elsevier; 2014. pp. 911-5.
30. Rakowska A, Slowinska M, Kowalska-Oledzka E, Rudnicka L. Trichoscopy in genetic hair shaft abnormalities. J Dermatol Case Rep. 2008;2(2):14-20.
31. Patel HP, Unis ME. Pili torti in association with citrullinemia. J Am Acad Dermatol. 1985;12(1 Pt 2):203-6.
32. Pauvels LSP, Dorn T, Cartell A, Boza JC, Cestari TF. Trichoscopy in acrodermatitis enteropathica. Int J Dermatol. 2022;61(4):480-3.
33. Utsumi D, Yasuda M, Amano H, Suga Y, Seishima M, Takahashi K. Hair abnormality in Netherton syndrome observed under polarized light microscopy. J Am Acad Dermatol. 2020;83(3):847-53.
34. Canda E, Uçar SK, Çoker M. Biotinidase deficiency: Prevalence, impact and management strategies. Pediatric Health Med Ther. 2020;11:127-33.
35. Ragunatha S, Kumar GV. Fluid, electrolyte and nutrition therapy in dermatological emergencies. In: Inamdar A, Palit A (Eds). Critical Care in Dermatology. India: Jaypee Brothers Medical Publishers; 2013. p. 115.
36. Mohd Noor N, Hussein SH. Transepidermal water loss in erythrodermic patients of various aetiologies. Skin Res Technol. 2013;19(3):320-3.
37. Ringer SA. Core concepts: Thermoregulation in the newborn part I basic mechanisms. Neo Rev. 2013;14(4):e161-e167.
38. Inamdar AC, Palit A. Acute skin failure: Concept, causes, consequences and care. Indian J Dermatol Venereol Leprol. 2005;71:379-85.
39. Fox RH, Shuster S, Williams R, Marks J, Goldsmith R, Condon RE. Cardiovascular, metabolic, and thermoregulatory disturbances in patients with erythrodermic skin diseases. Br Med J. 1965;1(5435):619-22.
40. O'Flaherty D, Boulton JE. Acute Care of At-risk Newborns: A Resource and Learning Tool for Health Care Professionals. Vancouver: ACoRN Group; 2012.
41. Kanthraj GR, Srinivas CR, Devi PU, Ganasoundari A, Shenoi SD, Deshmukh RP, et al. Quantitative estimation and recommendations for supplementation of protein lost through scaling in exfoliative dermatitis. Int J Dermatol. 1999;38(2):91-5.
42. Vaishampayan SS, Sharma YK, Das AL, Verma R. Emergencies in dermatology: Acute skin failure. Med J Armed Forces India. 2006;62(1):56-9.
43. Park SE, Kim S, Ouma C, Loha M, Wierzba TF, Beck NS. Community management of acute malnutrition in the developing world. Pediatr Gastroenterol Hepatol Nutr. 2012;15(4):210-9.
44. Oji V, Preil ML, Kleinow B, Wehr G, Fischer J, Hennies HC, et al. S1 guidelines for the diagnosis and treatment of ichthyoses - update. J Dtsch Dermatol Ges. 2017;15(10):1053-65.
45. Criton S, Gangadharan G. Non pharmacological management of atopic dermatitis. Indian J Paediatr Dermatol. 2017;18:166-73.
46. Mazereeuw-Hautier J, Vahlquist A, Traupe H, Bygum A, Amaro C, Aldwin M, et al. Management of congenital ichthyoses: European guidelines of care, part one. Br J Dermatol. 2019;180(2):272-81.
47. Edwards WH, Conner JM, Soll RF; Vermont Oxford Network Neonatal Skin Care Study Group. The effect of prophylactic ointment therapy on nosocomial sepsis rates and skin integrity in infants with birth weights of 501 to 1000 g. Pediatrics. 2004;113(5):1195-203.
48. Czarnowicki T, Malajian D, Khattri S, da Rosa JC, Dutt R, Finney R, et al. Petrolatum: Barrier repair and antimicrobial responses underlying this "inert" moisturizer. J Allergy Clin Immunol. 2016;137(4):1091-102.e7.
49. St. Jude Children's Research Hospital. (2022). Isotretinoin. [online] Available from https://stjude.org/treatment/patient-resources/caregiver-resources/medicines/a-z-list-of-medicines/isotretinoin.html [Last accessed November, 2022].
50. Glick JB, Craiglow BG, Choate KA, Kato H, Fleming RE, Siegfried E, et al. Improved management of harlequin ichthyosis with advances in neonatal intensive care. Pediatrics. 2017;139(1):e20161003.
51. Sonthalia S, Jakhar D, Jha AK. An extemporaneous approach for optimizing acitretin dosing in pediatric patients. J Am Acad Dermatol. 2018;78(5):e101-e102.
52. Sarkar R, Chugh Z, Garg VK. Acitretin in dermatology. Indian J Dermatol Venereol Leprol. 2013;79:759-71.
53. Ormerod AD, Campalani E, Goodfield MJD; BAD Clinical Standards Unit. British Association of Dermatologists guidelines on the efficacy and use of acitretin in dermatology. Br J Dermatol. 2010;162(5):952-63.
54. Zaenglein AL, Levy ML, Stefanko NS, Benjamin LT, Bruckner AL, Choate K, et al.; PeDRA Use of Retinoids in Ichthyosis Work Group. Consensus recommendations for the use of retinoids in ichthyosis and other disorders of cornification in children and adolescents. Pediatr Dermatol. 2021;38(1):164-80.
55. Vahlquist A, Blockhuys S, Steijlen P, van Rossem K, Didona B, Blanco D, et al. Oral liarozole in the treatment of patients with moderate/severe lamellar ichthyosis: Results of a randomized, double-blind, multinational, placebo-controlled phase II/III trial. Br J Dermatol. 2014;170:173-81.
56. Bassotti A, Moreno S, Criado E. Successful treatment with topical N-acetylcysteine in urea in five children with congenital lamellar ichthyosis. Pediatr Dermatol. 2011;28:451-5.
57. Yarmohammadi H, Cunningham-Rundles C. Primary Immunodeficiency Diseases. Treatment of Primary Immunodeficiency diseases, 1st edition; 2008. pp. 315-34.
58. Harrison SC, Tsilifis C, Slatter MA, Nademi Z, Worth A, Veys P, et al. Hematopoietic stem cell transplantation resolves the immune deficit associated with STAT3-dominant-negative hyper-IgE syndrome. J Clin Immunol. 2021;41(5):934-43.
59. Kulkarni H, Kansra S, Karande S. Cystic fibrosis revisited. J Postgrad Med. 2019;65:193-6.
60. Buch J, Ranganath P. Approach to inherited hypertrichosis: A brief review. Indian J Dermatol Venereol Leprol. 2021;88(1):11-21.

22
A Child with Fever and Rash

Sabha Neazee, Pooja Agarwal

INTRODUCTION

Fever accompanied with rash is one of the most common presentations in pediatric as well as dermatology clinics. As a dermatologist, one should be able to diagnose and treat the child and be aware of timely referral to pediatricians as some of the causes of fever with rash have high morbidity and mortality.

DEFINITIONS

- *Fever:* Elevation of body temperature above normal circadian variation (AM temperature >98.9°F/PM temperature >99.9°F).
- *Exanthem:* Skin eruption occurring as a symptom of a general disease, usually an infectious process.[1]
- *Enanthem:* Lesions in mucous membranes occurring with fever of infective etiology.

The causes may be broadly classified as infectious and noninfectious. Among them, viral exanthems are by far the most common cause of fever with rash in children.[1-5] Noninfectious causes include rash due to drug reactions, connective tissue diseases, Kawasaki disease, Gianotti–Crosti syndrome, pityriasis rosea, etc.; some of which have a presumed viral or bacterial trigger. Rash accompanying the fever may be varied in morphology and includes maculopapular, vesicular, purpuric, nodular, or diffuse erythema with desquamation **(Tables 1 and 2)**.

APPROACH TO A CHILD WITH FEVER AND RASH

As there are not many investigations available for diagnosis of causes of fever accompanied with rash in children, clinical history, and examination are of paramount significance.

Table 1: Morphology of rash in various infectious causes of fever.	
Bacterial	**Viral**
Fever with maculopapular rash	
Scarlet fever, disseminated gonococcal infection, enteric fever	Measles, rubella, exanthem subitum, erythema infectiosum, dengue, chikungunya, infectious mononucleosis
Fever with vesicular/pustular rash	
Impetigo, gonococcemia	Chicken pox, varicella zoster, hand, foot, and mouth disease
Fever with diffuse erythema with desquamation	
Scarlet fever, toxic shock syndrome, Staphylococcal scalded skin syndrome, Kawasaki disease	
Fever with petechial rash	
Meningococcemia, spotted fevers, leptospirosis	Dengue

History

- *Appearance of rash in relation with fever*: The day on which the rash appears in relation with fever can give an important clue to diagnosis of the exanthema in most cases **(Table 3)**.
- *Associated symptoms*: Many fevers are associated with various systemic complains which may help in the diagnosis of the disease **(Table 4)**.
- *Progression and location of rash*: Many exanthems have a typical onset and classic progression of rash over the body, which helps to differentiate between the various diseases **(Table 5)**.

Table 2: Morphology of rash in various noninfectious causes of fever.					
Maculopapular	**Vesicular**	**Urticarial**	**Hemorrhagic**	**Nodular**	**Diffuse erythema with desquamation**
• Drug eruption • Toxic erythema neonatorum • Erythema multiforme • Urticaria • Rheumatic fever • Lupus erythematosus • Gianotti–Crosti syndrome • Pityriasis rosea	• Eczema vaccinatum • Erythema multiforme	• Vasculitis • Malignancy • Still's disease • Idiopathic	• Acute allergic eruptions • Allergic purpura • Acute thrombocytopenia • Hematological malignancy • Acute rheumatic fever • Systemic Lupus erythematosus • Thrombotic thrombocytopenic purpura • Amyloidosis • Cutaneous small vessel vasculitis	• Sweets syndrome • Kaposi sarcoma • Erythema nodosum	• Graft-versus-host disease • Generalized pustular psoriasis • Steven–Johnson syndrome–toxic epidermal necrolysis • Cutaneous small vessel vasculitis

Table 3: Diagnosis on basis of days of appearance of rash.	
Day of appearance of rash after fever	**Probable diagnosis**
Day 1	**V**aricella
Day 2	**S**carlet fever
Day 3	Small **P**ox
Day 4	**M**easles
Day 5	**T**yphus
Day 6	**D**engue
Day 7	**E**nteric fever
(Mnemonic: **V**ery **S**ick **P**eople **M**ust **T**ake **D**ouble **E**ggs)	

- *Mucosal lesions*: Many diseases may present with oral ulcers along with fever. However, for the purpose of this chapter, only common diseases which present as febrile illness with rash and associated specific enanthems are summarized in **Table 6**.
- *History of drug ingestion within past 30 days*: Although any medication can cause a drug rash, the most common types of medications that trigger a drug rash include:
  ○ Antibiotics, such as penicillin or sulfa drugs
  ○ Anti-inflammatory medicines, such as ibuprofen, naproxen, or indomethacin
  ○ Anti-convulsants such as phenytoin or carbamazepine
  ○ Chemotherapy agents
  ○ Psychotropic medications
  ○ Diuretics
  ○ Iodine, especially that found in X-ray contrast dye
- *History of similar complaints in siblings, neighborhood or school*: Many diseases such as measles and chicken pox have high infectivity, so it is common to find clustering of cases.
- *Travel history*: In recent time, with increased travel and population movements, imported infections with secondary local transmission are of great concern and outbreaks in susceptible populations may present containment issues. In this aspect, imported viral infections such as chikungunya, dengue, Rocky Mountain spotted fever, and coronavirus disease 2019 (COVID-19) infection should be considered due to recent travel history.
- *Insect bite*: Vector-borne diseases such as dengue/chikungunya commonly present with generalized rash along with fever, so it is important to ask about any history of insect bites.
- *Immunizations*: Atypical presentations may be seen in vaccinated children like break out varicella or measles like illness.
- *Lymph node examination*: Significant in Kawasaki disease and many viral exanthems.

The salient systemic features of various common causes of fever accompanied by rash in a child are summarized in **Table 7**.

NUMBERED DISEASES OF CHILDHOOD

This is of historical significance only as the diseases were assigned numbers in chronology when they were identified **(Table 8)**.

COVID-19: A NOVEL CAUSE OF FEVER WITH RASH[20]

- *Infective agent:* Severe acute respiratory syndrome coronavirus 2 (SARS-CoV-2) virus.

Table 4: Differential diagnosis based on different associated symptoms.[6]	
Prodrome/associated symptoms	Differential diagnosis
Upper respiratory tract infection	Measles, rubella, erythema infectiosum, erythema subitum, varicella, scarlet fever
Fever of acute onset	Measles, rubella, erythema infectiosum, erythema subitum, varicella, infectious mononucleosis, scarlet fever, toxic shock syndrome, meningococcemia, bacterial endocarditis, Kawasaki disease, systemic onset juvenile chronic arthritis, acute rheumatic fever
Fever of insidious onset	Systemic lupus erythematosus (SLE), polyarteritis nodosa, Wegener's granulomatosis
Relapsing fever	*Borrelia, Bartonella quintana*
Polyarthritis of small joints/myalgia	Chikungunya fever, dengue fever, *Leptospira*, systemic onset juvenile chronic arthritis, systemic lupus erythematosus, vasculitis (rare in children)
Arthritis involving large joints	Acute rheumatic fever, Henoch–Schonlein purpura (HSP), disseminated gonococcal infection
Hepatosplenomegaly with lymphadenopathy	Infectious mononucleosis, leptospirosis, *Borrelia*, brucellosis
Hemorrhagic manifestations	Dengue fever, chikungunya fever, meningococcemia, HSP
Multiorgan failure, hypotension, shock	Dengue fever, meningococcemia, toxic shock syndrome, leptospirosis, chikungunya fever
Eye involvement	Measles (conjunctivitis/keratitis/retinopathy), Kawasaki disease (nonexudative conjunctivitis/anterior uveitis), hypocomplementemic urticarial vasculitis syndrome
Gastrointestinal features	Enteric fever, hypocomplementemic urticarial vasculitis syndrome, juvenile chronic arthritis, HSP

Table 5: Pattern of progression, characteristics and location of rash in common diseases.	
Diseases	Characteristics of rash
Measles[7]	• Erythematous blanchable maculopapular rash that may become confluent (**Figs. 1 and 2**) • Appears first near hairline and retroauricular area • Cephalocaudal spread to involve whole body • Sparing palms and soles
Rubella[8]	• Starts on face or neck and then spreads caudally • Light pink macules and papules. Individual lesions are small often with peripheral blanching
Erythema infectiosum/fifth disease/slapped cheek syndrome[9]	• The rash is biphasic • *First phase*: Confluent, erythematous plaques on cheeks, with sparing of nasal bridge and periorbital regions. So called *slapped cheek* (**Fig. 3**). Fades over 1–4 days • *Second phase*: The rash then spreads to the trunk and extensor extremities which undergoes patchy clearing with lacy reticular pattern (**Fig. 4**)
Exanthem subitum/sixth disease/roseola infantum[10]	• Generalized erythematous macules with some papules. Rash described as "rainbow following the storm" as the rash appears after fever has subsided • Face is usually spared, rash seen on trunk and neck, extremities are involved later
Varicella/chicken pox[11]	• Pleomorphic rash • Erythematous macules → papules → umbilicated vesicles/pustules → scabs (**Fig. 5**) • Tense vesicles surrounded by erythema give *dew drops on rose petals* appearance • Centripetal in distribution
Hand, foot, and mouth disease (HFMD)	• Prodrome of fever, malaise • Maculopapular rash → vesicle with erythematous halo → ulcer → scab • Over extremities/buttocks/perioral area (**Figs. 6 to 8**) • Hands/palm involvement → soles/feet involvement • Nail shedding may be seen after recovery from HFMD which reverts back on its own

Continued

Continued

Diseases	Characteristics of rash
Gianotti–Crosti syndrome/infantile papular acrodermatitis[12]	• Monomorphic, flat topped, pink brown papules, or papulovesicles 1–10 mm in diameter **(Fig. 9)** • Cheeks, buttocks, extensor surfaces of forearms, extensor surfaces of legs • Characteristic sparing of abdomen • Symmetrical
Kawasaki disease[13]	Widespread maculopapular rash on limbs and trunk, which later becomes localized over distal extremities
Pityriasis rosea[14]	• Discrete, oval or round, erythematous plaques with fine scales (*hanging curtain sign*—the scales tend to fold across the line of stretch when the skin is stretched across the long axis of a lesion of PR) • *Herald patch*: 2–10 cm, round to oval scaly patch or plaque with depressed center and elevated border, appears days to weeks before generalized rash • *Christmas tree pattern* over trunk • *Multiple morphology*: Papulosquamous/vesicular/pustular/erythema multiforme like/follicular/urticarial/purpuric
Dengue[15]	Transient facial erythema, maculopapular eruption, generalized erythema with islands of normal skin, purpura/ecchymosis **(Figs. 10 and 11)**
Chikungunya[16]	• Maculopapular eruption, transient generalized erythema, with islands of normal skin, palmoplantar desquamation • Hyperpigmentation over centrofacial area • Striking pigmentation of the nose, described as the "chik sign"
Scarlet fever[17]	• Punctuate erythema, becoming confluent, rash fading in 4–5 days followed by desquamation • *Pasti's sign*: Linear petechiae in antecubital and axillary folds
Morbilliform drug eruption[18]	• Annular, targetoid, urticaria-like or polymorphous morphology may occur • Lesions mostly blanch with pressure but may be nonblanchable (purpuric) on the lower legs • Discrete lesions may merge together to form large erythematous patches or plaques • Axilla, groin, hands, and feet are usually spared • Mucous membranes, hair, and nails are not affected in uncomplicated drug eruptions

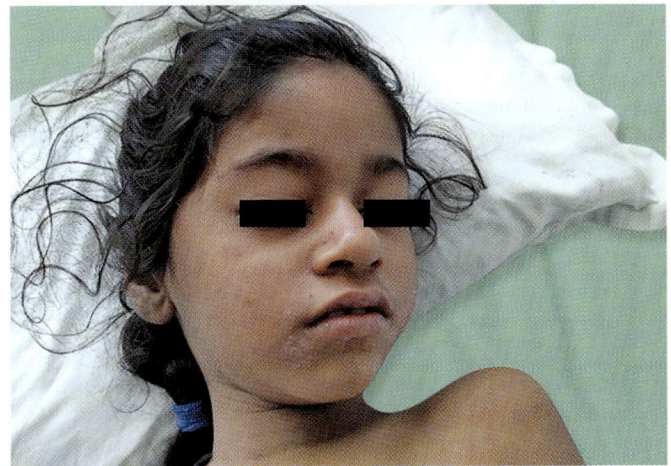

FIG. 1: Maculopapular lesions involving face in a child with measles.
Courtesy: Dr Nayan Patel.

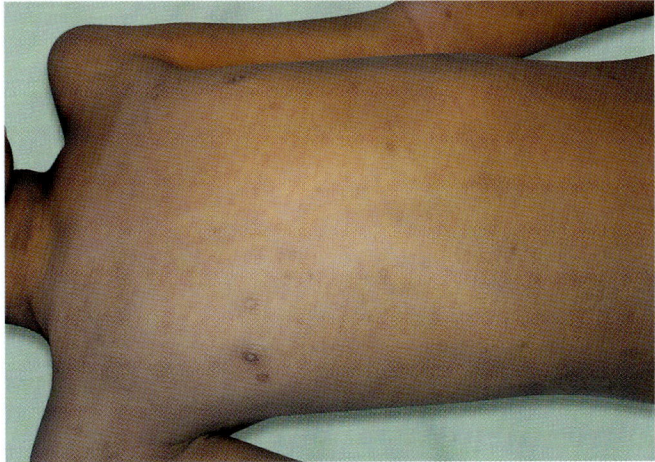

FIG. 2: Maculopapular lesions involving in a child with measles.
Courtesy: Dr Nayan Patel.

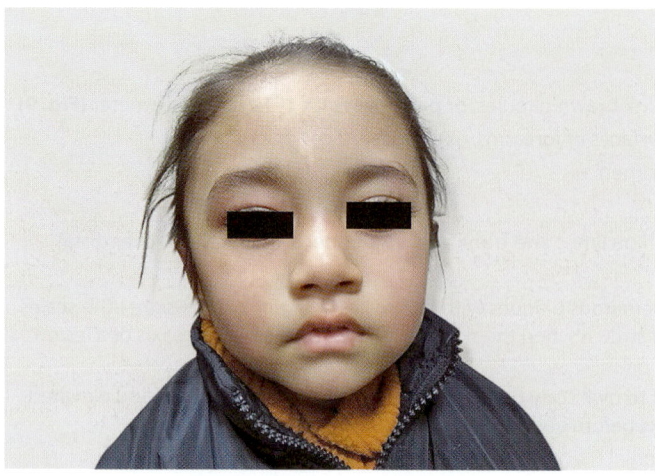

FIG. 3: Characteristic erythema over face showing accentuation over cheeks and sparing of perioral area seen in parvovirus B19 infection.
Courtesy: Dr Jigna Padhiyar.

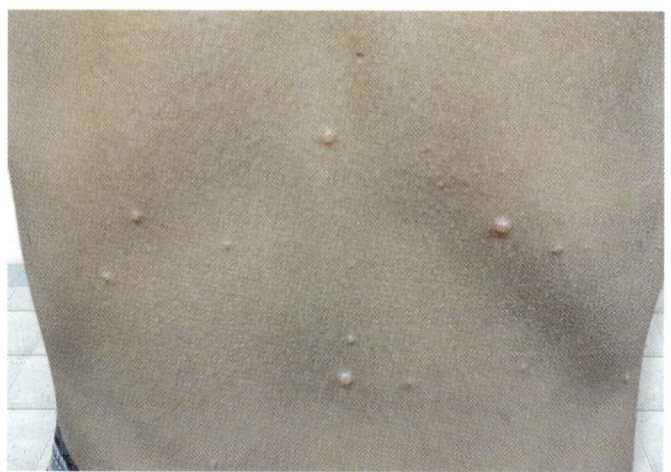

FIG. 5: Umbilicated vesicles in case of chickenpox.
Courtesy: Dr Ranjana Rawal.

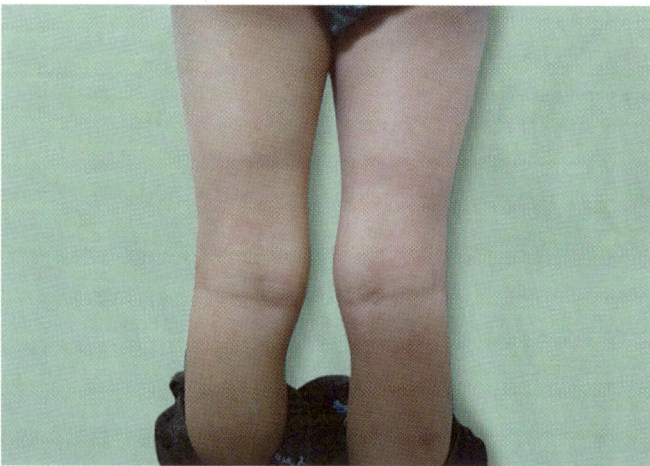

FIG. 4: Lacy pattern of erythema over extremities in Parvovirus B19 infection.
Courtesy: Dr Jigna Padhiyar.

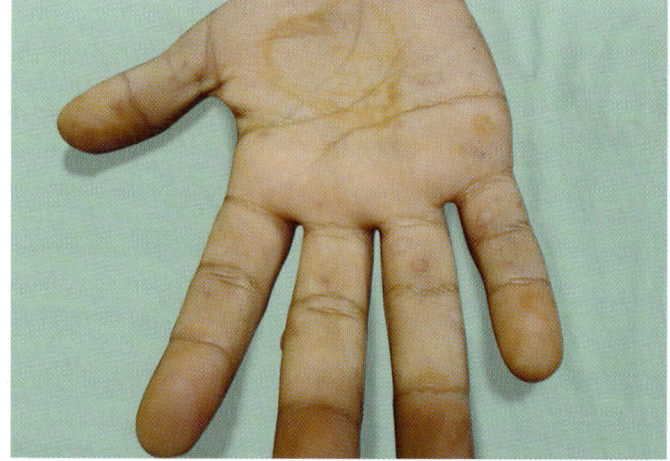

FIG. 6: Oval vesicles with perilesional erythema characteristic of hand, foot and mouth disease.
Courtesy: Dr Nayan Patel.

- *Epidemiology:*
    - Accounting for 1–8% of all COVID-19 cases
    - Increased morbidity in infants and young children, compared with older children.
- *History:* Rhinitis, cough, fever, and dyspnea:
    - Gastrointestinal clinical manifestations and pharyngeal erythema
- *Exanthem:* Six clinical patterns:
    - Urticaria
    - Maculopapular
    - Morbilliform eruption
    - Papulovesicular exanthem
    - Chilblain-like acral pattern
    - Livedo reticularis—livedo racemose pattern
    - Purpuric vasculitic pattern

  In children, the dermatologic features appear to occur before or concomitantly with other COVID-19 manifestations.
- Cutaneous manifestations of COVID-19 in both the adult and pediatric population are compared in **Table 9**.
    - *Complications*: COVID-19-induced multisystem inflammatory syndrome has been called the *pediatric inflammatory multisystem syndrome temporally associated with COVID-19* (PIMS-TS) or multisystem inflammatory syndrome in children (MIS-C) and has similarities to Kawasaki disease.

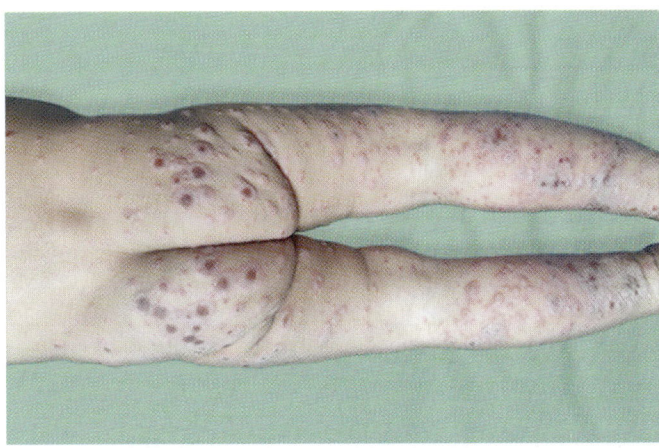

FIG. 7: Severe hand, foot and mouth disease in atopic child also known as eczema coxsackium.
Courtesy: Dr Jigna Padhiyar.

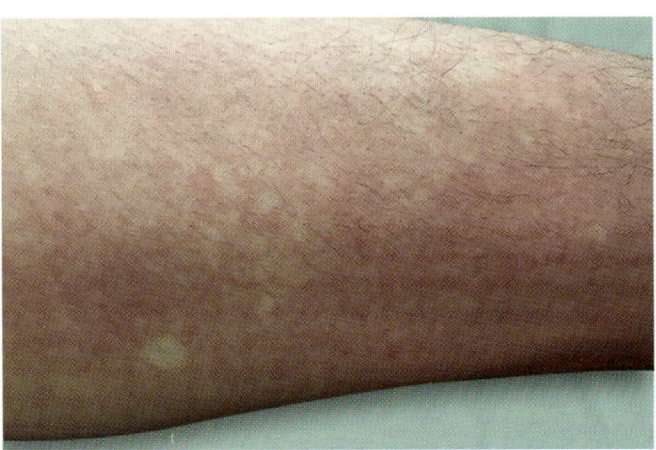

FIG. 10: Maculopapular rashes in patient of dengue fever with characteristic sparing of abdomen.
Courtesy: Dr Jigna Padhiyar.

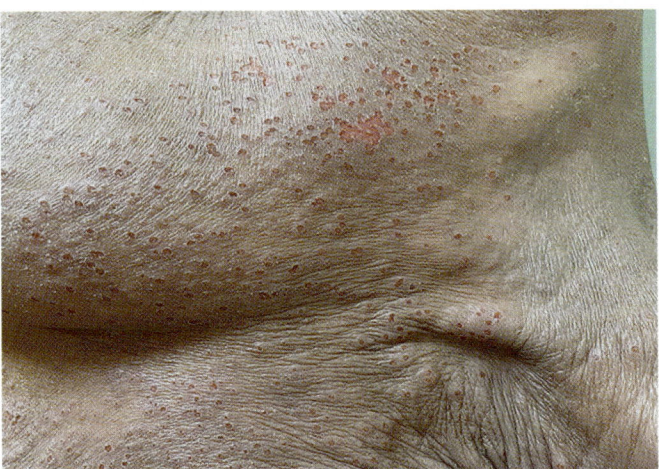

FIG. 8: Multiple grouped vesicles and erosion in adult patient with preexisting atopic dermatitis.
Courtesy: Dr Jigna Padhiyar.

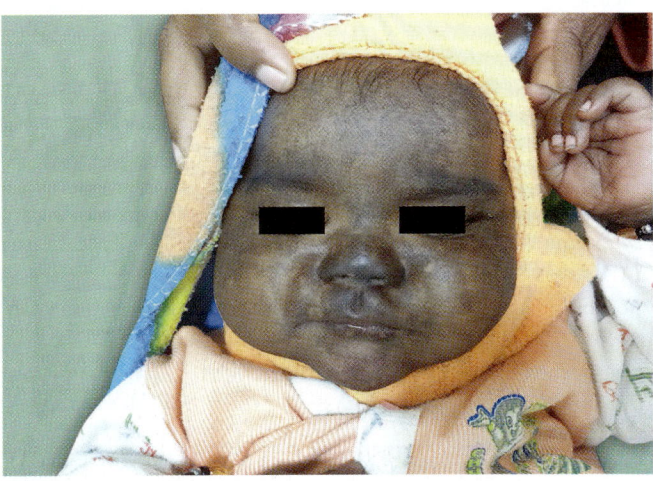

FIG. 11: Diffuse hyperpigmentation of face in child post chikungunya fever. Note the characteristic involvement on nose.

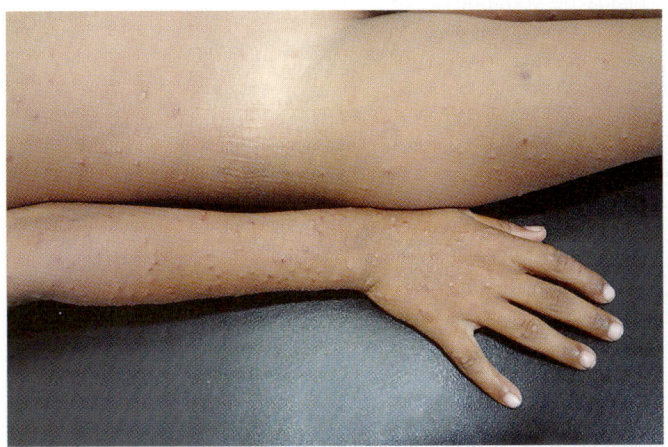

FIG. 9: Monomorphic papular lesions involving extensor of extremities with relative sparing of abdomen.
Courtesy: Dr Jigna Padhiyar.

Erythema Multiforme[21]

- Acute self-healing mucocutaneous disorder
- *Exanthem*: Characteristic target lesions with acral distribution and concentric color disparity:
    - *Typical targets*: Round regular lesions having classic three zones—the inner most purpuric or necrotic with or without blister, the middle pale edematous ring, and the outer erythematous ring.
    - *Raised atypical targets*: Round palpable edematous lesions that have two zones instead of three and/or an ill-defined border.
    - *Flat atypical targets*: Round nonpalpable lesions with two zones and/or a poorly defined border. Blister may be present in the center.
    - *Macules with or without blisters*: Nonpalpable erythematous macules of irregular size and shape with or without blisters.

Table 6: Common enanthems.

Disease	Enanthem
Measles	• *Koplik spots*—pathognomonic • Bluish white lesions opposite to the premolars • 24–48 hours before exanthem
Chicken pox	Erosions with erythematous halo
Rubella	*Forchheimer spots*—small, red spots (petechiae) on soft palate
Hand, foot, and mouth disease[19]	Vesicle—ulcer with erythematous halo
Kawasaki disease	Strawberry tongue, diffuse erythema of the oral mucosa or oropharynx
Scarlet fever	*Strawberry tongue*

Table 7: Summary of systemic features in common diseases which present with fever and exanthema.

Disease	Infective agent	Period of infectivity	Systemic	Complications
Measles	Paramyxovirus	4 days before up to 4 days after rash	Cough, coryza, conjunctivitis (3Cs)	Otitis media, pneumonia, diarrhea, subacute sclerosing pan encephalitis, thrombocytopenia
Rubella/German measles	Rubella virus	7 days before up to 7 days after rash	Cervical, occipital lymphadenopathy, conjunctivitis. Testalgia	Sensorineural hearing loss, cataract, glaucoma, hepatitis, and meningoencephalitis
Exanthem infectiosum/slapped cheek syndrome	Parvovirus B19	7 days before rash. Noncommunicable after appearance of rash	–	Chronic anemia, aplastic crisis
Roseola infantum	HHV-6 or 7	Noncommunicable	Cervical lymphadenopathy	Otitis media, eyelid edema, febrile convulsions, encephalopathy, myocarditis
Chicken pox	Varicella zoster virus	2 days before rash till all lesions are crusted		Pneumonia, encephalitis
HFMD	Coxsackie A16, A10, Echovirus 71	First 5 days after symptoms starts		Echovirus 71 is associated with HFMD with neurological complications
Scarlet fever	β-hemolytic streptococcus pyogenes	6 days before rash up to 2–3 weeks after (if antibiotics not started) until 24 hours after first dose of antibiotic	Fever with chills, upper respiratory tract infection (URTI), headache, vomiting	
Gianotti–Crosti syndrome/infantile papular acrodermatitis	EBV, *Enterovirus*, hepatitis C vaccinations	Noncontagious	Upper respiratory tract infection, diarrhea, fever, malaise	
Kawasaki disease		Noncontagious	Lymphadenitis	Cardiac complications, myocarditis
Pityriasis rosea	HHV-6, HHV-7	Noncontagious	Prodrome of fever, headache, arthralgias	
Papular purpuric gloves and socks syndrome		Noncontagious	Fatigue	
Dengue	DEN virus 1, 2, 3, and 4	Noncontagious	Fever, myalgia, arthralgia, headache, retrobulbar pain and rash	Thrombocytopenia, dengue shock syndrome, multiorgan dysfunction
Chikungunya	CHIK virus	Noncontagious		

(CHIK: chikungunya; EBV: Epstein–Barr virus; HHV: human herpesvirus; HFMD: hand, foot, and mouth disease)

Table 8: Historical names of exanthems.

Number	Name
First disease	**M**easles (rubeola)
Second disease	**S**carlet fever
Third disease	Rubella/**G**erman **m**easles
Fourth disease	**D**uke's disease
Fifth disease	**E**rythema infectiosum (butterfly pox)
Sixth disease	**R**oseola infantum (Pseudorubella)

(Mnemonic: MS GERMAN MD in ER)

Table 9: Cutaneous manifestations of COVID-19 in adult and pediatric population.

Features	Adult patients	Pediatric patients
Macules and papules	√	√
Vesicles/varicelliform-like eruption	√	√
Urticarial eruption	√	√
Acral pseudo-chilblain	√	√
Erythema multiforme		√
Half-moon nail sign	√	

- *Enanthem*: Erosive lesions of oral genital or ocular mucosa.

Morbilliform Drug Reactions[18]

- Most common form of adverse drug reactions
- Usually occur 2–3 weeks after drug administration
- Typically start on the trunk and spread peripherally in a symmetric fashion
- Relative sparing of face and pressure areas
- *Other features*: Fever, pruritus, and eosinophilia
- Resolution occurs by a change in color to brownish red, followed by scaling in 1–2 weeks.
  The distinguishing features between maculopapular drug rash versus viral exanthems are given in **Table 10**.

DIAGNOSIS AND TREATMENT

Viral exanthems are mostly self-limiting and require only supportive treatment but their diagnosis is crucial because of the potential systemic involvement as well as its contagiousness to the contacts. Diagnostic criteria have been set for few diseases which help in easy and early diagnosis **(Boxes 1 and 2)**. Recently, a burst in the incidence of viral exanthems has been noted in pediatric age group in spite of proper vaccination, which is sometimes referred to as *break through* cases or *atypical* infections.

Table 10: Differentiating features between maculopapular drug rash and viral exanthems.

	Drug rash	Viral exanthems
Age group	Adults > children	Mostly children
Site of onset	Usually trunk	Usually face/neck
Pruritus	Present	Absent
Temporal correlation with drug intake	Present	Usually absent
History to exposure to contact	Absent	Present
Fever and prodromal symptoms	Less common	Present
Mucosal involvement	Absent except SJS	Present
Lymphadenopathy	Absent	May be present

(SJS: Stevens–Johnson syndrome)

Box 1: Diagnostic criteria for Gianotti–Crosti syndrome (GCS) (Chuh et al.).[22]

Positive clinical features:
- Monomorphic, flat-topped, pink-brown papules or papulovesicles 1–10 mm in diameter
- At least three of the following four sites involved: (1) cheeks, (2) buttocks, (3) extensor surfaces of forearms, and (4) extensor surfaces of legs
- Symmetrical
- Lasting for at least 10 days

Negative clinical features:
- Extensive truncal lesions
- Scaly lesion

A patient is diagnosed as having Gianotti–Crosti syndrome if:
- On at least one occasion or clinical encounter, he/she exhibits all the positive clinical features
- On all occasions or clinical encounters related to the rash, he/she does not exhibit any of the negative clinical features
- None of the differential diagnoses is considered to be more likely than GCS on clinical judgment
- If lesional biopsy is performed and the findings are consistent with GCS

INVESTIGATIONS

Investigations needed to be ordered in few complicated cases. The various investigations and their interpretations are summarized in **Table 11**.

Red Flag Signs

Features suggestive of an unwell child are summarized in **Table 12**.

Box 2: Diagnostic criteria for Kawasaki disease.

- *Conjunctivitis*: Bilateral/painless/nonexudative
- *Lymphadenopathy*: Cervical, usually >1.5 cm/acute nonpurulent/at least one enlarged node
- *Skin rash*: Polymorphic nonvesicular
- *Extremity changes (one or more)*:
  ○ *Acute phase*: Erythema of palms and/or soles; induration of hands and/or feet
  ○ *Subacute phase*: Periungual desquamation
- *Mucosal changes (one or more)*: Red, cracked lips/glossitis with hyperplastic fungiform papillae seen as *strawberry tongue*/diffuse erythema of the oral and pharyngeal mucosa

(*Mnemonic: FEMaLE-R*: *f*ever, *e*yes, *m*ucous membrane, *l*ymphadenopathy, *e*xtremity, *r*ash)

The diagnosis of Kawasaki disease is confirmed when four out of these five criteria plus a high grade, persistent, unresponsive fever of >5 days is present, after excluding alternative clinical diagnosis

Table 11: Investigations in a child with fever and rash.

Findings	Interpretation
Leukocytosis	Bacterial or viral infections
Neutrophilia with lymphopenia	Bacterial infection
Neutropenia with lymphocytosis	Viral infection
Thrombocytopenia	Dengue
C-reactive protein	Marker of inflammation
Microscopic hematuria	Kidney involvement in vasculitis
Elevated liver enzymes	Many viruses can temporarily increase liver enzyme levels
Erythrocyte sedimentation rate	Marker of chronic infection
PCR test	For COVID infection, dengue, chikungunya
Nonstructural protein NS1 of dengue virus	For dengue fever

(PCR: polymerase chain reaction)

Table 12: Red flag signs in an unwell child.

Color	• Pallor (including parent/care taker report) • Mottled • Blue/Cyanosed
Activity	• Lethargy or decreased activity • Not responding normally to social cues • Does not wake or only with prolonged stimulation, or if roused, does not stay awake • Weak, high-pitched or continuous cry
Respiratory	• Grunting • Tachypnea • Increased work of breathing • Hypoxia
Circulation and hydration	• Poor feeding • Dry mucous membranes • Persistent tachycardia • Reduced skin turgor • Reduced urine output
Neurological	• Bulging fontanel • Neck stiffness • Focal neurological signs • Focal, complex, or prolonged seizures
Other	• Nonblanching rash • Fever for ≥5 days • Swelling of a limb or joint • Nonweight bearing/not using an extremity

Box 3: World Health Organization (WHO) recommended dose for vitamin A in measles.

- *<6 months*: 50,000 IU/day × two doses
- *6–11 months*: 100,000 IU/day × two doses
- *>1 year*: 200,000 IU/day × two doses
- *Children with clinical signs of vitamin A deficiency*: The first two doses are appropriate for age, then a third age-specific dose given 2–4 weeks later

If anyone of these red flag signs are present, patient should be referred to a pediatrician for further treatment.

TREATMENT

Treatment usually includes rest, proper hydration, soothing lotions, and symptomatic treatment for fever. Specific treatment is indicated in chicken pox in immunocompromised children (acyclovir @20 mg/kg PO qid for 5 days), scarlet fever (β-lactam antibiotics), Kawasaki disease (intravenous immunoglobulin @2 g/kg as a single IV infusion on diagnosis; aspirin @3–5 mg/kg orally as a daily dose until normal echo on follow-up or minimum 6 weeks and corticosteroids in high-risk groups). World Health Organization (WHO) recommends vitamin A supplementation for all children diagnosed with measles, regardless of country of their residence for prevention of blindness, and pulmonary complications (**Box 3**).

REFERENCES

1. Gelmetti C. Exanthema in pediatric dermatology: A confusing galaxy of myriad diseases. Indian J Paediatr Dermatol. 2021;22:100-6.
2. Mancini AJ. Exanthems in childhood: an update. Pediatr Ann. 1998;27:163-70.
3. Nelson JSB, Stone MS. Update on selected viral exanthems. Curr Opin Pediatr. 2000;12:359-64.
4. Fölster-Holst R, Kreth HW. Viral exanthems in childhood—infectious (direct) exanthems. Part 1: Classic exanthems. J Dtsch Dermatol Ges. 2009;7:309-16.
5. Knöpfel N, Noguera-Morel L, Latour I, Torrelo A. Viral exanthems in children: A great imitator. Clin Dermatol. 2019;37(3):213-26.
6. Sarkar R, Mishra K, Garg VK. Fever with rash in a child in India. Indian J Dermatol Venereol Leprol. 2012;78:251-62.
7. Misin A, Antonello RM, Di Bella S, Campisciano G, Zanotta N, Giacobbe DR, et al. Measles: An Overview of a Re-Emerging Disease in Children and Immunocompromised Patients. Microorganisms. 2020;8(2):276.
8. Lambert N, Strebel P, Orenstein W, Icenogle J, Poland GA. Rubella. Lancet. 2015;385(9984):2297-307.
9. Kostolansky S, Waymack JR. Erythema Infectiosum. In: StatPearls [Internet]. Treasure Island (FL): StatPearls Publishing; 2022.
10. Mullins TB, Krishnamurthy K. Roseola Infantum. In: StatPearls [Internet]. Treasure Island (FL): StatPearls Publishing; 2022.
11. Facts about chickenpox. Paediatr Child Health. 2005;10(7):413-4.
12. Pedreira RL, Leal JM, Silvestre KJ, Lisboa AP, Gripp AC. Gianotti-Crosti syndrome: a case report of a teenager. An Bras Dermatol. 2016;91(5 suppl 1):163-5.
13. Ramphul K, Mejias SG. Kawasaki disease: a comprehensive review. Arch Med Sci Atheroscler Dis. 2018;3:e41-e45.
14. Urbina F, Das A, Sudy E. Clinical variants of pityriasis rosea. World J Clin Cases. 2017;5(6):203-11.
15. Phakhounthong K, Chaovalit P, Jittamala P, Blacksell SD, Carter MJ, Turner P, et al. Predicting the severity of dengue fever in children on admission based on clinical features and laboratory indicators: application of classification tree analysis. BMC Pediatr. 2018;18(1):109.
16. Chandramathi J, Prabhu A, Kumar A. The "Chik Sign" in Neonatal Chikungunya. Rev Soc Bras Med Trop. 2020;53:e20200157.
17. Basetti S, Hodgson J, Rawson TM, Majeed A. Scarlet fever: a guide for general practitioners. London J Prim Care (Abingdon). 2017;9(5):77-9.
18. Stern RS. Clinical practice. Exanthematous drug eruptions. N Engl J Med. 2012;366:2492-501.
19. Kumar KB, Kiran AG, Kumar BU. Hand, foot and mouth disease in children: A clinicoepidemiological study. Indian J Paediatr Dermatol. 2016;17:7-12.
20. Lavery MJ, Bouvier CA, Thompson B. Cutaneous manifestations of COVID-19 in children (and adults): A virus that does not discriminate. Clin Dermatol. 2021;39(2):323-8.
21. Hasan S, Jangra J, Choudhary P, Mishra S. Erythema Multiforme: A Recent Update. Biomed Pharmacol J. 2018;11(1).
22. Chuh AA. Diagnostic criteria for Gianotti–Crosti syndrome: A prospective case-control study for validity assessment. Cutis. 2001;68:207-13.

23
A Child with Photosensitivity

Amit Mistry, Krishna Vivek Dave

INTRODUCTION

Photosensitivity is defined as an abnormal response to an ordinary light exposure of ultraviolet or visible lights. In children, there are a diverse group of photosensitivity disorders. Photosensitivity is quite rare in children than in adults, though there are some inherited genodermatoses and metabolic disorders which manifest photosensitivity in the early phase of life. Most common photodermatosis in pediatric age group is polymorphous light dermatosis followed by erythropoietic protoporphyria (EPP). Specific extracutaneous association may be the clue to diagnosis in this group of pediatric photodermatoses. Sunprotection strategies are required in all patients with evidence of photosensitivity. Early recognition and prompt diagnosis is essential to minimize the long-term complications associated with inadequate photoprotection.

WHEN TO SUSPECT PHOTOSENSITIVITY IN A CHILD?

If a child develops any type of lesions in photoexposed area, sunburn, intensive crying, burning or itching on limited exposure to light, photosensitivity should be suspected, and thorough evaluation of various diseases should be done. **Box 1** enumerates most possible causes of photosensitivity in a child. **Table 1** describes age predilection and disease to be suspected accordingly.

As photosensitivity in a child opens a wide variety of differential diagnosis, importance of history taking in such patients is that we can narrow down the list and relevant investigations can be ordered to confirm our suspicions.

Course of the disease: Idiopathic photodermatoses like PLE, nutritional deficiency disorders like pellagra, and

Box 1: Classification of photosensitivity disorders in children.

Idiopathic/immunologically mediated photodermatoses:
- Polymorphic light eruption (PLE)
- Juvenile spring eruption
- Actinic prurigo (AP)
- Hydroa vacciniforme (HV)
- Solar urticaria (SU)

Deoxyribonucleic acid (DNA) repair defective disorders and genodermatosis:
- Xeroderma pigmentosum
- Cockayne syndrome
- Rothmund–Thomson syndrome
- Trichothiodystrophy
- Bloom's syndrome
- Ataxia–telangiectasia
- Ultraviolet sensitive syndrome
- Smith–Lemli–Opitz syndrome
- Kindler syndrome

Photoexacerbated skin disorders:
- Atopic dermatitis
- Psoriasis
- Neonatal lupus erythematosus
- Systemic lupus erythematosus
- Dermatomyositis
- Pemphigus
- Lichen planus actinicus
- Darier's disease
- Dermatitis herpetiformis
- Herpes simplex infection

Continued

Continued

Nutritional and metabolic aberrations:
- Pellagra
- Hartnup disease
- Phenylketonuria
- Erythropoietic protoporphyria
- Congenital erythropoietic
- Porphyria cutanea tarda
- Hepatoerythropoietic porphyria

Pigmentary deficiencies:
- Albinism
- Vitiligo

Photosensitivity due to exogenous agents:
- Drug-induced phototoxicity
- Drug-induced photoallergy
- Phytophotodermatitis

Table 1: Age predilection.[1]

Age of presentation	Disorder with photosensitivity
At birth	- Neonatal lupus erythematosus (2/3rd cases) - Congenital erythropoietic porphyria and hepatoerythrocytic porphyria
≤1 year	- Rothmund–Thomson syndrome, Bloom's syndrome, Cockayne syndrome (3–6 months), xeroderma pigmentosum - Neonatal lupus erythematosus (1/3rd cases) - Childhood systemic lupus erythematosus (rarely) - Congenital erythropoietic porphyria - Phenylketonuria
1–5 years	- Ataxia telangiectasia - Hartnup disease (average 3 years of age) - Erythropoietic protoporphyria (mean age 4 years)
School going children	- Polymorphous light eruption (most common photodermatosis in children) - Actinic prurigo (average 9 years of age) - Hydroa vacciniforme (average 6 years of age) - Childhood systemic lupus erythematosus - Juvenile dermatomyositis

exogenous factor-related photodermatoses like drug-induced photosensitivity or phytophotodermatitis have an acute single episode. Disorders like PLE, solar urticaria (SU), actinic prurigo (AP), and hydroa vacciniforme (HV) may also have an intermittent course with complete clearing between episodes. Genodermatoses and metabolic disorders have a chronic course with acute exacerbation and the skin changes that occur during acute episode have tendency to persist. Conditions like collagen vascular disorders are aggravated by exposure to light. In patients with the photosensitivity and the skin changes become milder with age in patients with Hartnup disease.[2] In patients with HV, the condition either resolves or improves in adolescence.[3]

Exposure history to photosensitizing agents: Exposure to photosensitizers is common in school going children. Citrus fruits, mango, and extracts of a few common weeds containing furocoumarins are common sensitizing agents.[4] Lime juice is the most common offending agent.[5] Flowers of the Compositae group of plants (chrysanthemum, marigold, dahlia, and sunflower), contain oleoresins, may give rise to photosensitivity. Topical antimicrobials included in soaps, cosmetics, and medicaments such as halogenated salicylanilides, clioquinol, and sulfonamide derivatives are common photosensitizers and may go unnoticed. Some systemically administered drugs such as sulfonamides, nalidixic acid, chlorpromazine, ceftazidime, griseofulvin, ibuprofen, furosemide, and dapsone can cause photosensitivity.[5]

OTHER RELEVANT HISTORY

- History of seasonal variation is also important as it helps in differentiating with other diseases. Like in Hartnup disease there is an exacerbation of skin lesions in the spring or early summer.[2] Lesions of PLE and SU show hardening effect as they aggravate in the spring and early summer and gradually improve through the rest of the summer.[6,7] Hydroa vacciniforme, a very rare condition, occurs mostly during summer. AP aggravates in summer and persists through winter.[6]
- *Timing of development of lesions or symptoms after sun exposure*: As window glass shields filters ultraviolet B (UVB), development of lesions after exposure to filtered sunlight suggests UVA rays as etiological agent. Discussed and elaborated later in the chapter along with distribution of lesions.
- *Nature of the lesions*: Morphology of lesions can guide toward disease like development of freckles and sunburns might suggest xeroderma pigmentosum and vesicular lesions in cases of porphyria, Hydroa vacciniforme.
- Family history of consanguinity
- *History of drugs causing photosensitivity*: Doxycycline, retinoids, etc.
- *History of black discoloration of urine*: Phenylketonuria
- *History of bullous eruptions*: Kindler syndrome **(Fig. 1)**
- *Systemic complains* **(Table 2)**:
  - *Fever*: CTD, HSV
  - *Ataxia*: Ataxia telangiectasia, Hartnup disease
  - *Growth retardation and developmental delay*: Genodermatosis

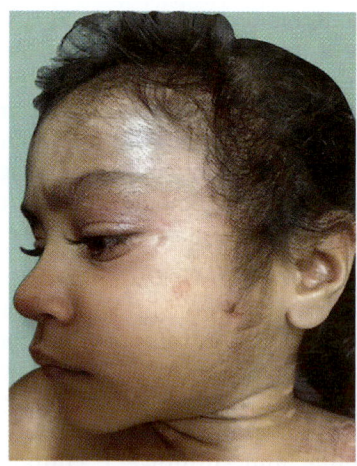

FIG. 1: Erythema over face because of photosensitivity in case of kindler syndrome. Notice the crusted lesion on cheek and postinflammatory hypopigmentation of healed blisters.

Courtesy: Dr Jigna Padhiyar.

Table 2: Associated systemic complaints.

Disorder	Findings
Idiopathic photodermatoses	Headache, nausea, bronchospasm, and syncope in case of inadvertent exposure to sunlight for a prolonged period[8]
Xeroderma pigmentosum	Mental retardation, cutaneous malignancies such as basal cell carcinoma, squamous cell carcinoma, and internal malignancy
Bloom syndrome	Growth retardation, recurrent infection due to immunodeficiency, internal malignancy like Hodgkin lymphoma[9]
Cockayne syndrome	Mental retardation, growth retardation, sensorineural deafness, decreased vision, and eventually blindness due to retinitis pigmentosa, dental caries
Rothmund–Thomson syndrome	Short stature, cataract, hypogonadism, osteogenic carcinoma
Hartnup disease	Cerebellar ataxia and psychiatric disturbances[2]
Ataxia telangiectasia	Mental retardation, prominent cerebellar ataxia, and nystagmus[10]
Phenylketonuria	Epilepsy and extrapyramidal disorders
Erythropoietic protoporphyria	Progressive liver failure
Neonatal lupus erythematosus	Congenital heart disease, neurological manifestations

CLINICAL FEATURES

Intolerance to sunlight of varying degrees is the presenting complaint in all the conditions. Infants and children with porphyrias experience burning and stinging pain on sun exposure and present with incessant crying even at night.[2] Children with idiopathic photodermatoses, drug-induced photosensitivity, and phytophotodermatitis may not have overt and significant sensitivity to sunlight. Following signs may be present in several of the disorders **(Table 3)**. **Table 4** distinguishing clinical features of photosensitive genodermatoses.[1]

- *Pigment dilution*: This can be observed in cases of phenylketonuria and albinism **(Fig. 2)**.
- *Periorbital erythematous rash*: Dermatomyositis **(Fig. 3)**.
- *Mottled hypo- and hyperpigmentation*: Xeroderma pigmentosum (XP—**Fig. 4**) and XP-Cockayne overlap **(Fig. 5)**.
- *Sunken eyes with microcephaly*: Cockayne syndrome (CS).
- *Cutaneous malignancy*: Xeroderma pigmentosus.
- *Burnt out skin on photoexposed parts*: Pellagra and Hartnup disease.
- *Micropapular lesions or lichenoid lesions on photoexposed parts*: Polymorphic light eruption.

Table 3: Various signs or clues in examination.

Butterfly erythema: It is the presenting feature in Bloom's syndrome (BS), Rothmund–Thomson syndrome (RTS), Cockayne syndrome (CS), systemic lupus erythematosus (SLE), pellagra, and Hartnup disease	*Vesicobullous lesions*: Present over photoexposed areas that heal by scarring and pigmentation resembling discoid lupus erythematosus (LE) are seen in RTS, BS, and porphyrias
Dermatitis: A sharply demarcated, erythematous, dry, scaly dermatitis over the face, neck, and other photoexposed areas is seen in pellagra and Hartnup disease.[2] Casal's necklace is one of the characteristic lesions of pellagra. Only photoexposed body parts are involved in these conditions. The presenting cutaneous feature of neonatal LE is an erythematous annular lesion involving periorbital area and trunk.[9] The skin lesions of phenylketonuria simulate atopic dermatitis, lesions are lichenified, scaly present over flexural aspect of body.[2] An eczematous eruption over the photoexposed parts may be found in patients with ataxia telangiectasia (AT)	
Telangiectasia: It is the prominent feature in genetic disorders such as RTS, BS, xeroderma pigmentosum (XP), and CS. In these patients, prominent conjunctival telangiectasia may also be seen.[9,11] Involvement of the bulbar conjunctiva is the initial presenting feature of AT.[10] Children with SLE and juvenile DM may show prominent facial telangiectasias[12]	
Poikiloderma: It is the predominant clinical feature in older children with RTS over photoexposed areas[13]	*Hypertrichosis*: Lanugo-like hair over the extremities and coarse facial hair are seen in congenital erythropoietic porphyria (CEP)[2]

Table 4: Distinguishing clinical features of photosensitive genodermatoses.	
Bloom syndrome (BS): • Photosensitivity • Skin atrophy • Narrow, keel-shaped, dolichocephalic facies • Recurrent infections • Deafness • Cutaneous and systemic malignancy	Cockayne syndrome (CS): • Photosensitivity eventually lost • Telangiectasia • Poikiloderma • Mottled pigmentation • Premature graying of hair • Skin atrophy • Loss of subcutaneous fat • Mickey mouse-like facies • Mental retardation • Neurological abnormality
Rothmund–Thomson syndrome (RTS): • Photosensitivity with involvement of covered body parts • Telangiectasia • Freckles • Mottled pigmentation • Skin atrophy • Bird-like facies • Recurrent infections • Deafness • Cutaneous and systemic malignancy	Xeroderma pigmentosum (XP): • Photosensitivity with involvement of covered body parts • Telangiectasia • Mottled pigmentation • Skin atrophy • Mental retardation • Neurological abnormality • Cutaneous malignancy
Ataxia telangiectasia (AT): • Photosensitivity with high sensitivity to ionizing radiation • Mottled pigmentation • Premature graying of hair • Recurrent infections • Neurological abnormality • Systemic malignancy	

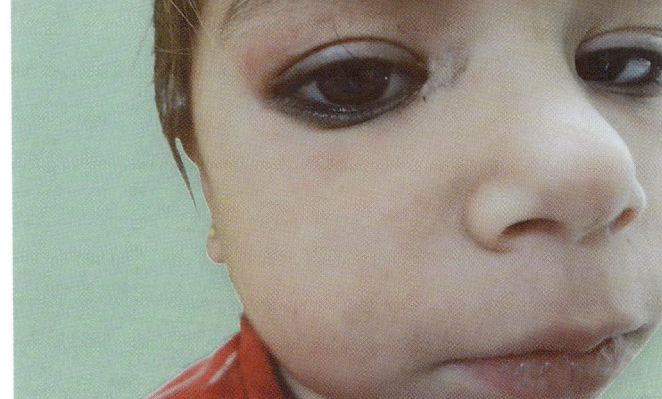

FIG. 3: Periorbital swelling and heliotrope rash along with telangiectasias in a case if dermatomyositis.
Courtesy: Dr Jigna Padhiyar.

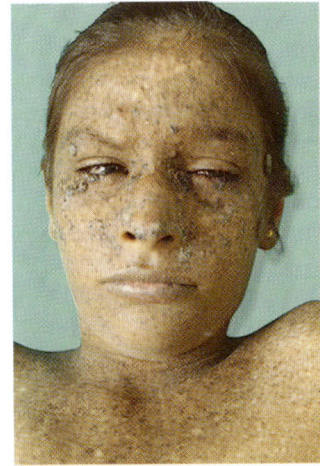

FIG. 4: Mottled hypo- and hyperpigmentations along with premalignant and malignant lesions over face in a case of xeroderma pigmentosum.
Courtesy: Dr Jigna Padhiyar.

IMPORTANCE OF DISTRIBUTION AND MORPHOLOGY OF LESIONS

Diseases might have overlapping clinical pictures but can be distinguished easily. PLE lesions usually appear 2 hours to 3 days following sun exposure. Grouped papules, vesicles, and eczematous plaques are commonly seen over the face, the "V" area of the chest, the back of the neck and the dorsolateral aspects of the forearms and persist for several days to weeks. Juvenile spring eruption observed in 5–12-year-old boys where, recurrent episodes of an itchy papulovesicular eruption occur over the helices of the ears and adjacent areas, followed by crusting and healing without scarring.[5]

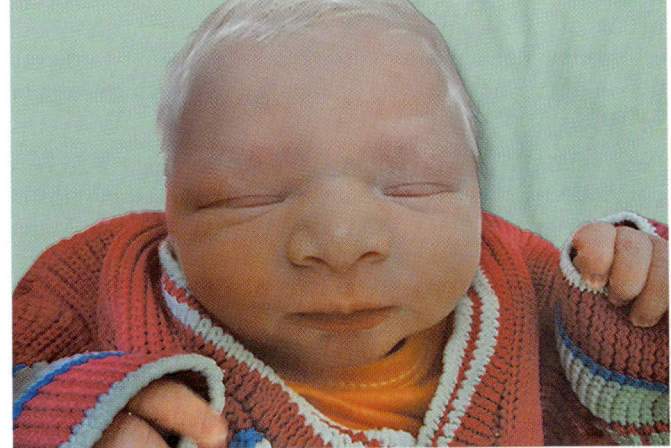

FIG. 2: A case of albinism.
Courtesy: Dr Jigna Padhiyar.

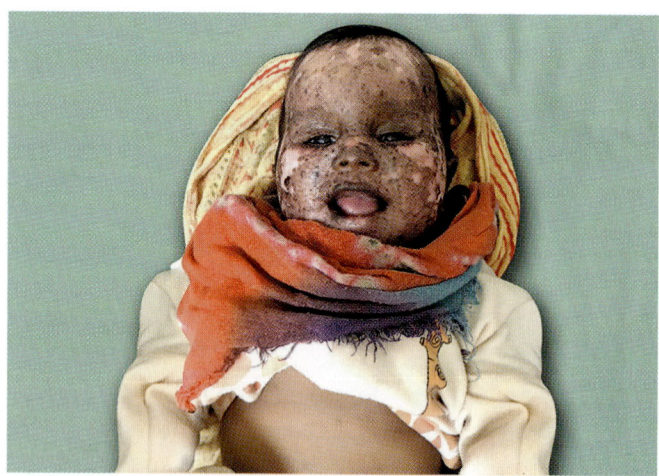

FIG. 5: Mottled hypo- and hyperpigmentations along with areas of depigmentation because of sunburn. Also notice the sunken eyes suggestive of XP-Cockayne overlap syndrome, which was confirmed with genetic analysis.

Courtesy: Dr Jigna Padhiyar.

Solar urticaria is a rare condition in young children, here urticarial wheals appear overexposed areas within seconds to minutes following sun exposure which generally resolve within 1–2 hours and almost always within 24 hours of avoidance of sun exposure.[4] Sunlight-induced urticaria may be a symptom of EPP, but it starts at an earlier age, with painful skin lesions, often have positive family history.[14]

Actinic prurigo is manifests by 9–10 years of age as pruritic excoriated papules and nodules on exposed body parts, commonly seen in girls.[5,15] Conjunctivitis and actinic cheilitis are characteristic features of AP.[12]

Hydroa vacciniforme is a very rare condition seen among school-going boys. Recurrent crops of deep-seated tense vesicles with surrounding erythema appear on exposed body parts within 1–2 days of sun exposure and heal with pock-like scars.[4]

Phytophotodermatitis is also common in school going children which is localized to the hands, lower legs, and around the lips.[4]

Xeroderma pigmentosum: First XP symptoms occur at a median age of 1–2 years.[16] Most of the XP patients tan normally without excessive burning while in few severe sunburn with blisters after a very short sun exposure, even through window glass. In later stages of infancy, pigmentary changes in sun-exposed skin develop, telangiectasia, and atrophic hyper- as well as hypopigmentation becomes apparent. It is a sign of premature skin aging. The risk of developing a cutaneous malignancy (basal cell carcinoma, squamous cell carcinoma), including melanoma, under 20 years of age is increased 1,000-fold in XP patients and is characterized by a typical UV mutation pattern predominantly in the *PTEN* gene.[17]

Ocular manifestations in XP photophobia, conjunctivitis, keratitis, pterygium, and neoplasia of the eyelids and conjunctiva may develop. The posterior portions of the eye, such as the retina, are usually unaffected because only visible light (400–800 nm) reaches the retina and UV light is absorbed by anterior portions of the eye.[18]

Neurological symptoms in XP may onset in early infancy or be delayed until puberty. The first neurological symptoms are reduction or loss of deep tendon reflexes, followed by progressive deafness then, mental deterioration with disabilities in speaking, hearing, walking, and balance may follow. Patients with De Sanctis–Cacchione syndrome have XP and severe neurological progressive deficiencies, including choreoathetosis, Achilles tendon shortening resulting from eventual quadriparesis, and immature sexual development. There is no marker or any method to predict the severity of the disease. The progression of disease cannot be predictable on the basis of age of onset of symptoms nor is the progression predictable within family members.[19]

Cockayne syndrome: Classic symptoms include growth retardation, neurological, and psychomotor impairment (tremor, incoordination, and dysarthric speech) with mental retardation, skin sensitivity to sunlight, progressive ophthalmological disorders including cataracts or retinitis pigmentosa, deafness, dental caries, and a characteristic facies including a thin face, flat cheeks, and prominent tapering nose (bird-like face). Early hallmarks for a clinical diagnosis are cachectic dwarfism and neurological disabilities. This leads to premature death at a mean age of 12 years.

Three clinical CS categories: CSI, a classic form in most CS patients; CSII, a severe form with early onset and rapid progression; CSIII, a mild form with late onset and slow progression.[20]

Pigmentary degeneration of the retina leading to a "salt and pepper" retinal change is a hallmark of CS and the most frequent ophthalmological complication. Cataracts, optic nerve atrophy, and optic disk pallor can be seen in some patients. Progressive sensorineural hearing loss may not manifest until the teenage years. Undescended testes occur in 30% of male CS patients. Kyphosis and contractures and a bird-like face caused by loss of subcutaneous fat tissue define the CS habitus. Most patients die of cachexia at 6 or 7 years of age.[20]

Rothmund–Thomson syndrome: The characteristic feature is poikiloderma, develops usually between 3 and 6 months of age,[21,22] appears first on the cheeks as erythema and later it spreads to the extensor surfaces of the arms and legs. Lesions may occur on the pinnae of the ears. The trunk, abdomen, and back tend to be spared. In the acute phase, the affected areas become inflamed with occasional blisters, but later inflammation settles into the chronic phase of poikiloderma. Transient photosensitivity has been reported in early childhood based on the typical distribution of lesions. Sparse hair affecting particularly the scalp, eyebrows, and eyelashes is commonly reported. The nails are slow growing and hypertrophic. Keratoses are often around the joints of the fingers or knee, and may be severe on the heels, commonly in older childrens.[22]

Dental anomalies such as short root anomaly, delayed or ectopic eruption of teeth, or hypoplastic teeth has been reported.[23,24] Subcapsular cataract usually occurs in all affected patients, are generally bilateral and of rapid onset.[25] Skeletal dysplasia is an important feature of RTS.[21,26] RTS is a cancer predisposition syndrome with very high risk of developing osteosarcoma, that arises in distal metaphyses of long bones. 5% of patients with RTS are also at increased risk of developing basal cell and squamous cell carcinomas.[25] Other forms of cancer such as squamous cell carcinoma of the oropharynx, myelodysplasia, and leukemia also been descirbed.[27-32] Patients are of normal intelligence with no neurological problems.

Bloom syndrome (BS): Affected patients have both pre- and postnatal growth deficiency.[33] The characteristic facies—underdeveloped malar and lower mandibular areas with resulting prominence of the nose (beaked nose) and ears.[34] Patients often have a high-pitched voice. Growth hormone levels are reported as normal. The butterfly rash usually appears during the first or second years of life after sun exposure. The rash becomes less severe with age and sometimes it can disappear completely. Café-au-lait spots are increased in BS.[33] Immunodeficiency has been reported as a feature of BS with reduced levels of immunoglobulin A (IgA) and IgM.[35] Infertility is impaired in BS; males are infertile (azoospermia or severe oligospermia), whereas females are fertile. Intelligence appears to be normal overall, although some patients have minor learning disabilities.[33]

Cancer is the most frequent medical complication and common cause of death. Major epithelial cancers such as lung, colorectal, breast, skin, genitourinary tract, and esophageal carcinomas, of which colorectal cancer is the most common in BS. Hematological malignancies including lymphomas, acute lymphoblastic leukemia and acute myelogenous leukemia, and myelodysplasia are common.[36,37] Life expectancy is reduced because of malignancy in early age, as well as other serious complications such as chronic obstructive pulmonary disease and diabetes mellitus.

Congenital erythropoietic porphyria (CEP): Manifests shortly after birth with severe cutaneous photosensitivity, blistering, erosions, excoriations, and ulcerations, which healed with extensive scarring and deformation, mainly of the hands. Loss of eyebrows, eyelashes, erythrodontia, and severe mutilation are frequently observed over face. Further, osteodystrophy and skeletal abnormalities are common clinical features.[38]

Erythropoietic protoporphyria: Characterized by photosensitivity manifesting early in life, with burning, stinging, and pruritus in sun-exposed skin, which later manifest as erythema, edema, and wax-like scarring. Symptoms start early in spring time, continuing through the summer and diminishing in autumn and winter.[38-40] The most important concern in here is development of cholestasis, due to accumulation of protoporphyrin hepatobiliary system, which resulting in severe liver damage. Progressive liver failure is rare but a well-recognized complication.[38,39,41,42]

Neonatal lupus: It affects skin, heart, blood, liver, brain, and bones. Cutaneous lesions are highly variable and polymorphous.[43] Lesions usually develop around the sixth week after birth. Typical lesions are erythematous, arcuate, polycyclic or annular macules, patches, and papules, which typically show slight central atrophy, with or without a fine scale, seen mainly over scalp and periorbital area, giving the baby an "owl eyes", "raccoon eyes" or "owl mask" appearance.[44] Mucosal ulceration has been seen in several patients. Although, lesions tend to be aggravated with sun exposure or phototherapy, they can appear in nonexposed areas such as the feet or napkin area and even be present at birth, before there is any sun exposure.[45]

Systemic features include, congenital heart disease (including persistent ductus arteriosus, atrial and ventricular septal defects, semilunar and atrioventricular valve abnormalities), liver disease (transaminitis, hepatomegaly, transient hepatitis, hyperbilirubinemia or, rarely, liver failure[46]), and hematological manifestations (thrombocytopenia, hemolytic or aplastic anemia and neutropenia[46]). Neurological manifestations (hydrocephalus, macrocephaly and neuropsychiatric dysfunction, calcification of the basal ganglia, and subependymal cysts[47]) and chondrodysplasia punctata.

INVESTIGATIONS

Phototesting and photopatch test: These are not commonly performed in children. It is indicated when idiopathic acquired photodermatoses are suspected[6] and if history and examination suggest the influence of a photo allergen. These tests are not helpful in diagnosing genodermatoses, porphyrias, and nutritional disorders.[6] Patient motivation and cooperation are needed in these tests, therefore difficult to conduct in children.

All patients without definitive clinical diagnosis should be evaluated for antinuclear (ANA), anti-Ro (SSA), and anti-La (SSB) antibodies and porphyrin levels.[48]

Patients with systemic lupus erythematosus (SLE) and diabetes mellitus (DM) need a thorough evaluation for systemic involvement such as muscle biopsy, muscle enzyme estimation, and electromyographic study in the presence of proximal myopathy and muscle tenderness.[12] ECG and echocardiography should be performed in all suspected cases of neonatal lupus erythematosus (NLE) to rule out congenital heart block or other anomalies.[12] Direct immunofluorescence study of the skin biopsy specimen is helpful in diagnosing SLE (complement and immune deposits at the dermoepidermal junction).

Table 5: Laboratory investigation and histopathology in genodermatoses.			
BS	**XP**	**CS**	**RTS**
• Molecular genetic testing identifying biallelic pathogenic variants in the *BLM* gene • Plasma levels of immunoglobulins	• Functional assessment of cellular repair capacity • Molecular genetic testing of the *XPA, XPC, ERCC2, ERCC3,* and *ERCC5* genes[20]	• Molecular genetic testing of CSA and CSB • Fundus examination of eye • CT scan of brain to see intracranial calcification	• Molecular testing for RECQL4 mutations • Ophthalmological evaluation to screen for cataracts. • Skeletal surveys to define underlying bone defects
Histopathological finding			
Nonspecific, showing epidermal atrophy, telangiectasia and a mild perivascular inflammatory infiltrate[49]	• Hyperkeratosis, atrophy of the epidermis and irregular elongation or atrophy of the rete ridges • Irregular hyperpigmentation of the basal layer, with or without an increase in the number of melanocytes is often present. Hypopigmented macules in between show decreased numbers of melanocytes	Appears as nonspecific dermatitis	Skin is edematous, with a perivascular lymphocytic infiltrate initially, later, skin shows hyperkeratosis, epidermal atrophy with dyskeratotic cells, dilation of the superficial vessels in the papillary dermis, pigmentary incontinence, basal cell vacuolization, fragmentation of elastic tissue, and loss of appendages[50]

(BS: Bloom syndrome; CT: computed tomography; CS: Cockayne syndrome; RTS: Rothmund–Thomson syndrome; XP: xeroderma pigmentosum)

Wood's lamp examination helps in demonstrating erythrodontia in CEP and hepatoerythropoietic porphyria (HEP).[48] Also in detecting the reddish pink fluorescence of serum, erythrocytes, urine, and stool in patients with different types of porphyrias.[2,48]

Screening of suspected neonates with phenylketonuria (PKU) by a blood test (serum level of phenylalanine >20 mg/dL) or Guthrie test is advised.[48] Urine chromatography for detection of amino acids is useful in children with PKU and Hartnup disease.[2]

Histopathological examination in porphyrias commonly reveals subepidermal, cell-poor blisters with a characteristic festooning of dermal papillae that is most likely due to the deposition of periodic acid-Schiff (PAS)-positive glycoproteins in and around the wall of vessels localized in the upper dermis. **Table 5** describes histopathological findings and other laboratory investigation in genodermatoses. In direct immunofluorescence, mainly IgG, complement, and fibrinogen can be detected at the dermoepidermal junction and around blood vessels of the papillary dermis.

MANAGEMENT

Counseling the parents plays a major part in treating a child with photosensitivity, regarding specific light avoidance, photoprotection and sometimes, change of lifestyle.[4] Outdoor activities of such children should be curtailed as much as possible. Environment in tropical countries and socioeconomic status are prohibitive factors for complete sun avoidance. General measures such as use of tightly woven, dark colored, full-sleeved clothing and a hat need to be encouraged.[4] Window glass filters out most of the UVB in sunlight but transmits UVA and visible light readily.[7] Strict sun avoidance is a must for children with porphyria, BS, XP, and RTS. Shades or filters can provide protection from fluorescent lights.[4]

Habitual use of sunscreens on all exposed areas is helpful. Topical agents, especially conventional chemical sunscreens for UVA and UVB, are ineffective in patients with porphyrias.[2] Physical sunscreen containing titanium dioxide and zinc oxide are more effective, since these patients are sensitive to the visible range.[2]

In addition to sunscreens, topical steroids, and antihistamines are used in idiopathic photodermatoses. Prophylactic use of low-dose UVA/PUVA/UVB is helpful in preventing recurrence in this group of disorders.[4] Regular surveillance should be done of children with albinisms, XP, and RTS for early diagnosis of cutaneous and systemic malignancies.

A low-phenylalanine diet continued lifelong is the mainstay of therapy in patients with PKU.[2] Skin color, photosensitivity, foul odor, and eczema are reversible with such treatment.[48] Children with HD and pellagra need supplementation with nicotinamide.[2]

In patients of XP having actively developed a large number of skin cancers, high dose of oral isotretinoin significantly reduces the frequency of cutaneous malignancies.[20] However, after cessation of isotretinoin the skin cancer frequency may recure. The topical use of T4 endonuclease V, a prokaryotic DNA repair enzyme that has been shown to reduce the rate of skin cancers. However, it is still subject to research and has not been approved for clinical use.[20]

There is currently no specific or causal treatment for CS available, patients can only be treated symptomatically. Patient needs to be followed up for assessment of neurological symptoms, social, auditory, and visual function. Exercise and physical therapy to compensate for deteriorating neurological function are also important.

Retinoids may improve the hyperkeratoses[51] in RTS. Pulsed dye laser can be used cosmetically for the telangiectatic portion of the rash.[52]

In CEP frequent blood transfusions can suppress erythropoiesis, thereby decreasing porphyrin production and photosensitivity. Bone marrow or stem cell transplantation has been reported to be curative in CEP which markedly reduces porphyrin levels.[53]

Synthetic α-melanocyte-stimulating hormone analog afamelanotide has been a breakthrough in treatment of EPP. After binding to the melanocortin-1 receptor, afamelanotide induces the tyrosine-mediated pathway in epidermal melanocytes. Thus, it enables physiological melanogenesis, this leads to increased skin pigmentation and UV quenching, which confer photoprotection and marked decrease of phototoxic reactions. Treatment consists of subcutaneous implants containing 16 mg of afamelanotide in a slow-release formulation, to be administered every 2 months.[54-56] Beta carotene improves light tolerance in patients with porphyria. A daily dosage of 50–200 mg/day to achieve a serum level of 500 µg/dL is effective and benefit is observed by 1–3 months.[2]

As cutaneous lesions are usually transient, sun avoidance is the only recommended intervention in NLE. Topical calcineurin inhibitors or topical corticosteroids might be considered in some cases.[57] Hydroxychloroquine during pregnancy was demonstrated to decrease the risk of fetal cardiac abnormalities.[58] Hydroxychloroquine inhibits the endosomal acidification required for optimal toll-like receptor (TLR) signaling, whose activation is known to promote cardiac inflammation and scarring. In mothers with neonate having LE, subsequent pregnancies should be strictly monitored, and maternal prophylactic systemic therapy may be considered.[59]

REFERENCES

1. Inamadar AC, Palit A. Photosensitivity in children: an approach to diagnosis and management. Indian J Dermatol Venereol Leprol. 2005;71(2):73-9.
2. Black MM, Gawkrodger DJ, Seymour CA, Weismann K. Metabolic and nutritional disorders. In: Champion RH, Burton JL, Burns DA, Breathnach SM (Eds). Textbook of Dermatology, 6th edition. Oxford: Blackwell-Science; 1998. pp. 2577-677.
3. Gupta G, Man I, Kemmett D. Hydroa vaccineforme: A clinical and follow-up study of 17 cases. J Am Acad Dermatol. 2000;42:208-13.
4. Hensley DR, Hebert AA. Pediatric photosensitivity disorders. Dermatol Clin. 1998;16:571-8.
5. Raimer SS, Raimer BG, Durate AM, Pruksachatkunakoru C, Boyer L. Physical injury and environmental hazards. In: Schachner LA, Hansen RC (Eds). Pediatric Dermatology, 3rd edition. Edinburgh: Mosby; 2003. pp. 1227-65.
6. Kim JJ, Lim HW. Evaluation of the photosensitive patient. Semin Cutan Med Surg. 1999;18:253-6.
7. Van Pragg MC, Boom BW, Vermeez BJ. Diagnosis and treatment of polymorphous light eruption. Int J Dermatol. 1994;33:233-9.
8. Ryckaert S, Roelandts R. Solar urticaria: A report of 25 cases and difficulties in phototesting. Arch Dermatol. 1998;134:71-4.
9. Harper JI. Genetics and genodermatoses. In: Champion RH, Burton JL, Burns DA, Breathnach SM (Eds). Textbook of Dermatology, 6th edition. Oxford: Blackwell-Science; 1998. pp. 357-436.
10. Cohen LE, Tanner DJ, Schaefer HG, Levis WR. Common and uncommon cutaneous findings in patients with ataxia telangiectasia. J Am Acad Dermatol. 1984;10:431-8.
11. Inamadar AC, Palit A. Bloom's syndrome in an Indian child. Pediatr Dermatol. 2005;22(2):147-50.
12. Barnett NK, Wright DA, Kawasaki T, Treadwell PA. Collagen vascular, connective tissue disease and selected systemic diseases with skin manifestations. In: Schachner LA, Hansen RC (Eds). Pediatric Dermatology, 3rd edition. Edinburgh: Mosby; 2003. pp. 943-88.
13. Inamadar AC, Palit A, Athanikar SB, Sampagavi VV, Deshmukh NS. Rothmund-Thomson syndrome: Report of 3 cases. Indian J Dermatol Venereol Leprol. 2003;69:67-9.
14. Fotiades J, Soter NA, Lim HW. Results of evaluation of 203 patients for photosensitivity in a 7.3-year period. J Am Acad Dermatol. 1995;33:597-602.
15. Lane PR, Hogan DJ, Martel MJ, Reeder B, Irvine J. Actinic prurigo. Clinical features and prognosis. J Am Acad Dermatol. 1992;26;683-91.
16. Kraemer KH, Lee MM, Scotto J. Xeroderma pigmentosum. Cutaneous, ocular, and neurologic abnormalities in 830 published cases. Arch Dermatol. 1987;123:241-50.
17. Masaki T, Wang Y, DiGiovanna JJ, et al. High frequency of PTEN mutations in nevi and melanomas from xeroderma pigmentosum patients. Pigment Cell Melanoma Res. 2014;27:454-64.
18. Bootsma D, Kraemer KH, Cleaver JE, Hoeijmakers JHJ. Nucleotide excision repair syndromes: xeroderma pigmentosum, Cockayne syndrome, and trichothiodystrophy. In: Vogelstein B, Kinzler KW (Eds). The Genetic Basis of Human Cancer. McGraw-Hill: New York; 2002. pp. 211-37.
19. Kraemer KH, Sander M, Bohr VA. New areas of focus at workshop on human diseases involving DNA repair deficiency and premature aging. Mech Ageing Dev. 2007;128:229-35.
20. Schubert S, Emmert S. Xeroderma Pigmentosum and Related Diseases. In: Hoeger P, Kinsler V, Yan A (Eds). Harper's Textbook of Pediatric Dermatology, 4th edition. Hoboken, NJ; Chichester: Wiley-Blackwell; 2020. pp. 1756-58.
21. Wang LL, Levy ML, Lewis RA, Chintagumpala MM, Lev D, Rogers M, et al. Clinical manifestations in a cohort of 41 Rothmund–Thomson syndrome patients. Am J Med Genet. 2001;102:11-7.
22. Wang LL, Plon SE. Rothmund-Thomson Syndrome. In: Adam MP, Everman DB, Mirzaa GM, Pagon RA, Wallace SE, Bean LJH, Gripp KW, Amemiya A (Eds). GeneReviews® [Internet]. Seattle (WA): University of Washington, Seattle; 1993.

23. Roinioti TD, Stefanopoulos PK. Short root anomaly associated with Rothmund–Thomson syndrome. Oral Surg Oral Med Oral Pathol Oral Radiol Endod. 2007;103:e19-22.
24. Haytaç MC, Oztunç H, Mete UO, Kaya M. Rothmund-Thomson syndrome: a case report. Oral Surg Oral Med Oral Pathol Oral Radiol Endod. 2002;94:479-84.
25. Vennos EM, Collins M, James WD. Rothmund–Thomson syndrome: review of the world literature. J Am Acad Dermatol. 1992;27:750-62.
26. Mehollin-Ray AR, Kozinetz CA, Schlesinger AE, Guillerman RP, Wang LL. Radiographic abnormalities in Rothmund–Thomson syndrome and genotype-phenotype correlation with RECQL4 mutation status. Am J Roentgenol. 2008;191:W62-6.
27. Borg MF, Olver IN, Hill MP. Rothmund-Thomson syndrome and tolerance of chemoradiotherapy. Australas Radiol. 1998;42:216-8.
28. Rizzari C, Bacchiocchi D, Rovelli A, Biondi A, Cantu'-Rajnoldi A, Uderzo C, et al. Myelodysplastic syndrome in a child with Rothmund-Thomson syndrome: a case report. J Pediatr Hematol Oncol. 1996;18:96-7.
29. Ilhan I, Arikan Ü, Büyükpamukçu M. Myelodysplatic syndrome and RTS. Pediatr Hematol Oncol. 1996;13:197.
30. Pianigiani E, de Aloe G, Andreassi A, Rubegni P, Fimiani M. Rothmund–Thomson syndrome (Thomson-type) and myelodysplasia. Pediatr Dermatol. 2001;18:422-5.
31. Narayan S, Fleming C, Trainer AH, Craig JA. Rothmund-Thomson syndrome with myelodysplasia. Pediatr Dermatol. 2001;18:210-2.
32. Porter WM, Hardman CM, Abdalla SH, Powles AV. Haematological disease in siblings with Rothmund-Thomson syndrome. Clin Exp Dermatol. 1999;24:452-4.
33. Keller C, Keller KR, Shew SB, Plon SE. Growth deficiency and malnutrition in Bloom syndrome. J Pediatr. 1999;134:472-9.
34. Sanz MM, German J, Cunniff C. Bloom's syndrome. In: Pagon RA, Adam MP, Ardinger HH (Eds). GeneReviews® [Internet]. Seattle (WA): University of Washington, Seattle; 1993.
35. Babbe H, McMenamin J, Hobeika E, Wang J, Rodig SJ, Reth M, et al. Genomic instability resulting from Blm deficiency compromises development, maintenance, and function of the B cell lineage. J Immunol. 2009;182:347-60.
36. de Renty C, Ellis NA. Bloom's syndrome: why not premature aging? A comparison of the BLM and WRN helicases. Ageing Res Rev. 2017;33:36-51.
37. Shi W, Zauber A, Sanz M, German J. Analysis of the markedly increased incidence of cancer in individuals with Bloom's syndrome (Abstract). In: 56th Annual Meeting of the American Society of Human Genetics, New Orleans; 2006.
38. Bickers DR, Frank J. The porphyrias. In: Wolff K, Goldsmith LA, Katz SI (Eds). Fitzpatrick's Dermatology in General Medicine, 8th edition. New York: McGraw Hill; 2012. pp. 1538-73.
39. Karim Z, Lyoumi S, Nicolas G, Deybach JC, Gouya L, Puy H. Porphyrias: A 2015 update. Clin Res Hepatol Gastroenterol. 2015;39:412-25.
40. Lecha M, Puy H, Deybach JC. Erythropoietic protoporphyria. Orphanet J Rare Dis. 2009;4:19.
41. Frank J, Poblete-Gutierrez P. Delayed diagnosis and diminished quality of life in erythropoietic protoporphyria: results of a cross-sectional study in Sweden. J Intern Med. 2011;269(3):270-4.
42. Karim Z, Lyoumi S, Nicolas G, Deybach JC, Gouya L, Puy H. Porphyrias: A 2015 update. Clin Res Hepatol Gastroenterol. 2015;39(4):412-25.
43. Silverman E, Jaeggi E. Non-cardiac manifestations of neonatal lupus erythematosus. Scand J Immunol. 2010;72:223-5.
44. Lee L. The clinical spectrum of neonatal lupus. Arch Dermatol Res. 2009;301:107-10.
45. Admani S, Krakowski A. Neonatal lupus erythematosus presenting as atypical targetoid-like lesions involving genitals and soles of feet following brief sun exposure. J Clin Aesthet Dermatol. 2013;6:19-23.
46. Kim KR, Yoon T. A case of neonatal lupus erythematosus showing transient anemia and hepatitis. Ann Dermatol. 2009;21:315-18.
47. Prendiville JS, Cabral DA, Poskitt KJ, Au S, Sargent MA. Central nervous system involvement in neonatal lupus erythematosus. Pediatr Dermatol. 2003;20:60-7.
48. Pierini A. Photosensitivity disorders. In: Schachner LA, Hansen RC (Eds). Pediatric Dermatology, 3rd edition. Edinburgh: Mosby; 2003. pp. 316-37.
49. McGowan J, Maize J, Cook J. Lupus-like histopathology in Bloom syndrome: Reexamining the clinical and histopathologic implications of photosensitivity. Am J Dermatopathol. 2009;31:786-91.
50. Shuttleworth D, Marks R. Epidermal dysplasia and skeletal deformity in congenital poikiloderma (Rothmund–Thomson syndrome). Br J Dermatol. 1987;117:377-84.
51. Shuttleworth D, Marks R. Congenital poikiloderma: treatment with etretinate. Br J Dermatol. 1988;118:729-30.
52. Potozkin JR, Geronemus RG. Treatment of the poikilodermatous component of the Rothmund-Thomson syndrome with the flashlamp-pumped pulsed dye laser: a case report. Pediatr Dermatol. 1991;8:162-5.
53. Katugampola RP, Anstey AV, Finlay AY, Whatley S, Woolf J, Mason N, et al. A management algorithm for congenital erythropoietic porphyria derived from a study of 29 cases. Br J Dermatol. 2012;167(4):888-900.
54. Biolcati G, Marchesini E, Sorge F, Barbieri L, Schneider-Yin X, Minder EI. Long-term observational study of afamelanotide in 115 patients with erythropoietic protoporphyria. Br J Dermatol. 2015;172(6):1601-12.
55. Minder EI. Afamelanotide, an agonistic analog of alpha-melanocyte-stimulating hormone, in dermal phototoxicity of erythropoietic protoporphyria. Expert Opin Invest Drugs. 2010;19(12):1591-602.
56. Harms JH, Lautenschlager S, Minder CE, Minder EI. Mitigating photosensitivity of erythropoietic protoporphyria patients by an agonistic analog of alpha-melanocyte stimulating hormone. Photochem Photobiol. 2009;85(6):1434-9.
57. Boh EE. Neonatal lupus erythematosus. Clin Dermatol. 2004;22:125-8.
58. Izmirly PM, Kim MY, Llanos C, Le PU, Guerra MM, Askanase AD, et al. Evaluation of the risk of anti-SSA/Ro-SSB/La antibody-associated cardiac manifestations of neonatal lupus in fetuses of mothers with systemic lupus erythematosus exposed to hydroxychloroquine. Ann Rheum Dis. 2010;69:1827-30.
59. Monari P, Gualdi G, Fantini F, Giannetti A. Cutaneous neonatal lupus erythematosus in four siblings. Br J Dermatol. 2008;158:626-8.

24
A Child with Suspected Primary Immunodeficiency: A Dermatologist's Perspective

Bhumesh Kumar Katakam, Nita Radhakrishnan

INTRODUCTION

Primary immunodeficiencies (PIDs) are a group of over 400 monogenic disorders that result in derangement in the immunological defense of the body. This predisposes an individual to repeated, unusual or prolonged infections, many of which may involve the dermatological system. In addition to infections, immune dysregulation manifesting as autoimmunity, allergies, atopy, and malignancies are other features. With the advent of next generation sequencing, many new mutations are being discovered each year, thus increasing the estimated prevalence to 1 in 1,200 population in the USA.[1] These group of disorders are thus more commonly expected than other genetic disorders such as hemophilias, cystic fibrosis, albinism, etc. However due to reduced awareness, reduced facilities for testing and treatment, many of these patients are not detected early and they either succumb to the disease or have organ-threatening complications.

Primary immunodeficiency disorders are usually monogenic disorders; they result from genetic defects affecting one or more arms of the immune system. Secondary immunodeficiency disorders on the other hand, result from infections [human immunodeficiency virus (HIV)], malignancy, malnutrition, immunosuppressive medications such as steroids, calcineurin inhibitors, tumor necrosis factor (TNF) inhibitors, etc.

Dermatological manifestations are common presenting features in PIDs. In a recent survey of skin manifestations in children with PIDs presenting to a center in Colombia, out of 306 patients under 18 years, 83 (27%) had cutaneous manifestations such as atopic dermatitis, infections, seborrhea, hair-nail changes, etc.[2] Most dermatological manifestations seen in PIDs are not pathognomonic and may be seen in patients with normal immunity as well.

Because of this, it is vital to have a wholesome approach with emphasis on past illnesses, family history, growth parameters, and other system involvement while evaluating any patient. In addition, the age at presentation, the degree of skin involvement, the evolution of the skin lesion, response to treatment, refractoriness, etc. can also help in differentiating these lesions in those with PID compared to those with normal immunity.[2]

Primary immunodeficiencies have now been renamed as human inborn errors of immunity. As per the International Union of Immunological Societies 2019 update, there are 10 categories under which these diseases can be classified.[3] These monogenic germline mutations could cause either loss of gain function of the encoded protein which could alter the phenotype of the disease. Based on the pathogenesis, these diseases are classified as:

- Immunodeficiencies affected cellular and humoral immunity
- Combined immunodeficiencies with associated or syndromic features
- Predominantly antibody deficiencies
- Diseases of immune dysregulation
- Congenital defects of phagocyte number, function or both
- Defects in intrinsic and innate immunity
- Autoinflammatory disorders
- Complement deficiencies
- Bone marrow failure
- Phenocopies of PIDs

The detailed description of each of these groups of diseases is beyond the scope of this chapter. The decision-making process aimed for physicians is available as open access both with the journal and as a smartphone application.[3,4] When encountering dermatological lesions that are unusual as mentioned above, keeping PIDs in differential diagnoses and encouraging consultation with specialists and referral to a tertiary center with diagnostic facilities is recommended.

WARNING SIGNS FOR PRIMARY IMMUNODEFICIENCIES

The warning signs for PIDs include: (a) four or more new ear infections within 1 year; (b) two or more serious sinus infections within 1 year; (c) two or more months on antibiotics with little effect; (d) two or more pneumonias within 1 year; (e) failure of an infant to gain weight or grow normally; (f) recurrent deep skin or organ abscesses; (g) persistent oral thrush (beyond 2 weeks of treatment) or fungal infection on skin; (h) need for intravenous antibiotics to clear infections; (i) two or more deep-seated infections including septicemia; and (j) a family history of PID. These warning signs although meant for lay public can also help physicians in considering immunological evaluation for children who present with features other than infections.

In addition, a close watch for phenotypic features such as delayed cord separation, congenital heart disease, hypopigmentation, failure to thrive, and investigations such as absent thymus on chest X-ray or hypocalcemia should be kept in mind.

As dermatology is a science of observing visible changes in skin, it also becomes more feasible to examine skin first followed by focused history taking pertaining to various observed findings. This chapter also flows same way.

DERMATOLOGICAL MANIFESTATIONS IN PRIMARY IMMUNODEFICIENCIES

Skin Infections

Chronic infections are the most common dermatological manifestation of PIDs. Depending on the immune compartment involved, this could be bacterial, fungal, viral, or parasitic. It could be either limited to the skin or associated with multisystem involvement. It has also been observed that skin colonization with species not normally observed in healthy controls was seen in patients with PIDs (dysbiosis of skin flora).

Bacterial Infections

Bacterial skin infections include follicular pyodermas (folliculitis, furunculosis, carbuncle abscesses) and nonfollicular pyodermas (impetigo, ecthyma, erysipelas, and cellulitis). This is often observed to be disseminated and refractory/resistant to treatment. PIDs with phagocytic dysfunction or combined immunodeficiencies are mostly associated with bacterial skin infections. In children with phagocytic disorders, those with severe congenital neutropenia (often with absolute neutrophil count <500 cells/µL) are associated with bacterial infections that become disseminated and often fatal.

In most neutrophil disorders (either neutropenic disorders or neutrophil function disorders such as leukocyte adhesion disorders) pus formation is not observed in the lesion. The skin lesions usually contain serosanguineous fluid which when cultured is often positive for the infective organism **(Fig. 1)**. Absence of pus or conventional signs of inflammation should not deter us from a diagnosis of bacterial infections and a low threshold for culturing the discharge or the lesion per se after a skin biopsy should be encouraged. In chronic granulomatous disease (CGD), there are defects in nicotinamide adenine dinucleotide phosphate (NADPH) oxidase complex that results in phagocytes that are unable to destroy the intracellular microbes such as *Staphylococcus aureus*, *Serratia*, *Klebsiella*, *Pseudomonas*, *Chromobacterium*, etc. CGD therefore presets with soft tissue abscesses as well as lymph node and deep abscesses affecting the liver and spleen along with nonresponding pneumonias **(Fig. 2)**. They also may present similar to Crohn's disease with inflammatory bowel disease and perianal fistulae.[1]

Leukocyte adhesion disorder is another category of neutrophil dysfunction that presents with severe bacterial infections affecting the skin and mucosae. Despite white blood cell (WBC) count and absolute neutrophil count being elevated (often >20,000/µL), these lesions are characteristically devoid of pus since the defect is in migration of neutrophils to the site of inflammation.

Bacterial skin infections may also be observed in autosomal dominant hyperimmunoglobulin E (IgE) (HIGE) syndrome (STAT3 deficiency) where cold abscesses (abscess with minimal inflammation) are noticed. *S. aureus* infections associated with PIDs have been reported with HIGE syndrome.[5]

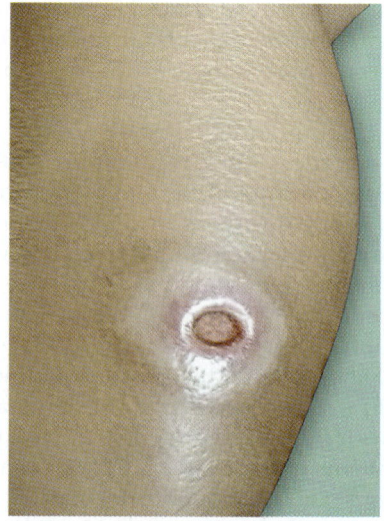

FIG. 1: Punched out lesion with no pus in a child with severe congenital neutropenia.

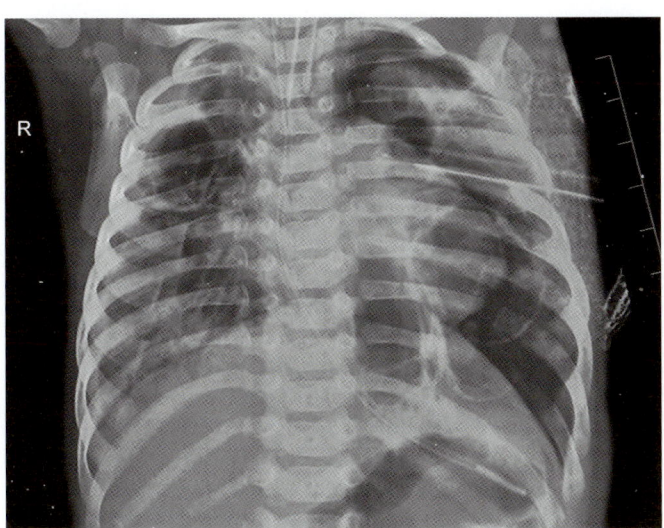

FIG. 2: Bronchopneumonia with multiple pneumatoceles in congenital granulomatous disease.

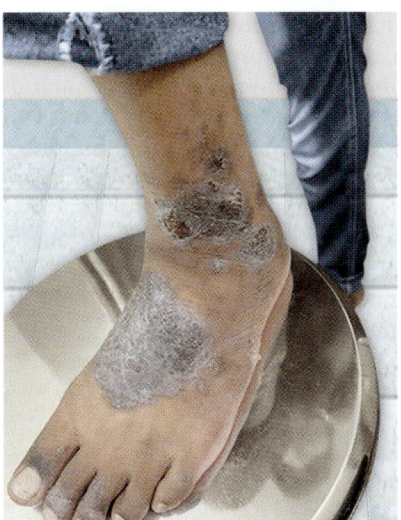

FIG. 3: Hyper-IgE syndrome (HIES) in a 10-year-old male child [chronic recurrent eczema, elevated IgE levels (>2,000 U/mL), history of atopy, eosinophilia].

Mycobacterial Infections

Disseminated BCG infections with involvement of skin and reticuloendothelial system are observed in patients with combined immunodeficiencies. Severe combined immunodeficiency (SCID) is the prototype of this group where children are born with severe T cell lymphopenia. In countries, where there is no newborn screening to detect children with this fatal condition at birth, all receive live vaccines such as BCG. The attenuated bacteria in the vaccine are capable of presenting as disseminated infection in children with SCID and is often life-threatening. Children with SCID present with failure to thrive, recurrent pneumonia, diarrhea, oral thrush, and other severe infections. Diagnosis of BCG infection can be made only on skin biopsy with appropriate microbiological investigations.

Mutations in interferon γ, interleukin 12 (IL-12) or their signaling pathways cause another group of diseases in the innate immune system named Mendelian susceptibility to mycobacterial diseases (MSMDs). They present with predilection to cutaneous mycobacterial infections, recurrent skin/bone infections, and susceptibility to *Salmonella*, *Nocardia*, *Histoplasma*, etc. Unlike SCID, children with MSMD are usually thriving well and live into adulthood with predilection only for this narrow spectrum of infections.

Viral Infections

Viral infections are less common in PIDs affecting the skin. They present as warts usually due to herpes or human papilloma virus. Children with autosomal recessive HIGE syndrome **(Fig. 3)** (DOCK8 deficiency) present with predilection for viral infections. This includes herpes zoster, herpes simplex, and molluscum contagiosum.

Recurrent and severe warts are also observed in patients with GATA2 deficiency (a disorder presenting with

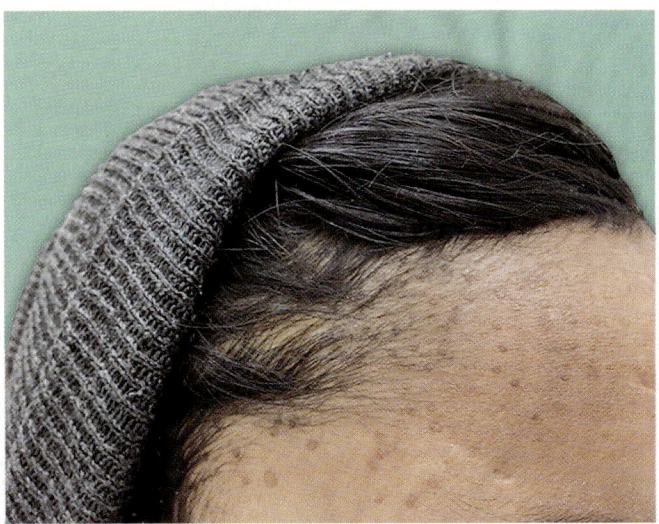

FIG. 4: Warts noticed in a child with GATA2 syndrome with acute myeloid leukemia.

myelodysplasia and myeloid leukemia) **(Fig. 4)**, WHIM syndrome (Warts, Hypogammaglobulinemia, Infections, and Myelokathexis), and WILD syndrome (Warts, Immunodeficiency, Lymphedema, and Dysplasia) among others. Any child who presents with recurrent/recalcitrant warts requires extensive immunological evaluation even if preliminary screening evaluation is reported as normal.

Fungal Infections

The most common fungal infections are of the *Candida* species and it presents as intertrigo, oral thrush, and perineal infections **(Fig. 5)**. Children with combined immunodeficiencies such as SCID, present with extensive nappy rash that is often difficult to treat. In addition, skin and soft tissue fungal infections such as *Fusarium*, mucormycosis, etc. may be noted in patients with neutrophil function disorders. Chronic granulomatous disease also presents with predilection for *Aspergillus* species.

Chronic mucocutaneous candidiasis (CMC) has been described in patients with Th17 pathway including gain of function STAT1 mutation, mutations in IL-17F, IL-17RA, etc. In these disorders, patients present with chronic infections limited to mucosal surfaces, skin, and nails. An approach to CMC is presented in **Flowchart 1**.[6]

Parasitic Infections

Occasionally, parasitic infections such as disseminated scabies (Norwegian or crusted scabies) may be noted in children with immunodeficiencies.

Eczema and Erythroderma

Eczematous skin lesions or atopic skin lesions are very frequently observed in certain categories of PIDs. It is observed in up to 25% of children with PIDs. Since atopy is commonly observed in children (clinically may present after 10 weeks of age), a close watch on associated symptoms, growth, and other system involvement should prompt immunological evaluation **(Fig. 6)**.

Eczema in association with thrombocytopenia and recurrent infections is observed characteristically in Wiskott–Aldrich syndrome (WAS). Although many patients do not have the classical triad of symptoms, a variety of skin manifestations from dry ichtyotic skin, recurrent skin infections to eczema is observed. Other features include recurrent infections, mucosal and deep bleeding, autoimmune manifestations such as nephritis and vasculitis, and malignancies. The eczema in WAS resembles atopic dermatitis closely (but eczema is early onset, severe, and poor response to treatment); the hemorrhagic component helps it differentiate from atopic dermatitis.[7] The presence of an underlying PID should explain the reason for poorly responding atopic dermatitis in some patients.[8,9]

Eczema is also noted in immunodeficiencies such as Omenn syndrome, HIGE syndromes and IPEX syndrome. IPEX syndrome is an X-linked disorder characterized by immune dysregulation, polyendocrinopathy, enteritis with severe diarrhea and X-linked inheritance. These children present with eczema, early onset diarrhea and neonatal

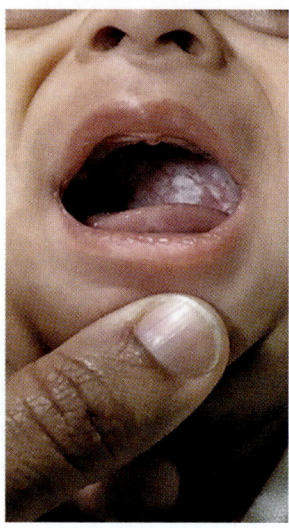

FIG. 5: Oral thrush in a child with severe combined immunodeficiency.

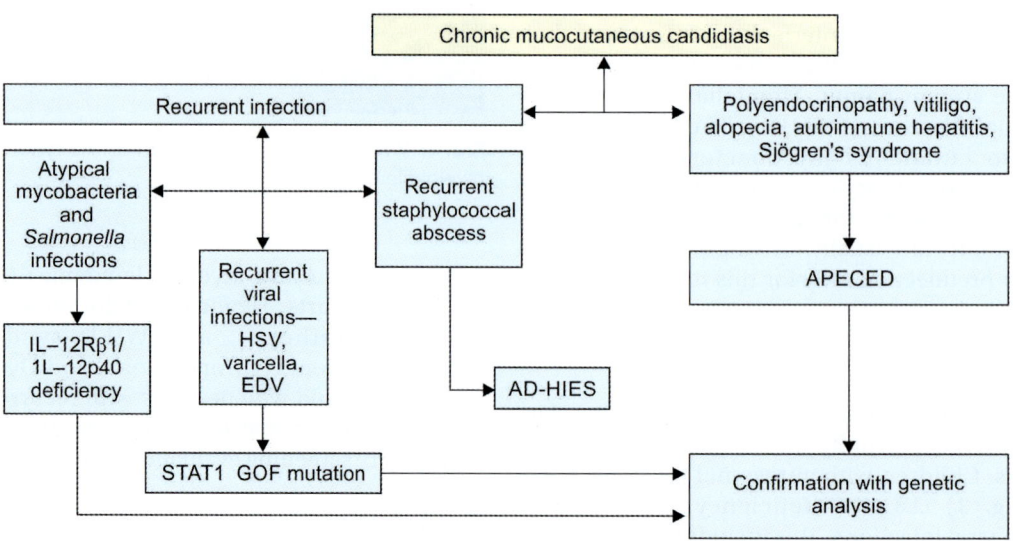

FLOWCHART 1: Clinical approach to the patient presenting with chronic mucocutaneous candidiasis.

(AD-HIES: autosomal dominant hyper-IgE syndrome; APECED: autoimmune polyendocrinopathy candidiasis ectodermal dysplasia; EDV: epidermodysplasia verruciformis; GOF: gain of function; HSV: herpes simplex virus)

onset type 1 diabetes mellitus. They have severe failure to thrive and are typically resistant to usual treatment unless hematopoietic stem cell transplantation is instituted early. An approach to causes of severe eczema in children is provided in **Flowchart 2**.[6]

Omenn syndrome is a condition characterized by hypomorphic mutations in causing severe combined immunodeficiencies. Unlike in SCID, T cells are not absent; they are present in an oligoclonal repertoire which is usually activated resulting in inflammatory phenotype and autoimmunity. These children present with erythematous skin rash (erythroderma) with alopecia often resembling inborn errors of metabolism such as biotinidase deficiency.

Omenn syndrome also presents with hepatosplenomegaly, lymphadenopathy, and infections.

Erythroderma is defined as involvement of >90% of the body surface area with erythema or scaling of skin. This is observed in Omenn syndrome as well as in Netherton syndrome (triad of congenital ichthyosiform erythroderma, trichorrhexis invaginata, and an atopic diathesis), which is another autosomal recessive disorder that presents with alopecia, bamboo hair, and congenital ichthyosis. Erythroderma is reported in around 7% of PIDs.[10,11] Skin biopsy in Omenn syndrome shows massive infiltration of T cells (mostly CD8 subset) with restricted repertoire of T cell receptors. Erythroderma may also be observed as a manifestation of graft-versus-host disease in patients with SCID following maternal engraftment. In this case, maternal cells are to be ruled out on skin biopsy by microsatellite analysis.

Granuloma

Granulomatous lesions are classically observed in chronic granulomatous disease, which is a phagocytic disease that presents with recurrent and persistent infections. Chronic granulomas may also be observed in the skin, gut, and lungs in these children. Common variable immunodeficiency (CVID) is a PID that presents with frequent granulomas in the same locations. CVID patients present with sinopulmonary infections and autoimmune manifestations. In granulomatous lesions, tissue biopsy for culture, staining, and polymerase chain reaction (PCR) can help reach a diagnosis. Ataxia telangiectasia is another antibody deficiency that presents with granulomas over the limbs and trunk in addition to telangiectasia **(Fig. 7)**. They seem to be related to immune dysregulation.[10]

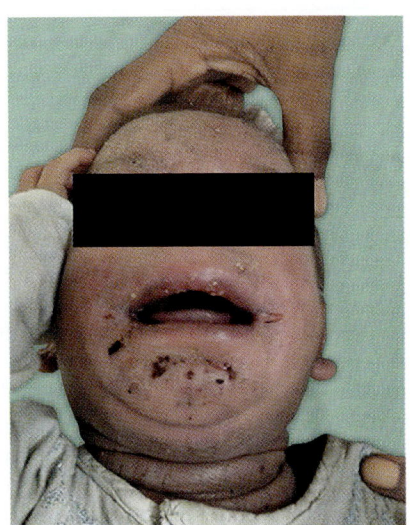

FIG. 6: Extensive eczema in a child with Wiskott–Aldrich syndrome.

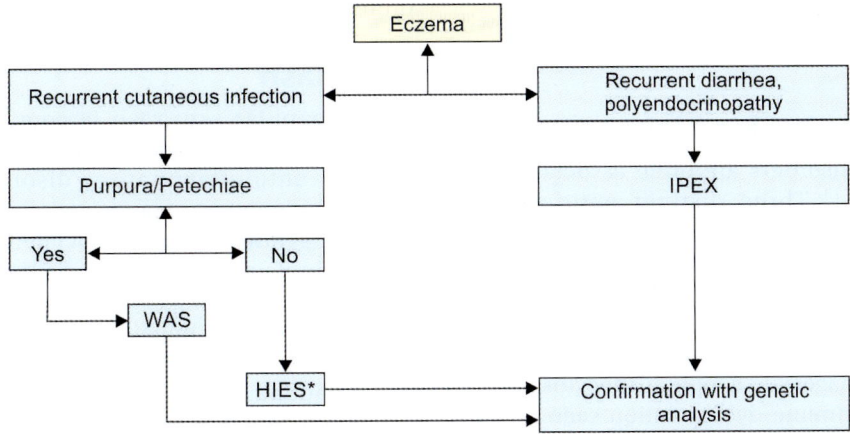

*History of recurrent viral infections and asthma suggests possibility of AR-HIES.

FLOWCHART 2: Approach to a child presenting with eczema.

(AR: autosomal recessive; HIES: hyper-IgE syndrome; IPEX: immunodysregulation, polyendocrinopathy, enteropathy, X-linked syndrome; WAS: Wiskott–Aldrich syndrome)

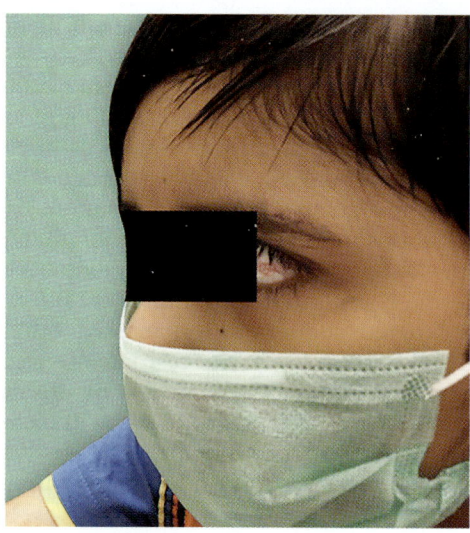

FIG. 7: Conjunctival telangiectasia in a child with ataxia telangiectasia.

	Griscelli 2	Chediak–Higashi	HPS	
Trafficking of secretory lysozymes defective affects hair, skin neurons, platelets, T and NK cells, neutrophils				
	Rab27a	LYST	AP3B1	
			Platelet dysfunction	
		Granules in neutrophils		
	Irregular melanin clumps	Regular small melanin clumps		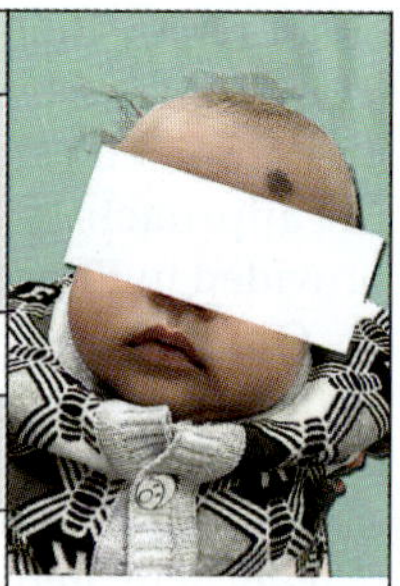 Griscelli syndrome

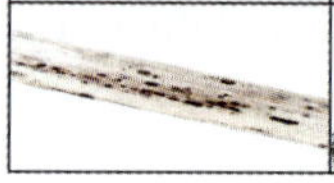

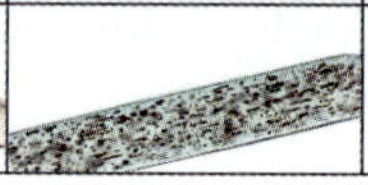

FIG. 8: Trichogram features which can help in differentiating primary immunodeficiency (PID) associated with pigment dilution in skin and hair.

Hair/Skin/Nail Dysplasia

Bone marrow failure syndromes have been included as a class of PIDs recently. Dyskeratosis congenita is a class of inherited bone marrow failure that presents with premature graying of hair, abnormal skin pigmentation, oral leukoplakia, and nail dystrophy. They also present with pulmonary fibrosis, idiopathic portal fibrosis, and malignancies such as myeloid leukemia.[12]

Cartilage hair hypoplasia is another autosomal recessive disease with dwarfism, scant hair, short finger, and toenails along with combined immunodeficiencies. Ectodermal dysplasia with immunodeficiency could be X-linked (NEMO mutations) or autosomal recessive (ORAI-1 mutations).[6] These patients present with atopic dermatitis, hypohidrosis, conical incisors, alopecia, and scant hair. Patients with autoimmune polyendocrinopathy can also present with dystrophic hair and nails.

Pigment Dilution in Skin/Hair

Pigmentary dilution disorders are often associated with immunodeficiencies.[13] Three distinct entities cause pigmentary abnormalities associated with immune dysregulation are Griscelli syndrome type II, Chediak-Higashi syndrome, and Hermansky–Pudlak syndrome type II. In resource-constrained settings, clinical examination of hair, and peripheral blood smear can help differentiate these entities. Hemophagocytic lymphohistiocytosis (HLH) is the predominant immune dysregulation seen in these patients. This manifests as prolonged fever, jaundice, pancytopenia, and hepatosplenomegaly with multiorgan dysfunction. Differentiating features of these three disorders on trichogram are illustrated in **(Fig. 8)**.

Angioedema

Hereditary angioedema (HAE) is characterized by recurrent episodes of swelling of face, airway, limbs, and often the intestinal tract. It is triggered by minor trauma, stress, and often can occur without a cause. Patients can have severe pain abdomen, nausea, vomiting, and often life-threatening airway edema. The frequency of attacks can be as frequent as 1–2 per week to once in few months. Depending on the level of C1 inhibitor, there are three different types of HAE. Mutations in *SERPING1* gene, causes HAE types I and II characterized by either reduced production or abnormally functioning C1 inhibitor respectively.[1,3] Without the production of C1 inhibitor, excessive amounts of bradykinin are generated, which promotes inflammation by leakage of fluids through the blood vessel wall. Type III HAE results from mutations in *F12* gene which produces coagulation protein factor XII.

Skin Rash

Maculopapular skin rash is common in immune dysregulation disorders such as HLH. There are many recently defined autoinflammatory disorders that also have pathognomonic skin manifestations. Cryopyrin-associated periodic syndromes are associated with fever, urticarial rash, arthralgia, and amyloidosis.[14] They may also develop sensorineural hearing loss, aseptic meningitis, hearing loss, myalgia, and visual impairment. In other autoinflammatory disorders such as Muckle–Wells syndrome, familial cold autoinflammatory syndrome, chronic infantile neurologic cutaneous articular syndrome, etc., patients present with fever, joint pain, and rash. Some are triggered by cold. Vasculitis may also present with skin rash in many PIDs **(Fig. 9)**.

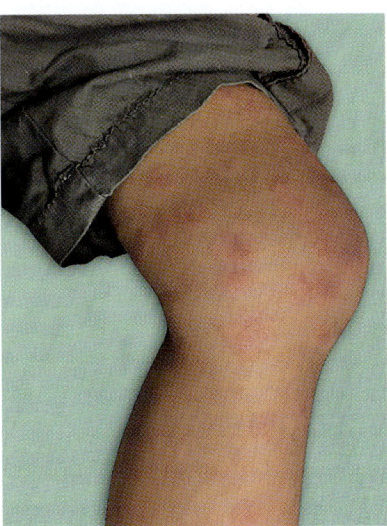

FIG. 9: Vasculitis in a child with severe combined immunodeficiency.

When to suspect PID in cases of systemic lupus erythematosus (SLE)?
Predominantly cutaneous lesions in a child of age <5 years should arise suspicion for PID. Antinuclear antibody (ANA) in such patients show speckled pattern with normal double-stranded deoxyribonucleic acid (dsDNA) antibody levels.

APPROACH TO A SUSPECTED CASE OF PRIMARY IMMUNODEFICIENCY

Focused history points:
- Age-based differential diagnosis is summarized in **Table 1**
- *History of similar disorders in siblings or family members*: Pedigree chart may help in understanding the inheritance pattern and hence list of differential diagnosis can be shortened.
- History of consanguinity
- *History regarding neonatal onset of rash*: Eczematous rash in hyper-IgE syndrome (HIES) starts from neonatal period while in rest of PID it starts later. Erythroderma of Omenn's syndrome also manifests within first few weeks of life. Seborrheic dermatitis like eczema in cases of SCID starts in neonatal period.
- History of hospitalization for severe infections
- History of recurrent cutaneous boils, recurrent upper respiratory tract infections, and otitis media
- *History of recurrent diarrhea*: SCID and IPEX
- *History of fracture*: AD-HIES
- *History of loss of tooth*: Leukocyte adhesion defects
- *History of bleeding*: WAS, Hermansky–Pudlak syndrome, HLH in cases of Chediak–Higashi syndrome

Table 1: Age-based approach to primary immunodeficiency.

Onset	Suggestive of
Before 6 months of age	**Usually innate immune defects and T-cell defects present very early in life.** Since maternal antibodies are usually protective for the first 6–9 months, primary antibody deficiencies present later • Combined immune deficiency (SCID, DGS, CD40L deficiency) • Phagocytic disorders: Leukocyte adhesion defect, X-chronic granulomatous disease • Innate immune defects (TLR signaling, IRAK4 deficiency) • BM failure: Severe congenital neutropenia, reticular dysgenesis
Between the age of 6 and 12 months	• Combined immune deficiencies • Antibody deficiencies (XLA) • WAS/Ataxia telangiectasia • AR and X-Chronic granulomatous disease • Immune dysregulation
Later than 12 months	CVID, specific antibody deficiency, complement disorders, immune dysregulation

- History of failure to thrive and developmental delay
- *History of atopy*: AR-HIES, Netherton syndrome

General and systemic examination:
- Growth chart
- *Lymphadenopathy*: CGD, Omenn's syndrome
- *Absence of lymphoid tissue*: SCID (except Omenn's syndrome)
- Hepatosplenomegaly
- Systemic examination as per history and cutaneous findings

Screening investigations:
- *Complete blood count (CBC)*: Platelet defects and cellular defects reflect in complete blood count.
- *IgE*: Elevated levels have been reported in various PID associated with eczema. Very high levels >2,000 can be found in HIES.
- *Absolute eosinophil count (AEC)*: This might be elevated in cases of HIES and is one of the criteria in NIH scoring for HIES.
- *X-rays*: Long bone in HIES and to rule out osteomyelitis if suspected
- *Antibodies levels*: Levels of IgM, IgG, and IgA can be obtained in suspected cases of severe combined immunodeficiency and deficiency of particular antibody.
- *T cell and B cell count*: This can be obtained SCID and antibody defects
- Complement levels
- *Nitro blue tetrazolium (NBT) reduction assay*: CGD

Additional investigations:
Additional investigations should be based on clinical suspicion and outcome of screening tests.
- Skin biopsy
- ANA and ANA profile
- *Computed tomography (CT) scan*: In HIES for lungs
- *Bone marrow examination*: It should be ordered when defects in phagocytosis is suspected.
- *Genetic testing for mutation*: This is the diagnostic test as many PID has overlapping features.
- *Endocrinological inventions*: Blood sugar levels and hormone assays.

CONCLUSION

Primary immune disorders are a spectrum of disorders characterized by multiorgan involvement, early onset of disease and are often fatal unless diagnosed early and referred to centers capable of delivering specific treatment such as gene therapy or hematopoietic stem cell transplantation.[15] Dermatological manifestations are a leading symptom complex in these disorders. Awareness regarding the various presentations can help us reach a diagnosis at the earliest. With advancements in the field of diagnosis, more and more disorders affecting immune system are being reported each year. The inclusion of skin manifestations can aid us immensely in identifying these diseases early and initiation of specific treatment.

ACKNOWLEDGMENTS

We would like to acknowledge Dr Manideepa Maji and Dr Sunki Karthik.

REFERENCES

1. Relan M, Lehman HK. Common dermatologic manifestations of primary immune deficiencies. Curr Allergy Asthma Rep. 2014;14(12):480.
2. López-Quintero W, Cleves D, Gomez-Vasco JD, Pérez P, Patiño J, Medina-Valencia D, et al. Skin manifestations in pediatric patients with primary immunodeficiency diseases (PIDs) in a tertiary care hospital in Colombia. World Allergy Organ J. 2021;14(3):100527.
3. Bousfiha A, Jeddane L, Picard C, Al-Herz W, Ailal F, Chatila T, et al. Human Inborn Errors of Immunity: 2019 Update of the IUIS Phenotypical Classification. J Clin Immunol. 2020;40(1):66-81.
4. Jeddane L, Ouair H, Benhsaien I, Bakkouri JE, Bousfiha AA. Primary Immunodeficiency Classification on Smartphone. J Clin Immunol. 2017;37(1):1-2.
5. de Wit J, Brada RJK, van Veldhuizen J, Dalm VASH, Pasmans SGMA. Skin disorders are prominent features in primary immunodeficiency diseases: A systematic overview of current data. Allergy. 2019;74(3):464-82.
6. Sharma D, Jindal AK, Rawat A, Singh S. Approach to child with primary immunodeficiency made simple. Indian Dermatol Online J. 2017;8:391-405.
7. Lehman H. Skin manifestations of primary immune deficiency. Clin Rev Allergy Immunol. 2014;46(2):112-9.
8. Aghamohammadi A, Moghaddam ZG, Abolhassani H, Hallaji Z, Mortazavi H, Pourhamdi S, et al. Investigation of underlying primary immunodeficiencies in patients with severe atopic dermatitis. Allergol Immunopathol (Madr). 2014;42(4):336-41.
9. Lehman H, Gordon C. The Skin as a Window into Primary Immune Deficiency Diseases: Atopic Dermatitis and Chronic Mucocutaneous Candidiasis. J Allergy Clin Immunol Pract. 2019;7(3):788-98.
10. Sillevis Smitt JH, Kuijpers TW. Cutaneous manifestations of primary immunodeficiency. Curr Opin Pediatr. 2013;25(4):492-7.
11. Pichard DC, Freeman AF, Cowen EW. Primary immunodeficiency update: Part I. Syndromes associated with eczematous dermatitis. J Am Acad Dermatol. 2015;73(3):355-64; quiz 365-6.
12. Karalis A, Tischkowitz M, Millington GW. Dermatological manifestations of inherited cancer syndromes in children. Br J Dermatol. 2011;164(2):245-56.
13. Dotta L, Parolini S, Prandini A, Tabellini G, Antolini M, Kingsmore SF, Badolato R. Clinical, laboratory and molecular signs of immunodeficiency in patients with partial oculo-cutaneous albinism. Orphanet J Rare Dis. 2013;8:168.
14. Keddie S, Parker T, Lachmann HJ, Ginsberg L. Cryopyrin-Associated Periodic Fever Syndrome and the Nervous System. Curr Treat Options Neurol. 2018;20(10):43.
15. Al-Herz W, Nanda A. Skin manifestations in primary immunodeficient children. Pediatr Dermatol. 2011;28(5):494-501.

Part 5: Special Considerations in Dermatology

25
Systemic Steroid in Patient with Comorbidities

Nayan Patel

INTRODUCTION

Systemic glucocorticoids (GCs) are one of the most widely prescribed molecules by dermatologist in management variety of autoimmune, autoinflammatory, connective tissue, vesiculobullous, and eczematous dermatosis. On one hand, GC without doubt hold a unique place in management of many life-threatening disorders where it considerably reduces the mortality and morbidity, unfortunately this comes along with plethora of adverse drug reactions (ADRs) associated with its use. Over the year, use of GC by dermatologist shows declining trend in secondary to availability of effective steroid-sparing agents and biologics, GC still holds important place in management of many dermatological conditions owing to its low cost and excellent anti-inflammatory and immunosuppressive effects. In day-to-day practice, dermatologist comes across a situation where judicious use of GC becomes unavoidable. In this regard, it becomes extremely important on the part of dermatologist to remain aware about prevention, early identification, and management of ADR associated with systemic steroid. This chapter will focus on approach to GC therapy in context of its ADRs. Only systemic GC therapy will be discussed here. **Table 1** describes the important adverse events related to GC.

APPROACH TO USE OF GC IN RELATION TO ITS ADRS AND PREEXISTING COMORBIDITIES

Dermatologist must go through following steps of consideration before and after commencing GC therapy in any patient.
1. Is use of systemic GC necessary?
2. How much and how long systemic GC is required?

Table 1: Important adverse events related to glucocorticoid therapy.[1]	
Metabolic: • Hyperglycemia • Increased appetite and weight • Hypokalemia • Hypertriglyceridemia • Cushingoid changes	*Cardiovascular*: • Hypertension • Congestive heart failure • Myocardial ischemia
Bone: • Osteoporosis • Osteonecrosis • Hypocalcemia	*Gastrointestinal*: • Peptic ulcer disease • Bowel perforation • Fatty liver changes • Esophageal reflux
Ocular: • Cataract • Glaucoma • Infections	*Psychiatric*: • Psychosis • Agitation • Personality changes • Depression
Infection: • Tuberculosis reactivation • Opportunistic deep fungal infection • Prolonged herpes virus infection	*Musculoskeletal*: • Myopathy
In pediatric population: • Growth retardation • Cataract • Hyperglycemia	

3. Selecting the right GC.
4. Is patient at risk of developing GC-related ADRs?
5. How to prevent GC-related ADRs?
6. How to identify developing ADRs to GC therapy early?
7. How to manage ADRs to GC if develop?
8. How to manage ongoing systemic GC therapy if patient develops ADRs.

1. Is use of systemic GC necessary?
First thing, a dermatologist ponders upon before prescribing systemic GC is whether it is necessary to prescribe systemic steroid? With few dermatological conditions where systemic GC has lifesaving potential or they are used as first-line therapy, answer to this question is straightforward. One must use systemic GC in necessary dose and for necessary duration with all precaution to minimize ADRs and if at all one develops, be prepared to manage it. Classic example of such scenario is listed in **Table 2**.

Stay abreast with emerging evidence for alternative therapies.

Even for conditions traditionally considered to be GC responsive, knowledge of recent advances in field of therapeutics will help dermatologist to consider alternative safer or effective modalities for treatment or at least minimize the use of systemic GC in terms of dose and duration. **Table 3** enumerates emerging evidences in management of skin conditions traditionally treated with systemic GC.

Short course for rapid control of symptoms where "dermatologist is best judge": Dermatologist will every now and then comes across conditions where GC is not considered as mainstay of treatment or established as robust "evidence-based" treatment but rapid short burst of systemic GC is considered clinically useful to alleviate suffering of patient. Without doubt, dermatologist remains the best judge for use of GC with all necessary precautions in such case. In author's view, such decision of dermatologist must be respected by peers. Such consideration should always be based on principal of "primum non nocere" (first, do no harm) and patient should be well aware and part of that decision-making. In addition, for medicolegal safety, it is advisable to document dermatologist's own rationale for use of systemic GC in case record. For example, "severe contact dermatitis not responding to topical therapy and severely compromising patient's quality of life" should be mentioned in case record if dermatologist decides to use systemic GC in case of severe contact dermatitis. **Box 1** enumerates few of such conditions.

Resisting the temptation (this paragraph is author's view): There are situations in clinical practice where dermatologist is dealing with a potentially self-limiting dermatosis or where evidence for use of systemic GC is poor. Dermatologist should resist the temptation of using systemic GC with view of exploiting potential anti-inflammatory effect of GC and temporary sense of general well-being it provides to patient **(Box 2)**.

Table 2: Conditions where GC therapy remains mainstay of treatment.

Pemphigus vulgaris*	Bullous pemphigoid*
Mucous membrane pemphigoid	Herpes gestationis
Epidermolysis bullosa acquisita	Linear IgA bullous dermatosis
Lupus erythematosus*	Dermatomyositis*
Mixed connective tissue disease	Relapsing polychondritis
Systemic vasculitis involving skin	Pyoderma gangrenosum
Behçet's disease	Sweet syndrome
DRESS syndrome	Sarcoidosis
Stevens–Johnson syndrome*	Erythema multiforme major*

*US FDA approved uses.
(DRESS: drug reaction with eosinophilia and systemic symptoms; FDA: Food and Drug Administration; GC: glucocorticoid; IgA: immunoglobulin A)

Table 3: Dermatological conditions where use of GC can be minimized.

Dermatological conditions where use of GC was widespread	Emerging evidence for use of alternative therapies
Antihistamine refractory chronic spontaneous urticaria	Up-dosing of second-generation antihistamine, omalizumab cyclosporine[2]
Severe atopic dermatitis (AD) not controlled with topical medications or acute flare	Long-term use of GC is not recommended in AD. Alternatives are cyclosporine and biologics[3]
Eruptive or extensive lichen planus	Low-quality evidence for prolonged GC therapy. Alternatives are cyclosporine and acitretin[4]
Neutrophilic dermatosis	Alternative are cyclosporine, anti-TNF, and anti-IL17 biologics
Large or function compromising infantile hemangioma	Propranolol is FDA-approved therapy
Stevens–Johnson syndrome and toxic epidermal necrolysis	Cyclosporine is being used as first-line therapy[5,6]
Alopecia totalis and universalis	JAK-STAT inhibitor, cyclosporine[7]
Erythroderma	Retinoids, biologics, and immunosuppressive depending on etiology

(FDA: Food and Drug Administration; GC: glucocorticoid; IgA: immunoglobulin A; IL: interleukin; TNF: tumor necrosis factor)

2. How much and how long systemic GC is required?

Once the decision to use systemic steroid is made next important point to deliberate is the dose of GC and expected length of GC therapy. As many ADRs of systemic GC are directly proportional to dose and duration of therapy. Normally, response of GC therapy on disease activity and development of ADRs is variable in individual patient and consequently it is difficult to quantify dose as high or low and duration as short or long. Following classification is used for dose and duration of GC therapy for academic and research purpose **(Table 4)**.

Clinical implications of this for dermatologist are clear, if you are planning to use high or very high dose of GC or therapy is expected to last medium to long term, one has to more thoroughly screen patient for possible ADRs, remain more vigilant to identify one during course of treatment, and be prepared to manage ADRs without seriously compromising outcome of underlying condition being treated if one develops.

3. Choose your GC wisely.

Detailed understanding of various pharmacodynamics and pharmacokinetic properties of various GC molecule **(Table 5)** will help dermatologist to decide selection of correct molecule depending upon condition being treated.

Box 1: Conditions where use of short-term glucocorticoi therapy can be utilized based on dermatologist's judgment of risk and benefit.

- Severe contact dermatitis
- Acne fulminans and isotretinoin-induced acne flare
- Rapidly progressive vitiligo
- Severe aphthous stomatitis
- Severe pain of herpes zoster and postherpetic neuralgia
- Progressive alopecia areata
- Severe insect bite reaction
- Erythema multiforme minor

Box 2: Situations where use of systemic glucocorticoi should be avoided.

- Mild eczema
- Pruritus of unknown origin
- First episode of skin-limited small-vessel vasculitis
- Maculopapular exanthema of uncertain origin
- Localized fixed drug reaction
- Severe pruritus of infective dermatosis
- Diffused hair loss of unknown etiology

Table 4: EULAR Standing Committee on International Clinical Studies including Therapeutic Trials describes following classification for dose and duration of corticosteroid.[8,9]

Dose classification	
Low	7.5 mg prednisone equivalent per day
Medium	>7.5 mg but <30 mg prednisone equivalent per day
High	>30 mg but <100 mg prednisone equivalent per day
Very high	≥100 mg prednisone equivalent per day
Pulse dose	≥250 mg prednisone equivalent per day for 1 or a few days
Duration classification	
Short term	<3 months
Medium term	3–6 months
Long term	>6 months

(EULAR: European Alliance of Associations for Rheumatology)

Table 5: Major pharmacodynamics and pharmacokinetic properties of various steroid molecules.[1]

Corticosteroid	Equivalent dose (mg)	Glucocorticoid potency	Mineralocorticoid potency	Plasma half-life (min)	Biologic half-life (hours)
Short acting					
Cortisone	25	0.8	+2	30–90	8–12
Hydrocortisone	20	1	+2	60–120	8–12
Intermediate acting					
Prednisone	5	4	+1	60	24–36
Prednisolone	5	4	+1	115–212	24–36
Methylprednisolone	4	5	0	180	24–36
Triamcinolone	4	5	0	78–118	24–36
Long acting					
Dexamethasone	0.75	2–30	0	100–300	36–72
Betamethasone	0.6–0.75	20–30	0	100–300	36–72

In clinical practice, choice of GC molecule will depend on many factors, most important being conversance of physician with particular molecule. Relative GC and mineralocorticoid (MC) potency of particular molecule can be matched with other at appropriate dose traditionally described as "equivalent of prednisolone". Here, one has to remember that effect of systemic GC is exerted through genomic and nongenomic mechanism. Genomic effect is exerted through cytosolic GC receptors and can be matched with other molecule at equivalent dose. Conversely nongenomic effect is exerted through direct action of GC on cell membrane, membrane-bound GC receptors and, to some extent, through cytosolic GC receptors. They are more rapid in onset and differ considerably for various GC molecules particularly at higher doses (possibly due to saturation of cytosolic GC receptors).[10] Nongenomic effects of GC are increasingly being recognized and studied in recent time. Preference of methylprednisolone for pulse therapy and less preference of betamethasone for systemic use are based on their nongenomic effects.[1] Though systemic steroids are classified in short acting, intermediate acting, and long acting based on their biological effect on hypothalamus pituitary axis, their effect at cellular level can last much longer.[11] Shorter acting steroid is preferred for treatment of acute condition such as anaphylaxis; requirement for frequent dosing makes them unsuitable for prolonged use. Medium-acting steroid such as prednisolone is most widely used in practice when long-term therapy is planned owing to its high GC potency and desirable biological half-life. Methylprednisolone has comparable GC potency to prednisolone with minimal MC activity, which makes it preferred systemic steroid when MC effect (salt and water retention) is particularly undesirable (e.g., preexisting hypertension and congestive heart failure).[12] In addition to pharmacokinetic and pharmacodynamic characteristic, available published evidences for particular molecule are also factored into consideration while selecting the GC, dexamethasone–cyclophosphamide pulse therapy used in pemphigus vulgaris being classic example.

4. Is your patient at risk of developing GC-related ADRs?

As a general rule, majority of ADRs related to systemic use of GC correlate positively with dose (high vs. low) and cumulative duration (short vs. long) of exposure, yet no particular threshold in term of dose or duration can be defined for any particular ADRs. Dermatologist must remain extra vigilant while planning long-term or high-dose GC therapy. Identification of particular baseline characteristic or risk factor in patient may help to foresee possible ADRs in due course of therapy. **Table 6** enumerates "at risk" patient for development of major systemic steroid-related ADRs.

5. How to prevent GC-related ADRs?

Next step in approach is an attempt at prevention of GC-related ADRs before they develop. Few general precautions on part of dermatologist can prevent some of the ADRs of GC if not all **(Table 7)**.

6. How to identify and manage GC-related ADRs early?

Key to early identification of developing ADRs to GC remains with thorough history taking which should include evaluation of any comorbidities, inquiry about past history of event similar to GC-related ADRs (for example, history of gestational hyperglycemia, glaucoma, etc.), family history of disorders similar to GC-related ADRs (family history of DM, IHD, etc.) before starting GC therapy. This will identify the patient at risk. Thorough baseline laboratory, radiological and microbiological evaluation as per standard guidelines to identify risk factors which may not be apparent on history taking and examination particularly in patients identified at "high risk" on initial clinical evaluation should be undertaken. Another important factor is periodic clinical and laboratory monitoring for any emergent ADRs. If any patient develops GC-related ADRs, prompt management and referral to required specialist are essential. Dermatologist's role is vital in modulation of ongoing steroid therapy to balance remission of disease being treated and minimize further adverse events. Following section discusses early identification, management of major GC-related ADRs.

GLUCOCORTICOID-INDUCED HYPERGLYCEMIA

When planning for medium- to long-term GC therapy, it is important to educate patient about warning signs of developing hyperglycemia; this should also be part of clinical evaluation by dermatologist during every follow-up visit of patient who is on high-dose prolonged GC therapy **(Table 8)**.

Baseline laboratory evaluation should include fasting blood glucose (FBG), postprandial blood glucose (PPBG), and HbA1c estimation to screen preexisting DM. GC-induced hyperglycemia develops more commonly after meal, particularly when intermediate-acting GCs are administered. For screening and monitoring purpose, relying solely on FBG or random blood glucose (RBG) is not advisable.[37] Steroid-induced hyperglycemia will reflect into HbA1c monitoring only after 3 months of therapy so it is only useful when long-term steroid use is contemplated. PPBG remains the most sensitive investigation to detect the GC-induced hyperglycemia earliest.

Frequency of monitoring: Frequency of monitoring will depend on presence of risk factors **(see Table 6)** and outcome of initial assessment. There are no uniform guidelines for frequency of monitoring **(Box 3)**.

If during screening or monitoring, patient is detected with hyperglycemia, criteria for diagnosis of diabetes mellitus (DM) remain same as for patient without GC therapy **(Box 4)**.

What if patient develops hyperglycemia?[37]
1. If patient is nondiabetic before starting the GC therapy and first time detected with GC-induced hyperglycemia (asymptomatic), effect of GC on endocrine system is

Table 6: Risk factors for developing GC-related ADRs.		
GC-induced osteoporosis (GIOP):[13] • Expected exposure >3 months, cumulative exposure >1 g equivalent of prednisolone in year[14,15] • Current use > prior use • Higher current daily dose > cumulative dose[16] • Low body mass index • Underlying chronic disease (particularly rheumatoid arthritis) • Hypogonadism, secondary hyperparathyroidism • Smoking • Excessive alcohol use (≥3 units/day) • Past history of fracture • Family history of hip fracture **GC-induced osteonecrosis:**[6] • High dose, longer exposure • Can occur over short exposure also[17] • Underlying disorder (SLE and renal failure) • Presence of Cushingoid features • Dexamethasone has higher chances over prednisolone[18]	**GC-induced hyperglycemia:** • Preexisting DM • High BMI[19] • Family history of DM • History of gestational DM • Old age[20] • Longer duration of exposure • High dose of exposure	**GC-induced acid peptic disease and GI bleed:**[21] • Age >65 years • High-dose GC therapy • Concomitant use of NSAIDs (including low-dose aspirin with high-dose GC) • Hospitalized patient[22] • Past history of peptic ulcer disease • Heavy smoking • Heavy use of alcohol
GC-induced ophthalmic side effects: **Glaucoma:**[23] • Patient with primary open-angle glaucoma • Family history of glaucoma • High myopia • Patient with DM and RA on GC therapy • Eye with pigment dispersion syndrome • Common with intravitreal GC therapy followed by inhaled GC • Least likely with systemic GC, if develops, risk increases with dose and duration of GC exposure[24] **GC-related posterior subcapsular cataract:** • Higher dose and longer therapy[25]	**GC-induced HT and CVS side effects:**[13] • Higher dose and continuous exposure • Patient already having risk factor for CV event (obesity, HT, smoking, hyperlipidemia, and family history) • Preexisting underlying condition-related increased risk (RA SLE)[26] • Use of pulse dose (sudden death)[27] • Presence of Cushingoid features • Association with hyperlipidemia is not conclusive	**GC-induced psychiatric events:**[13] • Past history or underlying undiagnosed psychiatric illness[28] • Mood and behavioral symptoms are associated with moderate-to-high-dose steroid • Depression with long-term use[29]
Others: *Reactivation of TB risk*: Prednisolone (or equivalent) > 15 mg for >1 month (CDC).[30] Evaluation of past history of TB and completion of AKT therapy is extremely important in Indian context. *Reactivation of hepatitis B*: GC therapy can reactivate and increase viral load.[31]		

(ADR: adverse drug reaction; CVS: cardiovascular system; DM: diabetes mellitus; HT: hypertension; GC: glucocorticoid; SLE: systemic lupus erythematosus; TB: tuberculosis)

reversible initially (not in all patient).[39] If dermatologist decides no prolonged therapy with GC is required in patient, blood glucose levels of patient can be monitored closely with emphasis on lifestyle modification. Monitoring should not discontinue till levels return to nondiabetic range postdiscontinuation of GC therapy, if remain high, patient should be referred to physician or endocrinologist for further management.

2. If patient is nondiabetic before starting GC therapy and detected with hyperglycemia and fulfill the criteria for DM, initiation of antidiabetic therapy is necessary particularly when GC therapy cannot be stopped.

Table 7: Various measures for prevention of GC-related ADRs.

GC-induced osteoporosis (GIOP):	GC-induced hyperglycemia:[33]	GC-induced acid peptic disease and GI bleed:[14]
• Judicious use of GC, tapering when disease activity allows • Early use of steroid-sparing agents • Optimizing calcium intake (1,000–1,200 mg/day) and vitamin D intake (600–800 IU/day; serum level >20 ng/mL) • Balanced diet • Maintaining weight in the recommended range • Smoking cessation • Regular weight bearing or resistance training exercise • Limiting alcohol intake to 1–2 alcoholic beverages/day *GC-induced osteonecrosis:* • Avoid use of alcohol • Be extra careful while using pulse steroid[32]	• Judicious use of GC, tapering when disease activity allows • Early use of steroid-sparing agents • Use of medium-acting steroid over long acting[34] • Use of single morning dose over divided dose • Weight reduction • Diet low in saturated fat and sugar • Diet rich in fiber • Increase in physical activity	• Avoid taking GC on empty stomach • Avoid use of concomitant use of NSAIDs whenever possible • Prescribe proton pump inhibitor (PPI) when coprescribed with NSAIDs (even low-dose aspirin) or patient with risk factors • Balanced diet • Avoidance of smoking • Limit alcohol use
GC-induced ophthalmic side effects:	*GC-induced HT and CVS side effects:*	*GC-induced psychiatric events:*[13]
• Baseline ophthalmic evaluation before initiation of long-term or high-dose steroid or as early as possible after staring therapy • Periodic ophthalmic evaluation if preexisting risk factors present or identified during initial work up • Monitoring and management of hyperglycemia to prevent DM-related ocular complications	• Baseline blood pressure, lipid profile, and blood sugar monitoring • If baseline values are abnormal, more frequent monitoring of blood pressure (2–3 times) and lipid profile (every 3 months) • Emphasis on all lifestyle-related changes for cardiovascular event in general such as weight reduction, cessation of smoking, and regular exercise	• Baseline evaluation of history or preexisting psychiatric disorder particularly tendency to self-harm • Use of single morning dose (avoid night-time dose to prevent insomnia)

(ADR: adverse drug reaction; CVS: cardiovascular system; DM: diabetes mellitus; HT: hypertension; GC: glucocorticoid; NSAIDs: nonsteroidal anti-inflammatory drugs)

Table 8: Early clinical signs of developing hyperglycemia.[35,36]

Polyphagia	Dry mouth
Polydipsia	Blurred vision
Polyuria	
Unexplained weight loss	Numbness in hand and feet
Unexplained fatigue	Recurrent pyoderma
Recurrent balanoposthitis	Recurrent vaginitis

Box 3: Practical points in blood glucose monitoring in patient on high-dose GC therapy.[11,23,38]

- Encourage all patients on long-term steroid therapy to monitor their blood glucose frequently
- Home monitoring of glucose using glucometer should be encouraged
- PPBG twice or thrice should be monitored any reading above 200 should prompt visit to doctor
- Low-risk patient who is not willing or unable to home monitor blood glucose should be checked on every follow-up assessment visit (more frequently initially)
- For hospitalized nondiabetic patient on high-dose steroid daily monitoring of PPBG via glucometer is advisable
- For patient with preexisting DM, who is put on high-dose or long-term steroid, frequency of monitoring increases (preferably daily via glucometer) till effect of GC on glycemia is established and necessary changes in drug and insulin regimen is made. This has to be done in cooperation with primary physician

(DM: diabetes mellitus; GC: glucocorticoid; PPBG: postprandial blood glucose)

3. Both nondiabetic and known diabetic patients (nonhospitalized) before GC therapy who are poorly controlled with OHT (blood glucose >200) should be shifted to insulin therapy.
4. Two insulin schemes, prandial (0.1 U/kg regular insulin) and steroid dose and BMI based (0.4 U/kg of NPH in morning), are utilized to calculate the insulin requirement.

> **Box 4: Diagnostic criteria for DM.**
>
> - HbA1c ≥ 6.5
> - FBG ≥ 126 mg/dL
> - Two hours' plasma glucose ≥ 200 mg/dL during oral glucose tolerance test
> - RBG ≥ 200 mg/dL
>
> First three criteria need to be repeated if abnormal. Two abnormal readings suggest diagnosis of DM.
>
> (DM: diabetes mellitus; HbA1c: glycated hemoglobin; FBG: fasting blood glucose; RBG: random blood glucose)

> **Box 5: Management of ongoing GC therapy in patient with GC-induced hyperglycemia.**
>
> - Control of disease activity of condition being treated needs to be taken into consideration while adjusting the dose of ongoing GC therapy
> - Effort should be made to use of lowest possible dose of GC to maintain remission of disease if discontinuation is not possible
> - Switch to single morning dose should be made if patient is on divided dose of GC
> - Intermediate acting GC (such as prednisolone, methylprednisolone) should be preferred over long-acting one (e.g., dexamethasone)
> - Use of steroid-sparing molecules or biologics should be maximized if not already done
>
> (GC: glucocorticoid)

5. Patients who are poorly controlled on prandial scheme on regular insulin basal insulin (NPH or glargine) can be added for better glycemic control.
6. In hospitalized patients who have preexisting DM or detected to have hyperglycemia on GC therapy, management approach for hyperglycemia remains similar to nonhospitalized patient keeping strict glycemic control as underlying goal.
7. Patient with preexisting DM with insulin use prior to admission, requirement of insulin increases by 20%.
8. Hospitalized patient with very high blood glucose ≥ 400 mg/dL on GC therapy should be managed with insulin infusion pump particularly when pulse GC is used as insulin requirement is difficult to predict with pulse GC therapy.
9. Patients with dermatological conditions which produce acute stress and increase insulin demand (e.g., TEN, erythroderma, *Pemphigus vulgaris*) need stricter glycemic control for rapid recovery of disease and prevention of other complications related to hyperglycemia (e.g., infection).

What happens with GC therapy? **(Box 5)**

> **Box 6: Warning signs of OP.[41]**
>
> - OP may remain silent till patient develops OP fracture
> - Any back pain acute or chronic in patient on long-term or high-dose GC should be thoroughly investigated
> - Loss of height
> - Change in posture
> - Paresthesia in limb
>
> (OP: osteoporosis)

GLUCOCORTICOID-INDUCED OSTEOPOROSIS AND OSTEONECROSIS

Glucocorticoid-induced Osteoporosis[40]

Glucocorticoid-induced osteoporosis (GIO) is common and preventable ADR of GC therapy. Detailed assessment of patient for systemic and lifestyle-related risk factor and radiological screening can identify at-risk patient **(Table 6 and Box 6)**

Initial Assessment

When GC dose above 7.5 mg equivalent of prednisolone or higher and duration of 6 months or higher is contemplated by dermatologist, all patients should be evaluated for GIO.

Low risk: If patient is ≤40 years of age and there is no additional risk factor **(see Box 2)**, no further work-up is required except for preventive measures **(see Flowchart 1)**.

Moderate-to-high risk: If patient is ≥ 40 years of age, assessment of fracture risk must be done using fracture risk assessment tool available freely online (*https://www.sheffield.ac.uk/FRAX/tool.aspx*).

> For people receiving doses of >7.5 mg/day, the fracture risk generated with FRAX should be increased by a relative 15% for major osteoporotic fracture and 20% for hip fracture risk. For example, if the 10-year hip fracture risk is 2.0% with GC use entered in FRAX, the risk estimate should be increased to 2.4% if the prednisone dose is >7.5 mg.

In addition to FRAX score, baseline bone mineral density assessment using dual X-ray absorptiometry (DEXA) should be undertaken whenever it is available in this group of patients. For patient ≤40 years of age, if additional risk factors are present **(see Table 6)**, BMD should be evaluated at baseline or within first 6 months of starting GC therapy. Additionally, BMD study should be repeated within 2–3 years in this group of patients to evaluate the loss of bone density post-GC therapy. This assessment will identify the group of patients who will require additional antiosteoporotic treatment in addition to routine calcium and vitamin D supplementation **(see Flowchart 1)**.

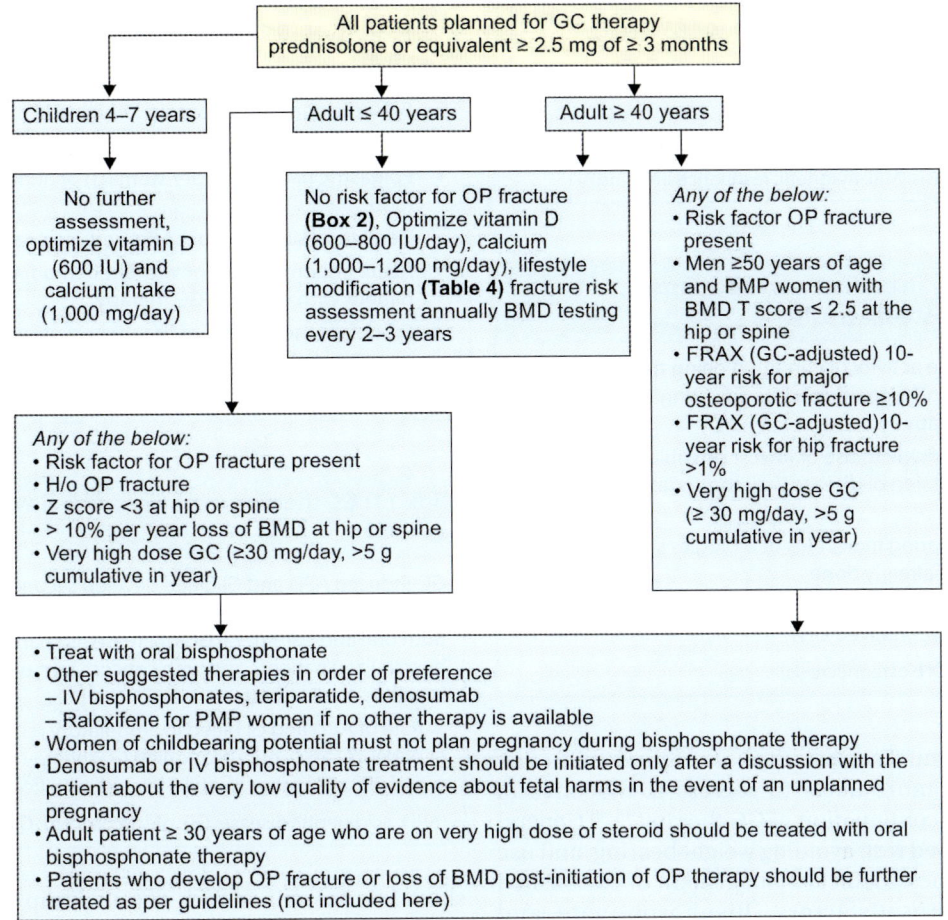

FLOWCHART 1: Recommendation for management of GC-induced osteoporosis.
(BMD: bone mineral density; GC: glucocorticoid; GI: gastrointestinal; IV: intravenous; OP: osteoporosis; PMP: postmenopausal pregnancy)

Box 7 shows precaution and common adverse events related to oral bisphosphonate therapy.[42,43]

Glucocorticoid-induced Osteonecrosis

Glucocorticoid-induced osteonecrosis is considered to be idiosyncratic ADR by some studies and can occur at any dose of steroid,[44] yet higher dose and longer duration defiantly increase the incidence of osteonecrosis.[45] Avascular necrosis (AVN) of femoral head is most common site of involvement; other bone too can be affected. High index of suspicion is required on part of dermatologist as early changes may be missed on X-ray, pain may be brushed aside by patient as routine weakness related to underlying disease and restriction of movement may not be apparent till advance stage. Inquiry about the symptoms of AVN should be made on every visit of the patient **(Box 8)**.

Management

Few studies show that variable percentage of patients who develop GC-induced osteonecrosis may undergo complete

Box 7: Precautions and common adverse events related to oral bisphosphonate therapy.

Precautions:
- Should be taken in the morning with a full glass of water on an empty stomach in an upright position
- Individuals should remain in an upright position for 30 minutes after intake to decrease the risk of adverse reactions
- Do not chew, suck, or crush the tablet

Common adverse events:
- Transient hypocalcemia
- Transient hypophosphatemia
- *GI side effects*: Abdominal pain, heartburn, nausea, constipation, diarrhea, flatulence, and esophagitis

Rare side effects:
- Toxic epidermal necrolysis
- Osteonecrosis of mandible (associated with tooth extraction or local infection)
- Esophageal ulceration

> **Box 8: Symptoms and investigation for AVN.**
>
> - Pain in hip which is usually insidious in onset and aggregates with activity and weight-bearing
> - MRI is the most sensitive modality in diagnosing AVN
>
> (AVN: avascular necrosis; MRI: magnetic resonance imaging)

> **Box 9: GC therapy in patient who develops osteoporosis or osteonecrosis.**
>
> - Control of disease activity of condition being treated needs to be taken into consideration while adjusting the dose of ongoing GC therapy
> - Effort should be made to use of lowest possible dose of GC to maintain remission of disease if discontinuation is not possible
> - Use of steroid-sparing molecules or biologics should be maximized if not already done
> - Pulse GC therapy should be avoided whenever possible (particularly for GC-induced ON)
>
> (GC: glucocorticoid; ON: osteonecrosis)

> **Box 10: Warning signs for acid peptic disease and GI bleed.[55,56]**
>
> - Episodic gnawing or burning epigastric pain
> - Aggravation of epigastric pain 2–5 hours after meal
> - Epigastric pain on empty stomach or at night relieved by food
> - Hematemesis, hematochezia, and melena
> - Acute abdomen with or without hemodynamic instability in patient with ongoing GC therapy
> - GC delays the healing of preexisting ulcer and masks early symptoms of ulcers. High index of suspicions is required
>
> (GC: glucocorticoid; GI: gastrointestinal)

> **Box 11: GC therapy in patient who develops GI adverse events.**
>
> GC-induced APD and GI bleed develop secondary to complex effect on gastric mucosa, acid secretion, and vascular component. Both oral and parenteral GCs increase risk particularly in hospitalized patients and with concomitant use of other gastric irritating medications.
>
> Rate of APD and GI bleed in ambulatory patient is low and most of patients can continue ongoing GC therapy with concomitant use of PPIs and other lifestyle-related modifications.
>
> (APD: acid peptic disease; GC: glucocorticoid; GI: gastrointestinal)

or partial regression. These studies also found that early stage of AVN are more likely to regress irrespective of continuation or discontinuation of GC therapy.[46-48] General measures include bed rest, avoiding weight bearing, and use of crutches and canes. Medical management of established AVN is usually unsatisfactory. Bisphosphonate and hyperbaric oxygen have been tried with variable success.[49-51] Surgical treatments including joint replacement remain mainstay of treatment particularly in advance stages of AVN.

What happens with ongoing GC therapy if patient develops GC-induced OP or ON? **(Box 9)**

GLUCOCORTICOID-INDUCED ACID PEPTIC DISEASE AND GI BLEEDING

There is conflicting evidence weather GC monotherapy increases the incidence of acid peptic disease (APD) or gastrointestinal (GI) bleeding. However, concomitant use of high-dose GC and nonsteroidal anti-inflammatory drugs (NSAIDs) increases the rate of both APD and GI bleed including low-dose aspirin.[52-54] All patients undergoing high-dose or prolonged GC therapy should be evaluated for risk factors for development of APD and GI bleeding **(see Table 6)**. Patient should be educated for warning sign of developing APD and GI bleed and evaluation of same should be included at every follow-up visit of patient **(see Box 10)**.

Management of APD and GI Bleed

For dermatologist's perspective, any patient who is on GC therapy and showing clinical symptoms and signs of APD should be prescribed with proton pump inhibitors (PPIs) as single morning dose before breakfast. Omeprazole reduced antiplatelet effect of clopidogrel and in such scenario, other PPIs should be selected. If symptoms are not adequately controlled with single morning dose of PPIs, twice-a-day dose can be prescribed. For patient having any signs and symptoms of GI bleed or persistent symptoms of APD, immediate reference to physician or gastroenterologist is recommended for further endoscopic work-up and management.

What happens with ongoing GC therapy? **(Box 11)**

GLUCOCORTICOID-INDUCED OCULAR SIDE EFFECTS[57]

Posterior subcapsular cataract and glaucoma are two important ocular side effects of GC therapy. Identification of at-risk patient is essential before starting long-term or high-dose GC therapy **(see Table 6)**. Identification of clinical signs and ophthalmological evaluation are essential for early detection of GC-related ocular side effects **(See Box 12)**.

Management[16]

Glucocorticoid-induced glaucoma is reversible at early stage, discontinuation of GC therapy should be contemplated if patient's primary disease activity allows. In cases where

> **Box 12: Symptoms and signs of GC-related ocular side effects.**
>
> - Patient may remain unaware of loss of peripheral vision and increase in intraocular pressure may be asymptomatic. High index of suspicion and ophthalmic examination is essential for early detection of glaucoma
> - Loss of peripheral vision, tunnel vision rarely reported by patient in early stage of glaucoma
> - Dimness of vision, difficulty in near vision, and with bright light can be early symptom of posterior subcapsular cataract
> - Prompt reference to ophthalmologist for any ocular complaint is essential on part of dermatologist for early identification of developing ocular ADRs to GC
>
> (ADR: adverse drug reaction; GC: glucocorticoid)

> **Box 13: Management of ongoing GC therapy in patient who develops ocular ADRs.**
>
> - Changes of GC-related glaucoma are reversible if detected early; serious consideration must be given to discontinuation of GC therapy if patient's primary disease allows the same
> - Maximize the use of immunosuppressive and alternative therapy for management of primary disease and effort should be made to minimize the dose and duration of GC therapy if discontinuation is not possible
> - Use of GC with high mineralocorticoid (MC) activity (e.g., prednisolone) should be avoided in patient who develops glaucoma which can be replaced by GC with low MC activity (e.g., methylprednisolone)
> - For patient who develops cataract, surgical treatment is usually curative and patient can be continued on GC therapy as per discretion of dermatologist
>
> (ADR: adverse drug reaction; GC: glucocorticoid)

> **Box 14: GC therapy in patient with psychiatric adverse events.**
>
> - Attempt for discontinuation or reduction of GC dose should be made particularly if suicidal ideation or other severe symptoms are present
> - If patient's underlying condition doses not allow reduction of GC dose, therapy should be continued at lowest possible dose with simultaneous management of ADR in close cooperation with mental health physician
>
> (GC: glucocorticoid)

discontinuation is not possible, medical management using prostaglandin analog (e.g., bimatoprost), adrenergic agents (e.g., brimonidine), beta-blockers (e.g., timolol), carbonic anhydrase inhibitor (e.g., brinzolamide), cholinergic/parasympathomimetic agents (e.g., pilocarpine) topically or acetazolamide and mannitol systematically is attempted. For cases nonresponding to medical management and showing progression of disease activity, surgical modalities such as trabeculoplasty can be undertaken.

What happens with GC therapy? (***Box 13***)

GLUCOCORTICOID INDUCED PSYCHIATRIC ADVERSE EVENTS

Glucocorticoid therapy can precipitate mood disorders, anxiety, depression, panic disorder, psychosis, delirium, confusion, and suicide, and they can produce cognitive deficits. Steroid psychosis is a more serious complication that is marked by a range of symptoms, including psychosis, dementia, delirium, depression, and suicidality. This adverse event seems to be dose dependent, dose of prednisolone above 40 mg is more likely to precipitate GC-induced psychiatric event.[58] Secondly, chances of development of GC-induced psychiatric adverse event is highest in early period (first 3 months) of GC therapy and rapid tapering.[59,60]

> Early identification of GC-induced psychiatric adverse event will depend on observation by patient and relatives for any change in mood, emotional lability, increased energy, insomnia, and behavior.

Management

Immediate referral to psychiatrist is necessary for any GC-related adverse event. Immediate intensive management under observation under mental health physician for any suicidal tendency is a must. For other psychiatric adverse events, psychotherapy, medical management in form of antidepressive, anxiolytic, etc., can be added as deemed necessary by treating psychiatrist.

What happens with ongoing GC therapy? (***Box 14***)

GLUCOCORTICOID-RELATED CARDIOVASCULAR ADVERSE EVENTS

Glucocorticoid therapy can increase blood pressure; this effect is being increasingly identified secondary to effect of GC on vascular smooth muscle and not only due to MC effect of GC.[61] Avoidance of GC with high MC activity is still desirable in patients with preexisting CVS comorbidities. Pulse GC therapy is particularly associated with CVS events.[27] Cardiovascular stress secondary to inflammation caused by underlying disorder (e.g., SLE and RA) contributes to incidence of CVS adverse event and makes absolute quantification of contribution of GC in same difficult.

Management

Thorough baselines work-up in terms of blood pressure (BP) monitoring, lipid profile, blood sugar, and, if necessary, electrocardiogram and echocardiogram (in high-risk patients) evaluations are desirable when long-term, or high-dose GC therapy is contemplated. Periodic reevaluation of same based on initial assessment and presence of risk factor is also desirable. Dermatologist should at least take every follow-up visit as opportunity to measure BP, blood glucose monitoring, and evaluation of any signs of CV-related ADRs such as weight gain, pedal edema, and breathlessness on exertion. Patients who develop Cushing syndrome are at higher risk of developing CV adverse events.[62] Addition of antihypertensive should be contemplated in patient who develops persistent HT. Reduction of vascular resistance (calcium-channel blockers, angiotensin receptor blocker, etc.) or volume overload (diuretics) should be attempted in cooperation with physician.

What happens with GC therapy? **(Box 15)**

QUICK OVERVIEW OF OTHER GC-RELATED ADVERSE EVENTS (BOX 16)[63,64]

Glucocorticoid and Hypothalamic–Pituitary–Adrenal Axis Suppression (Box 17)

Glucocorticoid remains one of the most path-breaking discoveries of modern medical science. Satisfaction on

---

Box 15: GC therapy in patient who develops CVS adverse event.

- If patient develops HT or any other CV adverse event, dose reduction of GC should be attempted via maximizing use of steroid-sparing agents and alternative
- Use of pulse dose GC should be avoided if possible. If situation demands pulse GC therapy, rapid infusion should be avoided and infusion be given under intensive cardiovascular monitoring
- GC therapy can be continued in cooperation of physician with simultaneous address to adverse event and emphasis on lifestyle modification if deemed necessary by dermatologist

(CV: cardiovascular; HT: hypertension; GC: glucocorticoid)

Box 16: Overview of other GC-related adverse events.

- GC-induced myopathy is associated with high dose and prolonged GC exposure. It should be suspected in patient with unexplained weakness (can confuse with disease activity of dermatomyositis). Laboratory investigation is of little help in diagnosis as muscle enzymes are usually within limit but it can help to rule out other inflammatory myositis. Improvement in weakness with reduction of dose of GC can help to correlate clinical diagnosis
- Growth retardation and cataract are some of unique GC-related ADRs seen in pediatric population. Baseline ophthalmic checkup and regular growth charting should always be part of monitoring when long-term GC therapy is initiated in pediatric patient
- Use of long-acting GC and very high dose should be avoided in pediatric patients as growth retardation may not be reversible even after stoppage of GC therapy, attempt should always be made to stop GC therapy as soon as possible if use cannot be avoided completely. Alternative therapies (propranolol for IH), biologics (rituximab for pemphigus), and other immunosuppressive (cyclosporine for severe AD) are rapidly collecting evidence for efficacy and safety in pediatric population; dermatologist must acquaint themselves for use of these molecules in pediatric population

(ADR: adverse drug reaction; GC: glucocorticoid)

Box 17: GC and hypothalamic pituitary adrenal axis suppression.

- GC suppresses HPA axis and abrupt withdrawal of GC can precipitate symptoms of adrenal suppression particularly if patient is on ≥20 mg of prednisolone (or equivalent) for ≥3 months. Presence of Cushingoid features is strong indicator of underlying HPA axis suppression
- Weakness, fatigue, nausea, vomiting, diarrhea, abdominal pain, fever, weight loss, myalgias, arthralgias, and malaise are features of HPA axis suppression
- Hypotension, loss of consciousness, seizure, or comma is feature of adrenal crisis
- Response of HPA to withdrawal of exogenous GC is highly variable from patient to patient; not all patients will develop symptoms of HPA axis suppression
- When patient is on long-term GC therapy, tapering beyond 15 mg/day should be slow (1–2.5 mg/week) with close monitoring of any symptoms or signs of HPA axis suppression
- Any surgery or intercurrent illness may increase GC demand for patients who is on long-term GC therapy. Respective specialist should be informed about ongoing GC therapy in advance

(HPA: hypothalamic pituitary adrenal; GC: glucocorticoid)

dermatologist's face while seeing dramatic improvement in patient of systemic lupus erythematosus or pemphigus vulgaris who is put on systemic GC therapy is unparalleled to anything else. Practice of dermatology is slowly but gradually moving toward era of minimum systemic GC use with advent of newer molecules particularly targeted biologic therapies. Will we progress to the era of steroid-free dermatology? Answer is yet to come till then every dermatologist must master the fine intricacies of use of GC therapy.

REFERENCES

1. Wolverton SE, Rancour EA. Systemic Corticosteroid. In: Wolverton SE, WU JJ (Eds), 4th edition. Canada: Elsevier; pp. 133-55.
2. Zuberbier T, Aberer W, Asero R, Latiff AA, Baker D, Ballmer-Weber B, et al. The EAACI/GA²LEN/EDF/WAO guideline for the definition, classification, diagnosis and management of urticaria. Allergy. 2018;73(7):1393-414.
3. Ring J, Alomar A, Bieber T, Deleuran M, Fink-Wagner A, Gelmetti C, et al. Guidelines for treatment of atopic eczema (atopic dermatitis) Part II. J Eur Acad Dermatol Venereol. 2012;26(9):1176-93.
4. Cribier B, Frances C, Chosidow O. Treatment of lichen planus: an evidence-based medicine analysis of efficacy. Arch Dermatol. 1998;134(12):1521-30.
5. Ng QX, De Deyn ML, Venkatanarayanan N, Ho CY, Yeo WS. A meta-analysis of cyclosporine treatment for Stevens–Johnson syndrome/toxic epidermal necrolysis. J Inflamm Res. 2018;11:135.
6. Balai M, Meena M, Mittal A, Gupta LK, Khare AK, Mehta S. Cyclosporine in Stevens-Johnson syndrome and toxic epidermal necrolysis: Experience from a tertiary care centre of South Rajasthan. Indian Dermatol Online J. 2021;12(1):116.
7. Darwin E, Hirt PA, Fertig R, Doliner B, Delcanto G, Jimenez JJ. Alopecia areata: review of epidemiology, clinical features, pathogenesis, and new treatment options. Int J Trichol. 2018;10(2):51.
8. Buttgereit F, da Silva JA, Boers M, Burmester GR, Cutolo M, Jacobs J, et al. Standardised nomenclature for glucocorticoid dosages and glucocorticoid treatment regimens: current questions and tentative answers in rheumatology. Ann Rheum Dis. 2002;61(8):718-22.
9. Panoulas VF, Douglas KM, Stavropoulos-Kalinoglou A, Metsios GS, Nightingale P, Kita MD, et al. Long-term exposure to medium-dose glucocorticoid therapy associates with hypertension in patients with rheumatoid arthritis. Rheumatology. 2008;47(1):72-5.
10. Stahn C, Buttgereit F. Genomic and nongenomic effects of glucocorticoids. Nat Clin Pract Rheumatol. 2008;4(10):525-33.
11. Williams DM. Clinical pharmacology of corticosteroids. Respir Care. 2018;63(6):655-70.
12. Liu D, Ahmet A, Ward L, Krishnamoorthy P, Mandelcorn ED, Leigh R, et al. A practical guide to the monitoring and management of the complications of systemic corticosteroid therapy. Allerg Asthma Clin Immunol. 2013;9(1):1-25.
13. Caplan A, Fett N, Rosenbach M, Werth VP, Micheletti RG. Prevention and management of glucocorticoid-induced side effects: a comprehensive review: a review of glucocorticoid pharmacology and bone health. J Am Acad Dermatol. 2017;76(1):1-9.
14. Weinstein RS. Glucocorticoid-induced bone disease. N Eng J Med. 2011;365(1):62-70.
15. Dubois EF, Roïder E, Dekhuijzen PR, Zwinderman AE, Schweitzer DH. Dual energy X-ray absorptiometry outcomes in male COPD patients after treatment with different glucocorticoid regimens. Chest. 2002;121(5):1456-63.
16. Briot K, Roux C. Glucocorticoid-induced osteoporosis. RMD Open. 2015;1(1):e000014.
17. Yildiz N, Ardic F, Deniz S. Very early onset of steroid-induced avascular necrosis of the hip and knee in a patient with idiopathic thrombocytopenic purpura. Intern Med. 2008;44(22):1989-92.
18. Weinstein RS. Glucocorticoid-induced osteonecrosis. Endocrine. 2012;41(2):183-90.
19. Uzu T, Harada T, Sakaguchi M, Kanasaki M, Isshiki K, Araki S, et al. Glucocorticoid-induced diabetes mellitus: prevalence and risk factors in primary renal diseases. Nephron Clin Pract. 2007;105(2):c54-7.
20. Kim SY, Yoo CG, Lee CT, Chung HS, Kim YW, Han SK, et al. Incidence and risk factors of steroid-induced diabetes in patients with respiratory disease. J Korean Med Sci. 2011;26(2):264-7.
21. Caplan A, Fett N, Rosenbach M, Werth VP, Micheletti RG. Prevention and management of glucocorticoid-induced side effects: A comprehensive review: Gastrointestinal and endocrinologic side effects. J Am Acad Dermatol. 2017;76(1):11-6.
22. Narum S, Westergren T, Klemp M. Corticosteroids and risk of gastrointestinal bleeding: a systematic review and meta-analysis. BMJ Open. 2014;4(5):e004587.
23. Phulke S, Kaushik S, Kaur S, Pandav SS. Steroid-induced glaucoma: an avoidable irreversible blindness. J Curr Glaucoma Pract. 2017;11(2):67.
24. Garbe E, LeLorier J, Boivin JF, Suissa S. Risk of ocular hypertension or open-angle glaucoma in elderly patients on oral glucocorticoids. Lancet. 1997;350(9083):979-82.
25. Black RJ, Hill CL, Lester S, Dixon WG. The association between systemic glucocorticoid use and the risk of cataract and glaucoma in patients with rheumatoid arthritis: a systematic review and meta-analysis. PLoS One. 2016;11(11):e0166468.
26. Wei L, MacDonald TM, Walker BR. Taking glucocorticoids by prescription is associated with subsequent cardiovascular disease. Ann Intern Med. 2004;141(10):764-70.
27. White KP, Driscoll MS, Rothe MJ, Grant-Kels JM. Severe adverse cardiovascular effects of pulse steroid therapy: is continuous cardiac monitoring necessary? J Am Acad Dermatol. 1994;30(5 Pt 1):768-73.
28. Fardet L, Petersen I, Nazareth I. Suicidal behavior and severe neuropsychiatric disorders following glucocorticoid therapy in primary care. Am J Psychiatry. 2012;169(5):491-7.
29. Wolkowitz OM, Burke H, Epel ES, Reus VI. Glucocorticoids. Mood, memory, and mechanisms. Ann N Y Acad Sci. 2009;1179:19-40.
30. Jick SS, Lieberman ES, Rahman MU, Choi HK. Glucocorticoid use, other associated factors, and the risk of tuberculosis. Arthritis Rheum. 2006;55(1):19-26.

31. Sagnelli E, Manzillo G, Maio G, Pasquale G, Felaco FM, Filippini P, et al. Serum levels of hepatitis B surface and core antigens during immunosuppressive treatment of HBsAg-positive chronic active hepatitis. Lancet. 1980;2(8191):395-7.
32. Massardo L, Jacobelli S, Leissner M, González M, Villarroel L, Rivero S. High-dose intravenous methylprednisolone therapy associated with osteonecrosis in patients with systemic lupus erythematosus. Lupus. 1992;1(6):401-5.
33. Uusitupa M, Khan TA, Viguiliouk E, Kahleova H, Rivellese AA, Hermansen K, et al. Prevention of type 2 diabetes by lifestyle changes: a systematic review and meta-analysis. Nutrients. 2019;11(11):2611.
34. Strohmayer EA, Krakoff LR. Glucocorticoids and cardiovascular risk factors. Endocrinol Metab Clin. 2011;40(2):409-17.
35. Verma SB, Wollina U. Looking through the cracks of diabetic candidal balanoposthitis!. Int J Gen Med. 2011;4:511.
36. De Leon EM, Jacober SJ, Sobel JD, Foxman B. Prevalence and risk factors for vaginal Candida colonization in women with type 1 and type 2 diabetes. BMC Infect Dis. 2002;2(1):1-6.
37. Tamez-Pérez HE, Quintanilla-Flores DL, Rodríguez-Gutiérrez R, González-González JG, Tamez-Peña AL. Steroid hyperglycemia: prevalence, early detection and therapeutic recommendations: a narrative review. World J Diab. 2015;6(8):1073.
38. Fong AC, Cheung NW. The high incidence of steroid-induced hyperglycaemia in hospital. Diab Res Clin Prac. 2013;99(3):277-80.
39. Trence DL. Management of patients on chronic glucocorticoid therapy: an endocrine perspective. Prim Care. 2003;30(3):593-605.
40. Buckley L, Guyatt G, Fink HA, Cannon M, Grossman J, Hansen KE, et al. 2017 American College of Rheumatology guideline for the prevention and treatment of glucocorticoid-induced osteoporosis. Arthritis Rheumatol. 2017;69(8):1521-37.
41. Sözen T, Özışık L, Başaran NÇ. An overview and management of osteoporosis. Eur J Rheumatol. 2017;4(1):46.
42. Musette P, Kaufman JM, Rizzoli R, Cacoub P, Brandi ML, Reginster JY. Cutaneous side effects of antiosteoporosis treatments. Ther Adv Musculoskelet Dis. 2011;3(1):31-41.
43. De Groen PC, Lubbe DF, Hirsch LJ, Daifotis A, Stephenson W, Freedholm D, et al. Esophagitis associated with the use of alendronate. N Eng J Med. 1996;335(14):1016-21.
44. Nagasawa K, Tada Y, Koarada S, Horiuchi T, Tsukamoto H, Murai K, et al. Very early development of steroid-associated osteonecrosis of femoral head in systemic lupus erythematosus: prospective study by MRI. Lupus. 2005;14(5):385-90.
45. McAvoy S, Baker KS, Mulrooney D, Blaes A, Arora M, Burns LJ, et al. Corticosteroid dose as a risk factor for avascular necrosis of the bone after hematopoietic cell transplantation. Biol Blood Marrow Transplant. 2010;16(9):1231-6.
46. Oinuma K, Harada Y, Nawata Y, Takabayashi K, Abe I, Kamikawa K, et al. Osteonecrosis in patients with systemic lupus erythematosus develops very early after starting high dose corticosteroid treatment. Ann Rheum Dis. 2001;60(12):1145-8.
47. Sakamoto M, Shimizu K, Iida S, Akita T, Moriya H, Nawata YA. Osteonecrosis of the femoral head: a prospective study with MRI. J Bone Joint Surg. 1997;79(2):213-9.
48. Takao M, Sugano N, Nishii T, Miki H, Yoshikawa H. Spontaneous regression of steroid-related osteonecrosis of the knee. Clin Orthop Relat Res. 2006;452:210-5.
49. Lai KA, Shen WJ, Yang CY, Shao CJ, Hsu JT, Lin RM. The use of alendronate to prevent early collapse of the femoral head in patients with nontraumatic osteonecrosis: a randomized clinical study. JBJS. 2005;87(10):2155-9.
50. Chen CH, Chang JK, Lai KA, Hou SM, Chang CH, Wang GJ. Alendronate in the prevention of collapse of the femoral head in nontraumatic osteonecrosis: a two-year multicenter, prospective, randomized, double-blind, placebo-controlled study. Arthritis Rheum. 2012;64(5):1572-8.
51. Camporesi EM, Vezzani G, Bosco G, Mangar D, Bernasek TL. Hyperbaric oxygen therapy in femoral head necrosis. J Arthroplasty. 2010;25(6):118-23.
52. Conn HO, Poynard T. Corticosteroids and peptic ulcer: meta-analysis of adverse events during steroid therapy. J Intern Med. 1994;236(6):619-32.
53. Piper JM, Ray WA, Daugherty JR, Griffin MR. Corticosteroid use and peptic ulcer disease: role of nonsteroidal anti-inflammatory drugs. Ann Intern Med. 1991;114(9):735-40.
54. García Rodríguez LA, Lin KJ, Hernández-Díaz S, Johansson S. Risk of upper gastrointestinal bleeding with low-dose acetylsalicylic acid alone and in combination with clopidogrel and other medications. Circulation. 2011;123(10):1108-15.
55. Ramakrishnan K, Salinas RC. Peptic ulcer disease. Am Fam Physician. 2007;76(7):1005-12.
56. Kim BS, Li BT, Engel A, Samra JS, Clarke S, Norton ID, et al. Diagnosis of gastrointestinal bleeding: A practical guide for clinicians. World journal of gastrointestinal pathophysiology. 2014;5(4):467.
57. Caplan A, Fett N, Rosenbach M, Werth VP, Micheletti RG. Prevention and management of glucocorticoid-induced side effects: A comprehensive review: Ocular, cardiovascular, muscular, and psychiatric side effects and issues unique to pediatric patients. J Am Acad Dermatol. 2017;76(2):201-7.
58. Nishimura K, Harigai M, Omori M, Sato E, Hara M. Blood-brain barrier damage as a risk factor for corticosteroid-induced psychiatric disorders in systemic lupus erythematosus. Psychoneuroendocrinology. 2008;33(3):395-403.
59. Naber D, Sand P, Heigl B. Psychopathological and neuro-psychological effects of 8-days' corticosteroid treatment. A prospective study. Psychoneuroendocrinology. 1996;21(1):25-31.
60. Wolkowitz OM, Reus VI, Weingartner H, Thompson K, Breier A, Doran A, et al. Cognitive effects of corticosteroids. Am J Psychiatry. 1990;147(10):1297-303.
61. Baum M, Moe OW. Glucocorticoid-mediated hypertension: does the vascular smooth muscle hold all the answers? J Am Soc Nephrol. 2008;19(7):1251-3.
62. Fardet L, Petersen I, Nazareth I. Risk of cardiovascular events in people prescribed glucocorticoids with iatrogenic Cushing's syndrome: cohort study. BMJ. 2012;345:e4928.
63. Covar RA, Leung DY, McCormick D, Steelman J, Zeitler P, Spahn JD. Risk factors associated with glucocorticoid-induced adverse effects in children with severe asthma. J Allergy Clin Immunol. 2000;106(4):651-9.
64. Daley-Yates PT, Richards DH. Relationship between systemic corticosteroid exposure and growth velocity: development and validation of a pharmacokinetic/pharmacodynamic model. Clin Ther. 2004;26(11):1905-19.

A Patient with Recalcitrant Dermatophytosis

Pratik R Agarwal, Pragya Nair

INTRODUCTION

Human skin, in health, is a stealthy defense system, structurally, physiochemically, and immunologically, against noxae including microbes operating either synchronously or metachronously. The skin has, over years, been a rampart shielding the internal organs against the onslaught of the harsher terrestrial environment. This includes a barrage of conidia, arthrospores or chlamydospore of dermatophytes, especially geophiles, which, over time, have adapted to the animal hide and fur and thence human skin, hair, and nails. This process of adaptation,[1] rather than being a fight for attrition or predation, is an attempt by the fungi to find a niche space within the human skin where they can minimize the onslaught of body defenses and yet thrive.

Dermatophytosis, an invasion of the upper epidermis by any of the various obligate dermatophytes, may have a high lifetime global prevalence afflicting 20–25% of the population,[2] yet it not defined as a public health problem. Although the problem is visually ever-increasing and perceptible, isolated population-based epidemiological studies and nonrepresentative hospital-based studies have failed to define the burden of disease[3] as a public health problem of concern.

The last 15 years have witnessed a changing timeline and chronology of presentation, epidemiological determinants, distribution pattern, and possible speciation either through sympatric or allopatric evolution. Despite a paucity of large prospective representational studies, one observation seems to be strongly convincing—dermatophyte patterns and response to treatment have changed in the Indian landscape—a phenomenon known as recalcitrance.[4-6]

Whether an acute wound causes, Metchnikoff's theorized,[7] dysbiosis, whether dysbiosis causes dermatophyte colonization or vice versa is not known. An understanding of the niche space at the junction of the stratum corneum and granulosum where the water content, temperature, pH, osmolality, and tissue O_2 and CO_2 concentrations are conducive if not ideal for dermatophytes to thrive is critical to the understanding of dermatophytosis and recalcitrant dermatophytosis thereof **(Tables 1 and 2)**.

In the immunocompetent, dermatophytes evade human defenses by selectively thriving in the stratum corneum, more so in its disjunctum substrata. They try to express polyketides[14] to prevent themselves from the immune defense. However, two case scenarios arise in the situation of immune compromise:

1. Compromise in the local immune defense decreasing *locus minoris resistentiae*[15] may give an opportunity to the dermatophytes to expand their habitat:
   ○ Horizontally to newer and extensive areas on the surface from the center
   ○ Vertically into the infrainfundibulum of the vellus and terminal hair follicle causing folliculitis, a prototypical lesion being Majocchi granuloma on the legs or kerion celsii on the scalp
2. There may also be a generalized immune suppression,[16] either as a result of primary immunodeficiency (*CARD9* mutation) or secondary immunodeficiency. Under such conditions, the fungi invade deeper into tissues causing dermal perifolliculitis, subcutaneous granulomas, and invasive dermatophytosis.

India has been witnessing a new phenomenon in the last decade, a phenomenon of recalcitrance,[17-20] wherein the infection tends either not to disappear wholly or tends to reappear over a time span.

Based on the temporal reappearance,[17] the following conditions **(Flowchart 1)** can arise:

Table 1: Internal milieu of the skin.						
Thickness	Layer	Water	Temperature	pH	PtO$_2$	PtCO$_2$
10 μ	Stratum corneum Disjunctum Compactum	15%	35°C	4.5–5.5	8 ± 3.2 @ 5–10 μ	0.3 mm Hg
100 μ	S. granulosum S. spinosum S. basale	40%	37°C	7	24 ± 6.4 @ 45–65 μ	
	BMZ					
1 mm	Dermis Hypodermis	65–70%			35 ± 8 @ 100–120 μ	40 mm Hg

Table 2: Dermatophytes and the epidermal niche.		
Parameters	Dermatophyte requirements	Epidermis—potential culture environment
Temperature	25–35°C[8]**/***	S. corneum 35°C S. granulosum 37°C
pH	Usually neutral to alkaline	Acidic 4.5–5.5
Osmoreactivity[9]	• Anthropophiles—moderately osmosensitive and salt tolerant • Zoophiles—moderately osmoresistant • Geophiles—moderately osmoresistant	• Osmolyte gradient from epidermis to dermis is present[10] • This may increase during salt accumulation[11]
Iron	Inhibits growth	• Surface—unsaturated transferrin in sweat • S. corneum is deficient in iron • Unsaturated transferrin present in lower epidermis and dermis
Substrate	Amino acids[12] required for growth	• S. corneum is rich in amino acids • Lower epidermis is rich in peptides and keratin

*Skin has an extra renal counter current mechanism which may lead to tissue sodium storage.[11]

**Dermatophytes are moderately thermotolerant mostly growing at 37°C but growth ceases at 40°C, exception being M persicolor which shows poor growth.[13]

***Growth is uncommon at 40°C with nonpathogenic congeners not growing at 37°C.[13]

- Improper or inadequate treatment may lead to partial remission, or extension and persistence. Persistence beyond 6 months to a year regardless of therapy can be termed *chronic dermatophytosis*.
- Suboptimal treatment with the right drugs or treatment with combination drugs including topical corticosteroids may lead to transient remission and reoccurrence within 6 weeks of adequate treatment. Such a state can be termed *recurrent dermatophytosis*.
- Response to treatment is short lived and relapse occurs after 6-8 weeks of discontinuation of therapy, recrudescence being secondary to persistence. This state is termed a *relapsing dermatophytosis*.
- Adequate treatment using effective AFA for a given epidemiologic setting may show a poor response to therapy because the strains of dermatophytes may have developed resistance against a particular antifungal agent. Such infections are called *resistant dermatophytosis*.
- A case may arise when a particular patient may have been adequately treated both clinically and mycologically, may present with another episode of similar lesions after a varying and long period of time. This may be construed as *reinfection*.

APPROACH TO A PATIENT OF RECALCITRANT DERMATOPHYTOSIS

- Establish that the dermatosis is a possible superficial dermatophyte infection.
- Ascertain whether the condition is recalcitrant.
- Ascertain the extent of the disease.
- Evaluate the risk factors associated with the disease.
- Differentiate recalcitrant dermatophytosis from other dermatoses.

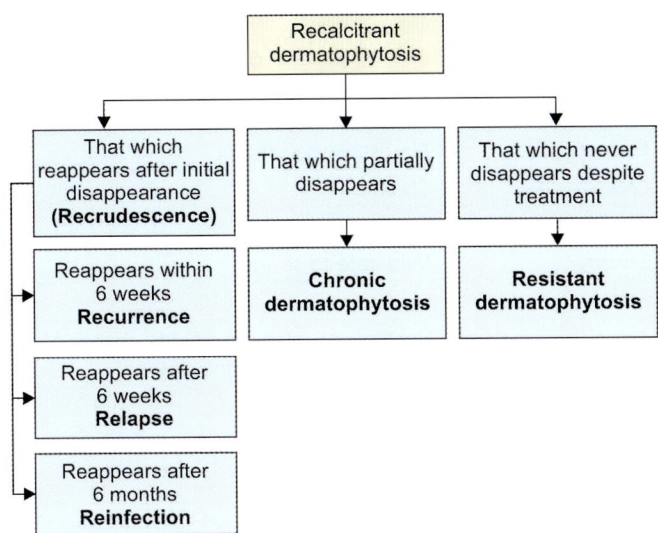

FLOWCHART 1: Schematic representation of recalcitrant dermatophytosis.

- Evaluate the patient's general medical condition for associated comorbidities.
- Document current medications and access drug interactions.
- Do a baseline laboratory investigation.
- Counsel the patient regarding the disease, precautions, and prevention.
- Generate a prescription, follow-up, monitor, and review.

Establishing the Dermatosis to be Possible Superficial Dermatophytosis

A careful history including personal data, presenting complaints, origin, duration, and progression of the disease, clinical examination, and laboratory findings are critical in establishing a dermatophyte infection.

History Taking

Age and gender: Although no age is a bar, Tinea infections are rare in the newborn. Naïve dermatophytosis, in India, is seen in young individuals in their twenties and thirties,[21,22] while recalcitrant dermatophytosis has been found often in fourth and fifth decade.[21] In contrast, naïve dermatophytosis is distributed among middle aged in the western countries[4] as a result of preponderance of Tinea unguium.

The distribution of dermatophytosis among genders, especially in India, was skewed toward a male predominance[23-27] till 2015. In the past 5 years, a parity among genders has been recorded.[21,28,29] However, in the present time, recalcitrant dermatophytosis is marginally skewed toward male predominance.[21]

Address: Tinea imbricata and favus were the only dermatophytosis known to be endemic to certain areas in the world. Today, we see clustering of cases in rural areas[30] more than urban areas.[25,26] Hospital-based studies in the past 5 years have pointed a shift with more urbanites reporting for treatment.

Occupation: Any occupation, which involves an increased susceptibility for microtrauma during physical work, hyperhidrosis, and clustering, especially in subtropics, makes an individual at-risk for developing a clinical infection. Recalcitrance has been noted in individuals engaged in farmlands,[22] manual labor,[20,27,28] in cooking, washing, and cleaning chores.[30]

Socioeconomic status: While the burden of disease is more among the lower socioeconomic strata,[31,32] hospital-based studies in India suggest that more individuals of high socioeconomic status[29] avail treatment. Furthermore, itching is more marked and severe among people belonging to higher socioeconomic group.[33]

Education: Recent data suggests that dermatophytosis is increasingly being reported by literates[26] and people with medium educational qualifications.[29] Furthermore, patient with higher education levels do report increased severity of pruritus.[33]

Marital status: With connubial dermatophytosis[18] being reported in recent times, it is necessary for the dermatologist to ask leading questions about it and examine the spouse if necessary.

Family history: Well-designed studies have found a significant correlation between chronic dermatophyte infection among individuals having a family member suffering from Tinea infection.[32,34] However, a significant correlation between overcrowding in a family as well as the presence of children <15 years seems to be elusive.[35]

Personal history: Chronicity of infection is often seen among people who engage in cooking, who infrequently wash their trousers, undergarments or jeans, and who do not bathe on a regular basis.[35] Frequent use of alkaline cleansers and exfoliants has the potential to breach the protective mantle of the skin and has been postulated to contribute to establishment of the infection on the skin. Similarly, it has been a fair observation that lesions abound in areas where garments snugly fit the body, a particular example being drawstrings.

Patients who partake diets rich in sugars are more predisposed to Tinea pedis.[36]

The sleep pattern is disturbed and difficulty in falling asleep or waking up after initiation of sleep are important parameters that need to be assessed to study the impact of recalcitrance on the quality of life.[33]

A history of self-medication is seen among, especially high-potency corticosteroid creams, an appreciable percentage of patients suffering from recurrence, relapse, or chronicity.[18,35,37]

Menstrual history is important in all women patient as the therapeutic armamentarium is largely curtailed and

Table 3: Important questions to record past history in recalcitrant dermatophytosis.	
Past history of medication	
Treatment in past	Yes/No
Topical antifungals	Yes/No
Fixed dose combination of topical antifungals and corticosteroids	Yes/No
Systemic antifungals	Yes/No
Topical corticosteroids	Yes/No
Intralesional corticosteroids	Yes/No
Systemic corticosteroids/immunosuppressives	Yes/No
Duration of response	Till clinical cure (√/×)
	Beyond clinical cure (record duration) (√/×)
	Till mycological cure (√/×)
Application accuracy	On the lesion (√/×)
	2 cm beyond lesional margin (√/×)
Concomitant medications	Record each and every medication

Table 4: Characteristics of pruritus in recalcitrant dermatophytosis.	
Pruritus in recalcitrant dermatophytosis	
Frequency	Almost always present
Course	Chronic
Type	Pruritoceptive
Severity	Moderate-to-severe
Extent	Lesion specific
Aggravating factors	Heat, sweat, relative humidity, change of clothes, and tight fitting clothes

the choice of drugs to treat dermatophytosis is limited in pregnancy.

There is no study incriminating alcohol abuse as a risk factor for recalcitrant dermatophytosis. The hazard risk for liver injury[38] due to fluconazole and itraconazole is low; however, the hazard risk of acute liver injury in alcoholics could be higher than normal and proper monitoring is recommended when administering azoles. Smoking,[36] on the other hand, has been found to have a protective effect, at least in Tinea pedis. A history of recent cessation of smoking may be worthwhile while evaluating a patient of dermatophytosis.

A history of atopic diathesis, casual exposure, and blood transfusion should be sought for.

Past history (**Table 3**) should be sought for diligently. Has there been a history of similar illness in the past? If yes, was it adequately treated? A record of the timeline, its course, and treatment, if documented, should be sought. If not available, every patient needs to be asked for past similar illness and treatment. Whether antifungal creams were used alone or in combination and if there was a corticosteroid in the preparation needs to be clarified. Whether systemic antifungals or intralesional corticosteroids were also administered needs documentation. Further, were the topicals properly applied and what was the duration till the treatment was continued need a thorough questioning. Also, if the treatment was stopped under medical advice or abruptly stopped on its own also needs to be questioned.

Chief Complaints

There is always an associated history of similar lesions in the past. While the history may suggest a fungal infection, it is the temporal distribution of the dermatosis that establishes recalcitrance.

Recalcitrant dermatophytosis differs from naïve dermatophytosis in the following ways:
- Speciation differences in the form of preponderance of anthropophiles being the causative.
- Morphological changes in form of larger size and variegated configurations as compared to the smaller sized and circinate and annular forms of naïve dermatophytosis.
- Distributional changes with extensive involvement of the glabrous skin.

Pruritus[33] (**Table 4**) is a *sine qua non* in dermatophytosis with recalcitrance. It is pruritoceptive, lesion-specific, and tends to assume a chronic course beyond 6 weeks.

The intensity of itching is severe in three out of four patients while the rest are moderate. The intensity of itch leads to difficulty in falling asleep or may compel the patient to wake up once he/she has fallen asleep.

One in two patients may complain of burning while two of five patients complain of isolated itching.[33] The rest may complain of both. The itch is aggravated with sweating, hot temperatures, and with wearing tight clothes. Alloknesis and punctate hyperknesis do not feature in recalcitrant infections.

The skin lesions, although the same prototype as in naïve dermatophytosis (**Table 5, Figs. 1 to 3**), differ in recalcitrant disease wherein they take a different course. The lesions are larger in size, greater in number, wider in distribution, and grotesque in configuration. Morphologically, the lesions retain their classic presentation in nine out of ten cases. Occasionally, they may present with papulosquamous, eczematous, pustular, pseudoimbricata, lichenoid, bullous and pityriasis rosea like morphologies (**Figs. 4 to 12**).[34]

They have been described in areas that are usually spared in adults, viz., scalp, eyelids,[19] oral lips,[19] penile shaft and scrotum.[19,39,40] Further, naïve lesions have a property to clear centrally and spread peripherally as the immune

Table 5: Comparative characteristics of naïve versus recalcitrant disease.		
Characteristics	***Naïve dermatophytosis***	***Recalcitrant dermatophytosis***
Primary morphology	Papule	Papule
Evolution of lesions	• Appearance • Phase of evolution • Phase of maturation • Phase of dissolution	• Appearance • Phase of evolution • Waxing and waning
Size	Small	Usually, larger
Morphology	Erythematoannular circinate patch	Erythematoannular circinate patch, papulosquamous psoriasiform, eczematous, pustular, pseudoimbricate, lichenoid, bullous and pityriasis rosea-like
Configurations	Discoid, circinate, annular, and imbricate (chronic)	Arcuate, incognita, annulogyrate, horseshoe shaped, pseudoimbricate
Distribution	Region specific (except in Tinea imbricata)	More than two regions, extensive or generalized
Sites	All body sites sparing scrotum, penile shaft, and scalp (in adults)	All body sites including penile shaft and scalp
Course of disease	Limited with eventual healing chronic and lifelong in Tinea imbricata	Chronic and smouldering (if left untreated or treated inadequately)
Response to treatment	Readily responds to local treatments or systemic treatments (if indicated)	Response is variable and requires prolonged systemic treatment as single, combination or sequential therapy
Prognosis	Good	Guarded

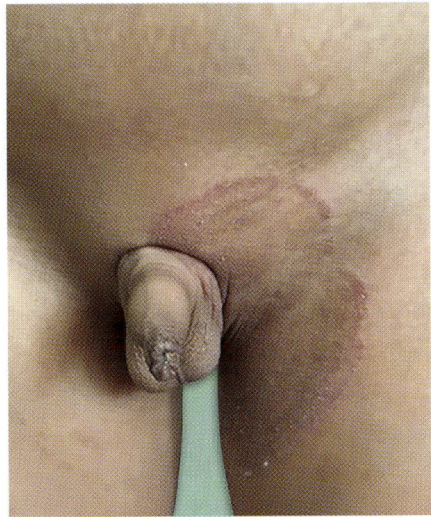

FIG. 1: Naïve Tinea inguinalis with asymmetrical unilateral presentation involving genitocrural fold, medial thigh, mons and a small part of scrotum.
Courtesy: Dr Pratik Agarwal.

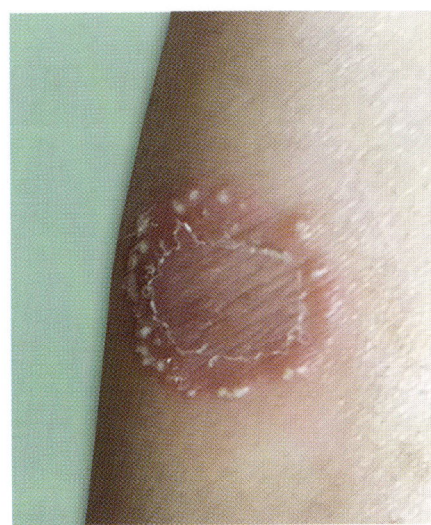

FIG. 2: Naïve Tinea corporis, inflammatory type with peripheral pustulation.
Courtesy: Dr Pratik Agarwal.

system tries to mount a defense, a phenomenon that may mirror acquired relative resistance to reinfection described in animals as "*le phenomene de la reaction acceleree*" or "*le phenomene de Bruno Bloch*".[41] This *locus minoris resistentiae* is disturbed resulting from immune suppression secondary to use of topical corticosteroids or immunosuppressants or other factors not known in present times. Hence, newer lesions continue to arise from the center of the lesion giving it multiannular or imbricata pattern, or else, arcuate or horseshoe pattern. The periphery of the lesions usually tends to be inflammatory but may be noninflammatory as well. The lesions in the genitocrural fold are also semiannular circinate rather than the classic erythema marginatum described in literature of the yore. The scall or squama, while it follows the erythematous margins in naïve disease, becomes interrupted, perifollicular, or presents as scruff throughout the patch. Pruritus is moderate-to-severe as compared to mild in naïve lesions, scratch marks are missing but occasionally may be found **(Figs. 13 to 21)**.

Telltale signs of previous therapy including dyschromia; striae secondary to use of potent steroids as monotherapy or combinations of antifungal, antibacterial, antipruritics;

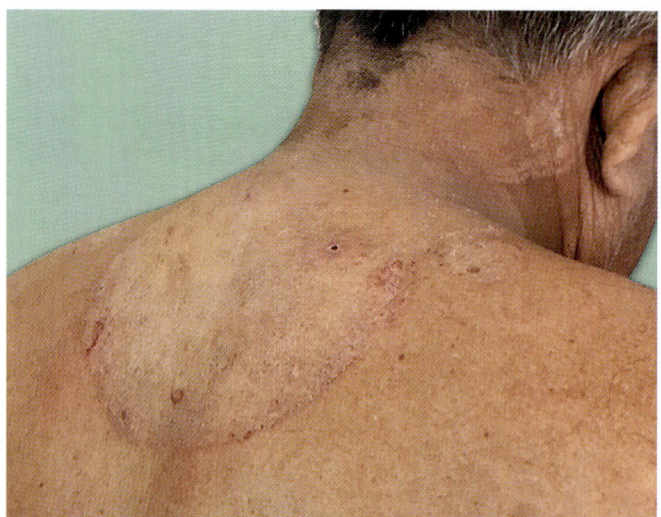

FIG. 3: Recalcitrant dermatophytosis over the posterior trunk in a diabetic patient.
Courtesy: Dr Pratik Agarwal.

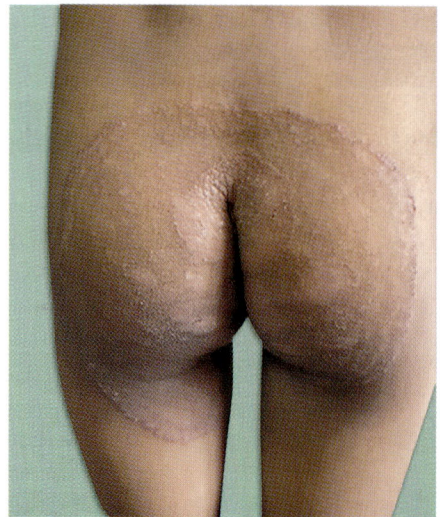

FIG. 5: Multi-annular rings, complete, and partial with minimal clearing.
Courtesy: Dr Pratik Agarwal.

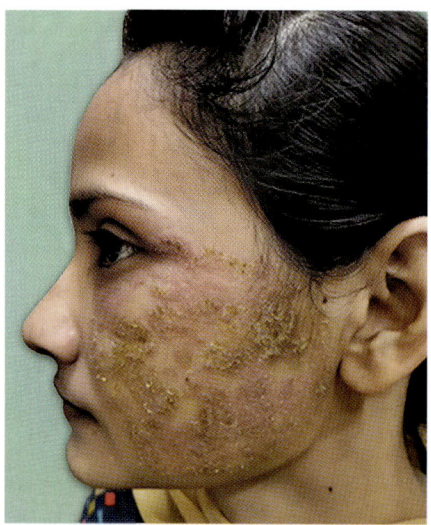

FIG. 4: Circumscription maintained in eczematous Tinea faciei.
Courtesy: Dr Pratik Agarwal.

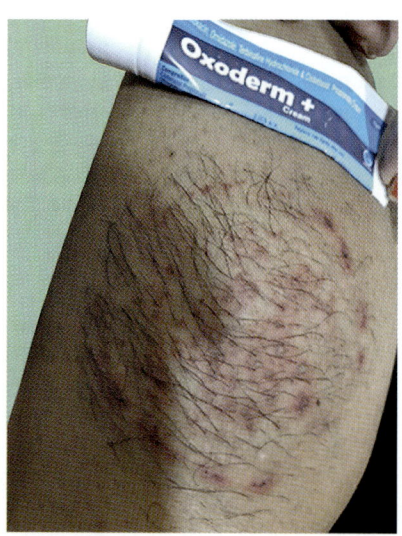

FIG. 6: Fixed combination containing corticosteroid leading to follicular pustulation while the circumscription is maintained.
Courtesy: Dr Pratik Agarwal.

and hypopigmented patches due to intralesional steroids **(Figs. 22 to 27)**.

General Examination of the Patient

Whether anemia is a risk factor for dermatophytosis, although described, is not validated in large studies. But the presence of pallor, iron deficiency anemia, and administration of iron supplements should be closely monitored. Presence of icterus should raise concern especially when systemic drugs such as terbinafine, fluconazole, or itraconazole are being prescribed. Further, icterus with occasional abdominal discomfort should raise a caution for Gilbert's syndrome[42] and caution should be exercised when administering H1 inverse agonists especially injectable pheniramine maleate.

Vital signs are important to assess the general health of the patient. Measuring blood pressure at every visit is especially important as patients on itraconazole occasionally may develop resistant hypertension.[43] Pedal edema may develop in patients administered itraconazole especially if cardiac decompensation is present.[44,45] It could also confound the edema caused by amlodipine[46] especially in

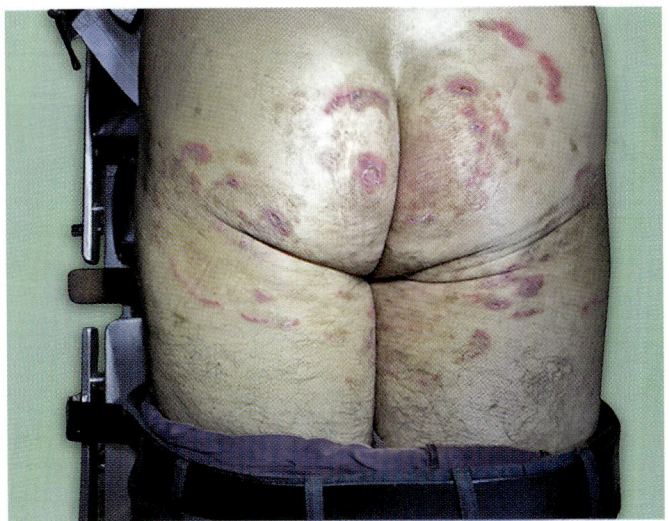

FIG. 7: Arcuate lesions arising out of circumscription as a result of partial treatment.
Courtesy: Dr Pratik Agarwal.

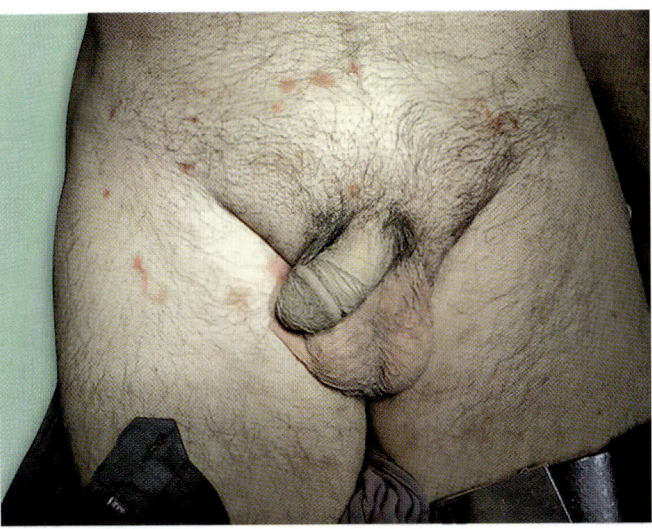

FIG. 9: Tinea incognita with minimal erythemtopapular lesions in a regional distribution.
Courtesy: Dr Pratik Agarwal.

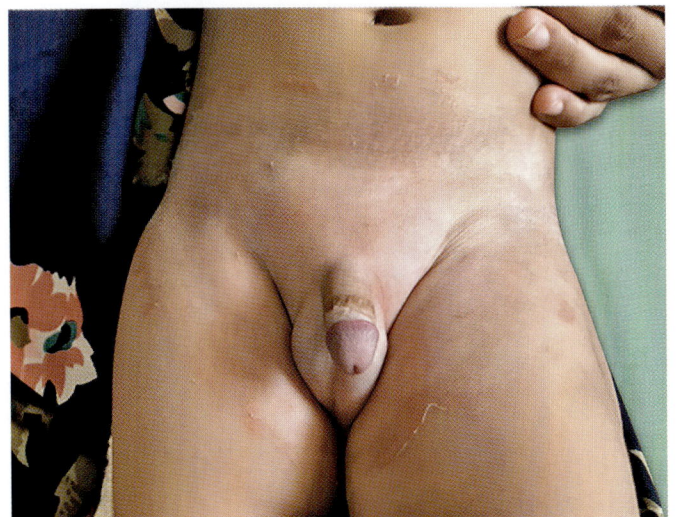

FIG. 8: Tinea incognita secondary to steroidal abuse leading to hypopigmentation, with broken partial arcs in the periphery and exfoliation.
Courtesy: Dr Pratik Agarwal.

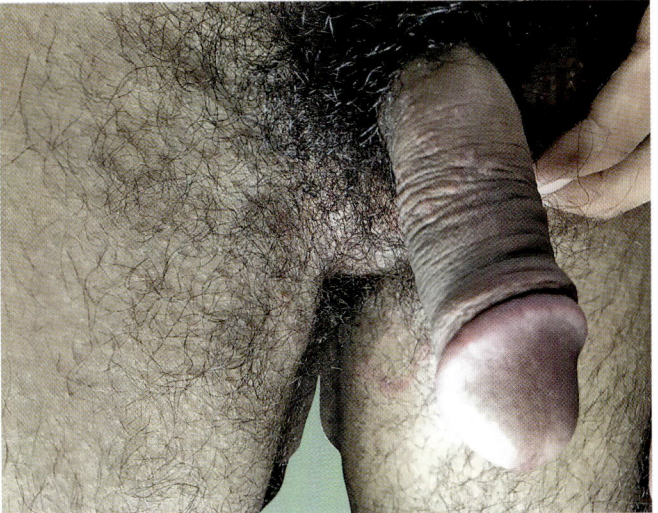

FIG. 10: Lichenoid lesions on the penile shaft and semi-annular lesions in the genitocrural fold.
Courtesy: Dr Pratik Agarwal.

hypertensives. Other causes of pedal edema should be ruled out. The edema will be bilateral and protracted. It may take 6 months or more to resolve despite discontinuation of therapy.

General examination of the cutaneous surface may reveal an endomorph with obesity in general and pendulous breasts among women. Further, dry skin,[47] evaluated clinically, has been recorded in a greater subset of patients in certain studies.

Ascertain Whether the Condition is Recalcitrant

The algorithm to assess for recalcitrance in dermatophytosis is schematically represented in **Flowchart 2**.

Ascertain the Extent of the Disease

The severity of the disease[17] needs to be assessed in terms of percentage of body surface area being involved. An

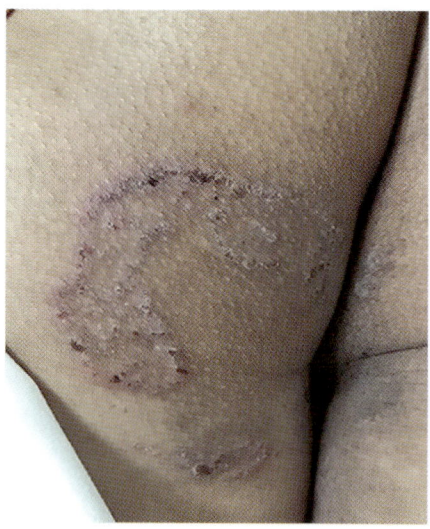

FIG. 11: Horseshoe-shaped lesion in recalcitrant dermatophytosis.
Courtesy: Dr Pratik Agarwal.

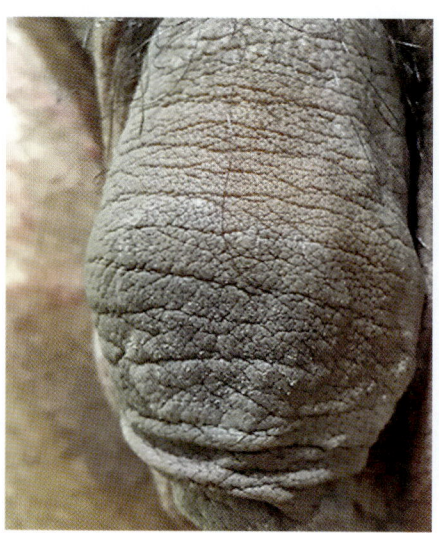

FIG. 13: Penile dermatophytosis.
Courtesy: Dr Pratik Agarwal.

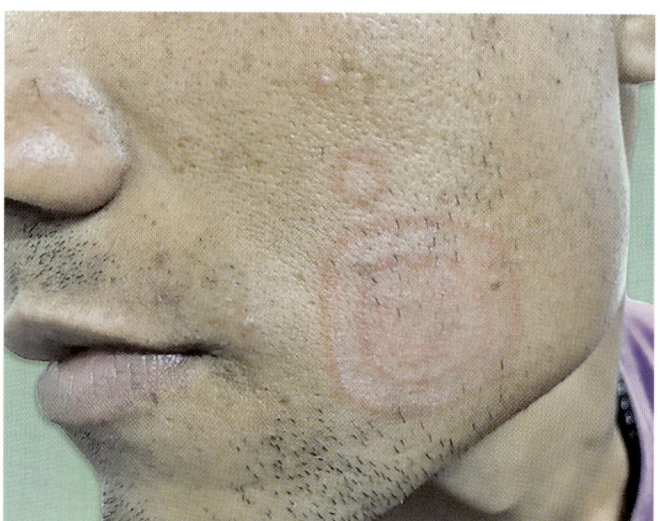

FIG. 12: Tinea pseudoimbricata over the face with complete multiple annular erythematous rings.
Courtesy: Dr Pratik Agarwal.

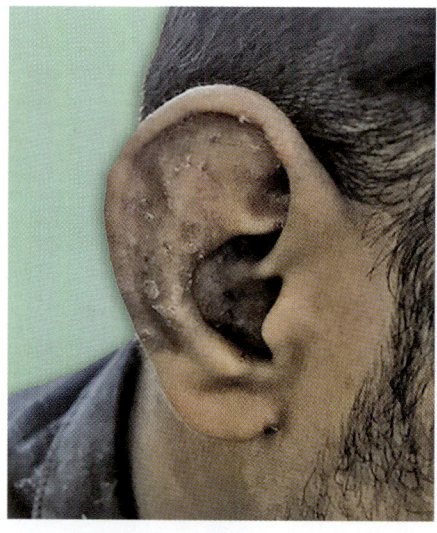

FIG. 14: Auricular dermatophytosis.
Courtesy: Dr Pratik Agarwal.

outstretched palm from the rascette to the tip of the finger is considered as 1% body surface area (BSA) **(Table 6)**.

At present, we are in want of studies that can tell us whether defining the extent of the disease shall offer help in predicting the course of the disease, prognosis of the disease, or the choice of antifungal therapy.

Evaluate the Risk Factors Associated with the Disease

While the risk factors for naïve dermatophytosis depend on the presentation of Tinea, there is lack of data and well-designed studies that can say whether the risk factors for recalcitrant dermatophytosis are the same or different. **Table 7** enlists the risk factors for each type of Tinea infection.

Differentiate Recalcitrant Dermatophytosis from Other Dermatoses

The differential set for naïve dermatophytosis differs from recalcitrant dermatophytosis. The differential set[49] for naïve Tinea lesions is given in **Table 8**.

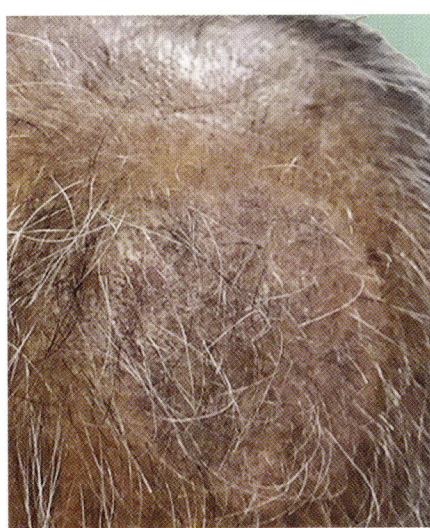

FIG. 15: Scalp dermatophytosis in adults.
Courtesy: Dr Pratik Agarwal.

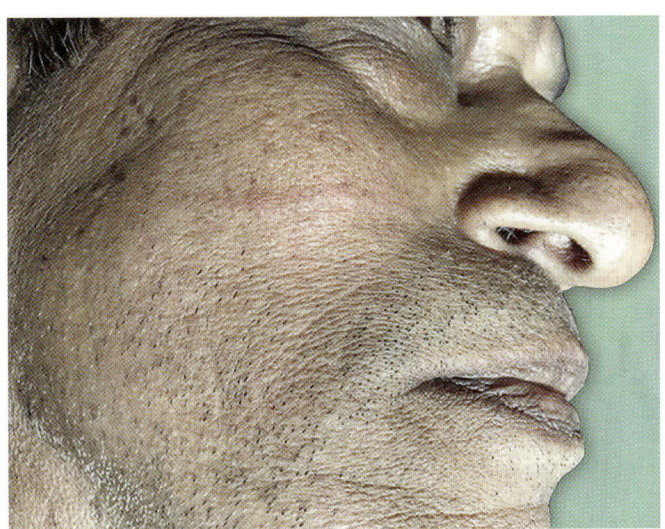

FIG. 17: Facial circinate—dermatophytic pattern.
Courtesy: Dr Pratik Agarwal.

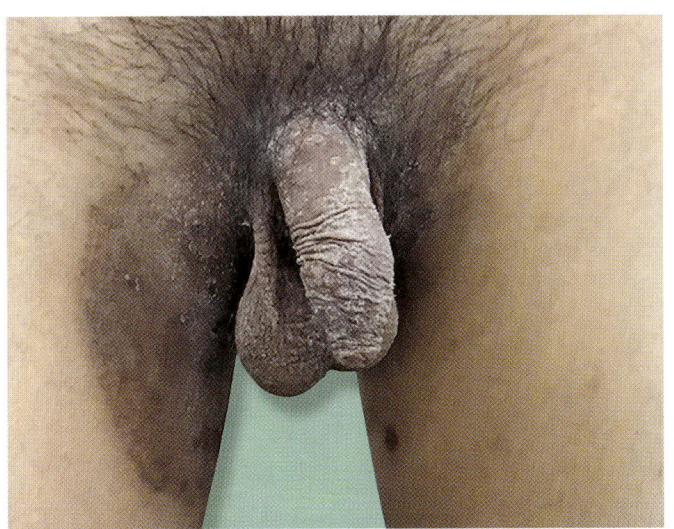

FIG. 16: Genitocrural with penile shaft involvement in recalcitrant dermatophytosis.
Courtesy: Dr Pratik Agarwal.

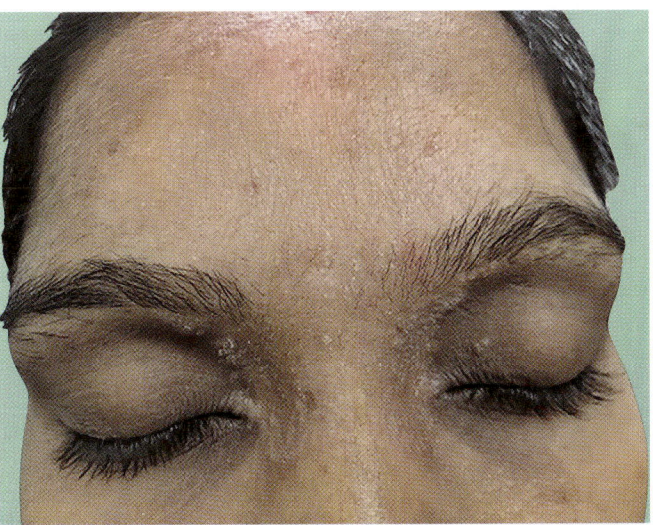

FIG. 18: Facial with eyelid involvement in recalcitrant dermatophytosis.
Courtesy: Dr Pratik Agarwal.

In recalcitrant dermatophytosis, while the differentials stated above may still apply, it is the extensive involvement that raises newer possibilities as given in **Box 1**.

Some of the differentials associated with unusual presentations in recalcitrant disease are pityriasiform Unna's disease, CTCL, annular erythemas, disseminated granuloma annulare, Tinea imbricata, and chronic trichophyton rubrum syndrome.

A few diagnostic dilemmas have been given in **Tables 9 and 10**. However, given a proper history, it is not difficult to clinically diagnose a case of recalcitrant disease.

Recalcitrant disease with large area involvement may be challenging and may masquerade as Miescher's granuloma or annular elastolytic actinic giant cell granuloma, O'Brien actinic granuloma, and subacute lupus erythematosus on the face, erythema marginatum, pityriasis rotunda, pityriasiform seborrheic dermatitis, superficial scaly dermatitis, and erythema annulare over the trunk.

Evaluate the Patient's General Medical Condition for Associated Comorbidities

Medical records or documentation, if available, should be carefully perused enlisting all comorbidities, hospitalization, and operations. If not available, a quest to rule out liver, renal and cardiac diseases should be actively

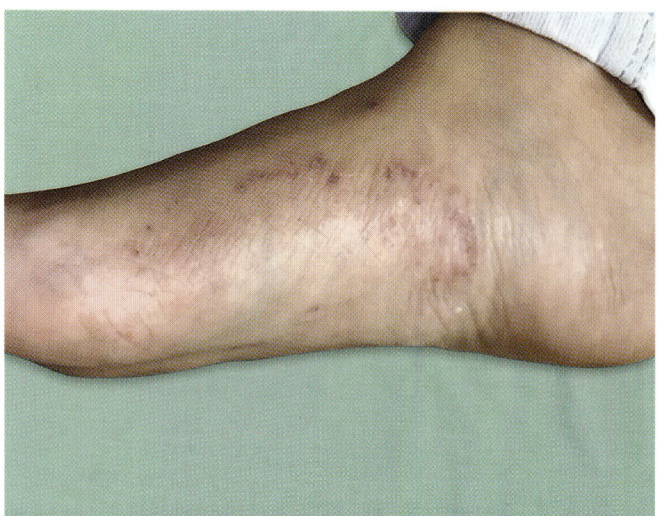

FIG. 19: Circumscribed pedal involvement in dermatophytosis.
Courtesy: Dr Pratik Agarwal.

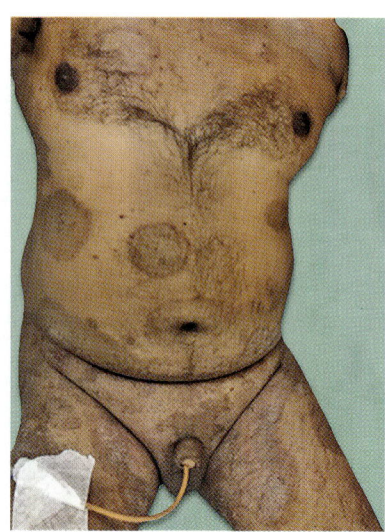

FIG. 21: Extensive Tinea corporis.
Courtesy: Dr Pratik Agarwal.

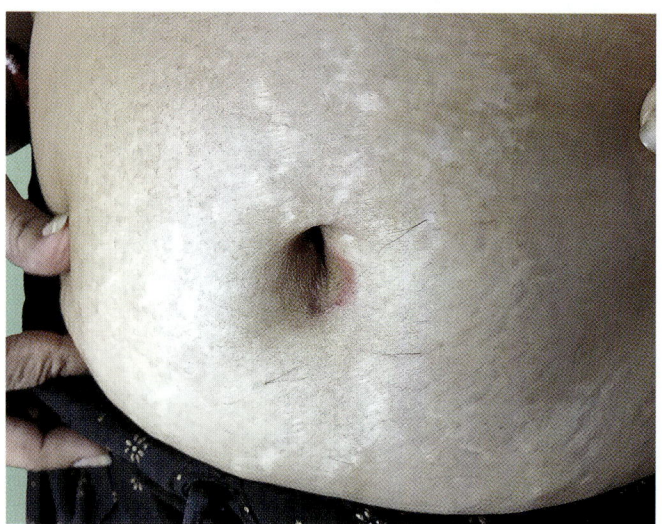

FIG. 20: Umbilical involvement in dermatophytosis.
Courtesy: Dr Pratik Agarwal.

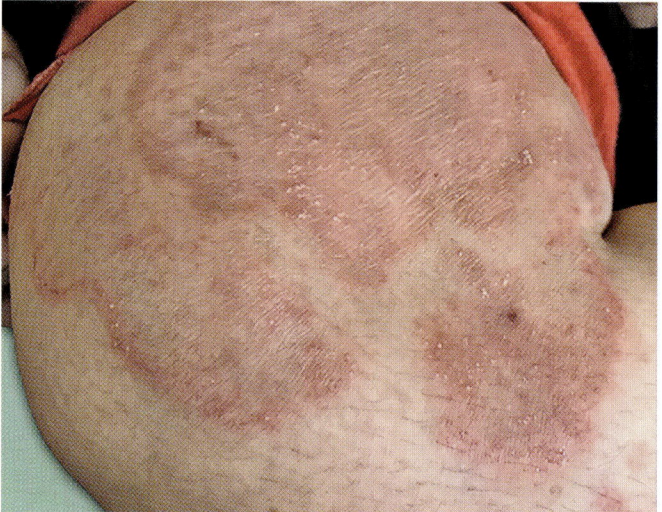

FIG. 22: Steroid-induced pustulation in dermatophytic lesion.
Courtesy: Dr Pratik Agarwal.

undertaken. History for blood transfusion, needlestick injury, and increased risk behavior for casual sex should be documented in all patients.

Document Current Medications

Patients with comorbidities are usually on multiple drugs which may be substrates or products of *p*-glycosylation, organic anion transporting polypeptide (OATP) transports, or cytochrome P450 (CYP) induction. There arises a need to predict the drug–drug interactions and the chances of adverse events before a prescription is rolled out.

Therapy in recalcitrant dermatophytosis is characterized by:
- Use of systemic antifungals
- Longer duration of oral medication

The plasma levels of fungicidal drugs need to be maintained above MIC levels around the clock. Moreover, as fungistatic inhibits further multiplication, its concentration in blood and tissue needs to be maintained.

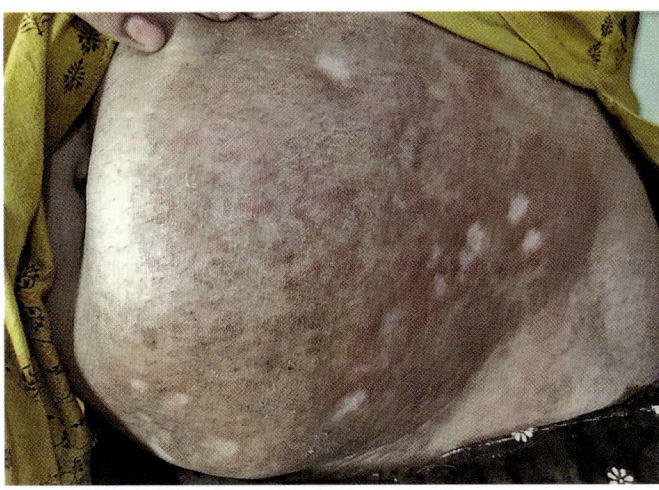

FIG. 23: Intralesional steroid-induced depigmentation in treated case of dermatophysotis.
Courtesy: Dr Pratik Agarwal.

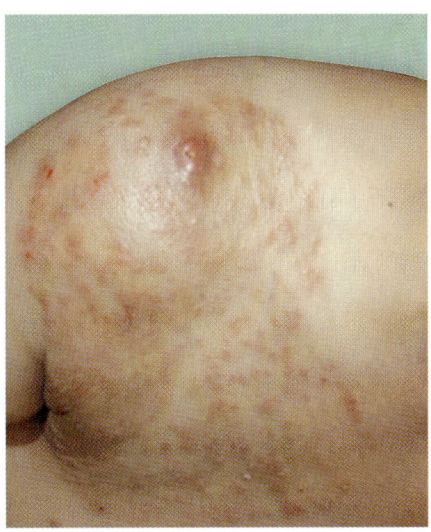

FIG. 25: Tinea corporis with furunculosis.
Courtesy: Dr Pratik Agarwal.

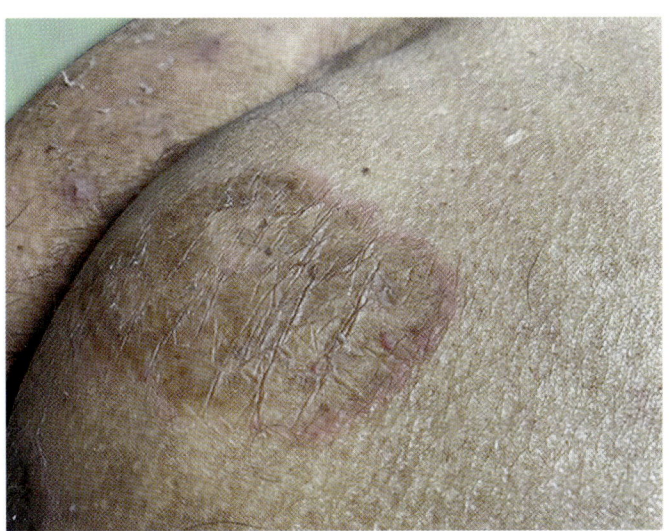

FIG. 24: Tinea corporis over ICD in COVID-19-positive patient.
(COVID-19: coronavirus disease 2019; ICD: irritant contact dermatitis)
Courtesy: Dr Pratik Agarwal.

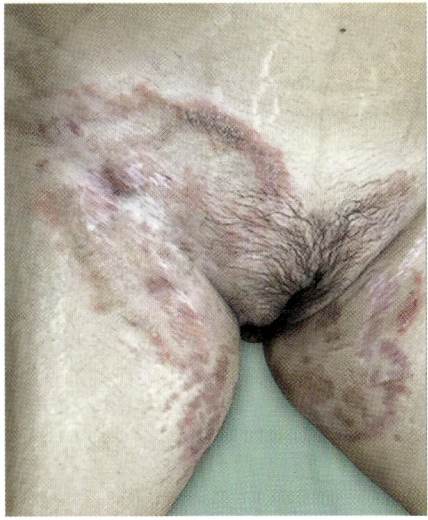

FIG. 26: Steroid-induced striae in Tinea inguinalis.
Courtesy: Dr Pratik Agarwal.

Do a Baseline Laboratory Investigation

Tests to establish the burden/quantum of disease

Clinical tests done at the physiological dermatology laboratory would include:
- Ascertain the presence of involvement of dermatophyte infection in vellus hair by dermoscopic[50] examination **(Box 2 and Figs. 28 to 30)**
- Ascertain barrier damage[51-53] by estimating pH and transepidermal water loss (TEWL)

Tests done in dermatology clinic and/or pathological laboratory:
- Ascertain the presence of dermatophyte by presence of hyaline septate hyphae in samples of squama **(Box 3)** taken from the edge of the lesion and doing on-site 10% KOH mount.[17,54,55]

Modifications in the form of 20% KOH with the addition of 36% DMSO or 25% KOH with 5% glycerol may yield better results. Congo red and Calcofluor white could be used along with a fluorescent microscopy.

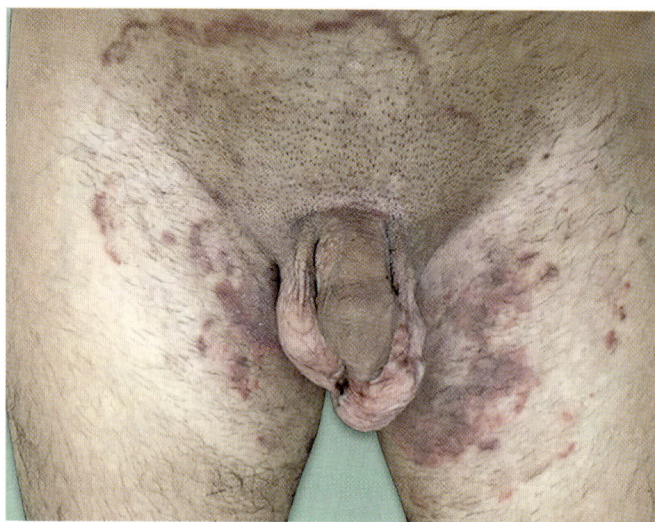

FIG. 27: Steroid-induced atrophy in Tinea cruris et corporis.
Courtesy: Dr Pratik Agarwal.

- Confirmation of dermatophytosis through culture in all cases of multisite Tinea and recalcitrant disease.
- Histological examination in cases where lesions are beyond cognition and can be labeled as Tinea incognita using GMS or PAS along with H&E stain **(Box 4 and Figs. 31 to 35)**.

Tests to ascertain the choice of drugs: Although chronic dermatophytosis is associated with immunoglobulin E (IgE) antibody (Ab)-mediated IH and a Th2 response characterized by presence of S IgE Ab, IgG Ab, and IgG4 Ab,[60] none of these require estimation in daily practice.
- Blood sugar estimations should be done to rule out diabetes mellitus.
- Liver function tests and renal function tests are indicated because there could arise a need or protracted therapy.[17]
- IgE measurements may indicate chronicity[61,62] in infection or an atopic epiphenomenon.[63]
- An EKG study in patients with history of cardiac decompensation especially elderly and all patients with cardiac comorbidities

Management of Recalcitrant Dermatophytosis

The ideal management of recalcitrant dermatophytosis **(Flowchart 3)** would entail:
- Eradication of the fungi, both in terms of clinical and mycological cure.
- Treatment of dormant arthrospores within the skin
- Address the putative role of biofilms in contributing to the recalcitrance.
- Disinfection of fomites and eradication of spores from the immediate environment.

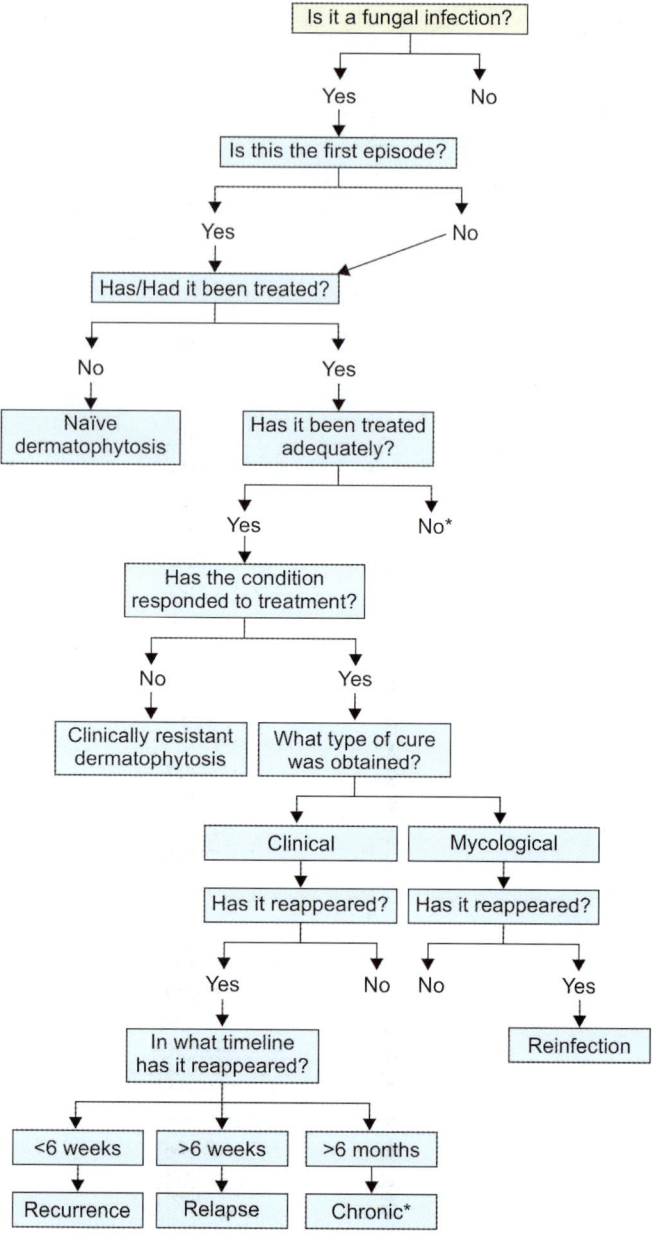

*Chronic dermatophytosis.

FLOWCHART 2: Algorithm to assess for recalcitrance in dermatophytosis.
Courtesy: Dr Pratik Agarwal.

Table 6: Severity grading of dermatophytosis.	
Severity	**Extent**
Mild dermatophytosis	<3% BSA
Moderate dermatophytosis	3–10% BSA
Severe dermatophytosis	>10% BSA
(BSA: body surface area)	

Table 7: Risk factors for naïve and recalcitrant dermatophytosis.

	Tinea cruris	Tinea pedis	Tinea corporis	Tinea barbae/capitis
Naïve dermatophytosis[48]	• Obesity • Hyperhidrosis • Manual laborers • Transport drivers	• Manual laborer • Farmers • Agriculturists • Use of public swimming pools • Psoriasis • Allergic rhinitis • Atopic dermatitis • High carbohydrate foods[37]	• Diabetes mellitus • Psoriasis • Ichthyosis • HIV infection • Sharing of towels and apparel	• Common use of trimmers • Sharing hats, combs • Contact with infected pets
Recalcitrant dermatophytosis[34,35]	• Indiscriminate use of topical corticosteroids • Infrequent bathing • Family history of Tinea infection • Preexisting diabetes mellitus • Cooking food • Infrequent washing of trousers and undergarments • High-carbohydrate diets[36]			

(HIV: human immunodeficiency virus)

Table 8: Differential diagnosis of naïve dermatophytosis.

Tinea corporis	Tinea cruris*	Tinea pedis	Tinea manuum
• Psoriasis • Pityriasis rosea • Annular erythemas • Granuloma annulare • Nummular eczema • Folliculitis • SCLE may be considered	• Candidiasis • Neurodermatitis • Erythrasma • Psoriasis	• Psoriasis • Pityriasis rubra pilaris • Keratoderma • Eczematous dermatoses	• Keratoderma • Psoriasis • Eczema

*Scrotal involvement generally includes a nondermatophyte infection.

Box 1: Differentials of recalcitrant dermatophytosis.

Mimicking dermatoses:
- Psoriasis
- Pityriasiform seborrheic dermatitis
- Subacute lupus erythematosus
- Parapsoriasis en mitis plaques poikilodermis
- Atopic eczema
- Annular erythemas
- Granuloma annulare disseminate
- Secondary annular syphilis
- Tinea imbricata
- Chronic trichophyton rubrum syndrome

Counsel the Patient Regarding Prevention of Disease (Table 11)

While treatment of recalcitrant dermatophytosis is largely administering systemic antifungals, an important part of the management is counseling with regards to prevention of reinfection and prevention of spread in community at large. Before a prescription is generated, a candid discussion should be forthcoming and counseling should be catered for each and every patient of recalcitrant dermatophytosis.

Arthroconidia may persist for months or years,[80] particularly when embedded in hair and/or skin scales, on floors, walls, and objects. Although the contact with a contaminated environment alone in the absence of infected

Table 9: Differentiating features of mimics of mild recalcitrant dermatophytosis.

Features	Annular LP	Granuloma annulare*	Recalcitrant annular Tinea lesion	Annular syphilides	EAC (superficial)
Genetic disposition	SNP, HLA, and epigenetic disposition	None	None	None	None
Age	30–50 years	20–40 years	30–40 years	Sexually active age	Early adulthood to middle age
Sex	Women 2:1	Women 2:1	Male 1.5–1	—	—
History	Infections, vaccination	Trauma	Manual labor, hyperhidrosis	Sexual exposure	Infection, infestation, drugs, food allergies
Clinical presentation:					
Morphology	Papule	Papule	Papule	Papule	Urticoid papule
Color	Purple red to violet	Discernible red	Skin colored to slight red	Skin colored	Red
Size	1–2 cm	1–2 inches	Variable	Variable	8–10 cm
Surface	Fine scale	Smooth	Scurfy	Smooth	Trailing scale, collarette
Shape	Circumscribed	Irregular	Polycyclic, geographic	Circumscribed	Circinate, archiform
Pattern	Annular	Annular	Annular circinate	Annular	Annular
Sensation	Normal	Hypoesthetic	Normal	Normal	Normal
Distribution	Glans, shaft, axilla, face*	Fingers, feet, elbow, ankle, and knee	Glabrous surface	Scrotum	Trunk, proximal extremities
Pruritus	Present	Absent	Moderate-to-severe	Absent	Absent
Course	Chronic	Up to 2 years	Long periods	None	Purpuric/residual pigmentation
Sequelae	Dyschromia	None	Dyschromia		
Histology	Lichenoid interface dermatitis	• Mucin in interstitium • Palisading granuloma • Curlicue collagen	• Sandwich sign • Neuts in the horn • Superficial perivascular infiltrate	Plasma cell infiltration	• Coat sleeve infiltrate with erythrocytosis • Parakeratosis • Spongiosis • Vacuolar alteration in basal cell • Erythrocytes

*Granuloma annulare has a cartilaginous glistening border

Table 10: Differentiating features of mimics of severe recalcitrant dermatophytosis.

	Recalcitrant dermatophytosis	Subacute lupus erythematosus	Parapsoriasis en grandes plaques
Gender	Males	Females	Males
Age	30–40 years		Middle aged
Pruritus	Moderate-to-severe	None	Often
Photoexposure	No change	• Increase with latency • Present in 63% cases	Relieves itching
Emotional stress	Secondary, may increase itch	No effect	No effect
Seasonal change	Increase with high relative humidity	No change	No change
Morphology	Papule	Papule Smooth, bright red, or violet	Irregular but sharply defined reddened plaques

Continued

Continued

	Recalcitrant dermatophytosis	**Subacute lupus erythematosus**	**Parapsoriasis en grandes plaques**
Configuration	Annular or circinate Gyrate, arcuate	Gyrate, annular, psoriasiform	Bizarre
Distribution	• No surface is immune. Most commonly in genitocrural, gluteal, truncal, auricular, and facial distribution • Palms and soles may be involved	• *Facial* rash*: Erythematous rash involving peripheral cheeks • <20% have coexistent malar rash of ACLE • *Truncal* rash*: Involves the shoulders, V neck, upper back and the extensors of upper limbs, spares the knuckles, elbows, knees and greater trochanters	Trunk, gluteal, and proximal limbs
Histology—Epidermis	• Hyperkeratosis • Acanthosis • Spongiosis • Parakeratosis with "neuts in the horn"	• Atrophy (+) • Hydropic degeneration of basal layer • Epidermal cleft • Civatte bodies numerous	• Acanthosis • Epidermal exocytosis • Pautrier's microabscess • Large cerebriform nucleated cells
Histology—Dermis	• Papillary edema • Superficial and deep lymphocytic infiltrate	• Edema (+++) • Lymphocytic infiltrate band like and top heavy • Mucin between interstitial tissue	• Edema (+) • Inflammatory infiltrate containing neutrophils • No appendageal involvement
*Spares upper eyelids and periorbital regions			

Box 2: Dermoscopic characteristics in recalcitrant disease.

Dermoscopic findings in long-standing dermatophytosis:
- Grayish black background replaces reddish background
- Follicular pustules, empty follicles, and black dots
- Translucent hairs, broken, corkscrew, and morse code like hairs

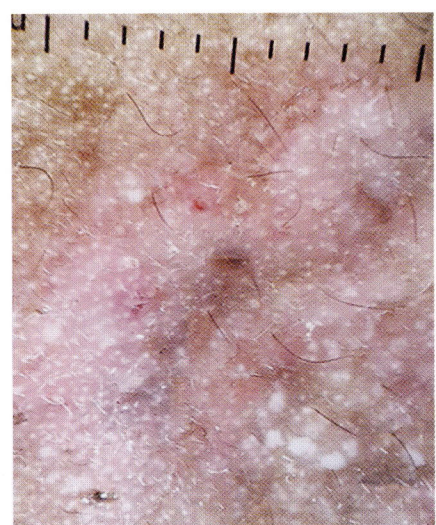

FIG. 29: Dermoscopic images in dermatophytosis.
Courtesy: Dr Pragya Nair.

animal is considered rare source of infection in animals and humans.[81] Decontamination is important to minimize the risk of reinfection and to reduce the treatment time required by animals. The same should apply to humans. Before the application of cleaning product, it is important to remove all debris by vacuuming or sweeping, since disinfectant does not work in the presence of organic material.[81]

Dermatophytes are susceptible to high heat. Moist heat for 20 minutes at 121° or 2 hours of dry heat at 165–170° is "cidal" for the dermatophyte.

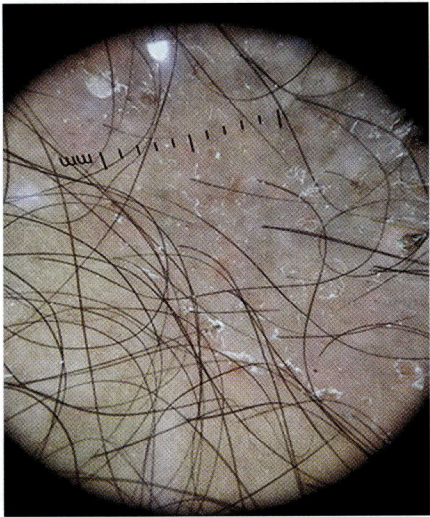

FIG. 28: Dermoscopic images in dermatophytosis.
Courtesy: Dr Pragya Nair.

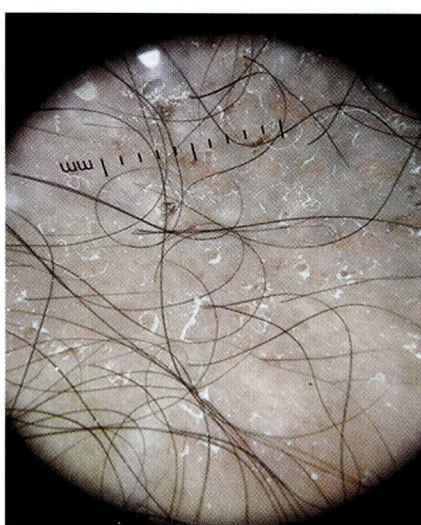

FIG. 30: Dermoscopic images in dermatophytosis.
Courtesy: Dr Pragya Nair.

Box 3: How to collect specimen for KOH mount?

Specimen collection in dermatophytosis:
- *Cutaneous lesion*: Advancing margin from center to edge across the margin
- *Vesicle or bulla*: Clip the roof and add to the specimen
- *Hair*: Basal root portion and proximal hair shaft
- *Nail*: Subungual debris or nail clips or white surface using nail drilling and/or skele curette

---

Box 4: Histological findings with H&E stain.

Histological findings in dermatophytosis:
- Spotty spongiosis, acanthosis, parakeratosis with occasional intraepidermal vesiculation[56]
- Mounds of parakeratosis contain neutrophils (neuts in the horn[49])
- Hyphae seen as long basophilic[57] structures (less as compared to *Candida* and *Malassezia species*) or refractile spaces in cornified layers (sandwich sign[58])
- Less common findings include superficial lymphocytic infiltrate[58] and occasionally deeper infiltrates[49]
- Presence of ectothrix and less often endothrix infection alongside surface infection[59]
- Occasional psoriasiform, vasculopathic, folliculitis involvement[49,59]

Note: Species identification and culture sensitivity studies may not be done as baseline and could be included only if resistance is suspected or multiple attempts to treat recalcitrant disease fails.

Generate a Prescription, Follow-up, Monitor, and Review

Prescription:
- Prescribe a "cidal" drug
- In absence or in case of contraindication, choose a fungistatic drug
- Avoid drugs that favor arthrospore formation
- Manage pruritus
- Manage barrier disruption or defect
- Do a dermatology life quality index (DLQI) baseline study.

While itraconazole and fluconazole have an extended spectrum of activity against yeasts, molds and dematiaceous fungi, they should, in principle, be used with restraint in the presence of another effective molecule; the relative efficacy of molecules is given in **Figure 36**.

Terbinafine[94] is a systemic allylamine with fungicidal activity against most dermatophytes. It is keratinophilic and lipophilic. Three points of concern with terbinafine are a variable range of MIC, low to fair C_{max}/MIC and AUC/MIC and high interindividual variability of C_{max} and AUC (0–24) values **(Table 12)**. It is indicated as a first line of systemic therapy especially for noninflammatory presentations of Tinea. Given at 5 mg/kg/day, it achieves concentrations above the MIC of most of dermatophytes. However, increasing it to 9 mg/kg increases the cure rate, in case of which a twice-daily dosing would be more appropriate. The T1/2 life of Terbinafine being in the range of 11.35–16.4 hours, coupled with the fact that the %T/MIC is 17.6 hours for T mentagrophytes with a MIC level above 0.001 μg/mL, it is compelling to dose the drug on a 12 hourly basis than at a 24 hourly interval especially when the up-dosing is indicated.[95]

Itraconazole is a triazole derivative that disrupts the synthesis of ergosterol. This highly lipophilic drug achieves a high bioavailability on a full meal. Capsules of itraconazole should be taken in a fed state or in patients with achlorhydria, it can be administered with a cola.[96] Paradoxically, a formulation consisting of solution should be administered in a fasting state wherein the bioavailability in more.[95] Despite being protein bound, it is extensively distributed in the cutaneous tissue. Having a high affinity for keratinized tissue, the tissue levels obtained after multiple doses are higher than the peak plasma levels. It is indicated as 5 mg/kg body weight per day over a period of 4–6 weeks.

There are proponents of fluconazole[97] and it may be good choice in patients with hyperhidrosis and Tinea pedis. This triazole blocks the synthesis of ergosterol by inhibiting cytochrome P450-dependent 14α-demethylase (Erg11). Fluconazole, being a small-sized molecule, it penetrates most tissues with exceptional penetrability in skin. With a bioavailability >90% and only 12% of the drug being bound to proteins and a long half-life of 24–30 hours, it can be dosed on a daily basis. >90% of the drug is excreted

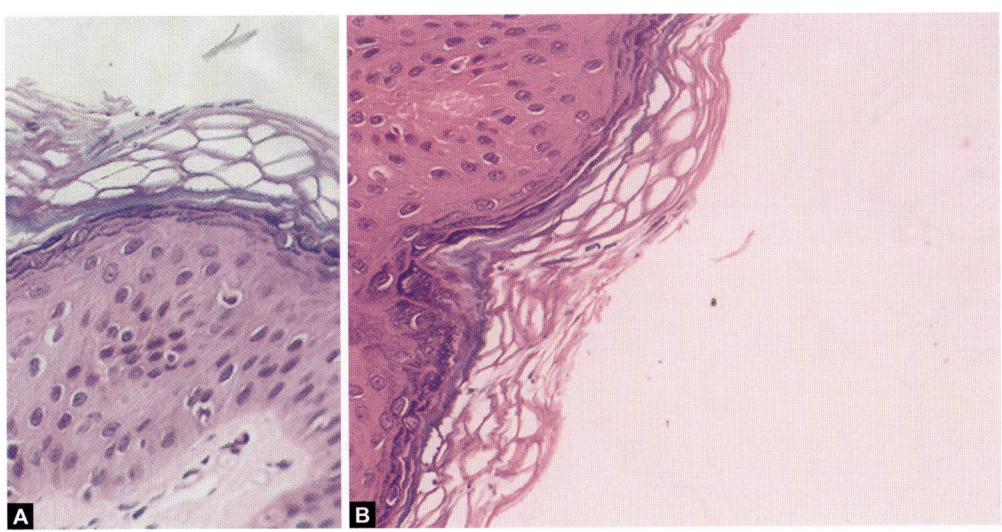

FIGS. 31A AND B: Hyphae high in stratum corneum disjunctum in Malassezia infection on H&E.
Courtesy: Dr Pratik Agarwal.

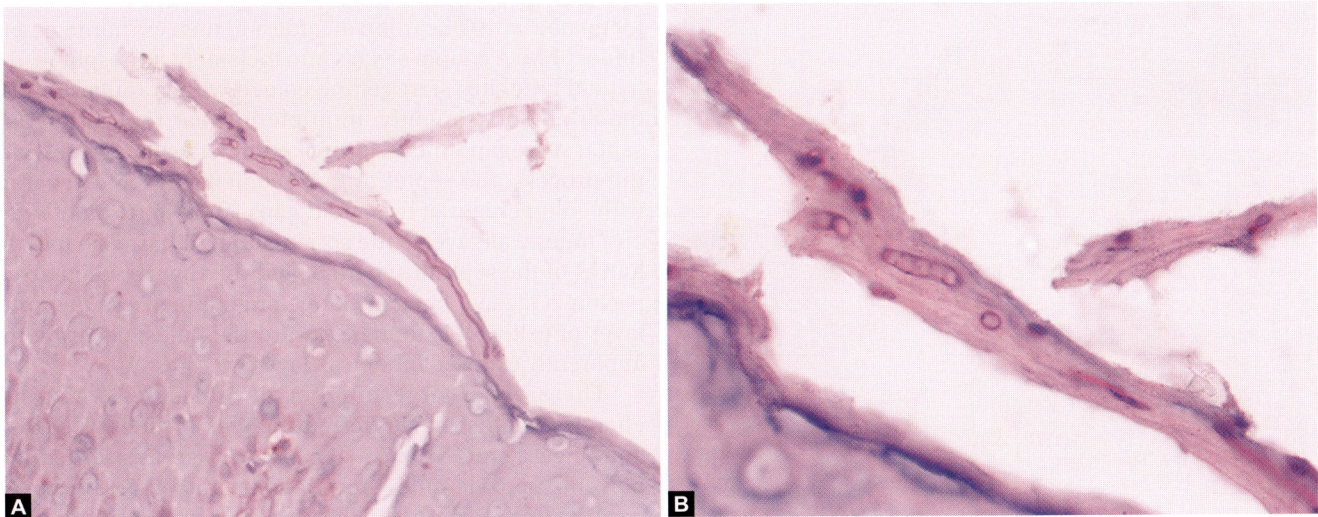

FIGS. 32A AND B: Red-stained hyphae with periodic acid Schiff.
Courtesy: Dr Pratik Agarwal.

via urine and the dose needs to be reduced in cases of renal insufficiency.

Table 13 depicts the recommended dosage schedule and the duration of treatment.[67] Following this, is tabulated (**Table 14**) the compatibility of these molecules.

COMBINATION THERAPY: A CAUTIOUS APPROACH

Attempts to study combination therapy in recalcitrant disease are underway but practitioners need to exercise caution while prescribing. There are certain pitfalls to combination therapy as under **Table 15**.

Drugs that Favor Arthrospore Formation

Whenever dermatophytes encounter a hostile environment, be it in vitro or in vivo, they change their form into metabolically inactive state. It has been shown that arthroconidia of T rubrum and T mentagrophytes appear to be more resistant to drugs than microconidia and may be one of the causes of therapeutic failure, mainly in patients whose lesions contain abundant arthrospores.

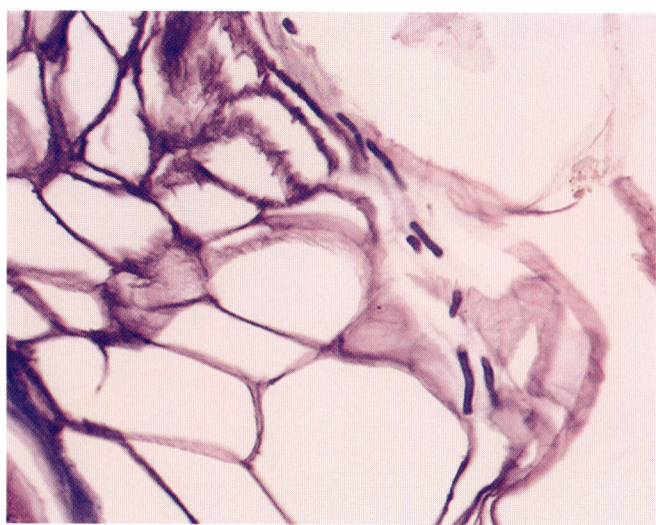

FIG. 33: Basophilic hyphae in S corneum seen in P versicolor with H&E stain.
Courtesy: Dr Pratik Agarwal.

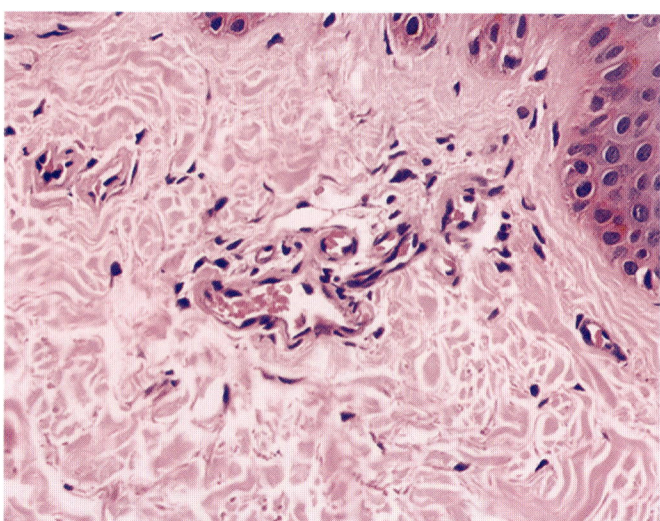

FIG. 35: Perivascular infiltrate in upper dermis with H&E stain in recurrent dermatophytosis.
Courtesy: Dr Pratik Agarwal.

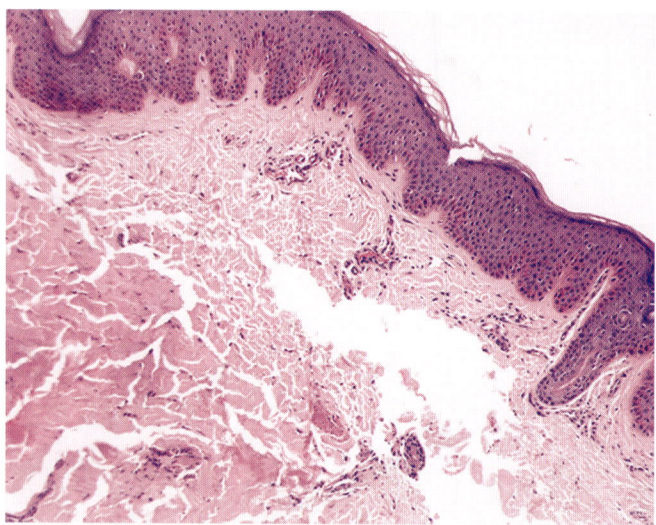

FIG. 34: Histological findings in recalcitrant dermatophytosis showing hyperkeratosis, zonal parakeratosis, acanthosis, spongiosis, exocytosis of neutrophils, and lymphocytes.
Courtesy: Dr Pratik Agarwal.

Antifungal molecules,[103] be they topical or oral preparations, which tend to favor arthrospore formation, should be best avoided **(Box 5)**.

Arthrosporogenesis[104] requires a temperature of 37°C with an increase in partial CO_2 tension. Temperature at the surface of the skin, around 33°C, is not conducive and any temperature <30°C stops the process of arthrosporogenesis.

Arthrospore formation of trichophyton mentagrophytes was studied by plating microconidia on SDA plates incubated with 8% carbon dioxide and then examining them under SEM. A couple of days into inclement atmosphere, the hyphal branches start getting coated with granular fibrillar material. Subsequently, multiple nuclear replication and septal segregation lead to thickening of walls. A week into the process, the septal units become round and separate with enlargement of triangular gaps at the junction of septa and outer wall layers. The sore assumes a barrel shape, the halves of the septum separate, and the ring is pulled apart, leaving a jagged, circular flange originating from the outer layer of cell wall extended toward the poles, covering the apparently exposed inner wall layer.[105]

There are a large number of molecules which are effective against naïve dermatophytes **(Table 16)**. These antifungal agents belong to the following groups: allylamine, polyene, benzylamine, morpholines, imidazoles, triazoles, oxaboroles, dimethoxycoumarin: griseofulvin and oxoborolehydroxamic acid: ciclopirox olamine.

While some molecules such as tioconazole, miconazole, butenafine, and terbinafine have shown mycological cure, others have provided with sustained cure. The molecules include like naftifine, miconazole, butenafine and terbinafine.[106] However, their role in recalcitrant dermatophytosis, if justified in mild disease, is recommended in most patients along with systemic agents not as a therapeutic molecule but as an agent that can prevent spread of the disease, something similar to the recommendation in Tinea capitis.

At the present time, dermatophytoma as a mass of hyphae resulting from biofilm has been demonstrated in Tinea unguium and further studies are needed to ascertain whether biofilm dispensers can be used on a day-to-day basis.

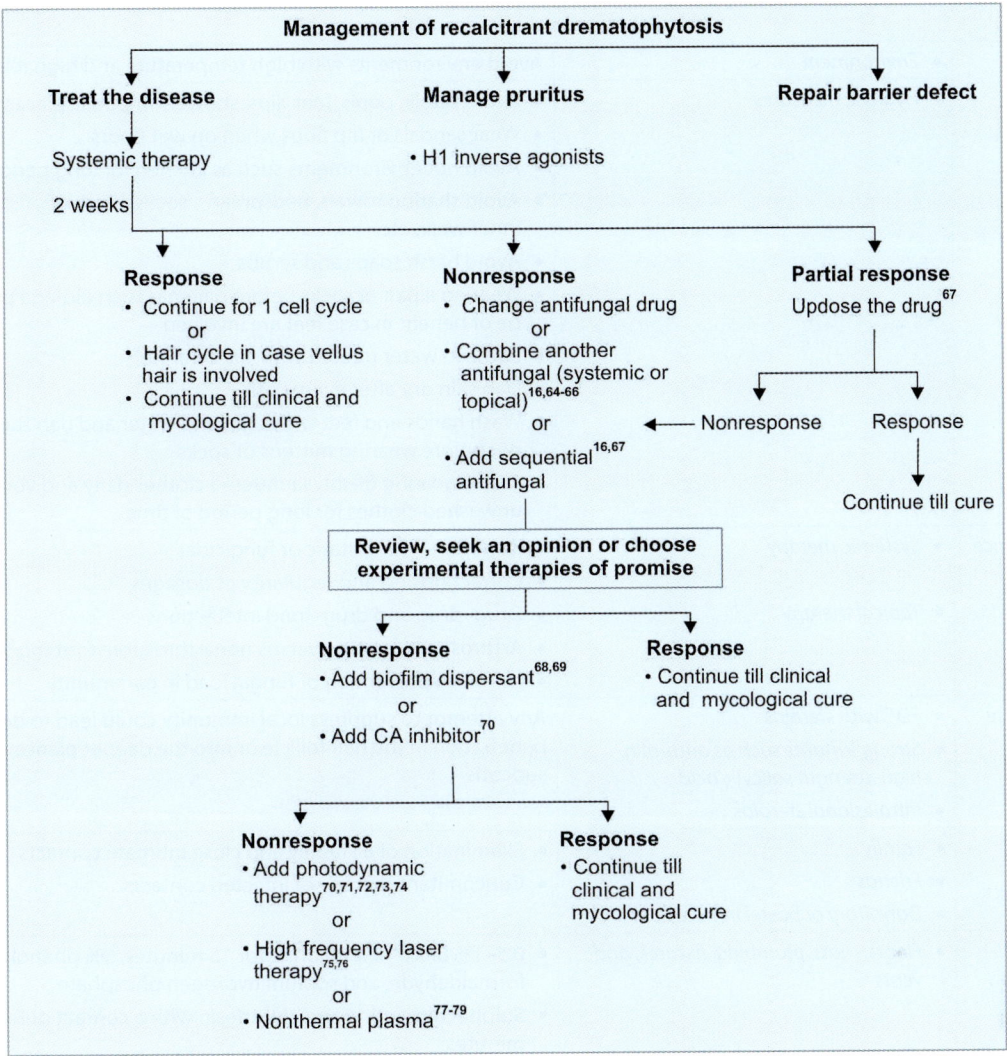

FLOWCHART 3: Schematic representation of the management of a case of Recalcitrant Dermatophytosis

Table 11: Preventive advice to patients with recalcitrant dermatophytosis.		
Inform	• *Diagnosis* • *Nature* • *Comorbidity* • *Duration of therapy* • *Outcome*	• Superficial dermatophytosis • Recalcitrance and purported difference with naïve disease • Specify comorbidity with leading questions for diabetes, atopy, thyroid dysfunction, hypertension, and renal disorders • Prolonged • Variable in treatment response and with possibility of recurrence
General measures	• *Clothing*	• Sweating for short duration (~20 minutes): Loose cottons • Prolonged sweating: Moisture management fabrics[82] such as Coolmax, Dri-FIT, and ClimaCool • Rainy or aquatic conditions: Gore-tex[83] • Prefer wearing loose clothes • Avoid tights, jockeys, leggings, and jeggings

Continued

Continued

	• Environment	Avoid environments with high temperature and high relative humidity
	• Hygiene measures	• Avoid public pools, feet dips, showers in public places • Wear sandals or flip flops when on wet floors • Avoid hot environments such as kitchen for long periods • Avoid sharing towels, bedspreads, socks, kerchiefs, footwear, inner wear, etc. • Avoid harsh soaps and scrubs • Wearing a pair of socks before pajamas is an old-age practice and may be of benefit in case feet are involved • Bathe in water treated with 1% chlorine[84] • Dab skin dry after every bath • Wash hands and feet with soap and water and dab them completely dry before wearing mittens or socks • Prefer wearing freshly laundered clothes daily and void wearing unwashed clothes for long period of time
Effective compliance of therapy	• Systemic therapy • Topical therapy	• Its nature—fungistatic or fungicidal • Correct dosing and regularity of dosages • Drug–drug and drug–food interactions • Arthrospore forming versus nonarthrospore forming topical agents • Its role in prevention of fungal load in community
Prevent drug abuse	• FDC with steroids • Strong irritants such as anthralin, high-strength salicylic acid • Intralesional steroids	Any attempt to suppress local immunity could lead to deeper penetration in the hair follicle or into the deeper planes of dermis or subcutis
Contact history	• Family • Friends • Dormitory or hostel inmates	• Examination of all family and close intimate contacts • Concomitant therapy of infected contacts

Disinfection	• Floors, mats, plumbing, fixtures, and vents
	
	Wooden surfaces
	• Animal contact
	   ○ Companion pets:
	
	   ○ Cattle:
	
	• Apparel:[85,86]
	   ○ Heavily soiled cotton or linen
	   ○ White cottons and linen
	   ○ Colored blends
	   ○ Silk and woolens
	
	• Accessories:[84]
	   ○ Hats
	   ○ Caps
		• 0.5–1% BAC,[84] 1% chlorine for 15 minutes, 5% phenol for 5 minutes, formaldehyde, and sodium hydrogen phosphate
		• Sulphochlorantine and chlordesin with a contact duration of 10–25 minutes[87]
		• 3% sulphochlorantine and chlordesin with a contact duration of 90 minutes[87]
		• Avoid clipping of hair coat with clippers, tack in infected dogs and cats
		• Avoid direct contact with infected pets
		• Lime sulfur 1:16 or enilconazole leave on rinse
		• Live-attenuated vaccine
		
		• Washing at 90° for 20–25 minutes, tumble dry, or sun dry
		• Washing at 60° for 20–25 minutes, tumble dry or sun dry
		• Avoid wearing or wash at 40° for 45 minutes with AOB detergent, tumble dry, and steam press
		• Avoid wearing or wash at 20° for 90 minutes with AOB* detergent, tumble dry, and steam press
		
		• 1% terbinafine spray, 1% bifonazole spray

Continued

Continued

	• *Footwear:*[87,88]	
	○ Socks	• White cotton socks at 80°, tumble dry
		• Colored socks and socks of other fabrics that cannot be treated at 80° can be treated in silver ion washing machine alone or in combination with UVA (395 nm) light[89]
	○ *Canvasses*[87]	• Sun dry for 3 days
		• Hexadecyl, mycodecidin, and Septonex spray with a contact 5–10 seconds every 7 days for 3 months after termination of therapy
		• Vapor heat treatment
	○ *Shoes, boots, tennis shoes, slippers, and gloves*[87]	• Chaotropic agents such as urea guanidinium salt
		• Dithiocarbamides, sulfonamides, benzothiazoles, and thiuramidodisulphides
		• Leather insoles of shoes and slippers treated with 8-hydroxyquinoline, parachlorometaxylenol, and chlorthymol[90]
		• In case of infection, it would be prudent to avoid wearing the same shoe daily after it has been dried in sunlight for a day after every wear
		• 5 liters of 0.1% formaldehyde formulated as formalin to be applied per meter square at temperatures ranging from 0 to 30°C for 3 consecutive days
	• *Soil decontamination*[87]	• Washed or wiped with 2% Amphyl
	• *Laboratory equipment:*	• Sealed in metal containers and discarded
	○ *Bench tops, capillary pipettes, microscopic slide preparations*[87]	
	○ *Petridish, test tubes*[87]	
Dietary advice	General counseling in the absence of therapeutic or preventive diet	• Patients with diabetes and foot involvement need to start low GI food.
		• Dietary restrictions for comorbidity, if any, to continue
		• β-*lactoferrin*-rich diet[91,92] may have a putative role
Occupation	Military personnel, miners and other who require wearing heavy boots for long hours	• Dusting feet with antifungal powder or undecylenic acid or with a combination of salicylic acid and benzoic acid or shoes and feet with a combination of hydroxyquinoline, sodium perborate, sodium borate, boric acid, and aluminum silicate twice daily before wearing socks[90]
		• 1% terbinafine spray (cidal effect),[84] 1% bifonazole spray (static effect)[84]
	Chefs and cooks	• Ensure cooking in well-ventilated kitchens so as to decrease perspiration
	Farmers exposed to conditions that favor sweating	• Wearing gumboots and avoid farm work barefooted
		• Taking a break during hours of intense sunlight, i.e., afternoons

*AOB: active oxygen bleach
(GI: gastrointestinal; UVA: ultraviolet A)

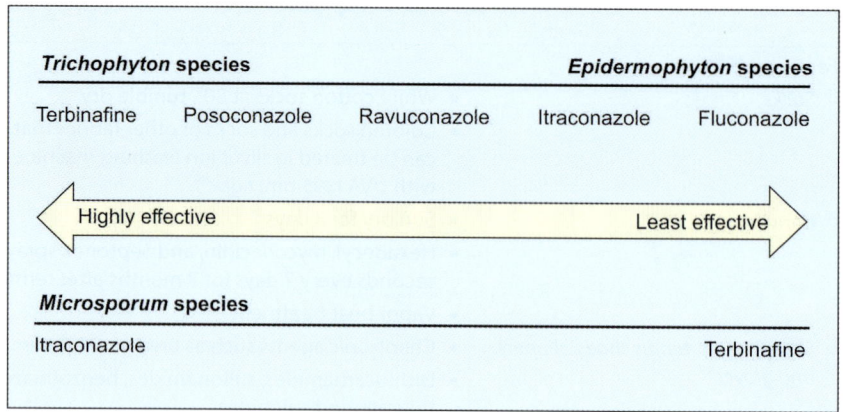

FIG. 36: Relative efficacy of antifungal drugs in dermatophytosis.

Table 12: The pharmacokinetics of systemic antifungal drugs.

Molecule	MIC	AUC	C_{max}	Tissue conc.				Drug class	Conc. dependent	Prolonged PAFE	PD index
				Sc	GT	GF	FN				
Terbinafine	0.0156–16	59.82	16.56	20				Polyene	Yes	Yes	C_{max}/MIC
Griseofulvin	0.032–256	86.18	6					Flucytosine	No	No	T>MIC
Itraconazole	0.009–4	154	22.8	0.5–8	1.6–20	0.1–0.5	0.6	Azole	No	Yes	AUC/MIC
Fluconazole	0.0625–256		2.9	11–40	0.8–1	X	1–2	Echinocandins	Yes	Yes	C_{max}/MIC; AUC/MIC
								Terbinafine	No	Yes	T/MIC

(AUC: area under the curve; MIC: minimum inhibitory concentration)

Table 13: Dosing Schedule in Recalcitrant disease.

Drug	Dosage	Schedule	Duration	Indication
Terbinafine**	5 mg/kg Up-dose till 9 mg/kg	Once daily[98] Twice, if up-dosed[95]	4–6 weeks	First-line therapy of choice
Itraconazole	3 mg/kg (solution)[61] 5 mg/kg	Once daily Twice daily[99]	4–6 weeks	First-line alternate therapy
Fluconazole*	2 mg/kg 3 mg/kg	Daily Biweekly	4–6 weeks	Add-on therapy or alternate T pedis with hyperhidrosis
Griseofulvin	20–25 mg/kg 10–15 mg/kg	q6 hourly q8 hourly	6–12 weeks	Add-on therapy

*Weekly administration of fluconazole shows inferior responses as compared to daily regimens.
**Relapse rate[100] after a short course of terbinafine has been found to be high.

Follow-up and review:
- Assess response treatment
- Keep a watch on adverse drug reactions **(Tables 17 and 18)**.
- In case of poor response titrate or change or add medication
- In case of no response, review diagnosis, sample for culture sensitivity and look out for resistance.
- Record clinical cure and mycological cure

An important aspect in management of recalcitrant disease is the judicious use of systemic antifungals, either alone or in combination, taking into account the comorbidities and the concomitant medicines used to manage them. We do not delve into the details as many authorities have dealt with the same in their articles.[94,111]

Dermatophytosis needs to be revisited in the wake of a surge in recalcitrant disease, newer reports of severe dermatophytosis in primarily and secondarily immuno-

Table 14: Compatibility of antifungal drugs with physiological and pathological states.					
	Compatibility in children	**Hepatic disease**	**Renal disease**	**Compatibility in pregnancy**[101]	**Side effects**
Terbinafine	Above 4 years	Halved	Avoided	Yes	*
Itraconazole	Caution	Reduction	No	Contraception recommended 2 months post-ITZ therapy	**
Fluconazole	6 months and above	No	Reduction avoided in dialysis patients	No	***

*Headache, gastrointestinal upset, SCLE, EM, AGEP, SJS, anterior optic neuropathy, dermatomyositis, autoimmune hepatitis, acute fulminant hepatic failure, and dysgeusia (protracted).
**Headache, rhinitis, sinusitis, upper respiratory tract infection, diarrhea, flatulence, abdominal pain, cystitis, myalgia, increased appetite, and liver function abnormality.
***Headache, transaminitis, AGEP, and TEN.
(AGEP: acute generalized exanthematous pustulosis; ITZ: itraconazole; SJS: Stevens–Johnson syndrome; TEN: toxic epidermal necrolysis)

Table 15: Pitfalls in combination therapy.	
Terbinafine and fluconazole[64]	A single dose of fluconazole at a strength of 100 mg per oral coadministered with terbinafine 250 mg is likely to increase the C_{max}, AUC (0–t_{last}) and AUC (0–∞) and at the same time decrease desmethyl terbinafine C_{max} to a significant degree that assumes statistical importance. Coadministration should be attempted with careful monitoring of liver enzymes especially AST and ALT
Further, CDR1 and -2 upregulated by terbinafine leading to fluconazole resistance in Candida infection. Whether it holds a similar potential for dermatophytes is not known
Terbinafine and griseofulvin[102]	No significant synergy noted in one trial
Terbinafine and itraconazole[65]	Synergistic effect on conidia and hyphae

(AUC: area under the curve; AST: aspartate aminotransferase; ALT: alanine aminotransferase)

Box 5: Efficacy of drugs against arthrospores.[103]

Drugs that are ineffective against dormant arthroconidia:
- Clotrimazole
- Nystatin
- Miconazole
- Griseofulvin

Drugs that favor arthroconidia at subinhibitory concentrations:
- Clotrimazole
- Amphotericin B
- Griseofulvin
- Betamethasone

Drugs that are effective against arthroconidia:
- **Terbinafine**
- **Itraconazole**

Table 16: Pharmacokinetics of topical antifungal agents.						
	MIC 90	**MIC GM**	**AUC**	**C_{max}**	**AUC/MIC90**	**Myco.cure**
Terbinafine	16	0.0156–16	17.38	313	1.08	95%(d84)92%
Luliconazole	0.004	0.00012–0.0025	0.0068	0.0004	1.7	
Eberconazole	2		28.03	1.684	14.015	
Oxiconazole	0.5		223.18	95.12	446	81%(d42)85%
Clotrimazole	4	0.0312–32	84.997	20.107	21.24	90%(d30)87%
Miconazole	4	0.03–>16	55.2	15.1	13.8	60%(60)58%
Tioconazole			455.964	12.242		
Bifonazole	>1	0.0078–32	45.5	0.713	45	93%(90)96%
Econazole	10	0.60–10	0.00344	0.000417	0.000344	
Sertaconazole	8	0.01–8	0.1114	0.011	0.001375	
Ketoconazole	1	0.016–0.13				
Amorolfine	4	0.0078–32		0.67		

Table 17: Monitoring of terbinafine.			
6–48 hours	Look for flare up and fever	• Paradoxical reaction[107] • Jarisch–Herxheimer-like reaction[108]	
At every visit	Look for vomiting, abdominal cramping, and cephalalgia		• Continue treatment if tolerable • Symptomatic treatment if needed
At 2 weeks	• Look for eye complaints • CBC and thin PS	• Anterior uveitis • Bilateral optic neuropathy • Leukopenia, neutropenia, pancytopenia, agranulocytosis	• Ophthalmologic reference • Discontinue treatment. Normalcy achieved within a month
At 4 weeks	• Liver function tests • CBC and thin PS	• Fulminant liver failure • Autoimmune hepatitis in patients with positive HbsAg • Leukopenia, neutropenia, pancytopenia, agranulocytosis	• Discontinue treatment • Levels normalize in 3 months-time[109] • Discontinue treatment • Normalcy achieved by the end of 1 week

(CBC: complete blood count; HBsAg: surface antigen of the hepatitis B; PS: peripheral smear)

Table 18: Monitoring of itraconazole.[110]			
At every visit	• Hypokalemia • Blood pressure • Look for muscular aches • Pedal edema • Complaints of neuropathy and tremors	• Resistant hypertension • Rhabdomyolysis • CCF • Peripheral neuropathy	• Continue treatment if tolerable • Symptomatic treatment if needed • Review for use of statins. Supplant statins • Stop medication • Pedal edema subsides by 6 months • Stop drug • Tremors continue for as long as 6 months
At 4 weeks	• Gastrointestinal disturbances • Liver function test	• Seen in 17.7% • Transaminitis • Raised alkaline phosphatase levels • Raised bilirubin levels	• Symptomatic treatment • Discontinue treatment • Normalcy achieved by the end of 3 weeks • Minimize by intermittent and short-term dosing

Note: Headache, rash, and injection site reactions need to be monitored in case itraconazole is administered intravenously.

deficient, discovery of dermatophytoma in nails, reports of resistance to systemic agents. Further, large-scale representative epidemiological studies need to be undertaken to measure the burden of disease, preventive strategies need to be designed for effective block on the dissemination of conidial, arthrospore, or chlamydospore forms.

REFERENCES

1. Naranjo-Ortiz MA, Gabaldón T. Fungal evolution: major ecological adaptations and evolutionary transitions. Biol Rev Camb Philos Soc. 2019;94(4):1443-76.
2. Havlickova B, Czaika VA, Friedrich M. Epidemiological trends in skin mycoses worldwide. Mycoses. 2008;51:2-15.
3. Cameron J, Jagals P, Hunter P, Pond K, World Health Organization, International Water Association. (2011). Valuing water, valuing livelihoods/edited by John Cameron… [et al]. [online] Available from https://apps.who.int/iris/bitstream/handle/10665/44635/9781843393108_eng.pdf?sequence=1&isAllowed=y. [Last accessed December, 2022]
4. Vena GA, Chieco P, Posa F, Garofalo A, Bosco A, Cassano N. Epidemiology of dermatophytoses: retrospective analysis from 2005 to 2010 and comparison with previous data from 1975. New Microbiol. 2012;35(2):207.
5. Balakumar S, Rajan S, Thirunalasundari T, Jeeva S. Epidemiology of dermatophytosis in and around Tiruchirapalli, Tamil Nadu, India. Asian Pacific J Trop Dis. 2012;2(4):286-9.
6. Kucheria M, Gupta SK, Chhina DK, Gupta V, Hans D, Singh K. Clinicomycological profile of dermatophytic infections at a tertiary care hospital in north India. Int J Com Health Med Res. 2016;2(2):17-22.

7. Iliev ID, Leonardi I. Fungal dysbiosis: immunity and interactions at mucosal barriers. Nat Rev Immunol. 2017;17(10):635-46.
8. Stockdale PM. Nutritional requirements of the dermatophytes. Biol Rev. 1953;28(1):84-104.
9. Kane J, Fisher JB. The effect of sodium chloride on the growth and morphology of dermatophytes and some other keratolytic fungi. Can J Microbiol. 1975;21:742-9.
10. Tokuda S, Yu AS. Regulation of epithelial cell functions by the osmolality and hydrostatic pressure gradients: a possible role of the tight junction as a sensor. Int J Mol Sci. 2019;20(14):3513.
11. Nikpey E, Karlsen TV, Rakova N, Titze JM, Tenstad O, Wiig H. High-salt diet causes osmotic gradients and hyperosmolality in skin without affecting interstitial fluid and lymph. Hypertension. 2017;69(4):660-8.
12. Martinez-Rossi NM, Peres NT, Bitencourt TA, Martins MP, Rossi A. State-of-the-Art Dermatophyte Infections: Epidemiology Aspects, Pathophysiology, and Resistance Mechanisms. J Fungi. 2021;7(8):629.
13. Kane JU, Sigler LY, Summerbell RC. Improved procedures for differentiating microsporumpersicolor from trichophyton mentagrophytes. J Clin Microbiol. 1987;25(12):2449-52.
14. Martinez DA, Oliver BG, Gräser Y, Goldberg JM, Li W, Martinez-Rossi NM, et al. Comparative genome analysis of Trichophyton rubrum and related dermatophytes reveals candidate genes involved in infection. MBio. 2012;3(5):e00259-12.
15. Verma S, Vasani R, Gupta S. Involvement of little discussed anatomical locations in superficial dermatophytosis sundry observations and musings. Indian Dermatol Online J. 2020;11(3):419.
16. Rouzaud C, Hay R, Chosidow O, Dupin N, Puel A, Lortholary O, et al. Severe dermatophytosis and acquired or innate immunodeficiency: a review. J Fungi. 2016;2(1):4.
17. Rajagopalan M, Inamadar A, Mittal A, Miskeen AK, Srinivas CR, Sardana K, et al. Expert consensus on the management of dermatophytosis in India (ECTODERM India). BMC Dermatol. 2018;18(1):1-1.
18. Verma S, Madhu R. The great Indian epidemic of superficial dermatophytosis: An appraisal. Indian J Dermatol. 2017;62(3):227.
19. Verma SB, Panda S, Nenoff P, Singal A, Rudramurthy SM, Uhrlass S, et al. The unprecedented epidemic-like scenario of dermatophytosis in India: I. Epidemiology, risk factors and clinical features. Indian J Dermatol Venereol Leprol. 2021;87(2):154-75.
20. Sharma R, Adhikari L, Sharma RL. Recurrent dermatophytosis: a rising problem in Sikkim, a Himalayan state of India. Indian J Pathol Microbiol. 2017;609(4):541-5.
21. Vineetha M, Sheeja S, Celine MI, Sadeep MS, Palackal S, Shanimole PE, et al. Profile of dermatophytosis in a tertiary care center. Indian J Dermatol. 2018;63(6):490.
22. Agarwal U, Saran J, Agarwal P. Clinico-mycological study of dermatophytes in a tertiary care centre in northwest India. Indian J Dermatol Venereol Leprol. 2014;80(2):194.
23. Bhagra S, Ganju SA, Kanga A, Sharma NL, Guleria RC. Mycological pattern of dermatophytosis in and around Shimla hills. Indian J Dermatol. 2014;59(3):268.
24. Bhatia VK, Sharma PC. Epidemiological studies on dermatophytosis in human patients in Himachal Pradesh, India. Springerplus. 2014;3(1):1-7.
25. Maulingkar SV, Pinto MJ, Rodrigues S. A clinico-mycological study of dermatophytoses in Goa, India. Mycopathologia. 2014;178(3-4):297-301.
26. Kaur R, Panda PS, Sardana K, Khan S. Mycological pattern of dermatomycoses in a tertiary care hospital. J Trop Med. 2015;2015:157828.
27. Poluri LV, Indugula JP, Kondapaneni SL. Clinicomycological study of dermatophytosis in South India. J Lab Physicians. 2015;7(02):084-9.
28. Hazarika D, Jahan N, Sharma A. Changing trend of superficial mycoses with increasing nondermatophyte mold infection: a clinicomycological study at a tertiary referral center in Assam. Indian J Dermatol. 2019;64(4):261.
29. Patro N, Panda M, Jena AK. The menace of superficial dermatophytosis on the quality of life of patients attending referral hospital in Eastern India: A cross-sectional observational study. Indian Dermatol Online J. 2019;10(3):262.
30. Hanumanthappa H, Sarojini K, Shilpashree P, Muddapur S. Clinicomycological study of 150 cases of dermatophytosis in a tertiary care hospital in South India. Indian J Dermatol. 2012;57(4):322.
31. Noronha TM, Tophakhane RS, Nadiger S. Clinico-microbiological study of dermatophytosis in a tertiary-care hospital in North Karnataka. Indian Dermatol Online J. 2016;7(4):264.
32. Olutoyin OO, Onayemi O, Gabriel AO. Risk factors associated with acquiring superficial fungal infections in school children in South Western Nigeria: a comparative study. African Health Sci. 2017;17(2):330-6.
33. Verma S, Vasani R, Reszke R, Matusiak Ł, Szepietowski JC. Prevalence and clinical characteristics of itch in epidemic-like scenario of dermatophytoses in India: a cross-sectional study. J Eur Acad Dermatol Venereol. 2020;34(1):180-3.
34. Pathania S, Rudramurthy SM, Narang T, Saikia UN, Dogra S. A prospective study of the epidemiological and clinical patterns of recurrent dermatophytosis at a tertiary care hospital in India. Indian J Dermatol Venereol Leprol. 2018;84(6):678-84.
35. Singh S, Verma P, Chandra U, Tiwary NK. Risk factors for chronic and chronic-relapsing tinea corporis, tinea cruris and tinea faciei: Results of a case-control study. Indian J Dermatol Venereol Leprol. 2019;85(2):197-200.
36. Daeschlein G, Rauch L, Haase H, Arnold A, Lutze S, von Podewils S, et al. Influence of nutrition, common autoimmune diseases and smoking on the incidence of foot mycoses. Hautarzt. 2019;70(8):581-93.
37. Mahajan S, Tilak R, Kaushal S, Mishra R, Pandey S. Clinico-mycological study of dermatophytic infections and their sensitivity to antifungal drugs in a tertiary care center. Indian J Dermatol Venereol Leprol. 2017;83(4):436-40.
38. Re III VL, Carbonari DM, Lewis JD, Forde KA, Goldberg DS, Reddy KR, et al. Oral azole antifungal medications and risk of acute liver injury, overall and by chronic liver disease status. Am J Med. 2016;129(3):283-91.
39. Das JK, Sengupta S, Gangopadhyay A. Dermatophyte infection of the male genitalia. Indian J Dermatol. 2009;54(5):21.
40. Thakur R, Kalsi AS. Updates on Genital Dermatophytosis. Clin Cosmet Investig Dermatol. 2020;13:743.
41. Grappel SF, Bishop CT, Blank F. Immunology of dermatophytes and dermatophytosis. Bacteriol Rev. 1974;38(2):222-50.
42. Bingol Kiziltunc P, Atilla H, Yalcindag FN. Accommodation Paralysis after Pheniramine Maleate Injection: A Case Report. Neuroophthalmology. 2013;37(6):257-9.

43. Denolle T, Azizi M, Massart C, Zennaro MC. Itraconazole: a new drug-related cause of hypertension. Ann Cardiol Angeiol (Paris). 2014;63(3):213-5.
44. Teaford HR, Saleh OM, Villarraga HR, Enzler MJ, Rivera CG. The many faces of itraconazole cardiac toxicity. Mayo Clin Proc Innov Qual Outcomes. 2020;4(5):588-94.
45. Karadi RL, Gow D, Kellett M, Denning DW, O'Driscoll RB. Itraconazole associated quadriparesis and edema: a case report. J Med Case Rep. 2011;5(1):1-4.
46. Khadka S, Joshi R, Shrestha DB, Shah D, Bhandari N, Maharjan M, et al. Amlodipine-Induced Pedal Edema and Its Relation to Other Variables in Patients at a Tertiary Level Hospital of Kathmandu, Nepal. J Pharm Tech. 2019;35(2):51-5.
47. HerizchiQadim H, Golforoushan F, Azimi H, Goldust M. Factors leading to dermatophytosis. Ann Parasitol. 2013;59(2):99-102.
48. Smith JD, BC-ADM CD. Cutaneous fungal infections. US Pharm. 2015;40(4):35-9.
49. Elewski BE. Chapter 118: The Dermatophytosis. In: Arndt KA, Leboit PE, Robinson JK, Wintroub BU (Editors). Cutaneous Medicine and Surgery, An integrated Programme in Dermatology. St. Louis: WB Saunders Co.; 1996; pp. 1043-55.
50. Ankad BS, Mukherjee SS, Nikam BP, Reshme AS, Sakhare PS, Mural PH. Dermoscopic characterization of dermatophytosis: A preliminary observation. Indian Dermatol Online J. 2020; 11(2):202.
51. Lee WJ, Kim JY, Song CH, Jung HD, Lee SH, Lee SJ, et al. Disruption of barrier function in dermatophytosis and pityriasis versicolor. J Dermatol. 2011;38(11):1049-53.
52. Jensen JM, Pfeiffer S, Akaki T, Schröder JM, Kleine M, Neumann C, et al. Barrier function, epidermal differentiation, and human β-defensin 2 expression in Tinea Corporis. J Invest Dermatol. 2007;127(7):1720-7.
53. Bhargava P, Nijhawan S, Singdia H, Mehta T. Skin barrier function defect-A marker of recalcitrant tinea infections. Indian Dermatol Online J. 2020;11(4):566.
54. Ardakani ME, Ghaderi N, Kafaei P. The diagnostic accuracy of potassium hydroxide test in dermatophytosis. J Basic Clin Med. 2016;5(2):4-6.
55. Levitt JO, Levitt BH, Akhavan A, Yanofsky H. The sensitivity and specificity of potassium hydroxide smear and fungal culture relative to clinical assessment in the evaluation of tinea pedis: a pooled analysis. Dermatol Res Pract. 2010;2010:764843.
56. Pinkus H, Mehregan AH. Chapter 13: Miscellaneous Papulosquamous Eruptions. A Guide to Dermatohistopathology, 3rd edition. New York: Appleton Century Crofts; 1981 pp. 151-62.
57. Guarner J, Brandt ME. Histopathologic diagnosis of fungal infections in the 21st century. Clin Microbiol Rev. 2011;24(2):247-80.
58. Gottlieb GJ, Ackerman AB. The "sandwich sign" of dermatophytosis. Am J Dermatopathol. 1986;8(4):347-50.
59. Patil PD, Pande S, Mahore S, Borkar M. Histopathology of hair follicle epithelium in patients of recurrent and recalcitrant dermatophytosis: A diagnostic cross-sectional study. Int J Trichol. 2019;11(4):159.
60. Woodfolk JA. Allergy and dermatophytes. Clin Microbiol Rev. 2005;18(1):30-43.
61. Patel NH, Padhiyar JK, Singh R, Patel T. Total serum IgE level in patients of dermatophytosis and its association with various clinical parameters. Indian J Dermatol Venereol Leprol. 2021;87(2):290-2.
62. Hay RJ. Chronic dermatophyte infections. I. Clinical and mycological features. Brit J Dermatol. 1982;106(1):1-7.
63. Shokri H, Mansouri P. Immediate hypersensitivity and serum IgE antibody responses in patients with dermatophytosis. Asian Pac J Allergy Immunol. 2012;30(1):40-7.
64. Nallani RS, Bhattaram A, Gobburu PT, Doddapaneni S. (2007). Clinical pharmacology review. [online] Available from https://www.accessdata.fda.gov/drugsatfda_docs/nda/2019/022075Orig1s000ClinPharmR.pdf. [Last accessed December, 2022]
65. Gupta AK, Konnikov N, Lynde CW. Single-blind, randomized, prospective study on terbinafine and itraconazole for treatment of dermatophyte toenail onychomycosis in the elderly. J Am Acad Dermatol. 2001;44(3):479-84.
66. Brescini L, Fioriti S, Morroni G, Barchiesi F. Antifungal combinations in dermatophytes. J Fungi. 2021;7(9):727.
67. Rengasamy M, Chellam J, Ganapati S. Systemic therapy of dermatophytosis: Practical and systematic approach. Clin Dermatol Rev. 2017;1(3):19-23.
68. Sen S, Borah SN, Bora A, Deka S. Rhamnolipid exhibits anti-biofilm activity against the dermatophytic fungi Trichophytonrubrum and Trichophyton mentagrophytes. Biotechnol Rep (Amst). 2020;27:e00516.
69. Pereira FD. A review of recent research on antifungal agents against dermatophyte biofilms. Med Mycol. 2021;59(4):313-26.
70. Supuran CT, Capasso C. A Highlight on the inhibition of fungal carbonic anhydrases as drug targets for the antifungal armamentarium. Int J Mol Sci. 2021;22(9):4324.
71. Chen B, Sun Y, Zhang J, Chen R, Zhong X, Wu X, et al. In vitro evaluation of photodynamic effects against biofilms of dermatophytes involved in onychomycosis. Front Microbiol. 2019;10:1228.
72. Calzavara-Pinton PG, Venturini M, Capezzera R, Sala R, Zane C. Photodynamic therapy of interdigital mycoses of the feet with topical application of 5-aminolevulinic acid. Photodermatol Photoimmunol Photomed. 2004;20(3):144-7.
73. Piraccini BM, Rech G, Tosti A. Photodynamic therapy of onychomycosis caused by Trichophyton rubrum. J Am Acad Dermatol. 2008;59(5):S75-6.
74. Baltazar LM, Ray A, Santos DA, Cisalpino PS, Friedman AJ, Nosanchuk JD. Antimicrobial photodynamic therapy: an effective alternative approach to control fungal infections. Front Microbiol. 2015;6:202.
75. Ghavam SA, Aref S, Mohajerani E, Shidfar MR, Moravvej H. Laser irradiation on growth of trichophyton rubrum: an in vitro study. J Lasers Med Sci. 2015;6(1):10.
76. Paasch U, Mock A, Grunewald S, Bodendorf MO, Kendler M, Seitz AT, et al. Antifungal efficacy of lasers against dermatophytes and yeasts in vitro. Int J Hyperthermia. 2013;29(6):544-50.
77. Švarcová M, Julák J, Hubka V, Soušková H, Scholtz V. Treatment of a superficial mycosis by low-temperature plasma: a case report. Prague Med Rep. 2015;115(1):73-8.
78. Lokajová E, Julák J, Khun J, Soušková H, Dobiáš R, Lux J, et al. Inactivation of dermatophytes causing onychomycosis using non-thermal plasma as a prerequisite for therapy. J Fungi. 2021;7(9):715.
79. Ouf SA, El-Adly AA, Mohamed AA. Inhibitory effect of silver nanoparticles mediated by atmospheric pressure air cold plasma jet against dermatophyte fungi. J Med Microbiol. 2015; 64(10):1151-61.
80. Šubelj M, Marinko JS, Učakar V. An outbreak of Microsporum canis in two elementary schools in a rural area around the

capital city of Slovenia, 2012. Epidemiol Infect. 2014;142(12): 2662-6.
81. Moriello KA, Coyner K, Paterson S, Mignon B. Diagnosis and treatment of dermatophytosis in dogs and cats. Clinical Consensus Guidelines of the World Association for Veterinary Dermatology. Vet Dermatol. 2017;28(3):266-8.
82. Ho CP, Fn J, Newton E, Au R. Improving thermal comfort in Apparel. In: Song G (Editors). Improving comfort in clothing. Amsterdam: Elsevier; 2011. pp. 165-81.
83. Elmogahzy YE. Finished fibrous assemblies. In: Elmogahzy YE (Editors). Engineering textiles: Integrating the design and manufacture of textile products. Sawston, United Kingdom: Woodhead Publishing; 2019. pp. 278-98.
84. Gupta AK, Ahmad I, Summerbell RC. Comparative efficacies of commonly used disinfectants and antifungal pharmaceutical spray preparations against dermatophytic fungi. Med Mycol. 2001;39(4):321-8.
85. Honisch M, Stamminger R, Bockmühl DP. Impact of wash cycle time, temperature and detergent formulation on the hygiene effectiveness of domestic laundering. J Appl Microbiol. 2014;117(6):1787-97.
86. Bockmühl DP, Schages J, Rehberg L. Laundry and textile hygiene in healthcare and beyond. Microbial Cell. 2019;6(7): 299.
87. Mackenzie DW, Loeffler W, Mantovani A, Fujikura T, World Health Organization. (1986). Guidelines for the diagnosis, prevention and control of dermatophytosis in man and animals/edited by DWR Mackenzie...[et al.]. [online] Available from https://apps.who.int/iris/bitstream/handle/10665/61519/WHO_CDS_VPH.86.67.pdf?sequence=1&isAllowed=y. [Last accessed December, 2022]
88. Gupta AK, Versteeg SG. The role of shoe and sock sanitization in the management of superficial fungal infections of the feet. J Am Podiatr Med Assoc. 2019;109(2):141-9.
89. Jung WK, Kim SH, Koo HC, Shin S, Kim JM, Park YK, et al. Antifungal activity of the silver ion against contaminated fabric. Mycoses. 2007;50:265.
90. Jamieson R, Mccrea A. Ringworm of the feet: shoes and slippers as a source of reinfection. Arch Dermatol. 1941;44:837.
91. Fernandes KE, Carter DA. The antifungal activity of lactoferrin and its derived peptides: mechanisms of action and synergy with drugs against fungal pathogens. Front Microbiol. 2017; 8:2.
92. Wakabayashi H, Uchida K, Yamauchi K, Teraguchi S, Hayasawa H, Yamaguchi H. Lactoferrin given in food facilitates dermatophytosis cure in guinea pig models. J Antimicrob Chemother. 2000;46(4):595-602.
93. Gupta AK, Kohli Y, Batra R. In vitro activities of posaconazole, ravuconazole, terbinafine, itraconazole and fluconazole against dermatophyte, yeast and non-dermatophyte species. Med Mycol. 2005;43(2):179-85.
94. Gupta AK, Ryder JE. The use of oral antifungal agents to treat onychomycosis. Dermatol Clin. 2003;21(3):469-79.
95. Sardana K, Gupta A. Rational for Drug Dosimetry and Duration of Terbinafine in the Context of Recalcitrant Dermatophytosis: Is 500 mg Better than 250 mg OD or BD? Indian J Dermatol. 2017;62(6):665-7.
96. Nett JE, Andes DR. Antifungal agents: spectrum of activity, pharmacology, and clinical indications. Infect Dis Clin. 2016; 30(1):51-83.
97. Felton T, Troke PF, Hope WW. Tissue penetration of antifungal agents. Clin Microbiol Rev. 2014;27(1):68-88.
98. Babu PR, Pravin AJ, Deshmukh G, Dhoot D, Samant A, Kotak B. Efficacy and safety of terbinafine 500 mg once daily in patients with dermatophytosis. Indian J Dermatol. 2017;62(4):395.
99. Mahajan H, Dhoot D, Barkate H. Clinical Assessment of Itraconazole in Dermatophytosis (CLEAR Study): A Retrospective Evaluation. Int J Sci Study. 2020;8(2):36-40.
100. Majid I, Sheikh G, Kanth F, Hakak R. Relapse after oral terbinafine therapy in dermatophytosis: a clinical and mycological study. Indian J Dermatol. 2016;61(5):529-33.
101. Pilmis B, Jullien V, Sobel J, Lecuit M, Lortholary O, Charlier C. Antifungal drugs during pregnancy: an updated review. J Antimicrob Chemother. 2015;70(1):14-22.
102. Singh S, Anchan VN, Raheja R. Futility of combining griseofulvin and terbinafine in current epidemic of altered dermatophytosis in India: Results of a randomized pragmatic trial. medRxiv. 2019. [online] Available from https://www.medrxiv.org/content/10.1101/19007617v1. [Last accessed December, 2022]
103. Farnoodian M, Yazdanparast SA, Sadri MF. Effects of environmental factors and selected antifungal agents on arthroconidia production in common species of Trichophyton genus and Epidermophytonfloccosum. J Biol Sci. 2009;9(6):561-6.
104. Emyanitoff RG, Hashimoto T. The effects of temperature, incubation atmosphere, and medium composition on arthrospore formation in the fungus Trichophyton mentagrophytes. Canadian journal of microbiology. 1979;25(3):362-6.
105. Bibel DJ, Crumrine DA, Yee K, King RD. Development of arthrospores of Trichophyton mentagrophytes. Infect Immunity. 1977;15(3):958-71.
106. Rotta I, Ziegelmann PK, Otuki MF, Riveros BS, Bernardo NL, Correr CJ. Efficacy of topical antifungals in the treatment of dermatophytosis: a mixed-treatment comparison meta-analysis involving 14 treatments. JAMA Dermatol. 2013;149(3):341-9.
107. Hryncewicz-Gwóźdź A, Wojciechowska-Zdrojowy M, Maj J, Baran W, Jagielski T. Paradoxical Reaction During a Course of Terbinafine Treatment of Trichophytoninterdigitale Infection in a Child. JAMA Dermatol. 2016;152(3):342-3.
108. Nikkels AF, Nikkels-Tassoudji N, Piérard GE. Oral Antifungal-Exacerbated Inflammatory Flare-Up Reactions of Dermatomycosis. Am J Clin Dermatol. 2006;7(5):327-31.
109. Maxfield L, Preuss CV, Bermudez R. (2020). Terbinafine. StatPearls [Internet]. [online] Available from https://www.ncbi.nlm.nih.gov/books/NBK545218/#:~:text=Terbinafine%20is%20an%20antifungal%20medication,for%20the%20treatment%20of%20onychomycosis. [Last accessed December, 2022]
110. Kurn H, Wadhwa R. (2021). Itraconazole. StatPearls [Internet]. [online] Available from https://www.ncbi.nlm.nih.gov/books/NBK557874/#:~:text=Itraconazole%20is%20a%20medication%20used,be%20detrimental%20to%20the%20immunocompromised. [Last accessed December, 2022]
111. Katz HI, Gupta AK. Oral antifungal drug interactions: a mechanistic approach to understanding their cause. Dermatol Clin. 2003;21(3):543-63.

SECTION 2

Observations in Dermatology: Signs, Faces and Phenomena in Dermatology

27
Cutaneous Signs in Dermatology

Vidya Kuntoji

INTRODUCTION

Clinical sign indicates observation or a physical finding made by the physician during examination of patients. It can most of the times be a signature mark left by a particular or group of conditions or diseases. While few of them are readily seen and can also be the presenting complaint of the patient, few others must be specifically looked for, keeping differential diagnosis in mind. Yet there are few signs which need to be elicited by certain maneuvers. While there are many signs that have been described many decades ago and are prevalent even today, the list of signs is increasing over the years which is in par with the varied presentation of skin disorders in the population and with the discovery of new dermatological conditions.

A total of 250 signs pertaining to skin have been described in the chapter, focusing mainly on clinical signs seen or elicited during examination. They are listed as per the category of dermatological disorders. Many are specific for a particular condition in the said category, yet there are few signs which are shared by multiple conditions. We have tried our best to include majority of the signs; however, an exhaustive description of all signs described in dermatology is beyond the purview of this chapter. Hence, additional reading has been suggested at the end of the chapter.

This chapter *excludes* the signs seen in dermoscopy, dermatopathology, and the majority of signs pertaining to hair, nails, and mucosa, which are described elsewhere in another chapter.

SIGNS IN DERMATOLOGY

Connective Tissue Disorder

Barnett's Sign (Scleroderma Neck Sign)[1,2]

Described by AJ Barnett.

It is observed in patients with *scleroderma*. The patient is made to sit in relaxed position with arms at sides and then asked to extend the head back by raising chin and looking upward. The sign is said to be positive if there is ridging and tightening of the neck skin that forms a visible and palpable tight band overlying the platysma.

Carpet Tack Sign (Tin Tack Sign or Cat Tongue Sign)[3,4]

The typical skin lesions of *discoid lupus erythematosus* include well-defined erythematous papules and plaques with partially adherent scales entering a patulous follicle. When scales are removed, their undersurface shows horny plugs that had previously occupied follicles. This clinical sign is described as Carpet Tack sign (tin tack sign or cat tongue sign). It is also observed in seborrheic dermatitis, pemphigus foliaceus, lymphoma, captopril-induced lichen planus, and cutaneous leishmaniasis.

Gottron Sign[5,6]

Described by Heinrich Adolf Gottron (1890–1974), a German dermatologist.

The sign refers to symmetric, occasionally scaling, violaceous, erythematous, or skin-colored macules or plaques over the extensor surfaces of the metacarpophalangeal and interphalangeal joints of the fingers in patients with *dermatomyositis*. Similar finding can also be seen over the bony prominences of the elbows, knees, and ankles and is considered to be the pathognomonic of dermatomyositis.

Heugh–Gottron Sign[7]

The sign refers to dystrophic and ragged cuticle seen in lupus erythematosus.

Heliotrope Sign[8]

The word heliotrope is derived from Greek (*Helio* meaning Sun and *Trepein* meaning to turn).

The sign refers to violaceous to dusky erythema with or without edema involving the periorbital skin symmetrically and is observed in patients with *dermatomyositis*. The heliotrope sign refers to the flower *Heliotropium*, a genus of flowering plants that includes the most representative species, *Heliotropium peruvianum*. The latter displays small fragrant purplish petals. The color heliotrope has been defined in relationship to this flower and has received specific color coordinates that are registered in A Dictionary of Color. The similarity between the hue of the periorbital rash of dermatomyositis and that of the petals of the flower justifies the use of the term heliotrope.

Holster Sign[9]

It refers to macular, erythematous to violaceous rash that affects the lateral aspects of hips and thighs with contour of a gun holster in patients with *dermatomyositis*.

Ingram's Sign[10]

It describes the inability to retract the lower eyelid in patients of progressive *systemic* sclerosis.

Inverse Gottron Sign[4]

The sign describes erythematous flat and ulcerated lesions on the palmar aspects of fingers, seen in *anti-melanoma differentiation-associated gene 5 (anti MDA5) antibody*-associated dermatomyositis. It is caused due to vasculopathy associated with the antibody-induced damage.

Keining Sign[11]

Named after Egon Keinig, German dermatologist (1892–1971).

The sign refers to bleeding nail fold in dermatomyositis.

Mizutani Sign (Round Finger Pad Sign)[12,13]

Described by Hitoshi Mizutani and Tomoko Mizutani.

The sign refers to the disappearance of the peaked contour on the finger pads and replacement with a hemisphere-like finger contour especially on ring fingers, observed in patients with Raynaud's phenomenon associated with *systemic sclerosis*.

Raccoon Sign[10]

The sign refers to erythematous, slightly scaly eruption on the face and periorbital skin, seen in *neonatal lupus erythematosus*. It is also termed as owl-eye/eye mask.

Periorbital hemorrhage seen after proctoscopic examination (postproctoscopic periorbital purpura) in patients with *systemic amyloidosis* is described as Raccoon eyes/sign/panda sign.

Raynaud Sign[6]

Described by Maurice Raynaud, French Physician (1834–1881).

It refers to the finding of digital cyanosis that occurs with exposure to cold temperatures or emotional stress. Raynaud sign is considered a physical manifestation of recurrent vasospasm of the fingers and toes, which is episodic and bilateral in nature. It is characteristic finding of Raynaud phenomenon. Secondary Raynaud phenomenon involves Raynaud sign in association with systemic disease. It is seen in systemic sclerosis, systemic lupus erythematosus (SLE), dermatomyositis, Buerger disease, arteriosclerosis, hematologic syndromes such as cryoglobulinemia, cold agglutinin disease, drugs such as beta-adrenergic blockers and nicotine.

Samitz Sign[14]

Described by Morris H Samitz.

The sign refers to thickening, roughness, hyperkeratosis, and irregularity of the cuticle with minimal or no redness nor inflammation.

Shawl Sign (Posterior Neck and Shoulder)[10]

The sign is observed in patients with *dermatomyositis*, and it refers to confluent, symmetric, macular violaceous erythema on the posterior shoulders and neck, which gives a distinctive shawl-like appearance.

Shuster's Sign[15]

Described by Sam Shuster in 1981.

It indicates cribriform scarring of the concha due to lesions of *discoid lupus erythematosus* (**Fig. 1**).

Stafne Sign[10,16]

It is seen in *progressive systemic sclerosis*. Widening of the periodontal ligament space secondary to increase in the collagen synthesis and increase in the bulk of the ligament, this is accommodated at the expense of alveolar bone, thus causing an increase in the width of the periodontal ligament space.

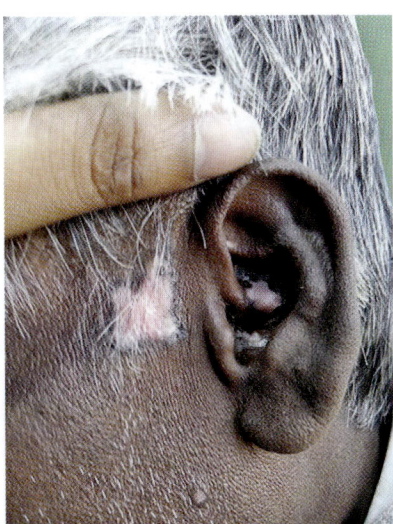

FIG. 1: Shuster's sign: Scarring of concha due to scaly depigmented scaly plaque of discoid lupus erythematosus (DLE). Similar plaque with hyperpigmented border is seen on face.
Courtesy: Dr Uttam Kumar Lenka, Consultant Dermatologist, Kolkata.

V Sign[17,18]

It refers to confluent macular erythema in a V shape over the lower anterior neck and upper anterior chest seen in patients with *dermatomyositis*.

Dermatitis/Eczema

Allergic Salute Sign[19,20]

The sign is seen in patients with atopic dermatitis, especially in children who develop atopic conditions such as allergic rhino conjunctivitis as they approach school age. The sign refers to transverse nasal crease caused by the upward hand rubbing or stroking of the nose precipitated by nasal symptoms such as itch.

Black Dot Sign[21]

Poison ivy dermatitis is characterized by a generalized erythematous pruritic rash in a linear distribution. Black spot poison ivy presents in a similar way. In addition, there will be black macules surrounded by erythema. Oleoresin in the sap of *Toxicodendron* plants, when exposed to air, produces the coal-black discoloration.

Butterfly Sign[22]

It denotes an area of normal or relatively hypopigmented skin over back owing to its inaccessibility to being scratched by patients of generalized pruritus. The sign has been described in cases of hepatobiliary disorders, atopic dermatitis, prurigo nodularis, Vagabond disease, and acne excoriee.

Dennie Sign, Dennie–Morgan Sign[23]

Described by Charles Clayton Dennie by American dermatologist (1883–1971).

A secondary crease in the lower eyelids. A sign of atopic dermatitis. Also known as Morgan's line.

Dirty Neck Sign[24]

It refers to reticulate pigmentation of the anterior or anterolateral aspect of neck seen in patients with *atopic eczema*. Due to its resemblance to unwashed skin, the label "dirty neck" was given. The pigmentary changes are secondary to melanin incontinence.

Earlobe Sign[25]

It is observed in patients who develop *contact dermatitis* to a substance applied with the hand to the face and neck. While the earlobe on the ipsilateral side is spared, the contralateral ear lobe is affected. This pattern is secondary to the hand-sweeping movement made during application of the substance.

Freund Sign[26]

Described by Emanule Freund, an Italian physician, 1869–1940.

It refers to brownish to reddish discoloration of the neck and sometimes the arms due to applying perfume or cologne to the skin and subsequent exposure to sunlight. Sometimes the skin first turns red before changing to a brownish color. Many perfumes and colognes contain oil of bergamot.

Synonym: Bergamot disease, Freund dermatitis, berloque dermatitis, eau de cologne dermatitis, photodermatitis pigmentaria, Pigmentation en coulée, breloque en collier, and toilet water dermatitis.

Headlight Sign[19]

It is seen in atopic dermatitis in children. Bilateral erythematous plaques on the cheeks with characteristic sparing of the nose give the appearance like a headlight due to prominence of nose.

Nose Sign (Pavithran Nose)[27]

Described by Pavithran K in 1988.

The sign refers to complete absence of erythema and scaling of the nose and perinasal areas in patients with *exfoliative dermatitis*.

Paget's Eczema Sign[28]

Named after Sir James Paget, English surgeon (1814–1899).

It refers to eczema of the areola, associated with breast cancer. Also known as eczema sign.

School Chair Sign[29]

The sign denotes the presentation of *allergic contact dermatitis* to nickel, when the rash occurs over the posterior thighs, corresponding to contact with a school chair.

Genodermatoses

Albright's Dimple Sign[30,31]

Described by Fuller Albright (1900–1969).

It is observed in *Albright's hereditary osteodystrophy* and refers to dimpling over the knuckles, enhanced by clenching of the fist. It results from underdeveloped metacarpal heads.

Buttonhole Sign[10,31]

It is mainly described in *type 1 neurofibromatosis (Von Recklinghausen's disease)*. It refers to the sensation of inserting the finger into a buttonhole after invaginating the cutaneous neurofibroma into the underlying dermal defect with digital pressure. This occurs owing to the soft myxoid stoma and dermal defect caused by the protruding tumor. The sign is also observed in *anetoderma, dermatofibroma, and old pigmented nevi*.

Crowe' Sign[6,32]

Described by Frank W Crowe, American physician in 20th century.

The sign refers to axillary freckling, which is one of the defining features of *type 1 neurofibromatosis*. It typically develops at a later age than café-au-lait macules.

Gorlin Sign[33]

The sign is accredited to Robert James Gorlin, an American oral pathologist and geneticist.

It is used to describe the ability to touch the tip of the nose with the extended tongue and is seen in patients with *Ehlers–Danlos syndrome*.

Molluscum Pendulum Necklace Sign[4,34]

It is seen in tuberous sclerosis complex (TSC). The sign refers to multiple molluscum pendulum (soft pedunculated growths; acrochordons) arranged linearly in a necklace pattern on the neck. Similar pedunculated growths can also be seen in axilla and groin in TSC.

Patrick Yesudian Sign[35]

Described by Yesudian et al. in 1984.

This sign is seen in *neurofibromatosis type 1* and refers to multiple palmar melanotic macules (palmar freckling) **(Fig. 2)**.

Reverse Namaskar Sign[36]

Described by Premalatha et al. in 2010.

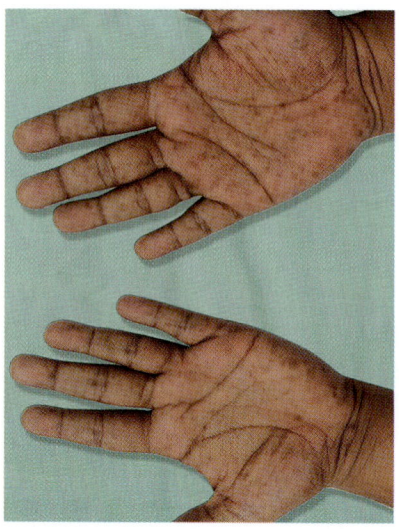

FIG. 2: Patrick Yesudian sign: Multiple melanotic macules involving both palms.
Courtesy: Dr Vijayalakshmi Kasiraman, Dermatologist.

The sign refers to the ability of patients with *Ehlers–Danlos syndrome* to fold the forearms at the back and palms facing each other in a way to do *Namaskar*.

Thumb Sign (Steinberg Sign)[37,38]

Described by Parker and Har in 1945, thumb sign was named as Steinberg sign in 1966, because he first proposed the thumb sign as a screening test for Marfan syndrome.

The sign confirms arachnodactyly in patients with *Marfan syndrome*. It is elicited by asking the patient to fold his thumb into the closed fist. If the thumb tip extends from the palm of the hand, the test is positive. It can also be seen in small proportion of normal children and in other collagen vascular diseases such as Ehlers–Danlos syndrome.

Umbilical Sign[10]

It is seen in *Marfan syndrome* and refers to the unusual ability to touch the umbilicus with the right hand, crossing the back, and approaching from the left side. It indicates increased length of upper extremity.

Wrist Sign (Walker-Murdoch Sign)[37,38]

Described by Bryan A Walker and J Lamont Murdoch in 1970.

The wrist sign indicates hypermobility and arachnodactyly, which is suggestive of *Marfan syndrome*.

It is elicited by asking the patient to grip his wrist with his opposite hand. If the thumb and fifth finger of the hand overlap with each other, the sign is positive.

Keratinization Disorders

Antenna Sign[10]

It is seen in *keratosis pilaris* in which individual follicles show a long strand of keratin glinting when examined in tangentially incident light **(Fig. 3)**.

Auspitz Sign[10,31]

It is named after Heinrich Auspitz, an Austrian dermatologist (1835-1886). Both Devergie Jeune [1860 and Hebra (1845)] observed this clinical sign before Auspitz, as did Robert Willan (1808), Joseph Plenck (1776), and Daniel Turner (1736).

The sign signifies the appearance of a red, glossy surface with pinpoint bleeding on removal of the scale in patients with *psoriasis* by scraping or scratching. It is also seen in *Darier's disease* and *actinic keratosis*.

Cornflake Sign[39]

The sign is observed in *Kyrle's and Flegel's disease* and it refers to the polygonal irregular configuration of the lesions that occur over the lower extremities

Fountain Sign[40]

Described by Dhar S in 1997.

This sign is mostly seen in *lichen planus hypertrophicus* lesions of <2 years' duration. While injecting intralesional steroids by a 26 G needle, it has been often found that the medicine comes out through the follicular openings in a jet mimicking a "fountain."

Igneous Rock Sign[21]

Hypertrophic lichen planus usually presents as verrucous plaque with scales at its edge on anterior shin. Superficial inspection of the lesion often suggests psoriasis or a keratinocyte neoplasm rather than lichen planus, but the typical appearance that resembles rapidly cooled igneous rock may be useful in suggesting lichen planus over a keratinocyte neoplasms.

Last Membrane Sign (Oblaten Sign)[41]

Described by Lucius Duncan Bulkley American physician, 1845-1928.

The sign is elicited in psoriasis. When all scales are removed, moist, thin, translucent layer of skin (de Duncan Buckley membrane) covering the lesions is seen.

Infections and Infestations

Arthropod Infections

Breakfast, Lunch and Dinner Sign[10]

The bites of bed bugs (*Cimex lectularius*) usually follow a linear pathway in a group of three to five blood meals and are often referred to as "breakfast, lunch, and dinner" or "breakfast, lunch, and supper" sign **(Fig. 4)**.

Comet Sign[42]

Dermatitis caused by *Pyemotes* species (a parasite of the furniture beetle) presents as erythematous pruritic macules or urticated plaques surmounted by vesicles; occasionally, they may be bullous. These lesions are sometimes associated with a specific linear erythematous macular tract and hence called the "comet sign."

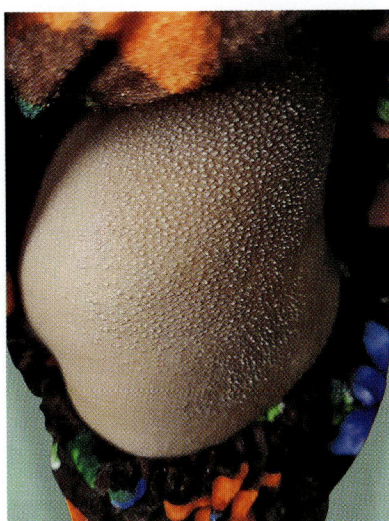

FIG. 3: Antenna sign: Individual follicles of keratosis pilaris showing a strand of keratin glinting when examined in tangentially incident light.
Courtesy: Dr Nitin Mishra, Associate Professor, Department of Dermatology, SRMS IMS Bareilly.

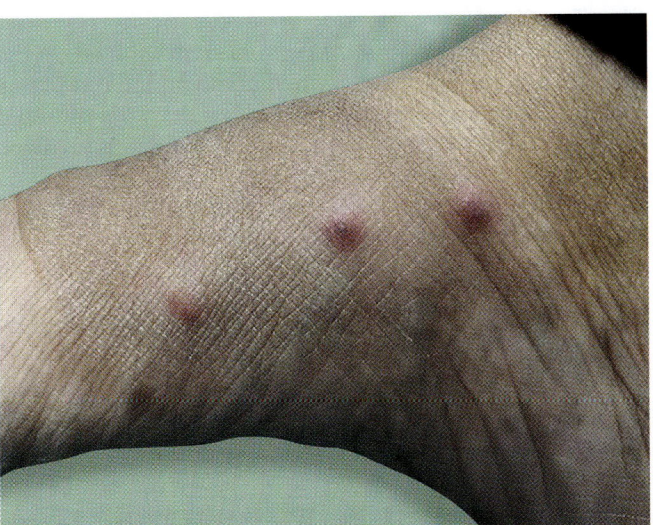

FIG. 4: Breakfast, lunch, and dinner sign: The bites of bedbugs following a linear pathway in a group of three blood meals.
Courtesy: Dr Bhushan Madke, Professor and Head, Department of Dermatology, MGIMS Wardha.

Eyelid Sign[43]
It is considered as a subtle clue to bedbugs as the culprit insect in *arthropod assaults* on children. The sign refers to a bite on the upper eyelid with associated erythema and ipsilateral upper eyelid edema.

Greenhow's Sign (Vagabond's Sign or Vagrant's Sign)[44]
It is also known as parasitic melanoderma, this sign represents excoriations and discoloration of skin caused by irritation of *body lice*.

Pullback Sign of Ashish[45]
In many cases of *blister beetle dermatitis*, even on mild touch over the affected area, patient will feel burning sensation and he will immediately pull back the touched body part. This sign is named as "Pullback sign of Ashish." This sign may be positive in few other conditions with localized hyperesthesia. It may be due to voluntary reaction due to hyperesthesia over inflamed area. This sign helps a lot in suspected cases of blister beetle dermatitis, where diagnosis is confusing.

Wake Sign[46]
Scabies burrows are the only pathognomonic lesion for *scabies*. They often occur on the creases of the palms and are followed by a pattern of scale reminiscent of the "wake" left on the surface of water by a moving bird or a ship. The wake sign is useful because (1) it is specific for scabies, (2) it is sufficiently large to be found by the naked eye, and (3) it points toward the location of the mite and its products.

Bacterial Infections

Blue Toe Sign[47,48]
In patients with *acrodermatitis chronica atrophicans* in the early stage, there is a vague erythema with minimal swelling. Usually the changes are sharply bordered, with a blue-red tint and slowly expand. Sometimes only digit is involved initially, it is termed as blue-term sign.

Blue toe sign has also been described as the initial manifestation of *popliteal artery aneurysm*.

Borsari's Sign[46,49]
Described by French physician Giovanni Battista Borsieri de Kanfield.

The sign is observed in the early stages of *scarlet fever* and it refers to white line produced by a fingernail being drawn along the skin quickly turning red.

Berliner Sign[21]
It is described in *roseola infantum* and refers to a characteristic "sleepy" appearance that results from associated palpebral edema. The latter is not related to ocular pathology and there is no periorbital swelling, the edema is confined only to eyelids. This sign is often useful in the pre-eruptive diagnosis of roseola infantum which disappears mostly 24 hours after an appearance of the rash.

Filipovitch-Skibnevski Sign[6]
Described by V Filipovitch, Odessa physician and Skibnevski, Russian physician in 1893.

It denotes yellowish discoloration of prominent parts of *palms and soles* seen in *typhoid fever*.

Hypopyon Sign[10,50]
It refers to the presence of small, discrete, vesicles either flaccid or tense that become secondarily infected and pus accumulates in the lower half of the pustule **(Fig. 5)** It is a clinical sign seen in *pyodermas and subcorneal pustular dermatosis (Sneddon–Wilkinson disease) and secondarily infected other vesiculobullous disorders* [e.g., pemphigus, bullous pemphigoid, and linear immunoglobulin A (IgA) dermatosis]. A transverse fluid level comprising purulent material at the bottom is seen when the patient is in erect position.

Milian's Ear Sign[51]
It refers to ear involvement in *erysipelas* and helps to distinguish erysipelas from cellulitis of the facial region. Ear does not contain deeper dermal tissue and subcutaneous fat and hence its involvement suggests erysipelas and not cellulitis.

Milk Sign (Scarlet Milk Sign)[52]
This sign indicates brightly flushed face with circumoral pallor seen in *scarlet fever*.

Myer Sign[52]
It denotes numbness and formication of both hands found in *scarlet fever*.

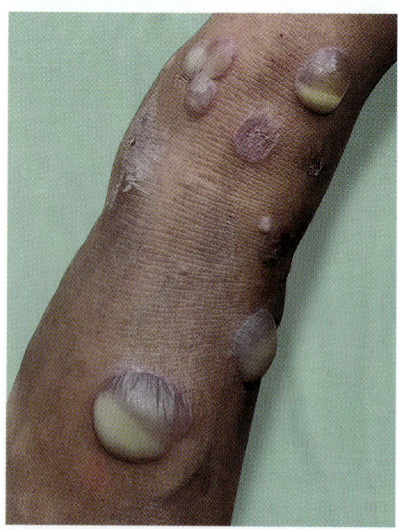

FIG. 5: Hypopyon sign: A transverse fluid level comprising purulent material in the lower half of tense and flaccid bullae.
Courtesy: Dr VK Chawla, Dermatologist, Skin and VD Institute, Bareilly.

Oyster Blister Sign[52]
This refers to the presence of bullous skin lesions, caused by the zoonotic *vibriosis* diseases (*Vibrio vulnificus*) contained in raw oysters, mussels, crabs, and shrimp.

Pastia's Sign (Thomson Sign)[31]
It is described by Constantin Chessec Pastia (1893-1926), a Roman physician. It is also known as Thomson sign, named after the British physician Frederick Holland Thomson (1867-1938).

It refers to pink or red transverse lines formed out of confluent petechiae seen in the antecubital fossae and axillary folds and are seen in the pre-eruptive stage of *scarlet fever*. These lines persist through the eruptive stage and remain as pigmented lines after desquamation.

Rudolph Sign[53]
It refers to recurrent exquisitely tender unilateral erythema and edema of the nasal tip observed in *nasal vestibular furunculosis*. The name of the sign refers to Rudolph, red-nosed reindeer.

Mycobacterial Infections

Apple Jelly Sign[54,55]
It denotes yellowish-brown granulomatous appearance seen on diascopy, resembling apple jelly and indicates collection of tubercles in dermis with degenerative changes. The sign is characteristically seen in *lupus vulgaris* and also has been described in sarcoidosis and lupoid cutaneous leishmaniasis.

Delmege Sign[52]
Deltoid flattening, most likely due to chronic cough, is said to be an early sign of *pulmonary tuberculosis*.

Turkey Ear Sign[56]
It refers to massively enlarged earlobe with bluish-red or violaceous indurated plaques or nodules. This sign is mainly described in *lupus vulgaris*, and is also seen in sarcoidosis, leprosy, and leishmaniasis.

Fungal Infections

Cayenne Pepper Pus Sign[52]
This sign indicates *actinomycosis* where cayenne pepper granules are observed with drops of pus.

Ear Sign[57]
The presence of erythematous and scaly well- to ill-defined papules and plaques over helix, antihelix, and retroauricular region in *tinea capitis* is described as ear sign.

Scratch Sign (Coup D'ongle Sign, Besnier's Sign, Stroke of the Nail)[58]
This sign is elicited in patients with *pityriasis versicolor*. It is characterized by asymptomatic hypopigmented or hyperpigmented macules and patches and produces fine scales (branny/furfuraceous). Often the scale is not visible. An important diagnostic clue may be the loosing of barely perceptible scale with a fingernail, which is called as the scratch sign. This sign may be negative if patient has taken recent bath or in case of treated lesion, in which case, only hypopigmentation persists.

Parasitic Diseases

Calabar Sign[59]
It refers to transient pruritic subcutaneous Calabar swellings, which mark the migratory course of the adult filarial eye worm, *Loa* through the tissues.

Chagas-Mazza Romana Sign or Romana Sign or Eye Sign[31]
The sign is named after Cecilio Romana (1899-1983), an Argentinian researcher. However, the credit for the recognition of this sign for its specificity in diagnosing Chagas' disease belongs to Emanuel Dias (1908-1962) and Evandro Chagas (1905-1940).

Romana sign refers to severe unilateral conjunctivitis and palpable, painless lid edema, which is the first clinical sign of sensitization response to the bite of the *Trypanosoma cruzi*. It is often associated with preauricular lymphadenopathy and inflammation of the tear gland.

Hanging Groin Sign[60]
It is seen in *onchocerciasis*. Progressive enlargement of lymph nodes in groin leads to inelastic and atrophic skin in the affected area which along with enlarged lymph nodes gives the appearance of hanging groins.

Leopard Skin Sign[52,61]
Repeated episodes of dermatitis associated with death of microfilariae leading to depigmentation is described as leopard skin sign in *onchocerciasis*.

Lizard Skin Sign[52,60,61]
It is seen in onchocerciasis and refers to appearance of skin like an old person, resembling lizard skin. It is due to the subcutaneous fibrosis, skin atrophy, and pigmentary changes in *onchocerciasis*.

Long Scar Sign[41]
It is seen in *onchocerciasis* and it refers to livid white blotches and scars on the shins and ankles from constantly scratching.

Pitaluga Sign[62]
It refers to trichomegaly (hypertrichosis of eyelashes) in patients of *visceral leishmaniasis (kala azar)*.

Seat Rash Sign[52]
It refers to urticarial lesion over buttocks seen in infection with strongyloides stercoralis.

Thumbprint Sign[39]

It is seen in patients with *disseminated strongyloidiasis* and refers to periumbilical purpura resembling multiple thumbprints. Respiratory assistance when given in such patients results in a transient rise in portal pressure, shunting portal blood through the periumbilical shunt. At this location, the larvae cause extravasation of red blood cells into the dermis, resulting in the characteristic petechiae and purpura.

Volcano Sign[52]

The classical appearance of evolved lesion of *old world cutaneous leishmaniasis (oriental sore)* is an enlarged nodule with central ulceration with crusting. The lesion is surrounded by the rim of erythema and is termed "volcano sign" due to its resemblance to an erupted volcano.

Winterbottom's Sign[63]

Described by Thomas Winterbottom, an English physician (1765–1859).

The sign refers to the occasionally visible enlargement of lymph nodes in the posterior cervical group, which is seen in the Gambian form of *African trypanosomiasis*. There are three stages of the infection, with Winterbottom's sign seen in the second stage that occurs 6–8 weeks into the disease.

Viral Infections

Blueberry Sign[64]

Synonym: Blueberry muffin baby or rash.

It refers to neonatal eruption characterized by non-blanching, blue red macules or firm dome-shaped papules (2–8 mm diameter) due to extramedullary (dermal) erythropoiesis. They are typically seen in infection with toxoplasma, rubella, cytomegalovirus, and herpes simplex virus. This sign is also observed in noninfectious conditions such as hematological dyscrasias, neonatal neuroblastoma, congenital alveolar rhabdomyosarcoma, neonatal lupus erythematosus, and congenital Langerhans cell histiocytosis.

Bote Sign[65,66]

It is an acronym for beginning of the end. The sign emphasizes that the inflammation in *molluscum contagiosum* represents a host response that often precedes resolution of the viral disease, rather than secondary bacterial superinfection and hence does not need additional antibacterial treatment.

Chik Sign[67,68]

Described by Riyaz N et al. in 2010.

A peculiar brownish hyperpigmentation in a centrofacial distribution, especially involving the nose, is seen in *chikungunya fever* (Fig. 6) It is also described as brownie nose appearance. Increased intraepidermal melanin dispersion/retention triggered by the chikungunya virus is postulated to be the cause of this hyperpigmentation.

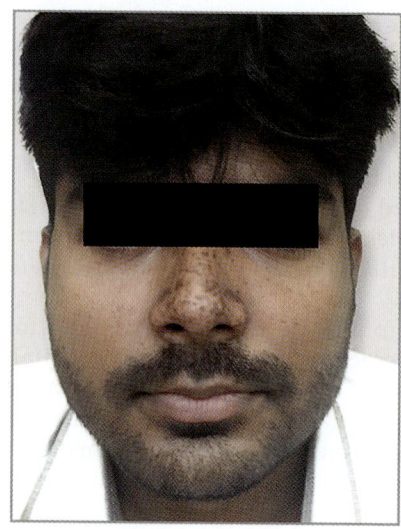

FIG. 6: Chik sign: Brownish hyperpigmentation on nose.
Courtesy: Dr Madhulika Mhatre, Chief Dermatologist, Skin Saga Centre for Dermatology.

Although it is said to be specifically seen in chikungunya fever, it has been recently observed in dengue fever.

Debre's Sign (Phenomenon of Debre)[23]

Named after Robert Debre, a French pediatrician and bacteriologist (1882–1978). The sign refers to the absence of measles rash at the site of injection of convalescent measles serum.

Filatov Sign[26]

Named after Nicolai Feodorovich Filatov Russian pediatrician (1847–1902). The sign refers to the occurrence of circumoral parlor in *scarlet fever*.

Goat Eye Sign[52,69]

It refers to the resemblance of horizontal, rectangular, iris-shaped areas at the center of lesions of *Orf* to goat's eye.

Grisolle Sign[70]

Described by Augustin Maurir Grisolle French physician, 1811–1869.

It helps to differentiate the papule of measles from that of smallpox. On stretching an affected portion of erupted skin, if the papule becomes impalpable to the touch, it is a sign of measles and if skin of the papule can still be felt, it is a sign of small pox.

Hatchcock Sign[52]

It refers to tenderness on running the finger along the angle of the jaw due to parotitis in *mumps*.

Hoagland Sign[71]

It was described by Hoagland in association with *infectious mononucleosis* in 1952.

The sign refers to early and transient bilateral upper lid edema occurring in patients with infectious mononucleosis. It precedes the occurrence of exudative pharyngitis or cervical lymphadenopathy. It is assumed that nasopharyngeal replication of virus, lymphoproliferation, or lymphatic obstruction contribute for the occurrence of this sign.

Hutchinson Eye Sign[72]

Described by Sir Jonathan Hutchinson (1828-1913) in 1885. He was a surgeon, pathologist, ophthalmologist, and dermatologist.

It refers to the presence of vesicles occurring on the tip of the nose or nasal mucosa on the ipsilateral side of *herpes zoster ophthalmicus*. This presentation signifies that the nasociliary branch of the ophthalmic division of trigeminal nerve is affected and hence corneal involvement may be present or forthcoming.

Knife-cut Sign[56]

It refers to linear ulcers and fissures in intertriginous areas such as the folds in the inguinal region, the vulva, and the abdomen, seen in *herpes simplex virus infection* and *Crohn disease*.

Statue of Liberty Sign[52]

It refers to unilateral laterothoracic exanthem (asymmetric periflexural exanthem of childhood) associated with infection due to *Epstein–Barr virus, adenovirus, or parvovirus B19*, the rash starts in the armpit or groin and gradually extends outward, remaining predominantly on one side of the body. This sign is demonstrated when the patient raises an arm to show the rash.

Tasleem Water Jet Sign[73]

The sign refers to spilling out of local anesthetic solution, like a jet of water, from the verrucous surface of wart while giving local anesthesia at the sight of wart. It is mainly seen as palmoplantar warts where the skin is rough and unyielding.

Endocrine, Nutritional, and Metabolic Disorders

Borda Sign[48]

Named after Borda Julio M.

It refers to the presence of marked actinic damage in a young patient with *porphyria cutanea tarda*.

Doughnut Sign[74]

The sign is seen in patients with *scleromyxedema*. It refers to the central depression surrounded by an elevated rim of skin on the extended proximal interphalangeal joint.

Dracula's Sign[23]

It refers to severe mutilating skin lesions caused by photosensitivity in addition to neurological disruptions, liver pathology, and purple urine, which are the indications of forms of *porphyria*. It is now suggested that Vlad Dracula, the 15th-century slayer prince, also known as Vlad the Impaler suffered from hereditary porphyria. Disease can be manifested with painful cutaneous photosensitivity, allowing some victims to only come out after dark caused them to be sadly mistaken for vampires. It is also called as Vampire's disease.

Enamel Paint Sign[39]

The sign consists of sharply demarcated hyperpigmented desquamating patches and plaques resembling enamel paint that occur on the skin, predominantly in areas of pressure and irritation. It is seen in patients with *kwashiorkor*.

Jellinek's Sign (Rasin's Sign)[75]

Described by Stefan Jellinek, Austrian Physician (1871-1968).

The sign refers to brownish eyelid pigmentation occasionally seen in *hyperthyroidism and hyperparathyroidism*.

Lantern Jaw Sign[41]

It refers to the enlargement of mandible that produces a lantern jaw appearance in *acromegaly*.

Liddle's Sign[21]

In *Cushing syndrome*, there is a severe thinning of the skin that gives rise to a cigarette paper appearance, especially on the dorsum of the hands. The skin may be easily pulled off when adhesive tape is removed from it. This is called as Liddle's sign.

Marshall's Sign[13]

Named after Geoffrey Marshall, British physician.

It is seen in *myxedema* and refers to the bagginess of the eyelids and bloated facies that give the patient an appearance of a wax doll. Also known as wax doll sign.

Necklace of Casal Sign[76,77]

Named after Don Gaspar Castle, Spanish Physician who described Pellagra in 1735.

The sign is seen in *pellagra* and refers to hyperpigmented rash (dermatitis) over the sun-exposed area of neck in the form of necklace **(Figs. 7A and B)**.

Prayer Sign[78]

It is a feature of *diabetic cheiroarthropathy*, also called diabetic stiff hand syndrome or limited joint mobility (LJM) syndrome. The sign is said to be positive if the patient is unable to completely close gaps between the opposed palms and fingers on pressing them together as at prayer.

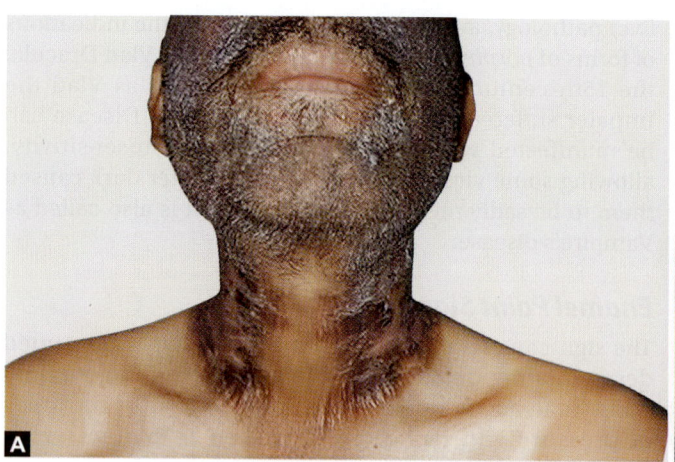
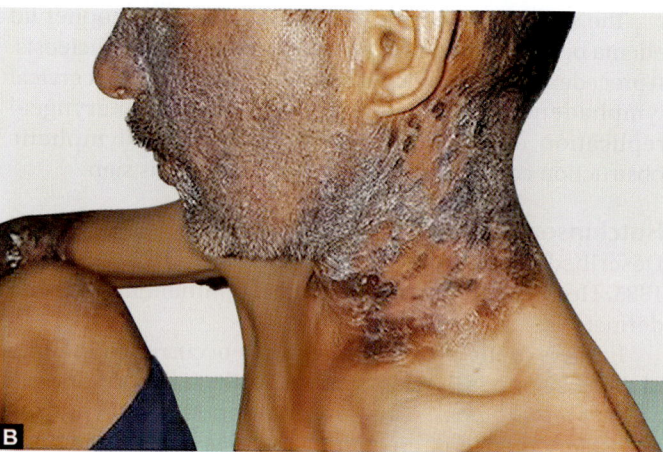

FIGS. 7A AND B: Necklace of Casal sign: Hyperpigmented plaque over the sun-exposed area of neck.
Courtesy: Dr Nitin Mishra, Associate Professor, Department of Dermatology, SRMS IMS Bareilly.

Sharpei Sign[73]

The sign is seen in *scleromyxedema*. It refers to deep furrows in the skin of back characteristic of the sharpie breed of dog.

Shoulder Pad Sign[21]

It is seen in *systemic amyloidosis* and refers to prominent deltoid muscles as a result of deposition of amyloid in the muscles and periarticular tissues.

Pigmentary Conditions

Punshi's Sign[79]

It refers to the color change of *vitiligo* macules in young women and girls from the original white color to red pink during menstruation and back to original color after menstruation.

Tumors

Albright's Sign[80]

It is used to refer to the short fourth metacarpal digits observed in *nevoid basal cell carcinoma syndrome*.

Brenner's Sign[6]

Described by Sarah Brenner in 1992.

It describes the presence of an erythematous eruption accompanying a *melanoma* lesion. The erythematous eruption typically has indistinct borders and appears adjacent to or in the vicinity of the primary lesion. Clinically, Brenner sign may serve as an additional cutaneous marker in the early detection of melanoma.

Clown Nose Sign[56]

It refers to the development of nodular *metastatic* lesion on the nasal tip. It is an indicator of cutaneous metastatic malignancy, mainly squamous cell carcinoma.

Central Dell Sign[21]

Desmoplastic trichoepithelioma is a firm tumor with an indented center and annular elevated border. This central indentation is called central dell sign.

Hildreth's Sign[56]

It is elicited in *glomus tumor*. It refers to relief of pain and tenderness on exsanguination and ischemia of the affected part by raising the extremity affected and inflating a sphygmomanometer applied to it above the systolic blood pressure, and sudden return of pain when the pressure on the cuff is released.

Leser–Trélat Sign[6,81]

Described by two European surgeons, Edmund Leser (1853-1916) and Ulysse Trélat (1828-1890). The sign is defined as the sudden eruption of multiple seborrheic keratosis (SK) with rapid increase in size and number, which are often pruritic, and are classically associated with *internal malignancy* **(Fig. 8)**. It is seen in adenocarcinomas of the gastrointestinal tract, nasopharyngeal carcinoma, and acute myeloid leukemia. Other reported associations include lung cancer, melanoma, and mycosis fungoides.

Pseudo Sign of Leser–Trélat

It refers to increase in size of SK after the use of cytarabine for the treatment of acute myelogenous leukemia. It is due to induction of inflammation of existing SK.

Love's Sign[56]

It refers to exact localization of tenderness with the help of pinhead in *glomus tumor*.

Nazzaro Sign[82]

Described by Paolo Nazzaro, Italian Dermatologist (1921-1975).

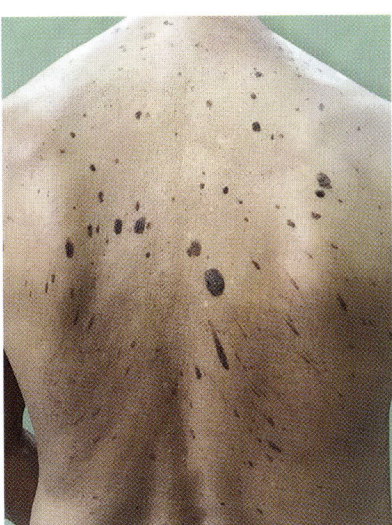

FIG. 8: Leser–Trélat sign: Sudden eruption of multiple seborrheic keratosis (SK) over back.
Courtesy: Dr VK Chawla, Dermatologist, Skin and VD Institute, Bareilly.

It is seen in *multiple myeloma* and consists of follicular hairy hyperkeratosis (horny follicular spicules) commonly located on the face which shows compact follicle bound hyperkeratosis.

Skin Crease Sign[83]

The sign is used to make a preoperative diagnosis of *pilomatricoma*.

It refers to the central longitudinal crease elicited within a lesion when it is squeezed lightly along its margins and perpendicular to the skin tension lines by using the thumb nail of each hand.

Teeter-Totter Sign[84]

It is seen in *pilomatricoma* on pressing one edge of the lesion the opposite edge protrudes from the skin like a Teeter-Totter.

Tent Sign[84]

Pilomatricoma usually presents as a solitary, asymptomatic, deeply seated firm, nontender subcutaneous masses adherent to skin but not fixed to underlying tissue. When the overlying skin is stretched, the lesion appears to be multifaceted and angulated, giving a "'tent" appearance.

Trousseau Sign of Malignancy (Trousseau Syndrome)[21,85]

Described by Armand Trousseau (1801–1867), a French physician.

It is a type of paraneoplastic syndrome, in which internal cancer gives rise to cutaneous manifestations that indicate its presence. This sign is also called migratory thrombophlebitis and is usually seen in *adenocarcinoma of the pancreas, stomach, and lung*.

Ugly Duckling Sign[31,86]

Described by Grob and Bonerandi in 1998.

Ugly duckling sign refers to the observation that nevi in the same individual tend to resemble one another and that *malignant melanoma* often deviates from individual's nevus pattern. This relates to the "ugly duckling" in Hans Christian Andersen's tale, which did not look like its siblings because it was not a duck but a swan.

Vesiculobullous Disorder

Asboe Hansen Sign (Bulla Spread Sign)[87]

Described by Gustav Asboe-Hansen (1917–1989), a Danish physician.

The sign refers to extension of a blister to adjacent unblistered skin when pressure is put on the top of the bulla. It is considered as variation of traditional bulla spread sign. In the traditional "bulla spread" sign also called Lutz sign, slow and careful unidirectional pressure applied by a finger to the bulla causes the bulla to extend beyond the marked margin.

The bulla spread sign is positive in all varieties of blistering diseases such as pemphigus group of disease and many cases of subepidermal acantholytic diseases including bullous pemphigoid, dermatitis herpetiformis, epidermolysis bullosa acquisita, cicatricial pemphigoid, dystrophic EB, bullous drug eruptions, Stevens–Johnson syndrome (SJS), and toxic epidermal necrolysis (TEN).

While irregular angulated border is seen in intraepidermal acantholytic diseases (e.g., pemphigus), rounded blister formation is associated with subepidermal acantholytic diseases.

Nikolsky Sign[87-89]

Described by Peter Vasiliyevich Nikolsky (1858–1940), a Russian dermatologist.

The sign refers to easy peeling of skin on applying tangential pressure over a bony prominence. Positive Nikolsky sign is the hallmark of pemphigus vulgaris and helps in the clinical diagnosis of pemphigus group of diseases. It includes the following subtypes.

Clinical Nikolsky Sign

- *Clinical Nikolsky sign:* When the tangential pressure is applied on apparently normal skin/mucosa, or on perilesional skin/mucosa or on affected skin/mucosa with the thumb or fingerpad, it results in a shearing force that dislodges the upper layers of epidermis from the lower epidermis resulting in formation of blisters.
- *Microscopic Nikolsky sign:* Upon exerting the tangential/lateral pressure, which is generally used for eliciting clinical Nikolsky sign, it produces the classical microscopic changes for pemphigus vulgaris or pemphigus foliaceus in the epidermis, which can be confirmed by a skin biopsy.

- *Marginal Nikolsky sign*: It refers to the ability to split the epidermis of the skin beyond the preexisting erosion by pulling the remnant of a ruptured blister or rubbing at the periphery of existing lesions.
- *Direct Nikolsky sign*: It refers to the ability to split the epidermis on skin areas distant from the lesions by lateral pressure with a finger. Both variants are observed in pemphigus vulgaris, pemphigus foliaceus, and staphylococcal scalded skin syndrome.
- *Wet and dry Nikolsky sign:* After exerting pressure on the skin, if the base is moist, glistening, and eroded, it is called wet Nikolsky sign and if the base is dry, it is called dry Nikolsky sign.
- *Modified Nikolsky sign:* The "modified Nikolsky" sign is described as the peripheral extension of blisters on applying pressure to their surface. This is helpful in patients in whom a new vesicle or bulla is not available for biopsy. The advantage here is that the artificially extended blister cannot show epithelial regeneration, which is sometimes seen in the floor of older subepidermal blisters making them appear as intraepidermal.
- *False Nikolsky sign or Sheklakov sign*: It is elicited by pulling the peripheral remnant roof of a ruptured blister, thus extending the erosion on the surrounding normal skin. It is positive for subepidermal blistering disorders and is seen in bullous pemphigoid, cicatricial pemphigoid, dermatitis herpetiformis, epidermolysis bullosa, porphyrias, and bullous SLE.
- *Pseudo Nikolsky sign or epidermal peeling sign*: It is elicited only on areas that are already involved and affected and also on erythematous areas. It is positive for SJS, TEN, and bullous ichthyosiform erythroderma. Here, the underlying pathophysiology is necrosis and not acantholysis, which is seen in the "true Nikolsky sign."

Cluster of Jewel Sign (String of Pearls or Rosettes Sign)[7]

It refers to an early stage of *chronic bullous disease of childhood (CBDC)*, when new lesions appear at the margin of older ones, resembling a cluster of jewels **(Fig. 9)**.

Premalatha Sign[87,90]

Described by Premalatha et al. in 1981.

The sign refers to the characteristic cerebriform changes seen on the tongue in patients with *pemphigus vegetans*. Cerebriform tongue is characterized by a pattern of sulci and gyri on the dorsum of the tongue and has been reported in up to 50% of cases of Neumann type.

Vascular Disorders

Bandaid Sign[48]

The "band aid sign" typically refers to one used to cover a pyogenic granuloma because it bleeds so easily. Typically, the bandaid has been on so long that its outline is easily

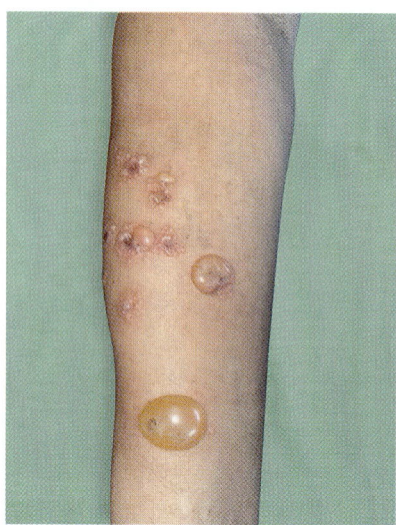

FIG. 9: Cluster of jewel sign: Appearance of new bullae and vesicles at the margin of older ones in chronic bullous disease of childhood (CBDC).
Courtesy: Dr Sachin Roy, Dermatologist, Skin Hair Clinic, Goregoan Mumbai.

visible when it is removed for the photograph to be taken. The net effect is a contact dermatitis.

Nicoladoni–Branham (Branham's) Sign[10]

It is to be elicited in cases of arteriovenous fistula where there is slowing of the heart rate in response to (manual) compression.

Miscellaneous Signs

Alcohol Wipe Sign[56]

The reticulated brown patches of *terra firma-forme dermatosis* appear dirt-like and they can be cleared by forceful rubbing with alcohol wipe. This is termed as alcohol wipe sign.

Axillary Ecchymosis Sign[91]

It is described in *acute pancreatitis* and refers to ecchymosis seen in axilla. It plays a role in early diagnosis and also signifies severity of pancreatitis. The deep blue color of ecchymosis is attributed to the formation of methemalbumin.

Ball-site Sign[56]

It refers to sports-induced targetoid erythema (annular red ring surrounding a central area of normal appearing skin) and is seen in cutaneous injury resulting from a high-velocity ball (paint ball and ping pong ball).

Battle's Sign[92]

Described by William Henry Battle (1855–1936), an English Surgeon.

The sign refers to postauricular or mastoid ecchymosis and is highly specific and predictive for the *basal skull fracture*.

Billard Sign[48]

It refers to bluish discoloration of the skin, covering the face, neck, and upper part of the chest. It is a sign of *toxic exposure to indigo*.

Blanch Sign[21]

This sign is used to differentiate the *weathering nodules* from tophaceous gout and other lesions that arise at the rim of the ear. Application of pressure to the adjacent helical rim will blanch the weathering nodules.

Blue Dot Sign[31]

It refers to blue or black nodule under the skin on the superior aspect of the testis or epididymis. It manifests as the *torsion of the testicular epididymis and appendices*.

Bryant Sign[93]

Described by John Henry Bryant (1867–1906).

Blue coloring appearing on the scrotum due to bleeding from the retroperitoneal space, produced, among other causes, by *acute pancreatitis*.

Coral Bead Sign[94]

The sign refers to small papules around nail folds resembling coral bead, seen in *multicentric reticulohistiocytosis*.

Cullen' Sign[93,95]

Described by Thomas Stephen Cullen (1868–1953), a Canadian gynecologist.

The sign is described mainly in patients with *acute pancreatitis*. It is described as superficial edema with bruising in the subcutaneous fatty tissue around the periumbilical region. It is also known as periumbilical ecchymosis.

This sign has also been described in *ruptured ectopic pregnancy, perforated duodenal ulcer, ruptured spleen, amoebic liver abscess, percutaneous liver biopsy*, and many other medical conditions.

Cyrano Sign[96,97]

It refers to destructive lesions of *juvenile xanthogranuloma* that involve the nose and distort the face.

Darier's Sign[81,98,99]

Described by Ferdinand-Jean Darier (1856–1938), a French dermatologist in 1905.

The sign consists of local wheal and erythema **(Fig. 10)** associated with pruritus within 2–5 minutes of stroking an existing lesion with a blunt object approximately five times

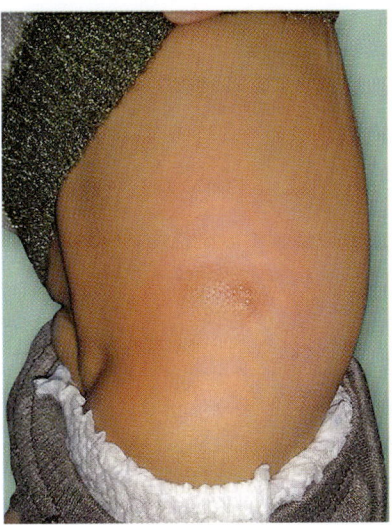

FIG. 10: Darier's sign: Erythema and swelling after stroking the lesion in solitary mastocytoma.

Courtesy: Dr Sourabh Jain, Assistant Professor, Department of Dermatology, ABV Government Medical College, Vidisha, Madhya Pradesh.

with moderate pressure. It occurs in conditions with an increase in the number of mast cells in the dermis, including *urticaria pigmentosa, systemic mastocytosis, insect bite reactions, neurofibroma, juvenile xanthogranuloma, acute neonatal lymphoblastic leukemia, histiocytosis X, leukemia cutis, lymphoma, anetoderma, cutaneous plasmocytosis,* and *Langerhans cell histiocytosis*.

Pseudo Darier Sign

It refers to transient induration with piloerection induced by stroking, rubbing, or cooling of the lesion. It is seen in *smooth muscle hamartoma* and signifies a functioning neural component.

Deck Chair Sign[100,101]

The sign refers to the distinctive pattern of sparing of the natural skin folds, resembling the slats of a deck chair **(Fig. 11)**. It is mainly observed in *papuloerythroderma of Ofuji*. Other conditions include *generalized acanthosis nigricans, Waldenstrom macroglobulinemia, large plaque parapsoriasis, angioimmunoblastic T-cell lymphoma, mycosis fungoides, diffuse leprosy,* and *erythroderma due to various causes*.

Dimple Sign (Fitzpatrick Sign, Pinch Sign)[102]

It is seen in *dermatofibroma*. On giving lateral pressure to the firm nodule with the thumb and index finger, the lesion dimples or becomes indented. The dimpling effect is seen due to the attachment of lesion to the subcutaneous fat. The sign is used in the diagnosis of dermatofibroma and may be useful in differentiating dermatofibromas from other lesions, including malignant melanoma.

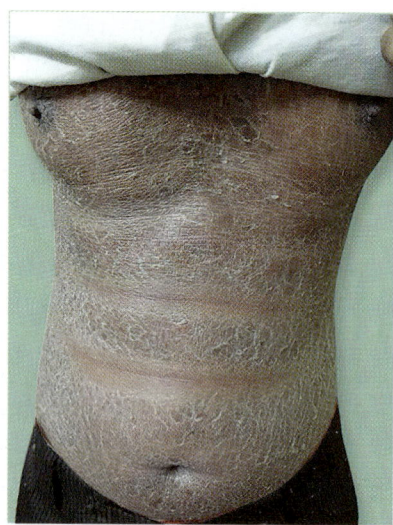

FIG. 11: Deck chair sign: Sparing of natural skin folds in erythroderma.

Courtesy: Dr Bala Ganpathy Ravindran, Dermatologist, Bengaluru.

Drip Sign[39,103]

The sign is found in *dermatitis artefacta* and consists of patterned burned areas corresponding to the areas of dripping of the corrosive liquid when applied by the patient.

Fox's Sign[93]

Described by JA Fox.

A characteristic sign of necrohemorrhagic *pancreatitis* consisting of ecchymosis at the level of the inguinal ligament secondary to the displacement of blood originating in the retroperitoneum through the fascia of the psoas muscle. It has also been associated with the rupture of an aortic aneurysm.

Frank's Sign[104]

Described by Dr Sanders T. Frank.

The sign refers to bilateral diagonal earlobe creases (DELCs), which have been associated with an increased risk for *coronary heart disease*. It is also described in association with *cerebrovascular disease* and *peripheral vascular disease*.

Goose Bumps Sign[105]

Presence of goose bumps or goose pimples without temperature cause, a sign of *hypothalamus disorder*.

Gubler Sign[68]

A distinct swelling on the wrist in *lead poisoning* paralysis.

Grey Turner Sign[93]

Described by George Grey Turner (1877–1951), a British surgeon.

The sign refers to cutaneous ecchymosis in the lumbar region and abdominal flanks due to extension of a retroperitoneal hematoma secondary to necrohemorrhagic *pancreatitis*.

Gulliver's Sign[106]

It is named after the eponymous character in Jonathan Swift's book Gulliver's Travels.

This sign helps in recognizing the transition of inflammatory stage of *pyoderma gangrenosum* (PG) to healing phase and hence serves as a guide to taper corticosteroids and other immunosuppressant therapies used in the treatment of PG. While the inflammatory stage is characterized by wound edges which are raised, erythematous, and sometimes necrotic, the healing phase shows the edges becoming more even with the surrounding skin and string-like growth of epithelium straddles the border between the ulcer bed and the normal surrounding skin.

Hair Collar Sign[10,31,107]

It is an important cutaneous marker for *neural tube closure defects* of the scalp. The sign consists of a ring of long, dark coarse hair surrounding a midline scalp nodule/malformation, such as aplasia cutis, encephalocele, meningocele, or heterotropic brain tissue. The defect is often in the midline, and the occipital or parietal scalp is typically affected.

Halsted's Sign[93]

Described by William Stewart Halsted (1852–1922), an American surgeon.

Ecchymotic spots spread across the abdomen, mainly in the periumbilical area, observed in the course of acute necrohemorrhagic *pancreatitis*.

Hanging Curtain Sign[108]

Described by Dhar S and others in 1995.

It is seen in patients with *pityriasis rosea*. When the skin is stretched across the long axis of the herald patch, the scale is noted to be finer, lighter, and attached at one end, which tends to fold across the line of stretch. This appearance resembles hanging curtain which is attached at one end (hanging string) and hangs with multiple folds along its long axis, gravitational force being the stretch factor.

Hertoghe's Sign[10,31,109,110]

The sign is described by Eugene Ludovic Christian Hertoghe (1860–1928), a Belgian physician. It is also called Queen Anne sign, named after Anne of Denmark.

The sign refers to the lack of the outer third of the eyebrows. Hanifin and Rajka included Hertoghe sign as part of the minor criteria for diagnosing *atopic dermatitis* in 1980. It is also seen in *trichotillomania, ectodermal dysplasia, alopecia* areata, alopecia mucinosa, leprosy, syphilis, ulerythema ophryogenes, systemic sclerosis, and hypothyroidism. It can also sometimes be seen in normal elderly patients.

Hiker's Feet Sign[111]

It refers to bilateral dryness, cracking, and hyperkeratosis predominantly on the plantar aspect of feet and toes seen in *inflammatory myositis*. The presentation resembles a callousing pattern more typical of avid hikers or long-distance walkers, hence the name.

The gross appearance of Hiker's feet is akin to mechanic's hands, which is also seen in inflammatory myopathy, most often in dermatomyositis and the antisynthetase syndrome.

I Love You Sign[112]

The appearance of this hand is very typical of infants with *trisomy 18*, occurring in about 50% of affected infants. The clenched hand with a tendency for the index finger to overlap the third and for the fifth finger to overlap the fourth. At times, these fingers are extended, giving the appearance of the sign for "I love you" in American Sign Language. Infants with trisomy 18 also commonly have hypoplasia of the nails on both the fingers (especially the fifth finger) and the toes.

Kaposi–Stemmer Sign[113]

Inability to pinch or pick up a fold of skin at the base of the second toe because of its thickness is seen in *chronic lymphedema*.

Kerr's Sign[6]

Described by William J Kerr in 1936.

The sign refers to palpable change in the skin below the level of a *spinal cord lesion*. Kerr described that the normal skin above the lesion felt smooth, soft, and pliable when compared with the stiff, dry, and tense skin found below that level.

Kirmisson Sign[11]

Described by *Edouard Francis Kirmisson* (1848-1927), a French pediatric surgeon, transverse striated ecchymoses at the elbow. A sign seen in fractures of the humerus with displacement of the proximal fragment.

Leathery Palm Sign[41]

A classic sign of *arsenical poisoning*, in which the palms and the soles of the feet have a leathery texture. It is also known as arsenic sign.

Limburger Sign[41]

Strong smell of Limburger cheese, present in wounds, bandages, or bed linens. An indication of *gangrene* infection.

Magnan's Sign[13]

Named after Valentin Jacques Joseph Magnan (1835-1916), a French psychiatrist.

It refers to a frightening illusory sensation of a foreign body under the skin, seen in cases of *cocaine addiction*.

Matchbox Sign[10,114]

Patient having *delusions of parasitosis* (acarophobia, entomophobia) collects skin debris with mistaken belief that such collected material contains alleged parasite in a matchbox, tissue paper, or small container. This whole exercise executed by the patient is referred to as matchbox sign. Freudenmann et al. proposed to use the name *specimen sign* since patients use other receptacles such as plastic bags, glasses, paper, tissue wraps, and adhesive tapes more than the matchbox.

Meffert Sign[10]

It is described in *Fordyce disease*, characterized by presence of ectopically located sebaceous glands on the lips, oral mucosa, and less commonly on gums. Prominent lip involvement can result in a lipstick-like mark left on the rim of a glass mug after consuming a hot beverage.

Osler Sign (Osler Nodes)[6,56]

Sir William Osler (1849-1919), an American and English physician, is credited with this cutaneous finding.

The sign describes the presence of areas of painful nodular erythema on the pads of fingers and toes in patients with *chronic or subacute bacterial endocarditis*.

These nodular lesions are a result of small emboli to typically the distal phalanges of the palms and soles, with associated swelling, vasculitis, and inflammation. They have also been observed in bacteremia and SLE. On the other hand, Janeway lesions seen in bacterial endocarditis are nontender and hemorrhagic lesions and are seen on the palms and soles.

Paired Ear Creases of the Helix Sign[115]

The sign refers to paired creases on the helix of the ear and signifies risk of *coronary artery disease and metabolic syndrome*, as does Frank's sign; DELCs. It is postulated that both DELC and PECH are the result of the ear being caught in between the rock of the cranium and the hard place of the mattress/pillow/hand. Another theory suggests that the diagonal ear lobe creases may be the consequence of fat cheeks inducing a gravity-mediated valgus deformity of the hang of the ear lobe to such a degree that creases supervene.

Panda Sign[116]

It refers to the periorbital under-response of *nevus of Ota* to laser therapy. While peripheral sites clear well and the nevus persists in periorbital area, it gives an appearance of a panda, hence the name of the sign Panda sign.

Pink Sign[117]

A 20-minute occlusive testing may be helpful in identifying urticarial reaction, which could be missed in conventional patch testing which is read at 72 hours. In cases of chronic urticaria, the adhesive patches are peeled off and the area is identified after 20 minutes, which reveals a pink rim around the allergen strips.

Plantar Ecchymosis Sign[118]

The sign refers to ecchymosis found on midfoot region on the plantar aspect, seen in *calcaneal or Lisfranc fracture*. It implies the potential for significant injury to the plantar tarsometatarsal ligaments.

Rope Sign[119]

The sign refers to palpable subcutaneous linear cords that typically occur in axilla. This sign occurs in *interstitial granulomatous dermatitis (Ackerman syndrome) with arthritis*.

Russell Sign[6]

Described by Gerald FM Russell, an English physician.

The sign is observed in patients with *bulimia nervosa*. It refers to the callosities that are found on the dorsum of the hand due to friction of fingers against teeth during self-induced vomiting.

Thinker's Sign[21]

It refers to asymptomatic, dry, and hyperpigmented keratotic plaques on the front of the lower third of the thighs seen in patients with chronic obstructive pulmonary disease.

Urschel Sign[120]

The sign refers to the presence of dilated superficial venous collateral vessels on the shoulder and the upper arm. It is seen in *Paget–Schroetter syndrome*.

Walzel Sign[93]

Described by P Walzel, an Austrian surgeon in 1927.

It seen in association with *acute and chronic pancreatitis*. Walzel sign refers to livedo reticularis in the thorax, abdomen, or flank due to the action of trypsin on the cutaneous vasculature which prevents it from having adequate vascularization.

Yoga Sign[121]

The sign refers to the *callosities* on the outer ankles and fifth toes due to the mechanical stress exerted by the characteristic yoga sitting position on plain and hard floor.

SIGNS IN VENEREOLOGY

Syphilis and Congenital Syphilis

Barber Pole Sign[52]

In congenital syphilis, necrotizing funisitis leads to typical appearance of interspersion of blue and pink areas along with the chalky white appearance in spiral course on umbilical cord, which resembles the barber pole.

Biett Sign[122,123]

Described by Laurent Thedore Biett, a French Dermatologist.

It refers to multiple discrete symmetrical hyperpigmented macules with collarette of scales on both palms **(Fig. 12)**.

Bulldog Jaw Sign[52,124]

It is seen in congenital syphilis and refers to the appearance of normal mandible relatively longer and bigger due to maxillary hypoplasia.

Buschke–Ollendorff Sign[125]

Described by Abraham Buschke (1868–1943), a Jewish-German dermatologist and Helene Ollendorff Curth (1899–1982), a German-American dermatologist.

It refers to extreme sensitivity of papular lesions of secondary syphilis to pressure with a dull probe and is due to cutaneous vasculitis.

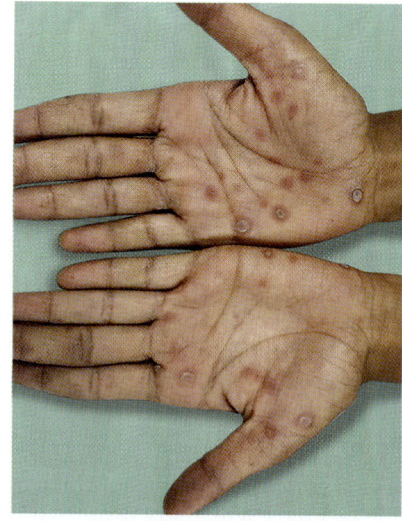

FIG. 12: Biett's sign: Multiple discrete symmetrical hyperpigmented macules with collarette of scales on both palms in secondary syphilis.

Courtesy: Dr Dharmendra Dave, Dermatologist, Dave Skin & Laser Clinic, Patan, Gujarat.

Dory Flop Sign[10,126]

Named by John Stokes, a dermatologist and syphilologist.

The sign is described in relation to the chancre that develops on undersurface of prepuce in primary syphilis. On retraction of foreskin, the affected area where the chancre is present, tips up slowly and then flips over all at once. It is attributed to the underlying button-like induration of chancre which makes it difficult to bend. The movement is akin to the movement of a dory, a small flat bottomed fishing boat which flips over all at once when overturned, hence the name of the sign Dory flop sign.

Dubois Sign[127]

It is named after the observations made by the Swiss dermatologist Charles du Bois (1874–1947) in connection with congenital syphilis.

It refers to shortening of the little finger associated with congenital syphilis which is occasionally seen as a late stigma of the disease.

Café-au-lait Tint Sign[124]

Typical brownish-yellow appearance of skin in congenital syphilis due to combined effect of hyperpigmentation, jaundice, and anemia.

Crown of Venus Sign[52]

It refers to scaly papules seen along hairline of scalp in secondary syphilis.

Elliot Sign[52]

It refers to the induration of the edge of a syphilitic skin lesion.

Fournier's Sign (Sabre Shin)[124]

It refers to the typical appearance of shins, resembling the sabre sword, in late congenital syphilis and is due to thickening of shaft of the middle third of tibia.

Higoumenakis Sign[125,128]

It was described in 1927 by Gregorios "George" Higoumenakis (1895–1983), a Greek dermatologist. It is also called clavicle sign of late congenital syphilis.

Enlargement of sternal end of (right) clavicle of frequently observed in patients with late congenital syphilis due to periostitis. It is appreciated on clinical examination and can be seen on X-ray.

Krisowski's Sign[11]

Described by Max Krisowski, a German physician.

It indicates the presence of cicatricial lines radiating from the mouth in congenital syphilis.

Natiform Skull Sign (Hot Cross Bun Skull)[52]

It refers to the frontoparietal bossing along with prominent suture lines of skull; stigmata due to healed gummatous osteoperiostitis in congenital syphilis.

Olympian Brow Sign[52,129]

It signifies the bony prominence of forehead seen in congenital syphilis due to periostitis involving the supraorbital area. It is also known as "beetled brow."

Omnibus Sign[130]

Eyebrow alopecia in secondary syphilis is termed the omnibus sign as it could be seen by a glance at a patient in an omnibus, from the sidewalk.

Opera Glass Nose Sign[52]

In congenital syphilis, due to nasal chondritis, the appearance of nose resembles opera glass as the lower part of nose appears to be pushed toward intact upper part.

Seeping Sign[52]

Bleeding from the mucous surfaces and navel, shortly after birth; a sign of syphilis hemorrhagic neonatorum.

Silex's Sign[16]

Described by Paul Silex (1858–1929), a German ophthalmologist.

A pathognomonic sign of congenital syphilis and is characterized by radial furrows around the mouth.

Virchow Sign[124,125]

Described by Rudolf Carl Virchow (1821–1902), the father of modern pathology.

It refers to tongue with a smooth base seen in patients with congenital syphilis.

Wimberger's Sign[125,131]

It is also known as Wimberger's corner sign.

The sign was named after Hans Wimberger (1887–1954), an Austrian pediatrician.

It is a radiological sign, and it refers to localized bony destruction of the medial portion of the proximal tibial metaphysis.

OTHER SEXUALLY TRANSMITTED DISEASES

Groove Sign of Greenblatt[56,80,132]

Described by Greenblatt in 1953.

It is observed in *lymphogranuloma venereum (LGV)*. The enlargement of both inguinal and femoral group of lymph nodes with their separation by Poupart's ligament produces a groove which is described as groove sign of Greenblatt. It is also described in Hodgkin and non-Hodgkin lymphomas. Groove sign is also used to describe eosinophilic fasciitis (Shulman syndrome) where there is linear groove or indentation along the superficial veins of the medial aspect of the upper extremity.

Pseudo Groove Sign

It is described in *Donovanosis* and it refers to subcutaneous swelling on either side of Poupart's ligament that gives the appearance of groove. Unlike the lymph nodes responsible for groove sign in LGV, here the groove sign is due to multiple abscesses formed due to invasion of skin by bacteria.

SIGNS IN LEPROSY

Benediction Sign (Pointing Index Sign)[133]

It denotes outstretched index finger with flexion of other fingers due to median nerve involvement at or above elbow in leprosy.

To test the median nerve involvement in leprosy, the muscles of upper extremity are tested. When flexor digitorum superficialis and profundus (lateral part) are tested by asking the patient to clasp both hands (Ochsner's clasping test), if there is median nerve involvement, the index finger of affected side does not flex and remains straight.

Elbow Sign[52]

Thickened ulnar nerve at the elbow in leprosy.

Fibula Sign[52]

Thickened common peroneal nerve in leprosy.

Fountain of Youth Sign[52]

In diffuse lepromatous leprosy, there is smoothening out of patient's facial wrinkles which restores the youthful appearance.

Froment Sign and Jeanne's Sign[52,134]

These signs indicate weakness of first palmar interossei and adductor pollicis (involvement of deep branch of ulnar nerve).

Froment sign refers to the flexion of the distal interphalangeal joint of the thumb when the patient tries to grasp a piece of paper between thumb and index finger. If this is associated with hyperextension of metacarpophalangeal (MP) joint of the thumb as well, it is known as Jeanne's sign. Some individuals have normal MP joint volar plate laxity, allowing hyperextension of the joint. Therefore, if Jeanne's sign is seen, one must determine whether it is related to a normally lax volar plate or to the absence of part or all (innervation is variable) of the flexor pollicis brevis or both.

Tap Sign[135]

It refers to deep pain felt upon percussion of lesions over bone in tuberculoid leprosy, despite superficial sensory impairment. It is a useful clinical sign in diagnosis of tuberculoid and borderline tuberculoid leprosy where a lesion overlies a bone.

Wartenberg's Sign[52]

It is one of the earliest signs of ulnar nerve involvement in leprosy and refers to subtle abducted position of little finger. It indicated paralysis of adductor digiti minimi, which is supplied by the ulnar nerve.

Most of the above mentioned signs in dermatology, venereology, and leprosy have been compiled in the following tables **(Tables 1 to 7)** according to the site where

Table 1: Signs seen in face.				
Involving/around eyes/eyelash/eyelid		*Involving eyebrow*	*Involving/around nose*	*Involving/around ears*
Berliner sign	Jellinek sign	Hertoghe sign	Allergic salute sign	Battle sign
Calabar sign	Panda sign	Omnibus sign	Chik sign	Ear sign
Chagas-Mazza	Pitaluga sign		Cyrano sign	Earlobe sign
Romana sign			Clown nose sign	
Dennie–Morgan sign	Pitaluga sign		Hutchinson eye	Franks sign
Eyelid sign	Raccoon sign		Nose sign	Milian ear sign
Heliotrope rash	Romana sign		Opera glass sign	Milian ear sign
Hoagland sign			Pavithran nose	Paired ear creases of the helix
Ingram sign			Rudolph sign	Shuster sign
				Turkey ear sign

Table 1: Signs seen in face (continued).

Involving forehead	Involving/ around jaw	Involving/ around mouth	Overall face
Olympian brow sign	Bulldog jaw sign	Filatov sign	Billard sign
	Hatchcock sign	Krisowski sign	Fountain of youth sign
	Lantern jaw	Meffert sign	Headlight sign
		Silex sign	Marshall sign
			Nazzaro sign
			Scarlet milk sign

Table 3: Signs seen in fingers/toes/hands/feet/palms/soles.

Fingers/Toes/Hands/Feet		Palms/Soles
• Albright's dimple sign	• I love you sign	• Biett sign
• Benediction sign	• Jeanne sign	• Filipovitch–Skibinski sign
• Blue toe	• Mizutani sign	• Leathery palm sign
• Doughnut sign	• Myer sign	• Osler sign
• Dubois sign	• Raynaud sign	• Patrick Yesudian sign
• Froment sign	• Russell sign	• Plantar ecchymosis sign
• Gottron sign	• Wartenberg sign	• Wake sign
• Hiker's feet	• Yoga sign	

Table 2: Signs seen in neck and chest/shoulder.

Neck/Chest/Shoulder		Flexures	Femoral and gluteal region
Barnett sign	Molluscum pendulum necklace sign	Axillary ecchymosis sign	Holster sign
Delmege sign	Necklace of casal sign	Crowe sign	School chair sign
Dirty neck	Shawl sign	Pastia sign	Seat rash sign
Freund sign	Shoulder pad sign	Rope sign	
Higoumenakis sign	V sign	Statue of Liberty sign	

Table 4: Signs seen around umbilicus/femoral/gluteal/back/lymph node involvement.

Around umbilicus	Femoral and gluteal region	Back	Lymph node involvement
Cullen sign	Holster sign	Butterfly sign	Groove sign of Greenblatt
Halsted sign	School chair sign	Sharpei sign	Hanging groin sign
Thumb print sign	Seat rash sign		Winterbottom sign

Table 5: Signs seen after elicitation.

Signs seen after elicitation by dermatologist			Signs seen with patient maneuvers
• Albright's Dimple sign	• Dimple sign (Fitzpatrick sign)	• Meffert sign	• Matchbox sign
• Alcohol wipe sign	• Dory flop sign	• Nikolsky sign	• Prayer sign
• Antenna sign	• Elbow sign	• Nicoladoni–Branham sign	• Reverse Namaskar
• Apple jelly sign	• Fibula sign	• Pink sign	• Thumb sign (Steinberg sign)
• Asboe Hansen (blister spread)	• Fountain sign	• Pullback sign of Ashish	• Umbilical sign
• Auspitz sign	• Grisolle sign	• Raccoon eyes/sign/panda sign	• Wrist sign (Walker–Murdoch sign)
• Barnett sign (scleroderma neck sign)	• Gorlin sign	• Raynaud sign	
• Blanch sign	• Hanging curtain sign	• Scratch sign	
• Borsari sign	• Hatchcock sign	• Skin crease sign	
• Branham sign	• Hilderth sign	• Tap sign	
• Buschke–Ollendorff sign	• Ingram sign	• Tasleem water jet sign	
• Buttonhole sign	• Kaposi–Stemmer sign	• Teeter totter sign	
• Carpet tack sign	• Kerr sign	• Tent sign	
• Darier sign and Pseudo-Darier sign	• Last membrane sign		
	• Love' sign		

Table 6: Multiple signs in single condition.

Dermatomyositis	Gottron sign, Holster sign, Heliotrope sign, Hiker's feet, inverse Gottron sign, Keining sign, Shawl sign, V sign
	Others: Secondary Raynaud's phenomenon
Discoid lupus erythematosus (DLE)	Carpet tack sign (Tin tack sign or Cat tongue sign), Shuster's sign
Ehlers–Danlos syndrome	Gorlin sign, Reverse Namaskar sign
Leishmaniasis	Pitaluga sign, volcano sign;
	Others: Carpet tack sign, apple jelly sign
Marfan syndrome	Thumb sign (Steinberg sign), umbilical sign
	Wrist sign (Walker–Murdoch sign)
	Others (less commonly reported)
Onchocerciasis	Hanging groin sign, leopard skin sign, lizard skin sign, long scar sign
Pancreatitis	Axillary ecchymosis sign, Bryant sign, Cullen sign, Fox sign, Grey Turner sign, Halsted sign, and Walzel sign
Scarlet fever	Borsari sign, Filatov sign, milk sign, Myer sign, Pastia sign
Strongyloidiasis	Seat rash sign, thumbprint sign
Systemic sclerosis/scleroderma	Barnett sign, Ingram sign, Mizutani sign (round finger pad sign), Stafne sign
	Others: Secondary Raynaud phenomenon
Trypanosomiasis	Chagas-Mazza Romana sign (Romana sign or eye sign)
	Winterbottom sign
Congenital syphilis	Barber pole sign, Bulldog sign, Café-au-lait tint sign, Dubois sign, Fournier sign (Sabre shin), Higoumenakis sign, Krisowski sign, Natiform skull sign (hot cross bun skull), Olympian brow sign, Opera glass nose sign, Seeping sign, Silex sign, Virchow sign, and Wimberger sign
Primary/secondary syphilis	Biett sign, Buschke Ollendorff sign, crown of Venus sign, dory flop sign, Elliot sign, and Omnibus sign

Table 7: Signs and Synonyms.

Sign	Synonym[11,16,23,26,28,41,44,48,70,112,136-143]
Bandy legs sign	A presentation of syphilis
Bartholinus's sign	Chromidrosis, perspiration with the color of black ink
	Named after Caspar Bartholin, a Danish anatomist and physician
Bateman sign	Molluscum contagiosum, epithelioma contagiosum, molluscum epitheliale, porcelaneus condyloma, and molluscum sebaceum
	Named after Thomas Bateman, an English dermatologist (1778–1821)
Bearded woman sign	Diabetes bearded woman syndrome, Achard-Thiers syndrome
	Type 2 diabetes and androgen excess in postmenopausal women
Borellus sign	Chromidrosis, perspiration with the color of green
Bowditch sign	Tinea imbricata found in the Bowditch, Union Islands
Brug sign	Skin lymphatic disease caused by nematodes transferred by the bite of an infected mosquito
	In 1927, Lichtenstein and Brug discovered a microfilaria in the Dutch East Indies (now Indonesia) which was morphologically different from W. Bancroft and called it filariasis malayi
Brussel sign	Mycosis fungoides
	Adam Thomson described a case of MF in a young girl of the age 14 whom he saw in Brussels in October 1893
Bull eye sign	Erythema migrans in Lyme disease
Danielssen sign	Danielssen disease, Danielssen–Boeck disease, dry leprosy, and trophoneurotic leprosy
	Named after Daniel Cornelius Danielssen (1815–1894)

Continued

Continued

Sign	Synonym[11,16,23,26,28,41,44,48,70,112,136-143]
De Morgan sign	Cherry angioma and senile angiomas Named after Campbell Greig De Morgan English physician (1811–1876)
Dercum sign	Adiposis dolorosa and Dercum disease Named after Francis Xavier Dercum, American neurologist (1856–1931)
Duhring sign	Dermatitis herpetiformis. Named after Louis Adolphus Duhring, American dermatologist (1845–1913)
Duke sign/Filatov-Duke sign/fourth sign	Fourth disease, rubeola scarlatina, Dukes' disease, Dukes-Filatov disease Named after Clement Dukes, an English physician (1845–1925)
East India sign	Furunculus orientalis, oriental boil, Aleppo boil, Delhi boil, and Biskra button
Farmer skin sign	Cutis rhomboidalis nuchae
Fish-skin sign	Ichthyosis
Fisherman sign	Zoonotic skin or systemic cellulitis disease caused by erysipelothrix rhusiopathiae
Fothergill sign	Facial pain brought on by gentlest touch
Francis sign	Deer-fly fever, rabbit fever, Ohara fever, and zoonotic tularemia Named after Edward Francis, an American microbiologist (1872–1957)
French sign	Syphilis. Also called morbus gallicus or the French disease
Frenchify sign	An English term translated as: A person with venereal disease
Frog neck sign/Frog sign	Cystic hygroma A remarkable translucent swelling of the neck/lesions in the oral cavity
Gambian plague sign (Africa)	Lymphadenopathy associated with smallpox lesions
Gilchrist sign	Blastomycosis, Blasto and Chicago disease
Gill sign	Myxedema
Gleich sign	Gleich syndrome or episodic angioedema with eosinophilia Body swells up episodically (angioedema), associated with raised antibodies of the IgM type and increased numbers of eosinophil in the blood (eosinophilia)
Gruby sign	Tinea capitis caused by *Trichophyton tonsurans* Named after David Gruby, a Hungarian physician, (1810–1898)
Holster sign	Endemic syphilis
Hand-and-foot sign	A trophoneurotic affection characterized by ulceration of the hands and feet
Haverhill sign	Epidemic arthritis erythema Rat bite fever with peripheral rash from zoonotic bacterium *Streptobacillus moniliformis*
Italian sign	Syphilis. Also called mal d'Italie
Kedani sign	Akamushi disease, flood fever, inundation fever, island disease, island fever, Japanese river fever, kedani fever, mite typhus, scrub typhus, shimamushi disease, tropic typhus, and tsutsugamushi An epidemic disease of Japan due to a zoonotic proteus implanted by the bite of a mite (kedani)
Little dragon's sign	Guinea or Medina worm infection Vesicular skin lesion that ruptures to reveal a worm. Caused by the zoonotic *Dracunculus medinensis* nematode
Lonestar sign	Southern tick associated rash illness, a zoonotic *Borrelia* disease in Southern USA
Lusitanus sign	Chromidrosis, perspiration resembling the color of sooty water Named after Abraham Zacutus Lusitanus, a Portuguese-Dutch physician and medical historian, 1557–1642
Paullini sign	Chromhidrosis, perspiration with a leek-green color Named after Christian Franz Paullini, German physician and theologian (1643–1712)

Continued

Continued

Sign	Synonym[11,16,23,26,28,41,44,48,70,112,136-143]
Pettigrew sign	Paternal hereditary ichthyosis, morbid development of the papillae, and thickening of the epidermic lamellae Also called Armadillo sign. Described by Pettigrew and Ascanius
Port-Light Nose sign	Rhinophyma, Also called bottle nose
Raspberry sign	Yaws, Frambesia
Saint Lazare sign, Spedalskhed sign	Leprosy
Saint Main's evil sign	The sign of a patient suffering from scabies. Also called Saint Main's disease
Saint Roch sign	Plague Saint Roch was a patron saint of plague victims
Saint Semen sign	Synonym of syphilis
Skunk boil sign	Leptospirosis infection. Also known as Possum sign
Sudoku sign	Japanese rat-bit fever
Sticker sign	Erythema infectiosum
Violet sweat sign	Chromidrosis, perspiration with a violet color
Weil sign also called Landouzy sign and Fiedler sign	Severe leptospirosis
Werewolf sign	A sign of congenital hypertrichosis lanuginosa Individuals are completely covered in hair except for their palms and soles Described by Paul Gottlieb Werlhof, a German physician, 1699–1767
Werlhof sign	Purpura hemorrhagica
Westberg sign	White spot disease, morphea alba
White leprosy sign	Leukoderma
White skin sign	Keratosis follicularis, also known as Darier disease, Darier–White disease, dyskeratosis follicularis
Willan sign	Psoriasis circinate. Also called Willan's lepra
Willan cheek sign	Lupus vulgaris of the cheek
Willard sign	Lupus vulgaris
Wilson sign	Dermatitis exfoliative
Wine sweat sign	Perspiration with the taste of wine
Zaufal sign	Samriti Sood. Saddle nose For example sign of ectodermal dysplasia Named after Emanuel Zaufal, a Czechoslovakian rhinologist (1833–1910)

the signs are seen, elicitation of signs either by dermatologist or by patient manoeuvre, conditions where multiple signs are seen and a list of synonyms and signs, few of which were used in the past.

REFERENCES

1. Barnett AJ. The "neck sign" in scleroderma. Arth Rheumat. 1989;32:209-11.
2. Weinstein CL, Miller MH, Kossard S, Littlejohn GO. The scleroderma neck sign. J Rheumatol. 1989;16(12):1533-5.
3. Inamadar, AC. Perforation of paper with pen: Simple technique to explain the carpet tack sign in discoid lupus erythematosus. J Am Acad Dermatol 2019;81(6):e159-60.
4. Das A, Toshniwal A, Madke B. Newer signs in dermatology [2016-2020]. Indian Dermatol Online J. 2020;12(2):342-5.
5. Gottron's sign. In: Moreland LW, (eds). Rheumatology and Immunology Therapy. Berlin, Heidelberg: Springer; 2004.
6. Patel LM, Lambert PJ, Gagna CE, Maghari A, Lambert WC. Cutaneous signs of systemic disease. Clin Dermatol. 2011;29(5):511-22.
7. Muthusamy D. Prototypical signs of the orofacial region-eyes see what the mind knows. Int J Develop Res. 2017;7(11): 16844-7.

8. Russo T, Piccolo V, Ruocco E, Baroni A. The heliotrope sign of dermatomyositis: the correct meaning of the term heliotrope. Arch Dermatol. 2012;148(10):1178.
9. Dugan EM, Huber AM, Miller FW, Rider LG; International Myositis Assessment and Clinical Studies Group. Photoessay of the cutaneous manifestations of the idiopathic inflammatory myopathies. Dermatol Online J. 2009;15(2):1.
10. Madke B, Nayak C. Eponymous signs in dermatology. Indian Dermatol Online J. 2012;3(3):159-65.
11. Brzezinski P, Fiorentino DF, Arunachalam P, Katafigiotis I, Matuszewski L, Narita M, et al. Dermatology eponyms–sign – Lexicon – (K). Our Dermatol Online. 2014;5(1):95-102.
12. Mizutani H, Mizutani T, Okada H, Kupper TS, Shimizu M. Round fingerpad sign: an early sign of scleroderma. J Am Acad Dermatol. 1991;24(1):67-9.
13. Brzezinski P, Bourée P, Chiriac A, Bouquot JE, Schepis C, Hofer T, et al. Dermatology eponyms – sign – Lexicon – (M). Our Dermatol Online. 2014;5(3):312-26.
14. Samitz, Morris H. Cuticular changes in dermatomyositis. Arch Dermatol. 1974;110(6):866.
15. Shuster S. A simple sign of discoid lupus erythematosus. Br J Dermatol. 1981;104(3):350-1.
16. Brzeziński P, Wollina U, Espinoza-Benavides L, Chang P, Mohamed M, Geller SA. Dermatology eponyms – sign – Lexicon (S). Part II. Our Dermatol Online. 2018;9(4):470-7.
17. Ravi D, Prabhu S. Dermatomyositis: A dermatological perspective. Clin Dermatol Rev. 2019;3:18-22.
18. Marvi U, Chung L, Fiorentino DF. Clinical presentation and evaluation of dermatomyositis. Indian J Dermatol. 2012;57(5):375-81.
19. Kiken DA, Silverberg NB. Atopic dermatitis in children, part 1: epidemiology, clinical features, and complications. Cutis. 2006;78(4):241-7.
20. Lakshmi DV, Shilpa K, Nataraja HV, Divya KG. Nose: Applied aspects in dermatology. Indian J Dermatol. 2016;61(2):234.
21. Mancy A. Handbook of Signs in Clinical Dermatology. 2021.
22. Verma SB. Revisiting the origin, evolution and morphological nuances of the "Butterfly sign". Indian Dermatol Online J. 2021;12(3):475-6.
23. Brzezinski P, Wollina U, Poklękowska K, Khamesipour A, Herrero Gonzalez JE, Bimbi C, et al. Dermatology eponyms –phenomen/sign –Lexicon (D). N Dermatol Online. 2011;2:158-70.
24. Colver GB, Mortimer PS, Millard PR, Dawber RPR, Ryan TJ. (The 'dirty neck'—a reticulate pigmentation in atopics. Clin Exp Dermatol. 1987;12(1):1-4.
25. Rotstein E, Rotstein H. The ear-lobe sign: a helpful sign in facial contact dermatitis. Australas J Dermatol. 1997;38(4):215-6.
26. Brzezinski P, Godoy Gijón E, López-López J, Toyokawa T, Scrimshaw NS, Malard O, et al. Dermatology eponyms ? phenomen/sign? Lexicon (F). Our Dermatol Online. 2012;3:66-78.
27. Gupta G, Reshma P, Naveen KN, Athanikar SB. Indian signs in dermatology. Med J DY Patil Univ 2014;7:261-2.
28. Brzezin´ski P, Chang P, Fan R-Y, Krishnan V, Peh WCG, Francès P, et al. Eponyms – sign –Lexicon (P). Part 1. Our Dermatol Online. 2016;7(2):244-52.
29. Samimi SS, Siegfried E, Belsito DV. A diagnostic pearl: the school chair sign. Cutis. 2004;74(1):27-8.
30. Venkatesh C, Devi J, Srinivasan S. Albright's dimpling sign. Indian J Endocrinol Metab. 2013;17(2):364-5.
31. Freiman A, Kalia S, O'Brien EA. Dermatologic signs. J Cutan Med Surg. 2006;10:175-82.
32. IADVL Textbook-Genodermatoses chapter.
33. Kulkarni AS, Birangane RS, Parkarwar PC, Kazi AZ. Clinical and radiological signs of importance for the oral physician and oral surgeon. J Indian Acad Oral Med Radiol. 2019;31:257-62.
34. Gaurav V, Grover C. "Molluscum" Conditions in Dermatology. Indian Dermatol Online J. 2021;12(6):962-5.
35. Yesudian P, Premalatha S, Thambiah AS. Palmar melanotic macules. Int J Dermatol. 1984;23:468-71.
36. Premalatha S, Sarveswari K N, Lahiri K. Reverse-namaskar: A new sign in Ehlers-Danlos syndrome: A family pedigree study of four generations. Indian J Dermatol. 2010;55:86-91.
37. Gupta S, Gupta N. Wrist (Walker–Murdoch) and Thumb (Steinberg) Signs. MAMC J Med Sci. 2017;3:111-2.
38. Walker BA, Murdoch JL. The wrist sign: A useful physical finding in the Marfan syndrome. Arch Intern Med. 1970;126(2):276-7.
39. Pradhan S, Madke B, Singh AL, Kabra P. Less-known clinical signs in dermatology. Indian Dermatol Online J. 2016;7:421-3.
40. Dhar S. "Fountain sign" in lichen planus hypertrophicus. Indian J Dermatol Venereol Leprol. 1997;63:210.
41. Brzezinski P, Chiriac A, Arenas R, Dori GU, Monteiro R, Cairncross S, et al. Dermatology eponyms –sign – Lexicon – (L). Our Dermatol Online. 2014;5:217-30.
42. Zelin E, Di Meo N, Maronese CA, Zalaudek I. Pyemotes ventricosus dermatitis: 'comet sign'. Clin Exp Dermatol. 2021; 46:980-3.
43. Quach KA, Zaenglein AL. The eyelid sign: a clue to bed bug bites. Pediatr Dermatol. 2014;31(3):353-5.
44. Brzeziński P, Martini L, Stawczyk-Macieja M. Dermatology eponyms – sign – Lexicon (V). Our Dermatol Online. 2019; 10(4):413-6.
45. Singh A, Singh AK, Singh D, Varghese A. Blister beetle dermatitis: few observations helping in diagnosis. Int J Prev Med. 2013;4(2):241.
46. Yoshizumi J, Harada T. 'Wake sign': an important clue for the diagnosis of scabies. Clin Exp Dermatol. 2009;34(6):711-4.
47. Martínez-Morán C, García-Donoso MC, Moreno A, Borbujo J. Blue finger sign as initial manifestation of popliteal artery aneurysm. Actas Dermosifiliogr. 2011;102(7):551-52.
48. Brzeziński P, Sanaei-Zadeh H, Shane T, Bonifaz A, Arenas R, Royer-Bégyn M. Dermatology eponym – phenomen/sign – Dictionary (B). N Dermatol Online. 2011;2:35-45.
49. Wikipedia. Borsari's sign. [online] Available from: https://en.wikipedia.org/wiki/Borsari%27s_sign#:~:text=Borsieri's%20sign%20or%20Borsieri's%20line,Giovanni%20Battista%20Borsieri%20de%20Kanifeld. [Last accessed December, 2022].
50. Singh S, Gupta S, Chaudhary R. Hypopyon sign in pemphigus vulgaris and pemphigus foliaceus. Int J Dermatol. 2009; 48(10):1100-2.
51. Sugimoto H, Furukawa K. Milian's ear sign: Erysipelas. IDCases. 2018;14:e00449.
52. Amrani A, Sil A, Das A. Cutaneous signs in infectious diseases. Indian J Dermatol Venereol Leprol. 2022;88(4):569-75.
53. Dahle KW, Sontheimer RD. The Rudolph sign of nasal vestibular furunculosis: questions raised by this common but under-recognized nasal mucocutaneous disorder. Dermatol Online J. 2012;18(3):6.
54. Matos DM, Coelho R. "Apple Jelly" Sign: Diascopy in Cutaneous Sarcoidosis. Acta Medica Portuguesa. 2015;28(3):394.
55. Ravikiran SP, Jaiswal AK, Syrti C, Madan Mohan NT, Aradhya SS. Granuloma faciale: An unusual diascopic finding. Indian Dermatol Online J. 2016;7:174-6.

56. Sharma S, Khaitan BK, Kumarasinghe SP. Cutaneous signs in dermatological diseases; an overview. Indian J Dermatol. 2021;66(5):530-9.
57. Agarwal US, Mathur D, Mathur D, Besarwal RK, Agarwal P. Ear sign. Indian Dermatol Online J. 2014;5:105-6.
58. Kangle S, Amladi S, Sawant S. Scaly signs in dermatology. Indian J Dermatol Venereol Leprol. 2006;72:161-4.
59. Khetan, Vijay D. Subconjunctival Loa Loa with calabar swelling. Indian J Ophthalmol. 2007;55(2):165-6.
60. Pasha MM, Patil CC, Tanuja M, Mitra D. A rare case of cutaneous onchocerciasis in North-East India, review of literature. Indian Dermatol Online J. 2020;11(4):600-3.
61. Afolabi OJ. Clinical signs of river blindness and the efficacy of ivermectin therapy in Idogun, Ondo State, Nigeria. J Infect Dis Epidemiol. 2020;6:157.
62. Modjtahedi BS, Alikhan A, Maibach HI, Schwab IR. Diseases of periocular hair. Surv Ophthalmol. 2011;56(5):416-32.
63. Khalid Al Aboud, Ahmad Al Aboud: Eponyms linked to "signs" in the dermatology literature. Our Dermatol Online. 2013;4(4):579-81.
64. Mehta V, Balachandran C, Lonikar V. Blueberry muffin baby: a pictoral differential diagnosis. Dermatol Online J. 2008;14(2):8.
65. Sil A, Bhanja DB, Chandra A, Biswas SK. BOTE sign in molluscum contagiosum. BMJ Case Reports CP. 2020;13:e239142.
66. Butala N, Siegfried E, Weissler A. Molluscum BOTE sign: a predictor of imminent resolution. Pediatrics. 2013;131(5):e1650-3.
67. Chakraborty U, Biswas P, Chandra A, Pal K, Ray AK. Chik sign: post-chikungunya hyperpigmentation. QJM Int J Med. 2021;114(2):137-8.
68. Bhatia SS, Shenoi SD, Hebbar SA, Kayarkatte MN. The chik sign in dengue. Pediatr Dermatol. 2019;36(5):737-8.
69. Turan E, Seremet S. "Goat eyes": Horizontal rectangular pupils: An unusual clinical presentation of Orf. Indian J Dermatol Venereol Leprol. 2015;81:327.
70. Brzezinski P, Sinjab AT, Masferrer E, Gopie P, Naraysingh V, Yamamoto T, et al. Dermatology Eponyms–sign–Lexicon (G). Our Dermatol Online. 2012;3:243-57.
71. Sawant SP. Hoagland sign: An early manifestation of acute infectious mononucleosis-A case report. Curr Pediatr Res. 2017;21(3):400-2.
72. Gautam M, Sheth P. Hutchinson's signs in dermatology. Indian J Paediatr Dermatol. 2018;19:371-4.
73. Arif T, Amin SS. Tasleem's water jet sign - A new sign in dermatology. Our Dermatol Online. 2015;6(3):382-3.
74. Kapoor P, Gonsalves WI. Of lions, shar-pei, and doughnuts: a tale retold. Blood. 2020;135(14):1074-6.
75. Brzeziński P, Chiriac A, Munsey C, Sinjab AT: Dermatology eponyms – sign – lexicon – (J). Our Dermatol Online. 2013;4(3):399-402.
76. Segula D, Banda P, Mulambia C, Kumwenda JJ. Case report–A forgotten dermatological disease. Malawi Med J. 2012;24(1):19-20.
77. Madhyastha SP, Shetty GV, Shetty VM, et al. The classic pellagra dermatitis. BMJ Case Reports CP. 2020;13(10):e239741.
78. Upreti V, Vasdev V, Dhull P, Patnaik SK. Prayer sign in diabetes mellitus. Indian J Endocrinol Metab. 2013;17(4):769-70.
79. Mudang J, George AE, Varghese SA. Major contributions to dermatology from India. J Skin Sex Transm Dis. 2020;2(2):79-85.
80. Kannan KS, Sundharam SB, Manikandan R. Nevoid basal cell carcinoma syndrome. Indian J Dent Res. 2006;17(1):50-3.
81. Kudur MH, Hulmani M. "Pseudo" conditions in dermatology: Need to know both real and unreal. Indian J Dermatol Venereol Leprol. 2012;78(6):763-73.
82. Brzezinski P, Chiriac A, Rath SK. Dermatology eponyms – sign – Lexicon – (N). Our Dermatol Online. 2014;5(4):442-7.
83. Kim IH, Lee SG. (2012). The skin crease sign: A diagnostic sign of pilomatricoma. J Am Acad Dermatol. 2012;67(5):e197-8.
84. Pant I, Joshi SC, Kaur G, Kumar G. Pilomatricoma as a diagnostic pitfall in clinical practice: report of two cases and review of literature. Indian J Dermatol. 2010;55(4):390-2.
85. Stoyanov G S, Dzhenkov D L, Tzaneva M. Thrombophlebitis migrans (Trousseau syndrome) in pancreatic adenocarcinoma: An autopsy report. Cureus. 2019;11(8):e5528.
86. Scope A, Dusza SW, Halpern AC, et al. The "ugly duckling" sign: Agreement between observers. Arch Dermatol. 2008;144(1):58-64.
87. Ganapati S. Eponymous dermatological signs in bullous dermatoses. Indian J Dermatol. 2014;59(1):21-3.
88. Soni AG. Nikolsky's sign - A clinical method to evaluate damage at epidermal-dermal junction. J Indian Acad Oral Med Radiol. 2018;30:68-72.
89. Sachdev D. Sign of Nikolsky and related signs. Indian J Dermatol Venereol Leprol. 2003;69:243-4.
90. Premalatha S. Cerebriform tongue, the history behind the sign. Indian J Dermatol. 2014;59(2):198-9.
91. Pandiaraja J. Another cutaneous sign of acute pancreatitis. Indian J Crit Care Med. 2016;20(5):313-4.
92. Tubbs RS, Shoja MM, Loukas M, Oakes WJ, Cohen-Gadol A. William Henry Battle and Battle's sign: mastoid ecchymosis as an indicator of basilar skull fracture. J Neurosurg. 2010;112(1):186-8.
93. Navarro S. Eponyms in pancreatology: The people behind the names. Gastroenterol Hepatol. 2017;40(4):317-26.
94. Sarkar S, Fung MA, Raychaudhuri SP. "Coral bead sign" in Multicentric Reticulohistiocytosis. Int J Dermatol. 2020;59(6):e203-4.
95. Rahbour G, Ullah MR, Yassin N, Thomas GP. Cullen's sign - Case report with a review of the literature. Int J Surg Case Rep. 2012;3(5):143-6.
96. Szczerkowska-Dobosz A, Kozicka D, Purzycka-Bohdan D, Biernat W, Stawczyk M, Nowicki R. Juvenile xanthogranuloma: A rare benign histiocytic disorder. Postępy dermatologii i alergologii. 2014;31:197-200.
97. Plastic Surgery Key. The Histiocytoses. [online] Available from: https://plasticsurgerykey.com/the-histiocytoses/. [Last accessed December, 2022].
98. Goyal T, Kohli S. Darier's sign. Indian J Paediatr Dermatol. 2018;19:277-9.
99. Surjushe A, Jindal S, Gote P, Saple DG. Darier's sign. Indian J Dermatol Venereol Leprol. 2007;73:363-4.
100. Pakran J. Sparing phenomena in dermatology. Indian J Dermatol Venereol Leprol. 2013;79:545-50.
101. Shenoy M M, Bendigeri MA, Kamath PR, Vishal B. Diffuse leprosy with "deck-chair" sign. Indian Dermatol Online J. 2015;6:204-6.
102. Fitzpatrick TB, Gilchrest BA. Dimple sign to differentiate benign from malignant pigmented cutaneous lesions. N Engl J Med. 1977;296(26):1518.
103. Yadav S, Narang T, Kumaran M S. Psychodermatology: A comprehensive review. Indian J Dermatol Venereol Leprol. 2013;79:176-92.

104. Lin AN, Lin K, Kyaw H, Abboud J. A myth still needs to be clarified: A case report of the Frank's sign. Cureus. 2018;10(1):e2080.
105. Wu F, Ng CY. The goosebump sign. J Hand Microsurg. 2019;11(1):57-8.
106. Landis ET, Taheri A, Jorizzo JL. Gulliver's sign: A recognizable transition from inflammatory to healing stages of pyoderma gangrenosum. J Dermatolog Treat. 2015;26(2):171-2.
107. Drolet BA, Clowry L Jr, McTigue MK, Esterly NB. The hair collar sign: marker for cranial dysraphism. Pediatrics. 1995;96(2 Pt 1):309-13.
108. Dhar S, Kanwar AJ, Handa S. 'Hanging curtain' sign in pityriasis rosea. Dermatology. 1995;190(3):252.
109. Borzutzky A, Tejos-Bravo M, Venegas LF, Iturriaga C. Hertoghe's sign in atopic dermatitis. J Pediatr. 2020;226:299.
110. Parrino D, Di Bella S. Hertoghe sign: a hallmark of lepromatous leprosy. QJM Int J Med. 2016;109(7):497.
111. Cox JT, Gullotti DM, Mecoli CA, Lahouti AH, Albayda J, Paik J, et al. "Hiker's feet": a novel cutaneous finding in the inflammatory myopathies. Clin Rheumatol. 2017;36(7):1683-6.
112. Brzezinski P, Hassan I, Chiriac A, Sinjab AT. Dermatology eponyms-sign-Lexicon-(I). Our Dermatol Online. 2013;4(2):256-9.
113. Goss JA, Greene AK. Sensitivity and specificity of the stemmer sign for lymphedema: A clinical lymphoscintigraphic study. Plast Reconstr Surg Glob Open. 2019;7(6):e2295.
114. Freudenmann RW, Kölle M, Schönfeldt-Lecuona C, Dieckmann S, Harth W, Lepping P. Delusional parasitosis and the matchbox sign revisited: the international perspective. Acta Derm Venereol. 2010;90(5):517-9.
115. Pathmarajah P, Rowland Payne C. Paired ear creases of the Helix (PECH): A possible physical sign. Cureus. 2017;9(11):e1884.
116. Chan HH, Lam LK, Wong DS, Leung RS, Ying SY, Lai CF, et al. Nevus of Ota: A new classification based on the response to laser treatment. Lasers Surg Med. 2001;28:267-72.
117. Isaac J, Goldminz AM, Scheinman PL. "Pink sign": The importance of short-term occlusive testing in suspected cases of contact urticaria. Dermatitis. 2019;30(2):168-9.
118. Sherman SC, Lee J. Plantar ecchymosis sign. J Emerg Med. 2019;57(2):e57-8.
119. Savoia F, Stinchi C, Gaddoni G, Patrizi A, Odorici G, Tengattini V, et al. The rope sign: a case of interstitial granulomatous dermatitis with arthritis. G Ital Dermatol Venereol. 2016;151(1):102-5.
120. Chi WK, Tan GM, Yan BP. Urschel's sign in Paget-Schroetter syndrome: Multimodality evaluation by extravascular and intravascular imaging. J Invasive Cardiol. 2020;32(2):E47-8.
121. Madke B, Kar S, Yadav N. Newly described signs in dermatology. Indian Dermatol Online J. 2015;6(3):220-1.
122. Zampetti A, Rotoli M, Tiberi S. Clinical diagnostic skill in dermatology: How to read palms: Learning points from a routine clinical case. Austin J Dermatolog. 2015;2(2):103.
123. Goutham SM, Karunanandhan M. The Biett collarette: Secondary syphilis. IDCases. 2020;19:e00615.
124. Saliny M, Joy B, Sridharan R. Laws and signs of congenital syphilis. J Skin Sex Transm Dis. 2020;2(1):62-4.
125. Vashisht D, Baveja S. Eponyms in syphilis. Indian J Sex Transm Dis AIDS. 2015;36(2):226-9.
126. Katz KA. Dory flop sign of syphilis. Arch Dermatol. 2010;146(5):572.
127. Voelpel JH, Muehlberger T. The du Bois sign. Ann Plast Surg. 2011;66(3):241-4.
128. Yang Kl. Clavicle sign of late congenital syphilis: Review of literature and report of six cases. Arch Derm Syphilol. 1940;41(6):1060-5.
129. Fiumara NJ. Manifestations of late congenital syphilis. Arch Dermatol. 1970;102(1):78-83.
130. Arnold HL. Eyebrow Alopecia: "The Omnibus Sign". Arch Dermatol. 1965;91(1):94.
131. Radiopaedia. (2022). [online] Available from: https://radiopaedia.org/articles/wimberger-sign-1. [Last accessed December, 2022].
132. Nair PS, Nanda Kumar G, Jayapalan S. The "sign of groove", a new cutaneous sign of internal malignancy. Indian J Dermatol Venereol Leprol. 2007;73:141.
133. Palit A, Raghunatha S, Inamadar AC. History taking and clinical examination. In: Kar HK, Kumar B, (eds). IAL Textbook of Leprosy, 1st edition. New Delhi: Jaypee Brothers Medical Publishers; 2010. pp. 121-43.
134. Colditz JC. Clinical pearls Difference between Froment's sign and Jeannes sign in ulnar palsy. HandLab. 2013;25.
135. Kumarasinghe SP, Kumarasinghe MP, Amarasinghe UT. "Tap sign" in tuberculoid and borderline tuberculoid leprosy. Int J Lepr Other Mycobact Dis. 2004;72(3):291-5.
136. Brzeziński P. Dermatology eponyms-phenomenon/sign-Lexicon(E). Our Dermatol Online. 2011:2(4):235-40.
137. Brzeziński P, Pessoa L, Galvão V, Barja Lopez JM, Adaskevich UP, Pascal A, et al. Dermatology eponyms – sign – Lexicon – (H). Our Dermatol Online. 2013;4(1):130-43.
138. Brzeziński P, Tanaka M, Husein-ElAhmed H, Castori M, Barro/Traoré F, Kashiram Punshi S, et al. Eponyms – sign –Lexicon (P). Part 2. Our Dermatol Online. 2016;7(3):359-65.
139. Brzeziński P, Senanayake MP, Karunaratne I, Chiriac A. Dermotology eponyms – sign – Lexicon (R): Part 1. Our Dermatology Online. 2017;8(1):114-20.
140. Brzeziński P, Satoh M, Adaskevich UP, Dhavalshankh A, Aby J, Arenas R, et al. Dermatology Eponyms – sign – Lexicon (S). Part I. Our Dermatol Online. 2018;9(3):346-54.
141. Brzeziński P, Martini L, Sharquie KE, Ahu Y, Al Aboud K, Rafiei R, et al. Dermatology Eponyms – sign – Lexicon (W). Our Dermatol Online. 2019;11(1):103-12.
142. Brzeziński P, Martini L, Sood S. Dermatology eponyms – sign – Lexicon (Y). Our Dermatol Online. 2020;11(e):e181.1-e181.2.
143. White FA. Physical signs in Medicine and Surgery, An Atlas Of Rare, Lost And Forgotten Physical Signs. Bloomington: Xlibris, Corp; 2009.

Hair, Nail, and Mucosal Signs and Appearance in Dermatology

Akash Kumar Shah

INTRODUCTION

Many diagnostic clues are obtained during hair, nail, and mucosal examination, which aids in cutaneous examination and history findings. Many signs pertaining to these structures are of vital importance and we have tried to include all possible named signs and appearance, but few might have been missed.

This chapter does not focus and include dermoscopic signs or appearance pertaining to these structures as they are discussed in another chapter.

NAIL SIGNS

- *Angel's wings*: The combination of fissuring plus atrophy can lead to a deformity likened to "angel's wings" **(Fig. 1)**. A characteristic nail deformity associated with lichen planus in which the central portion of the nail appears raised and the lateral portions are depressed.[1]
- *Beau's lines*: This refers to transverse groove because of temporary growth arrest in nail matrix **(Fig. 2)**. It can be seen in various disorders such as trauma, pregnancy, and paronychia.[2]
- *Coral bead sign*: Papules present around the nail folds seen in cases of multicentric reticulohistiocytosis.[3]
- *Half and half nail*: A nail with proximal white and distal pink part separated by sharp demarcation line. It is seen in hemodialysis patient and renal transplant patients.[4]
- *Hutchinson nail sign*: Periungual extension of longitudinal melanonychia from nail bed to nail fold and surrounding area is suggestive of nail melanoma. Similar finding on onychoscopy is known as micro–Hutchinson sign.[4]

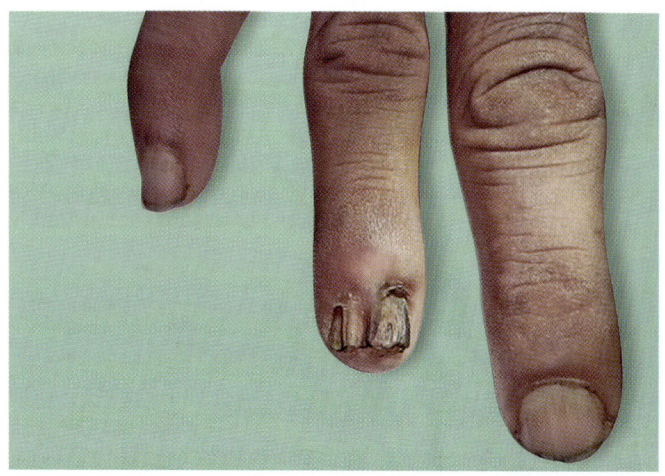

FIG. 1: Angel's wing sign.

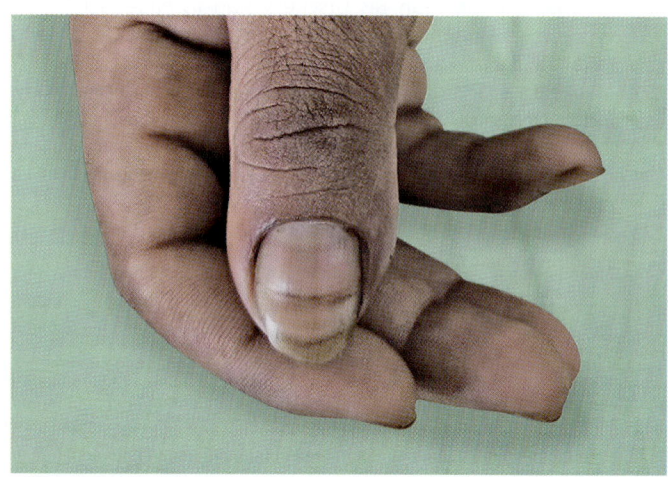

FIG. 2: Beau's line.

- *Love sign*: It refers to the tenderness localized over nail bed on giving vertical pressure over glomus tumor of nail with pin head or ball pen.[5]
- *Median canaliform dystrophy of Heller (solenonychia)/Inverted fir tree appearance*: A nail disorder characterized by paramedian canal or split in the nail plate with small fissures extending laterally from the central canal toward lateral nail edge giving it an inverted fir or Christmas tree appearance.[6]
- *Muehrcke's line*: Alternate transverse bands of white and pink lines which signifies chronic hypoalbuminemia.[4]
- *Nail floating on lake of pus appearance*: Localized form of pustular psoriasis involving nail bed, when the pustules coalesce which gives this appearance is seen in Acrodermatitis continua of Hallopeau.
- *Oil drop sign/Salmon patch*: Circular area of discoloration as a result of proximal subungual hyperkeratosis is observed in nail psoriasis.[7]
- *Pincer nail/Trumpet nails/Omega nail*: It is a common toenail disorder (rarely fingernails) in which lateral ends of the nail plate bends downward and inward, compressing the nail bed and underlying dermis. Seen in those wearing tight fitting shoes, trauma, Kawasaki disease, and renal disease, etc.[4]
- *Pseudo–Hutchinson sign*: Periungual pigmentation-like nail melanoma seen in Bowen's disease of nail and in many other benign conditions.[3]
- *Pup tent sign*: Tent-like elevation of nail plate (longitudinally) due to papule of nail bed in nail lichen planus.[8]
- *Racquet nail*: This refers to short, wide, and flattened thumbnails. Usually inherited but has also been reported in hyperparathyroidism and Erasmus syndrome.[4]
- *Ram's horn-like nail/Onychogryphosis*: It is thickening of nail plate with deformity [clawing/Ram's horn like; **(Fig. 3)**]. It may be seen in neglected nail, old age, due to trauma, or associated with peripheral vascular disease.[4]
- *Roller coaster nail*: Distal onycholysis as a result of manicure/pedicure along with edged whitish appearance of nail plate with an oscillating pattern resembles roller coaster.[9]
- *Samitz sign*: It refers to dystrophic and ragged cuticle seen in dermatomyositis.[3]
- *Schamroth's sign/Watch glass nail/Drumstick finger/Hippocratic finger*: Seen in nail clubbing where there is loss of diamond-shaped window when corresponding fingers of each hand opposed together. There is increase in Lovibond angle (>160°). It could be idiopathic or secondary to systemic diseases like, bronchogenic carcinoma of lungs, etc.
- *Scotch plaid pattern*: Fine and regular pitting over nails seen in alopecia areata.
- *Terry nail*: Whitish appearance of whole nail except distal 1–2 mm due to telangiectasia of nail bed. Seen in patients with cirrhosis, chronic congestive heart failure, and adult-onset diabetes.[4]
- *Thimble nail*: Irregular and course pitting of nail plate due to pathology of dorsal nail matrix, seen in nail psoriasis.
- *Yellow line of Pinkus*: A line or band formed by onychocorneal junction at proximal nail fold separating nail plate from the skin. Abnormality in this results in onycholysis, pachyonychia congenita, and pterygium inversum unguis.[10]

MUCOSAL SIGNS

- *Burton line*: This refers to very thin black-blue line present along the margin of gums in cases of chronic lead poisoning.[10]
- *Caviar tongue*: Purplish venous ectasias seen over ventral aspect of tongue, attributed to elastic tissue degeneration. Seen in elderly and can be associated with Fordyce angiokeratoma of scrotum.[11]
- *Dory flop sign*: Snapping back of retracted prepuce in case of lesion of primary syphilis [chancre; **(Fig. 4)**] present over inner surface of prepuce.[3]

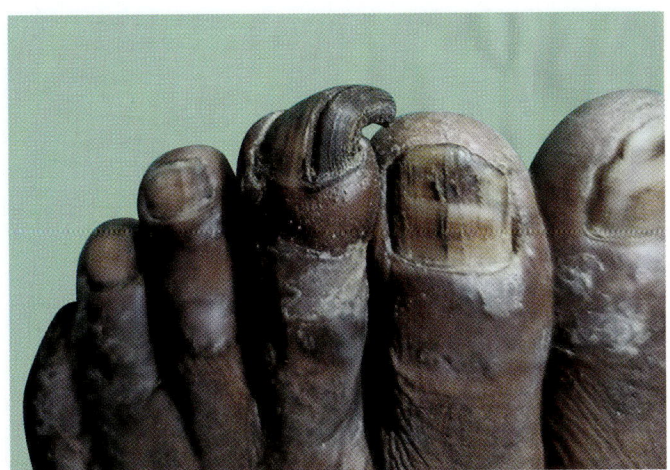

FIG. 3: Onychogryphosis.

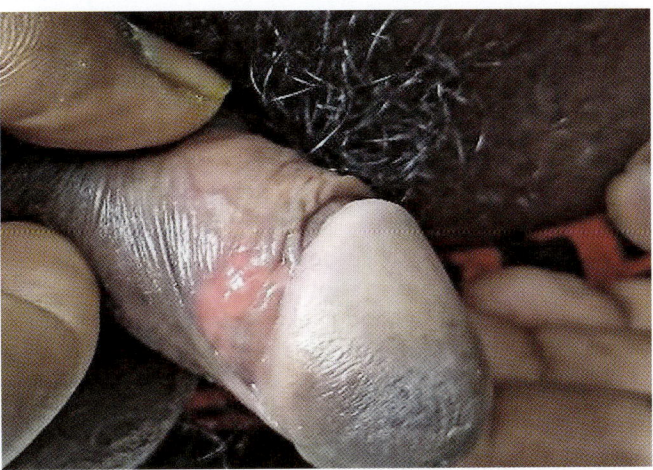

FIG. 4: Chancre with dory flop sign.

- *Figure-of-eight/Hourglass appearance*: In girls and women with lichen sclerosus et atrophicus, a figure-of-eight or hourglass configuration with vulvar and perianal involvement is common.[3]
- *Forchheimer's sign*: Fleeting enanthem seen as petechiae over the soft palate in 20% patients with rubella; can also been seen in scarlet fever and measles.[3]
- *Geographic tongue*: Sharply demarcated ringed or gyrate red dispersed patches with yellowish white border, making tongue look like a map. The patches may disappear at one site and appear on another. "Annulus migrans" term has been suggested for geographic tongue in reactive arthritis or pustular psoriasis.[4]
- *Hutchinson's teeth*: Peg-shaped incisors and is syphilitic stigmata. Seen as triad along with interstitial keratitis and sensorineural hearing loss.[3]
- *Koplik's spot*: Prodrome of viral enanthem seen as clustered white spots over buccal mucosa opposite first and second molar; 2–3 days before rash and is pathognomonic of measles.
- *Meffert's sign*: Seen in patients having Fordyce spots as lip marks over rim of cup while consuming a hot beverage.[3]
- *Mulberry molars*: Affected first molar has occlusive flat surface with only poorly enameled rudiments of the usual cusps. It is a syphilitic stigma.[12]
- *Premlatha sign*: It refers to cerebriform appearance of tongue seen in pemphigus vegetans.[13]
- *Stafne's sign*: Radiological sign of widening of periodontal ligament space seen in progressive systemic sclerosis due to bulk of ligament by increased collagen synthesis.[3]
- *Strawberry gums*: Petechial hemorrhage superimposed on friable micropapular surface of gingiva. Hypertrophic gums seen in Wegner's granulomatosis and mucosal sarcoidosis.[12]
- *Strawberry tongue (red)*: This term refers to a tongue that is swollen, bumpy (hypertrophic fungiform papillae) and bright red, resembling a strawberry. It generally occurs in children with medical conditions, such as scarlet fever and Kawasaki disease.[12]
- *Trumpeter's wart*: It is firm, fibrous, and pseudoepitheliomatous nodule of the upper lip of trumpet player.[4]
- *White strawberry tongue*: White coated tongue of scarlet fever.[12]

HAIR SIGNS

- *Bamboo hair*: Intussusception of hair shaft at the zone where keratinization begins, giving a bamboo appearance or ball and socket deformity. Sometimes, distal part of the hair breaks and proximal end has golf-tee appearance. In Netherton syndrome bamboo hair is associated with atopic dermatitis and ichthyosis linearis circumflexa with double border scale.[4]
- *Beaded hair*: Fusiform or spindle shaped swelling of hair shaft separated by narrow strophic segments seen in monilethrix. Hair breaks at internodes and is due to *desmoglein 4* gene mutation.[4]
- *Cadaverous hair*: These are remnant of broken hair in alopecia areata.[14]
- *Coudability sign*: Bending or kinking of hair on pushing the hair inward in alopecia areata **(Figs. 5 and 6)**. It is seen due to tapering of hair at the base.[14]
- *Exclamation point hair*: Tapering of hair follicle seen as thick distal end and thinning at proximal hair **(Fig. 7)** seen in alopecia areata.[14]
- *Flag sign*: Alternate band of depigmented hair and pigmented hair seen in protein energy malnutrition formed during the acute phase of deficiency.[15]
- *Frayed paintbrush hair*: Small white nodes present at hair shaft and breaks at the nodes seen in trichorrhexis nodosa.[4]
- *Friar tuck sign/Orentreich sign*: Patient with trichotillomania plucks his own hair either in a wave-like pattern across the scalp or centrifugally from a single starting point. This results in loss of vertex hair and sparing of the occipital area.[3]

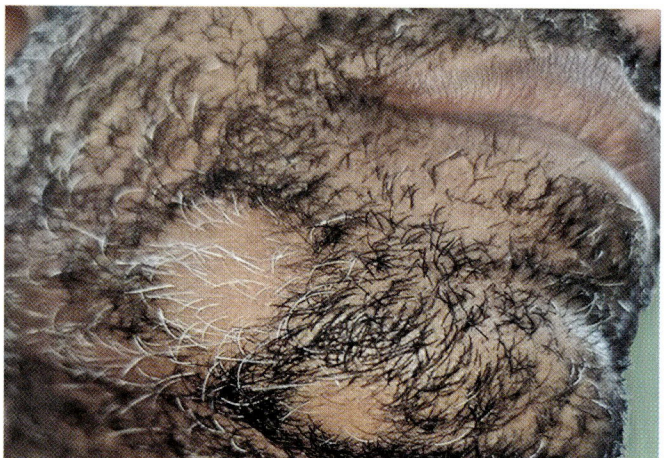

FIG. 5: Alopecia areata.

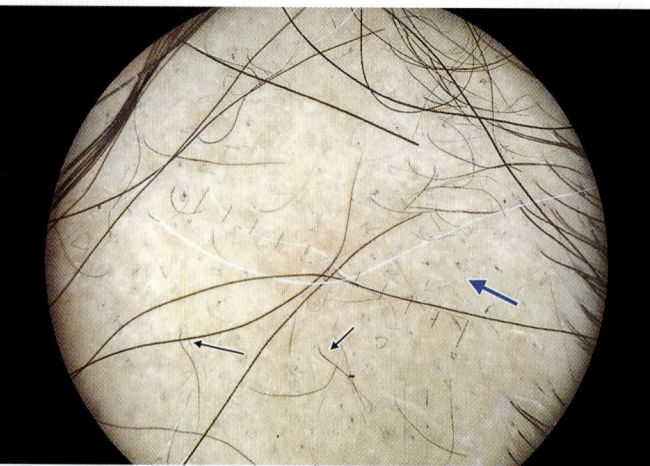

FIG. 6: Coudability sign (black); pigtail vellus hair (blue).

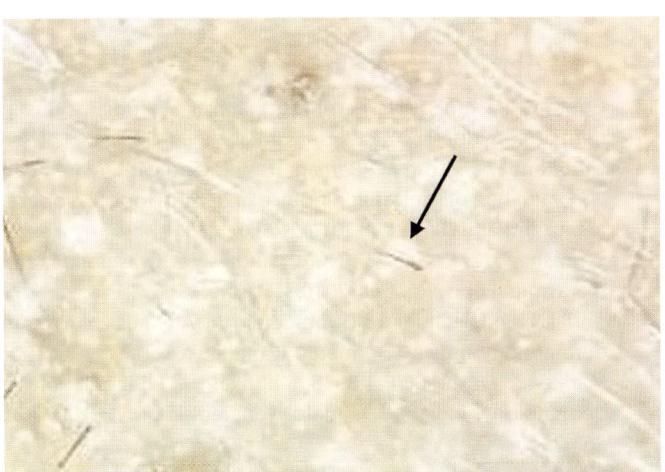

FIG. 7: Exclamation hair.

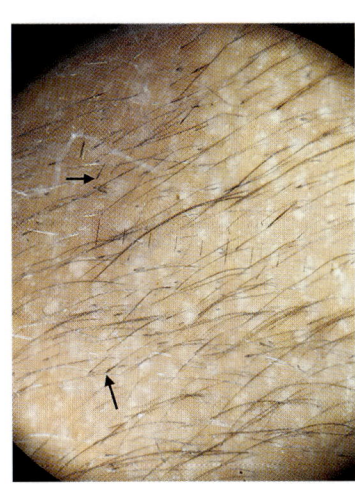

FIG. 8: Tulip sign.

- *Hair collar sign/Faun tail nevus*: It is seen in cranial dysraphism where the cranial defect is seen as hairless area and is surrounded by collar of hair. Similar appearance is noted as long hair over lower back in spinal dysraphism.[16]
- *Hamburger sign*: In trichotillomania, vertically oriented split of hair shafts and proteinaceous material and erythrocytes are present in the split resembling a hamburger within a bun.[3]
- *Lonely hair sign*: Presence of one or few terminal hair over middle of forehead seen in frontal fibrosing alopecia.[1]
- *Moth eaten alopecia*: Patches of nonscarring alopecia over occipital area, characteristically seen in secondary syphilis.
- *Paradoxical hair*: It is unwanted hair growth over areas other than scalp in patients using topical minoxidil preparations, it is also known as rochade or castling phenomenon. Paradoxical hair can also be seen after laser therapy for hair removal.[17]
- *Pig tail hair*: Seen in alopecia areata as short vellus hair signifying the remission of disease after treatment.[14] Also described in tinea capitis as short broken terminal hair that are coiled up like a pig tail or corkscrew.[18]
- *Pitaluga sign*: It refers to acquired hypertrichosis of eyelashes due to kala-azar.[3]
- *Pohl-Pinkus constriction*: It is progressive and irregular constrictions seen along the length of hair shaft, better viewed on dermoscopy. Pohl-Pinkus or monilethrix-like constrictions are the result of abrupt and repeated arrest of the metabolic and mitotic activity of the hair follicle caused by an internal or external factor and are observed in many congenital and acquired chronic processes, including alopecia areata, chemotherapy-induced alopecia, severe malnutrition, interferon alpha-2c treatment, and severe systemic infections.[19]
- *Pseudopelade of Brocq/footprint in snow*: Patchy areas of cicatricial alopecia in scalp. It has been classically described in pseudopelade of Brocq.[20]

- *Ringed or spangled hair*: Alternating segments of light and dark color of hair shaft when seen in reflected light. Light bands are seen due to air filled cavities seen in pili annulati.[4]
- *Rumpled sock appearance*: It is seen in anagen hair syndrome due to defect in hair cuticle of anagen hair, cuticle folds back as rumpled sock and can be easily plucked out.[4]
- *Spun glass appearance*: Triangular cross-sectional appearance of hair with longitudinal groove (pili trianguli et canaliculi) is observed in uncombable hair syndrome.[4]
- *Tiger tail appearance*: Alternating light and dark band seen over hair strand when seen under polarized light are observed in trichothiodystrophy/Tay syndrome.[16]
- *Tufted hair appearance (doll's hair)*: Seen in various cicatricial alopecia as bundling of follicular units seen in folliculitis decalvans, chronic lupus erythematosus (LE), lichen planopilaris, etc.[20]
- *Tulip sign*: Seen in trichotillomania as short hair with darker and tulip flower-shaped ends **(Fig. 8)**. These hair develop when a hair shaft fractures diagonally. When hair shafts are almost totally damaged by mechanical manipulation, only a sprinkled hair residue is visible. This finding is referred to as "hair powder".[21]
- *Whisker hair*: Short dark hair that grows anterior to the ears in young people who eventually develop androgenetic alopecia. Maybe a form of kinky hair.
- *White forelock*: A triangular flock of white depigmented hair present over the anterior scalp. Seen in Waardenburg syndrome and piebaldism.[4]
- *Woolly hair*: Uncommon congenital anomaly of scalp hair presenting with strongly curled hair with reduced diameter. Seen in Naxos syndrome and Carvajal syndrome.
- *Zigzag hair*: Short hair with several bends in them like a zigzag pattern in tinea capitis.[18]

REFERENCES

1. Bolognia JL, Schaffer JV, Cerroni L. Dermatology, 4th edition. Philadelphia: Elsevier; 2018.
2. Alobaida S, Lam JM. Beau lines associated with COVID-19. CMAJ. 2020;192(36):E1040.
3. Madke B, Nayak C. Eponymous signs in dermatology. Indian Dermatol Online J. 2012;3(3):159-65.
4. James WD, Elston DM, Treat JR, Rosenbach MA, Neuhaus IM. Andrew's Diseases of the Skin: Clinical Dermatology, 13th edition. Philadelphia: Elsevier; 2019.
5. Shukla A, Verma V, Shukla R, Chaudhary R, Sharma S, Sajid M. Love sign's love for glomus tumor. Hand Microsurg. 2018;7(2):105-8.
6. Kota R, Pilani A, Nair PA. Median Nail Dystrophy Involving the Thumb Nail. Indian J Dermatol. 2016;61(1):120.
7. Manhart R, Rich P. Nail psoriasis. Clin Exp Rheumatol. 2015;33(Suppl 93):S7-13.
8. Naveen KN. Pup tent sign. Indian Dermatol Online J. 2014;5(4):552-3.
9. Yarulmaz A, Yalcin B. A novel dermoscopic feature in traumatic onycholysis. Our Dermatol Online. 2018;9(3):307-9.
10. Savitha AS. Lines in dermatology. Clin Dermatol Rev. 2017;1(1):27-31.
11. Viswanath V, Nair S, Chavan N, Torsekar R. Caviar tongue. Indian J Dermatol Venereol Leprol. 2011;77(1):78-9.
12. Jindal N, Jindal P, Kumar J, Gupta S, Jain VK. Fruit and Food Eponyms in Dermatology. Indian J Dermatol. 2015;60(2):213.
13. Gupta G, Reshma P, Naveen KN, Athanikar SB. Indian signs in dermatology. Med j DY Patil Univ. 2014;7(2):261-2.
14. Guttikonda AS, Aruna C, Ramamurthy D, Sridevi K, Alagappan SL. Evaluation of clinical significance of dermoscopy in alopecia areata. Indian J Dermatol. 2016;61(6):628-33.
15. Scrimshaw NS, Viteri FE. INCAP studies of Kwashiorkor and marasmus. Food Nutr Bull. 2010;31(1):34-41.
16. Jindal N, Jindal P, Kumar J, Gupta S, Jain VK. Animals eponyms in dermatology. Indian J Dermatol. 2014;59(6):631.
17. Madke B, Doshi B, Pande S, Khopkar U. Phenomenon in dermatology. Indian J Dermatol Venereol Leprol. 2011;77(3):264-75.
18. Elghblawi E. Idiosyncratic Findings in Trichoscopy of Tinea Capitis: Comma, Zigzag Hairs, Corkscrew, and Morse Code-like Hair. Int J Trichology. 2016;8(4):180-3.
19. Lobato-Berezo A, Olmos-Alpiste F, Pujol RM, Saceda-Corralo. Pohl-Pinkus constrictions in Trichoscopy. Actas Dermosifiliorg. 2019;110(4):315-6.
20. Madke B, Chougule BD, Kar S, Khopkar U. Appearances in clinical dermatology. Indian J Dermatol Venereol Leprol. 2014;80(5):432-47.
21. Ankad BS, Naidu MV, Beergouder SL, Sujana L. Trichoscopy in Trichotillomania: A Useful Diagnostic Tool. Int J Trichology. 2014;6(4):160-3.

29. Facies in Dermatology

Avanitaben Dipakkumar Solanki, Ishan Asutosh Pandya

INTRODUCTION

We only see what we know. The process of vision is fairly simple. When we see something, the rods and cones situated in the retina transfers those signals to the brain. It is the brain in which the things get complex. The image received is processed and interpreted. Even though it is processed the same in everyone; interpretation differs from person to person. Our knowledge, past experiences, and beliefs play an important role in the interpretation of a specific image.

Reading face is an art. To differentiate a normal face from even a slightly abnormal one requires skills, knowledge, and experience on the part of a clinician. While we cannot impart skills and experience through literature, this is our humble attempt to spread the knowledge about recognition of various facies in dermatology.

TYPES OF FACIES

Acromegalic Facies (Fig. 1)[1]

- *Condition*: Acromegaly, familial partial lipodystrophy
- *Features*:
  - Large supraorbital ridge and frontal bossing
  - Protruding, edematous thick eyelids
  - Triangular large ears
  - Numerous skin tags ("fibroma molluscum")
  - Widely spaced teeth
  - Enlarged and furrowed tongue
  - Thickened lower-lip
  - Firm and square lower jaw (protruding jaw = prognathism)
  - Cutis gyrata of the scalp (extreme cases)
- *Cause*: Periosteal new bone formation of the facial bones and generalized thickening of the skin

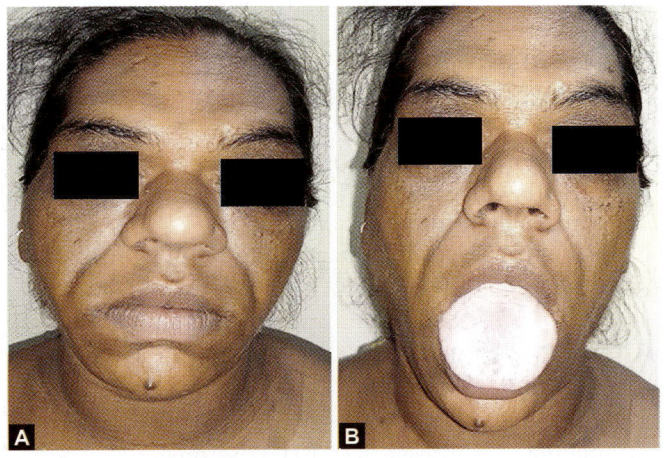

FIGS. 1A AND B: Acromegalic facies.

Adenoid Facies (Adenoid Hypertrophy) (Fig. 2)[2,3]

- *Conditions*: Hypertrophy of pharyngeal tonsils (adenoids), Cowden syndrome (multiple hamartoma syndrome), and Carney complex
- *Features*:
  - Underdeveloped thin nostrils
  - Short upper lip
  - Prominent upper teeth
  - Crowded teeth
  - Narrow upper alveolus
  - High-arched palate
  - Hypoplastic maxilla
  - Skin colored lichenoid papules tend to coalesce to give cobblestone appearance on and around the eyes and mouth (Cowden's syndrome)
  - Long, open-mouthed, dull and dumb-looking face

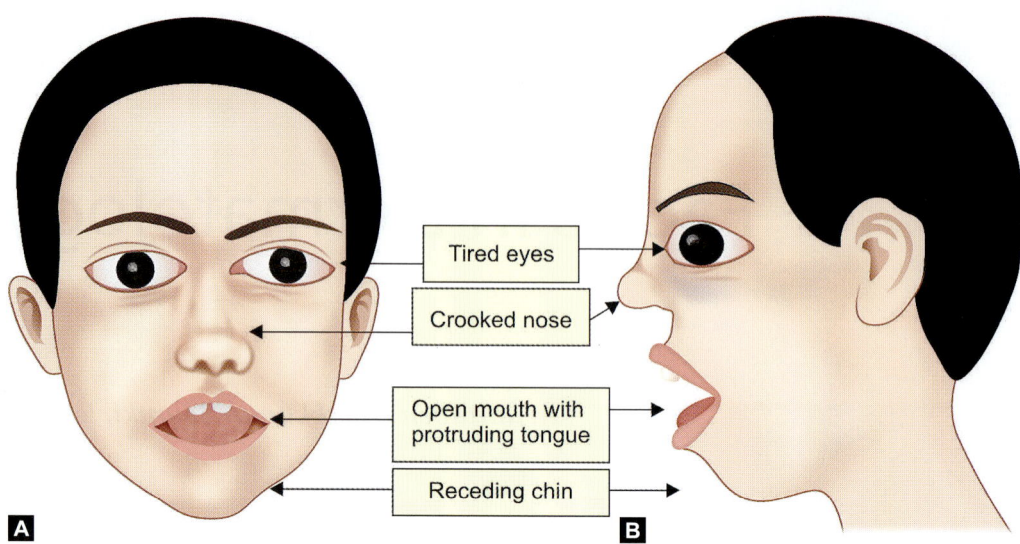

FIGS. 2A AND B: Adenoid facies.

Amiodarone Facies[4,5]
- *Condition*: Amiodarone administration
- *Features*:
  - Phototoxic eruption or a brown/blue-gray discoloration of sun-exposed skin, most commonly around malar area and nose
- *Cause*: Intralysosomal accumulation of lipids, amiodarone, and its metabolites in dermal macrophages

Angelic Facies[6,7]
- *Condition*: Chronic infantile neurological cutaneous and articular (CINCA) or neonatal onset multisystem inflammatory disease (NOMID) syndrome
- Nonpruritic urticarial erythema presents during first week of life
- *Features*:
  - Frontal bossing
  - Saddle-back nose
  - Midfacial hypoplasia

Antonine Facies/Facies in Facial Nerve Dysfunction (Fig. 3)[8,9]
- *Condition*: Bell's palsy, leprosy
- *Features*:
  - The eyelids on the paralyzed side cannot close (lagophthalmos)
  - Dry eye
  - The mouth is drawn to the unparalyzed side, producing a somewhat grotesque appearance.

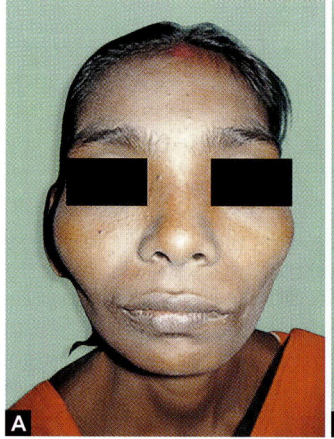 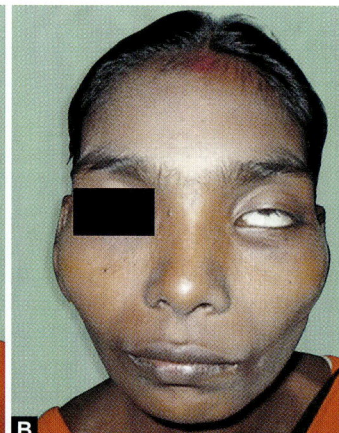

FIGS. 3A AND B: Antonine facies.

- Food and drink dribble from the mouth on the paralyzed side:
  - Face with blank expressions
- *Cause*: Involvement of facial nerves especially occipitotemporal and zygomatic branches

Asiatic Porcelain Doll Facies (Fig. 4)[10-12]
- *Condition*: Restrictive dermopathy (RD)
- Abnormal facies, tight and shiny skin, and secondary joint changes
- *Features*:
  - Small, fixed, and round open mouth
  - Micrognathia
  - Small nose

- Widely set ears
- Expressionless face
- Blurring of groove between nose and cheek
- Sparse or absent eyelashes

Asymmetric Crying Facies (Fig. 5)[13]
- *Condition*: Cayler cardiofacial syndrome
- *Features*:
    - Asymmetric appearance of the oral aperture and lips at rest
    - Significant depression of one side of the lower lip with animation (crying or smiling)

Bird-like Facies (Fig. 6)[14,15]
- *Conditions*: Pierre Robin malformation, Mulvihill-Smith syndrome, Hutchinson–Gilford progeria, Treacher Collins syndrome, Goldenhar syndrome, Miller syndrome, Nager syndrome, Nijmegen breakage syndrome, Familial partial lipodystrophy, and Hallermann–Streiff syndrome
- *Features*:
    - Small lower jaw (micrognathia) and retrognathia
    - A slit-like hole in the palate of mouth (cleft palate) with high arch
    - Tongue appears to fall into the throat (retroglosso-ptosis)

Bovine Facies (Fig. 7)[16]
- *Condition*: Craniofacial dysostosis or Crouzon syndrome
- *Features*:
    - Convex nasal profile
    - Shortened mandible
    - Macroglossia

Cachectic Facies (Fig. 8)[17]
- *Condition*: Human immunodeficiency virus (HIV) patients on highly active antiretroviral therapy (HAART)
- *Features*:
    - Prominent zygomata
    - Sunken eyes
    - Deepened redundant melolabial folds
- *Cause*: Peripheral lipoatrophy with loss of subcutaneous fat, particularly around buccal, parotid, and preauricular region

Cadaveric Facies (Fig. 9)[17]
- *Condition*: Congenital generalized lipodystrophy
- *Features*:
    - Slow symmetrical disappearance of metabolically active subcutaneous fat from face producing a cadaverous appearance
    - Distinctive muscular body habitus

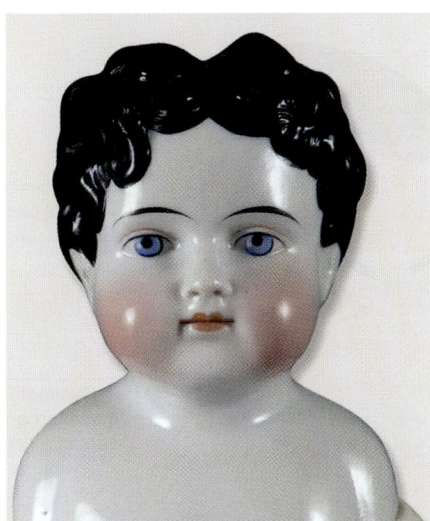

FIG. 4: Asiatic porcelain doll facies.

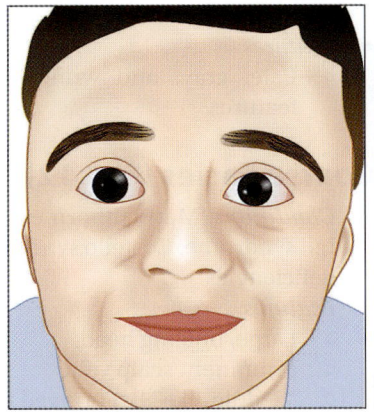 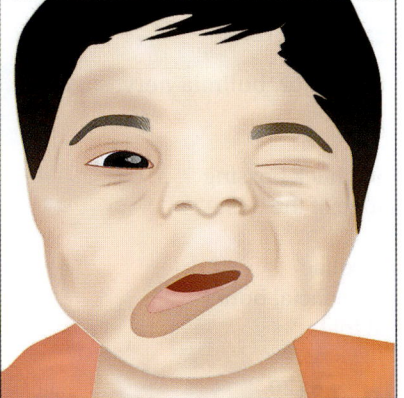

FIG. 5: Asymmetric crying facies.

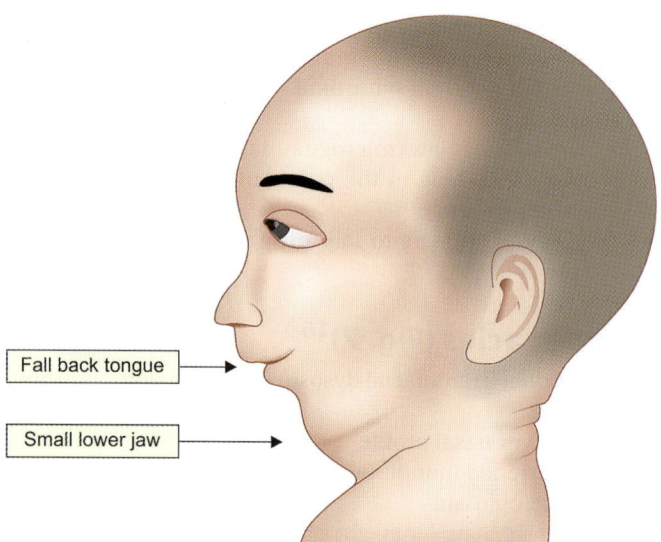

FIG. 6: Bird facies.

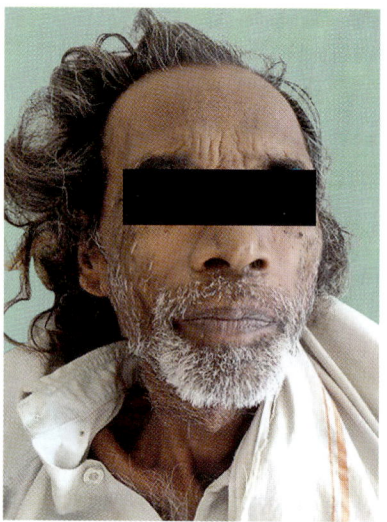

FIG. 8: Cachetic facies.

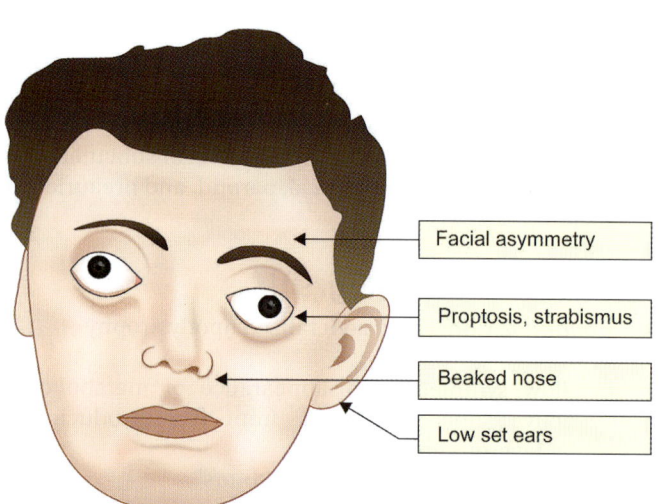

FIG. 7: Bovine facies.

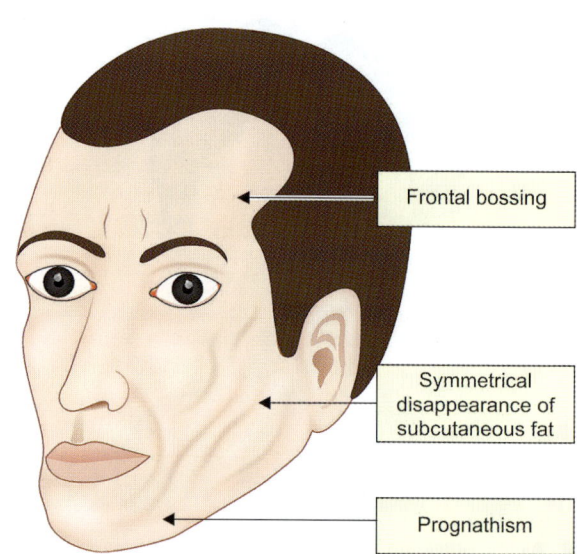

FIG. 9: Cadaveric facies.

Chipmunk Facies (Fig. 10)[18,19]

- *Conditions*: B-thalassemia major, bulimia nervosa, and parotid swelling
- *Features*:
  - Prominent frontal and cheek bossing
  - Depression of the bridge of the nose
  - Protrusive premaxilla
  - Expanded globular maxillae
  - BM hyperexpansion into facial bones
  - Prominent epicanthal folds

Cigarette Facies (Fig. 11)[20]

- *Condition*: Heavy smokers
- *Features*:
  - Pale, gray, and wrinkled skin with rather gaunt features

Coarse Facies (Fig. 12)[20-24]

- *Conditions*: Many inborn errors of metabolism, hyper-IgE syndrome, Costello syndrome, and multiple sulfatase deficiencies
- *Features*:
  - Large, bulging head
  - Prominent scalp veins
  - "Saddle-like" flat bridged nose with broad fleshy tip
  - Large lips and small tongue
  - Widely spaced and/or malformed teeth

CHAPTER 29 Facies in Dermatology

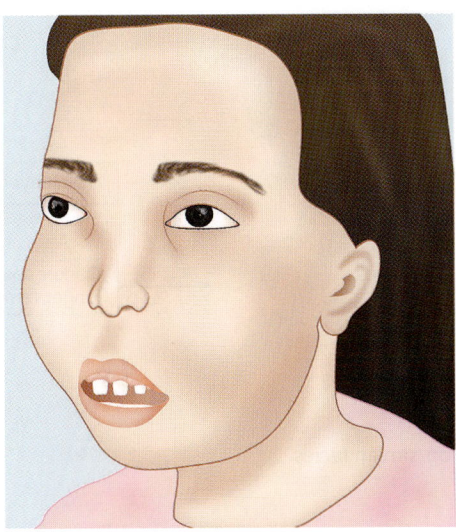

FIG. 10: Chipmunk facies.

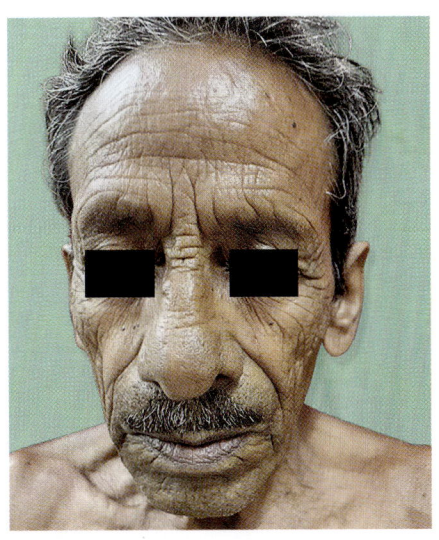

FIG. 11: Cigarette facies.

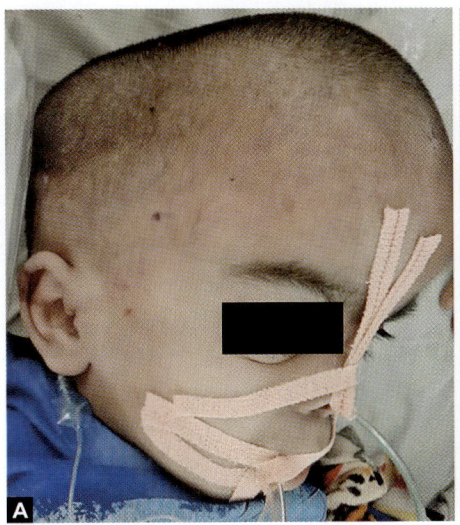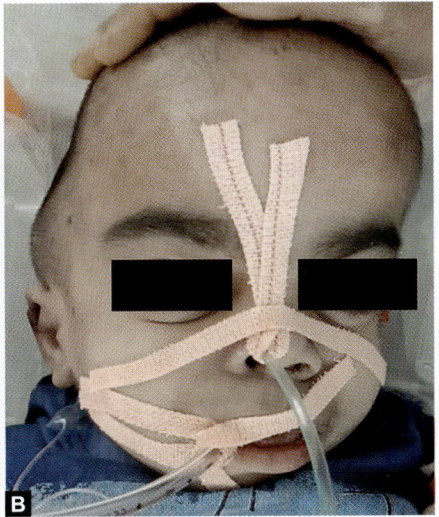

FIGS. 12A AND B: Coarse facies.
Courtesy: Pediatrics Department of LG Hospital, Ahmedabad, Gujarat, India.

- Hypertrophic alveolar ridges and/or gums
- Head tends to be longer than normal from front to back, with a bulging forehead due to premature fusion of skull bones

Cushingoid Facies (Moon Facies) (Fig. 13)[25]

- *Conditions*: Kwashiokor, Cushings disease, patients on corticosteroids therapy
- *Features*:
  - Round, full or puffy face
  - Double chin
  - Prominent flushed cheeks
  - Hirsutism

- *Cause*: Fat deposits in the temporal fossa and cheek leading to rounded appearance of face

Dengue Facies (Fig. 14)[26]

- *Condition*: Dengue fever
- *Features*:
  - Flushing
  - Palpebral edema
  - Conjunctival injection
  - Retro-ocular pain
  - Photophobia
  - On resolution of symptoms, morbilliform or scarlatiniform rash appears

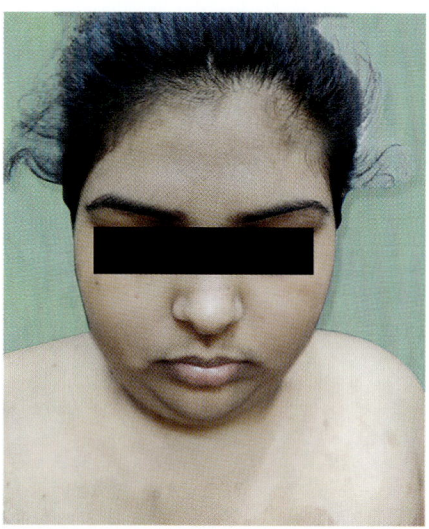

FIG. 13: Cushingoid facies.

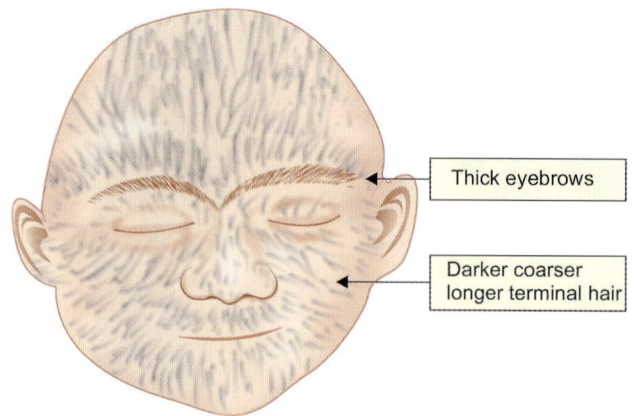

FIG. 15: Dog/simian facies.

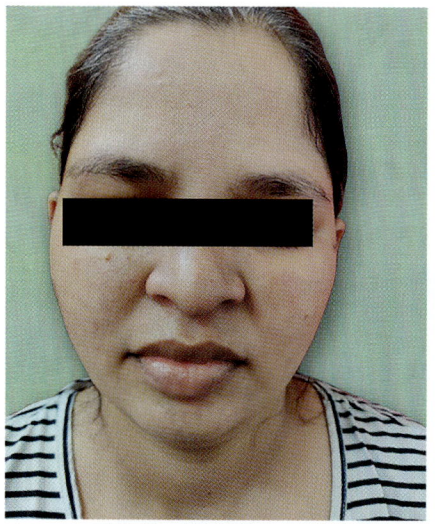

FIG. 14: Dengue facies.

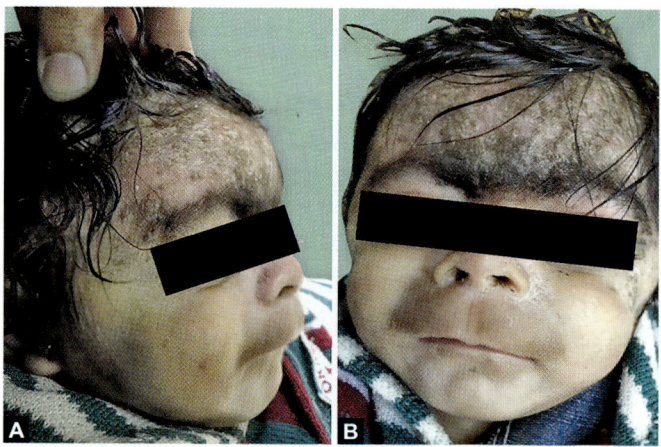

FIGS. 16A AND B: Dysmorphic facies.

Dog or Simian Facies (Fig. 15)[27]

- *Condition*: Congenital hypertrichosis lanuginosa
- *Features*:
  - The hair gradually lengthens till early childhood, the entire skin, apart from the palms and soles, covered by silky hair, which may be 10 cm or more long.
  - Long eyelashes and thick eyebrows
  - Whorls of hair noted around preauricular region, pinnae, and sacrum

Drawn Facies[28,29]

- *Condition*: Crow–Fukase syndrome
- *Commonly popular as acronym "POEMS syndrome"*:
  - Polyneuropathy
  - Organomegaly
  - Endocrine disorders
  - M protein
  - Skin changes
- *Features*:
  - Hyperpigmentation of predominantly sun-exposed areas
  - Pseudosclerodermiform skin thickening
  - Hypertrichosis affecting face and trunk
  - Hemangiomas

Dysmorphic Facies (Fig. 16)[30]

- *Condition*: DiGeorge syndrome, Cornelia de Lange syndrome, and fetal alcohol syndrome.
- *Features*:
  - Abnormally formed low-set ears
  - Hypertelorism
  - Antimongoloid slant
  - Micrognathia
  - Short philtrum to the upper lip
  - High-arched palate and cleft palate
  - Velopharyngeal insufficiency

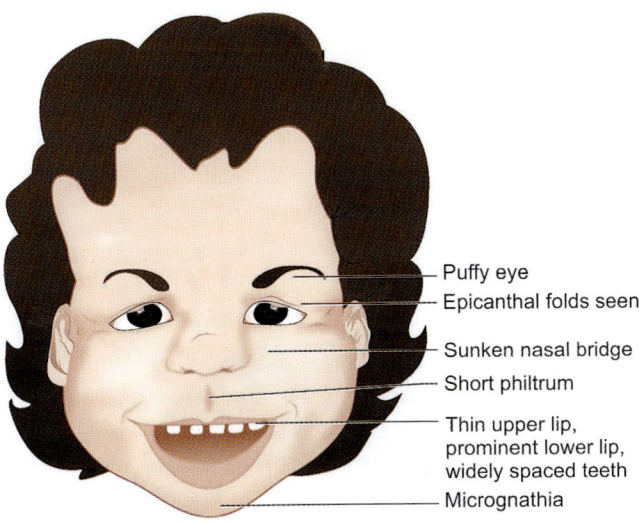

FIG. 17: Elfin/Williams facies.

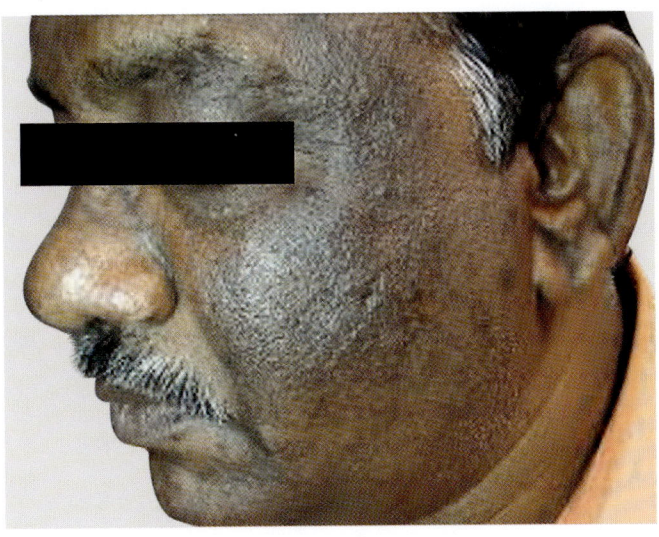

FIG. 18: Facies of acanthosis nigricans.

Elfin Facies (Fig. 17)[31]

- *Condition*: Williams syndrome
- *Features*: Facial characteristics similar to that of elves:
  - Sunken nasal bridge
  - Puffiness around eyes
  - Epicanthal fold
  - Blue starry eyes
  - Long upper lip length
  - Low-set ears
  - Small and widely spaced teeth
  - Small chin

Facies of Acanthosis Nigricans (Fig. 18)[32,33]

- *Condition*: Marfan syndrome
  - Mental retardation
  - Overgrowth
  - Remarkable facies
  - Extreme pigmentation
  - Acanthosis nigricans
- *Features*:
  - Triangular face
  - Prognathism
  - Abnormal teeth formation
  - Deep fissured large tongue
  - Posterior cervical and axillary acanthosis nigricans
  - Hair—dandruff

Facies of Addison's Disease (Fig. 19)[16]

- *Condition*: Addison's disease
- *Features*:
  - Generalized darkening of the skin of face
  - Pigmentation in the mucous membranes within the mouth

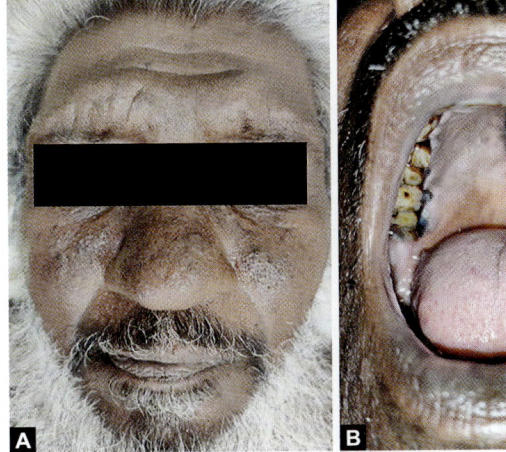

FIGS. 19A AND B: Facies in Addison's disease.

Facies of Argyria (Fig. 20)[34]

- *Condition*: Seen among people working with silver
- Also known as pseudo-ochronosis
- *Features*:
  - Even and uniform bluish gray discoloration; persists when pressure is applied on the skin
- *Cause*:
  - It is subcutaneous pigmentation rather than dermal pigmentation.

Facies of Cirrhosis of Liver (Fig. 21)[16]

- *Early stage*:
  - Telangiectasias over the cheek
  - Coarsening of tissues, especially on and around nose and mouth with purplish reddening in general
- *Later stage*:
  - Sallow, dull diffusely pigmented facies

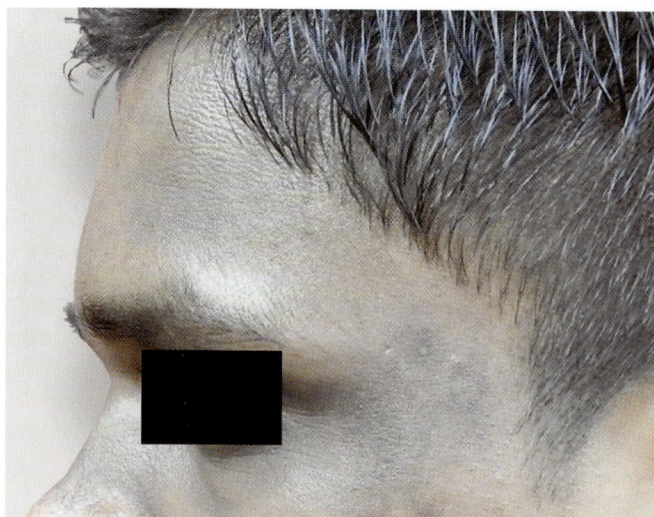

FIG. 20: Facies of argyria.

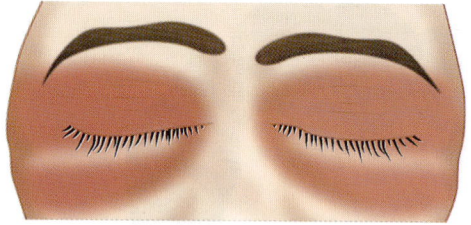

FIG. 22: Facies of dermatomyositis.

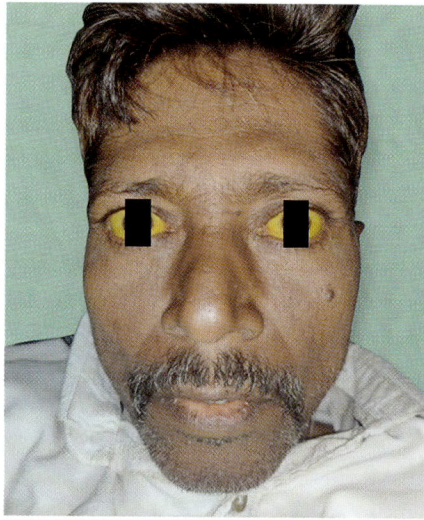

FIG. 21: Facies of cirrhosis of liver.
Courtesy: Medicine Department of LG Hospital, Ahmedabad, Gujarat, India.

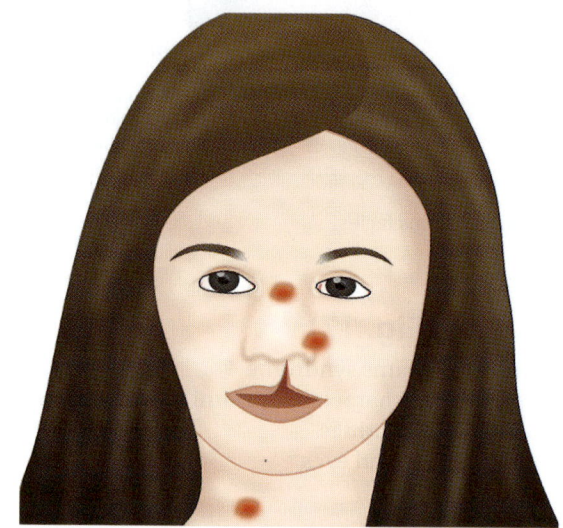

FIG. 23: Facies in Gorlin's syndrome.

Facies of Dermatomyositis (Fig. 22)[35]

- *Features*:
  - A purplish red heliotrope erythema on face especially involving the eyelids, upper cheeks, forehead, and temples
  - Edema of eyelids and periorbital tissues

Facies in Gorlin's Syndrome (Fig. 23)[36]

- *Condition*: Basal cell naevus syndrome and nevoid basal cell carcinoma syndrome
- *Features*:
  - Macrocephaly
  - Broad nasal root
  - Hypertelorism
  - Frontal and biparietal bossing
  - Exaggerated length of the mandible
  - Jaw cysts
  - Cleft lip
  - Abnormal dentition
  - Palate abnormalities
  - Bifid or otherwise misshapen ribs, vertebral and other skeletal anomalies
  - Pits of skin of palms and soles
  - Dysgenesis of the corpus callosum
  - Calcification of the falx cerebri (at an earlier age than seen in nonaffected individuals)
- *Cause*: Characteristic dysmorphic facies occur due to increased calvarial size

Facies of Hartnup Disease (Fig. 24)[37,38]

- *Condition*: Rare autosomal recessive light-sensitive disorder characterized by a pellagra-like cutaneous eruption, neurologic abnormalities, and a specific aminoaciduria
- *Features*:
  - Symmetrical distribution of erythematous macules that tend to coalesce and eventuate in well marginated red scaling lesions over light-exposed parts of the face and neck

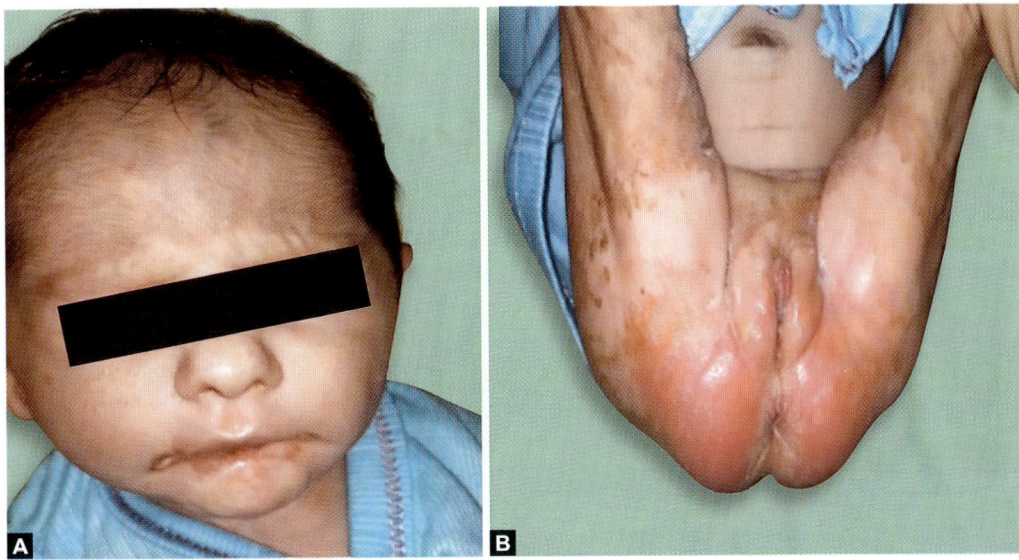

FIGS. 24A AND B: Facies in Hartnup disease.

- Acute dermatitis and blistering with secondary crusting and scarring following sun exposure
- Marked postinflammatory hyperpigmentation
- Glossitis
- Angular stomatitis
- Diffuse hair loss and fragility

Facies Lactrodectismica (Latrodectus Facies) (Fig. 25)[39,40]

- *Condition*: Blackwidow spider envenomation
- *Features*:
  - Facial swelling
  - Periorbital edema
  - Lacrimation
  - Blepharospasm and blepharitis
  - Painful grimace
  - Flushing
  - Diaphoresis
  - Trismus

Facies Leprosa (Fig. 26)[41,42]

- Seen as Bergen syndrome I (nasal leprosy) and Bergen syndrome II (leprogenic changes of the alveolar process of maxilla)
- *Features*:
  - Atrophy of anterior nasal spine; resorption of nasal bone, supraincisive alveolar region contributes to nasal collapse
  - Resorption of anterior alveolar process of maxillae associated with loss of upper central incisor teeth or of all four upper incisors

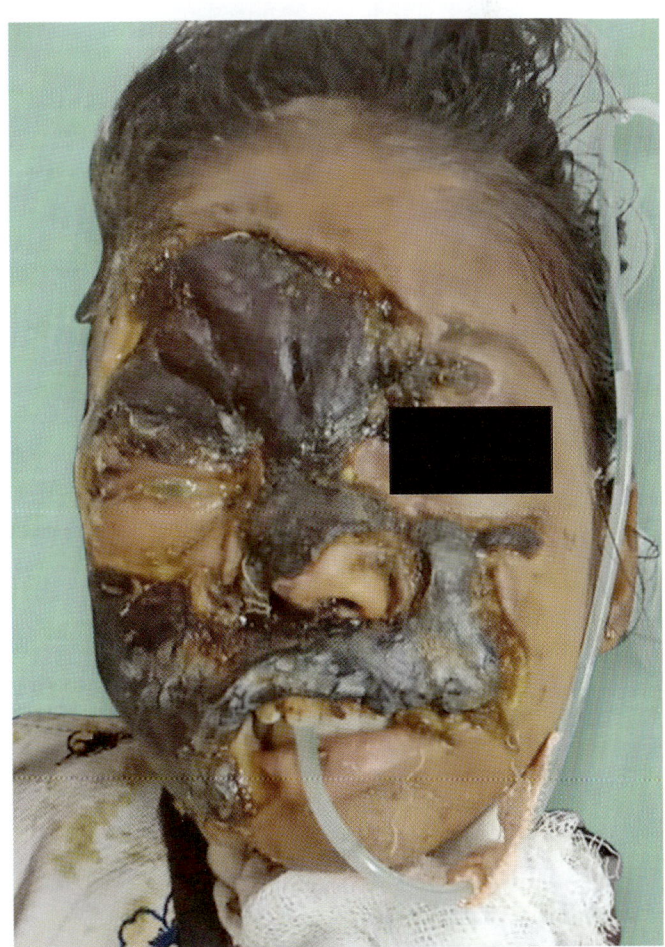

FIG. 25: Facies lactrodectismica (latrodectus facies).

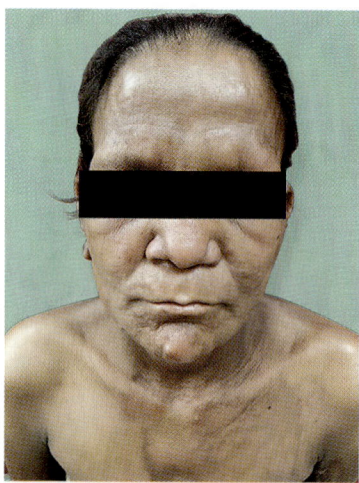

FIG. 26: Facies leprosa [Bergen syndrome I (nasal leprosy)].

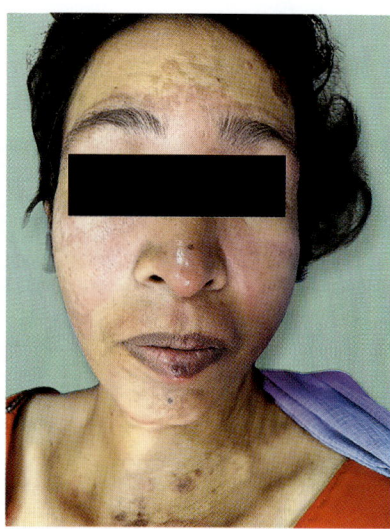

FIG. 27: Facies of lupus erythematosus.

Facies of Lupus Erythematosus (Fig. 27)[35]

- *Condition*: Acute cutaneous lupus erythematosus
- *Features*:
  o A confluent symmetrical bluish eruption with fine scaling
  o Edema centered over malar eminence with inflammation extending over bridge of nose
  o Resembles to the body of butterfly

Facies in Multiple Endocrine Neoplasia, Type 2B Syndrome[16]

- *Features*:
  o Numerous yellowish-white, sessile, painless nodules on the lips or tongue, with deeper lesions having normal coloration
  o Neuromas in the body of the lips to produce enlargement and a "blubbery lip" appearance
  o Nodules seen on the sclera and eyelids

Facies in Noonan Syndrome (Fig. 28)[43]

- *Features*:
  o Broad short webbed neck
  o Hypertelorism
  o Blepharoptosis
  o Epicanthic folds
  o Small chin
  o Widespread leukokeratosis of the lips and gingiva
  o Coarse, light colored and curly hair
  o Low posterior hairline
  o Downy hypertrichosis on the cheeks or shoulders
  o Short stature

Facies in Premature Aging Syndrome (Fig. 29)[44,45]

- *Acrogeria*:
  o Face appears pinched
  o *Features*:
    – Hollow cheeked, owl eyed
    – A beaked nose
    – Thin lips
    – Micrognathism
  o *Cause*: The loss of subcutaneous fat accentuates the appearance of premature senility.
- *Pangeria*:
  o *Features*:
    – Beaked nose
    – Atrophic and tightly bound skin of ears
    – Dry atrophic skin
    – Mottled hyperpigmentation and telangiectasias
- *Progeria*:
  o Facial appearance is reminiscent of a "fledging bird".
  o *Features*:
    – Disproportionately large cranium with patent fontanels
    – Frontal bossing
    – Prominent eyes and scalp veins
    – Very sparse scalp hair
    – Sparse or absent eyebrows and eyelashes
    – Centrofacial cyanosis
    – Micrognathia
    – Thin lips
    – A "beaked nose"

Facies of Systemic Sclerosis (Fig. 30)[46,47]

- *Grimace like facies*:
  o *Condition*: Seen in progressive systemic sclerosis
  o *Features*:
    – Forehead is smooth.
    – Fixed stare due to atrophy and tightening of the skin

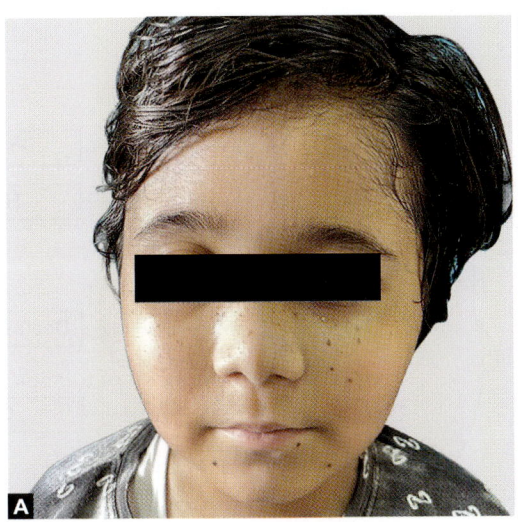
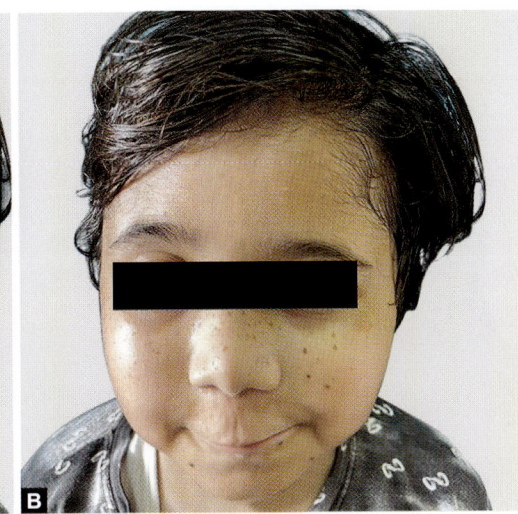

FIGS. 28A AND B: Facies in Noonan syndrome.

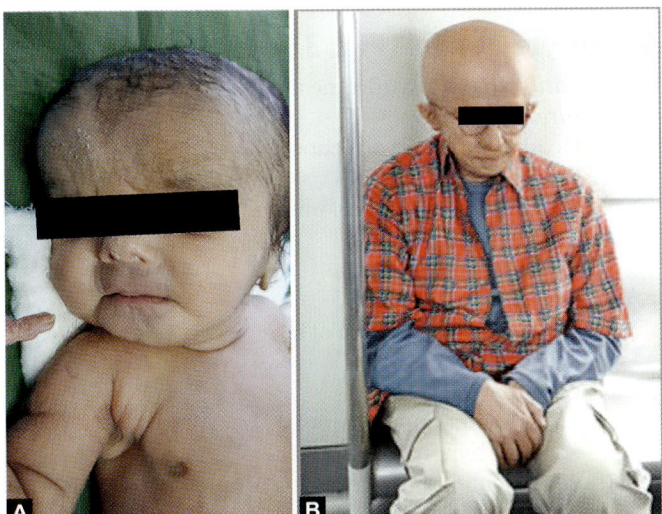

FIGS. 29A AND B: Facies in premature aging syndrome.

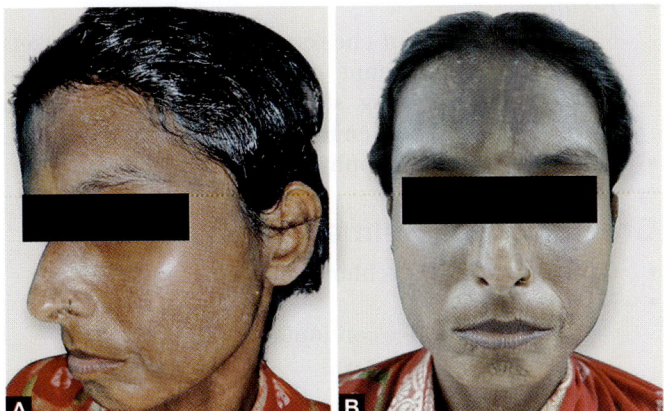

FIGS. 30A AND B: Facies of systemic sclerosis.

- Pinched nose
- Prominent teeth
- Pursed lips
- Reduced oral aperture
- *Mask like facies*:
  - *Other conditions with mask like facies*: Parkinsonism, psychotic conditions
  - *Features*:
    - Smooth and shiny forehead
    - The skin is bound down and hard, the lines of expression smoothed out
    - The lower eyelids cannot be depressed by the fingers to show the conjunctiva because of atrophy of tissues
    - Small and pinched nose
    - Constricted mouth opening with radial furrows giving a pursed appearance
    - Mat-like telangiectasias
    - Mandibular atrophy
- *Mouse like facies*:
  - *Features*: Nasal alae become atrophied resulting in pinched appearance of the nose.

Facies in Turner's Syndrome (Fig. 31)[43]

- *Features*:
  - Ptosis, strabismus
  - Epicanthal folds
  - Auricles posteriorly rotated or low set
  - High-arched palate, dental crowding or malocclusion
  - Webbed neck (pterygium colli)
  - Low posterior hair line
  - Loose folds of skin particularly in the neck

Flat Facies/Mongoloid Face (Fig. 32)[48]

- *Condition*: Down syndrome

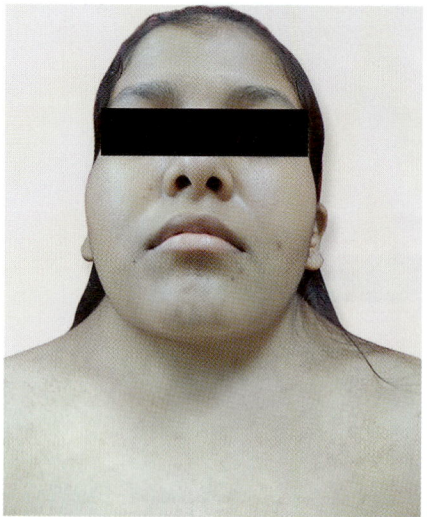

FIG. 31: Facies in Turner's syndrome.

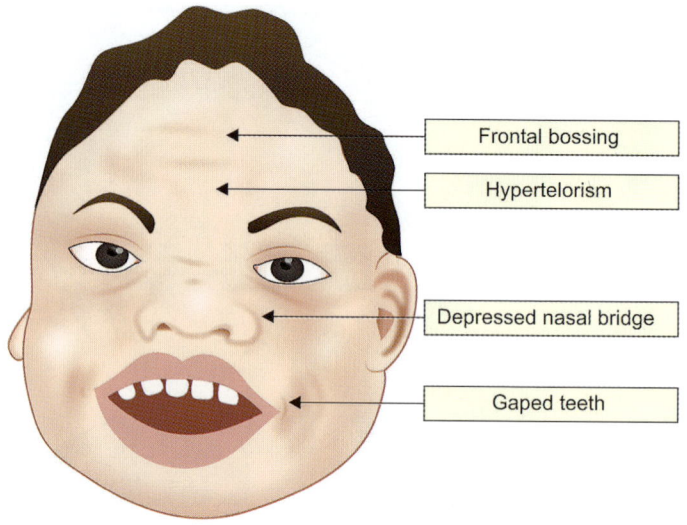

FIG. 33: Gargoyle facies.

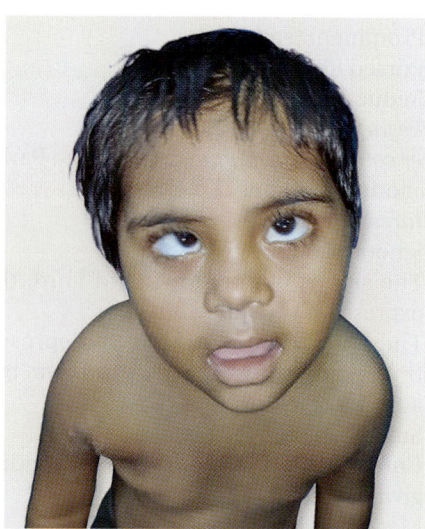

FIG. 32: Flat facies (Down syndrome).

- *Features*:
  - Brachycephalic head
  - Downy forehead
  - Hypertelorism
  - Mongoloid slant
  - Epicanthal folds
  - Brushfield spots on the iris
  - Saddle nose
  - Ears are larger and pitcher shaped
  - Fissured lips
  - Short, high-arched palate
  - Smaller teeth
  - Protruded and scrotal tongue
  - Scanty, wiry, mouse colored scalp hair
  - Florid and mottled complexion

Gargoyle Facies (Fig. 33)[49,50]

- *Condition*: Hurler syndrome and galactosialidosis
- *Features*:
  - Head is large and dolichocephalic
  - Frontal bossing
  - Prominent sagittal and metopic sutures
  - Midface hypoplasia
  - Depressed nasal bridge
  - Flared nares
  - Prominent lower third of face
  - Thickened facies
  - Widely spaced teeth
  - Attenuated dental enamel
  - Gingival hyperplasia
- *Cause*: Subcutaneous deposition of mucopolysaccharides

Gaunt Facies (Fig. 34)[51,52]

- *Condition*: Common cutaneous side effect of long-term use of highly active antiretroviral drugs (HAART)
- *Features*:
  - The hollowed-out cheeks, temples, and eye sockets often lead to gaunt cachectic facies which can be a disconcerting stigma of the disease and a psychological burden to the patient.
- *Cause*: Facial lipodystrophy

Greek Warrior Helmet Facies (Fig. 35)[53]

- *Condition*: Wolf–Hirschhorn syndrome
- *Features*:
  - Wide nasal bridge continuing to the forehead
  - High-arched eyebrows
  - Hypertelorism
  - Downslanting palpebral fissures
  - Microphthalmia

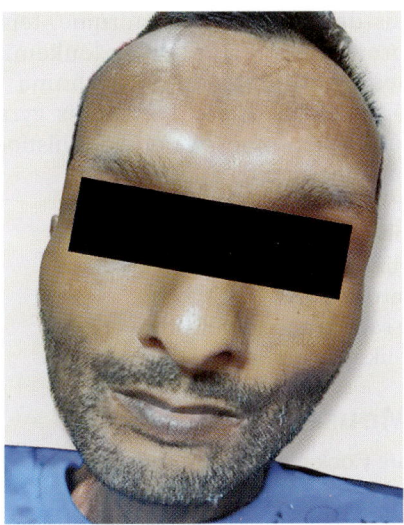

FIG. 34: Gaunt facies.

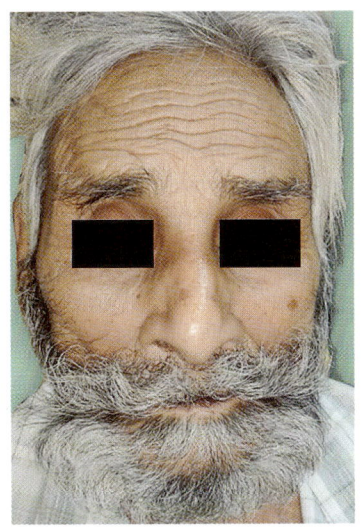

FIG. 36: Hippocratic facies.

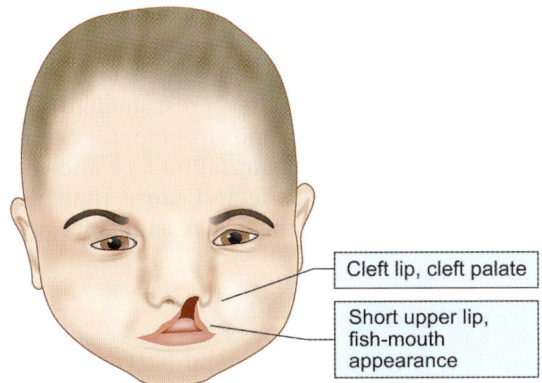

FIG. 35: Greek warrior helmet facies.

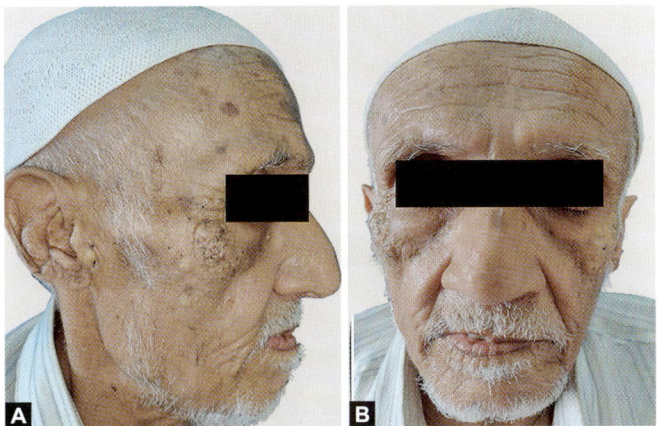

FIGS. 37A AND B: Hound dog facies.

- Epicanthal folds, proptosis, strabismus
- High anterior hairline
- Broad or beaked nose
- Short philtrum
- Short upper lip
- Micrognathia
- Taurodontism
- Downturned corner of the mouth
- Low-set ears with pits or tags
- Hemangioma over forehead or glabella
- Short stature and severe growth retardation
- Microcephaly
- Cleft lip or palate
- Scalp defect with or without underlying bony defect

Hippocratic Facies (Fig. 36)[54]

- *Seen in*: People close to death after severe and prolonged illness
- *Features*:
  - A pinched expression of the face
  - Sunken eyes
  - Concavity of cheeks and temples
  - Relaxed lips
  - Leaden complexion

Hound Dog/Blood Hound Facies (Fig. 37)[20,55]

- *Condition*: Cutis laxa
- *Features*:
  - Sagging jowls
  - Downward slanting palpebral fissures
  - A broad flat nose
  - Large ears
  - An aged appearance

Keel Like Facies (Fig. 38)[56]

- *Condition*: Bloom's syndrome
- *Features*:
  - Narrow, long, slender, delicate facies

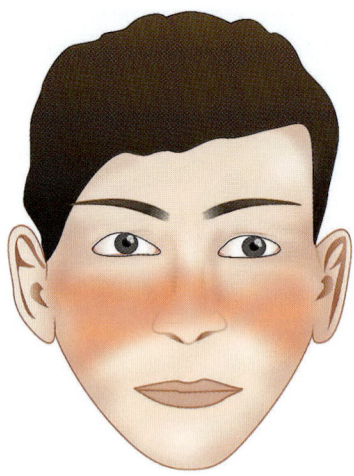

FIG. 38: Keel like facies.

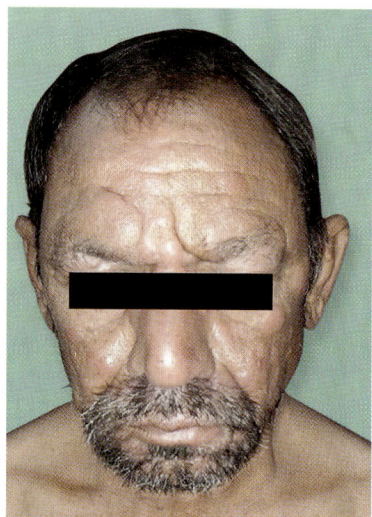

FIG. 39: Leonine facies.

ichthyosis-deafness (KID) syndrome, leishmaniasis, lipoid proteinosis, lymphoma, leukemia, mycosis fungoides, multiple keratoacanthoma syndrome, pachydermoperiostosis/cutis verticis gyrata, Paget's disease of bone, progressive nodular histiocytosis, and pseudophotodermatitis
- *Features*:
  ○ Deeply furrowed forehead and cheek
  ○ Prominent superciliary arches
  ○ Madarosis
  ○ Early saddle nose deformity
  ○ Lion-like appearance of the face

Mickey Mouse Facies[37,58,59]
- *Condition*: Cockayne syndrome
- *Features*:
  ○ Microcephaly
  ○ Pinched narrow face
  ○ Beaked nose
  ○ Sunken eyes giving premature senile appearance
  ○ Large protruding ears
  ○ Short stature
  ○ Facial erythema in a butterfly distribution
  ○ Mottled pigmentation and atrophic scars
- *Cause*: Loss of subcutaneous fat on face and cachectic look where weight is affected more than height—"cachectic dwarfism" with facial resemblance to Mickey mouse.

Monkey Like Facies[23,34]
- *Condition*: Porphyria cutanea tarda (PCT), marasmus (monkey facies)
- *Features*:
  ○ Hypertrichosis of face, involving cheeks, temples, and eyebrows giving monkey-like facies
  ○ Wrinkled, loose, and dry skin (marasmus) due to substantial loss of subcutaneous tissue

Myopathic Facies (Fig. 40)[16]
- *Condition*: Cerebrotendinous xanthomatosis (cholestanolosis), myotonic dystrophy
- *Features*:
  ○ An expressionless face
  ○ Sunken cheeks
  ○ Proptosis and juvenile onset cataract
  ○ Drooping lower lip, open mouth, and protuberant tongue
  ○ Yellowish discoloration of skin and mucosa

Parkinsonian Facies (Fig. 41)[16]
- *Condition*: Parkinson's disease
- *Features*:
  ○ Mask-like face
  ○ Tremor of head
  ○ Absence of blinking

○ Relatively prominent nose and/or ears
○ Eyebrow and eyelashes hair loss
○ High-arched palate
○ Retrognathia or micrognathia
○ Underdeveloped malar area
○ Head circumference is below the third percentile
○ Alopecia areata
○ Telangiectatic erythema on the face (butterfly distribution) and other photodistributed areas
○ Stunted growth (both prenatal and postnatal)

Leonine Facies (Fig. 39)[57]
- *Conditions*: Lepromatous leprosy, chronic actinic dermatitis, parthenium dermatitis, papular mucinosis, multicentric reticulohistiocytosis, pseudolymphoma, mycosis fungoides, scleromyxedema, chronic lymphedema as a complication of rosacea, carcinoid syndrome, focal facial dermal dysplasia, keratitis-

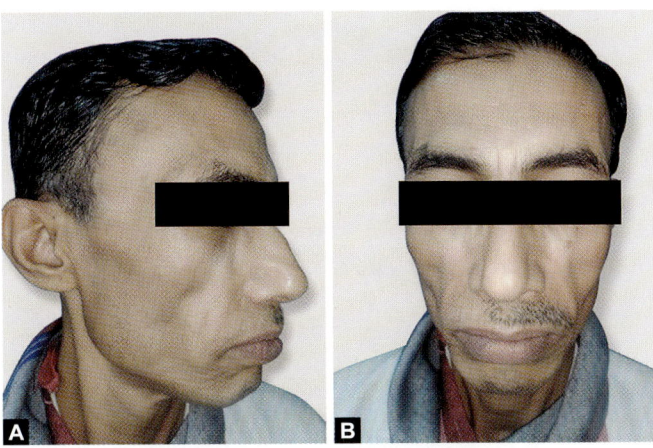

FIGS. 40A AND B: Myopathic facies.

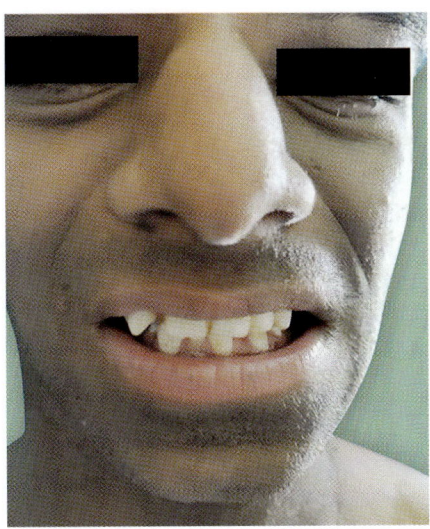

FIG. 42: Phenytoin facies.

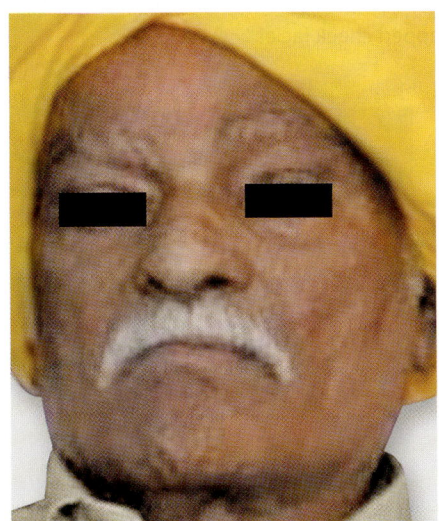

FIG. 41: Parkinsonian facies.

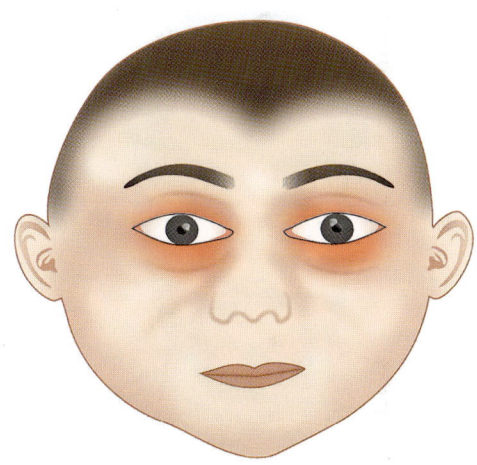

FIG. 43: Raccoon facies.

- Dribbling of saliva
- Weakness of upward gaze
- Seborrhea
- Sweatiness

Phenytoin Facies (Fig. 42)[60]
- *Condition*: Phenytoin in the long-term use
- *Features*:
  - Gingival hyperplasia
  - Coarsening of the facies
  - Enlargement of lips
  - Thickening of scalp and face
  - Hirsutism

Raccoon Facies (Fig. 43)[61,62]
- *Condition*: Neonatal systemic lupus erythematosus, primary systemic amyloidosis (following prolonged dependent positioning in a proctologist's chair)
- *Features*:
  - Erythematous scaly eruption on face and periorbital skin
  - Skin surrounding the eyes shows striking petechiae formation, resembling the mask-like facies of a raccoon

Rounded or Asymmetrical Facies[63]
- *Condition*: X-linked dominant ichthyosis Synonym: Conradi–Hünermann–Happle syndrome
- *Features*:
  - Frontal bossing
  - Broad flat nasal bridge
  - Congenital asymmetric cataracts
  - Coarse hairs with patches of cicatricial alopecia
  - Low-set ears
  - Yellow to white hyperkeratotic scales all over body

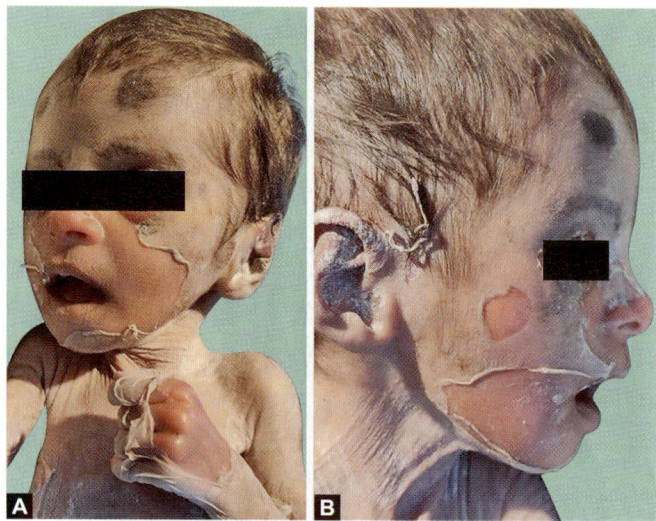

FIGS. 44A AND B: Sad man facies.

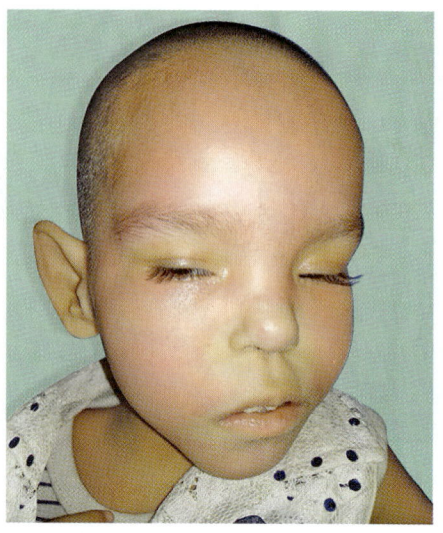

FIG. 46: Slapped cheek facies.

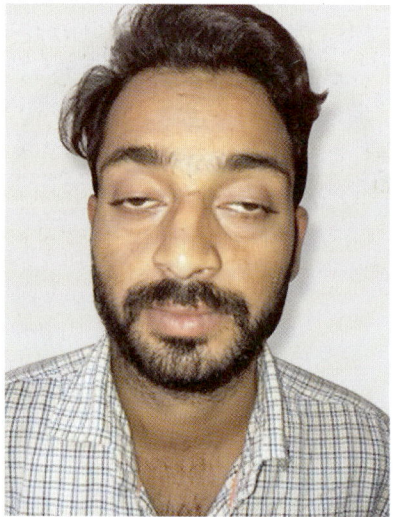

FIG. 45: Snarling or myasthenic facies (myasthenia gravis).

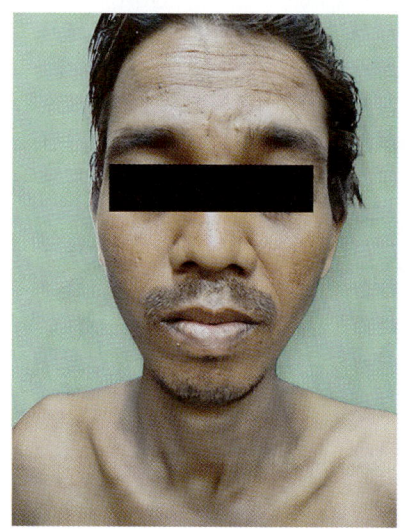

FIG. 47: Syphilitic facies.

Sad Man Facies (Fig. 44)[64]
- *Condition*: Staphylococcal scalded skin syndrome
- *Features*:
  - Wrinkled skin appearance (owing to formation of flaccid bullae within superficial epidermis)
  - Erythema first on head (within 24 hours). In 1–2 days, bullae are sloughed, varnish like crust.
  - Perioral crusting and radial fissuring
  - Mild facial edema

Snarling or Myasthenic Facies (Fig. 45)[16]
- *Condition*: Myasthenia gravis
- *Features*:
  - Drooping of the eyelids and corners of the mouth
  - Weakness of the facial muscles

Slapped Cheek Facies (Fig. 46)[65]
- *Condition*: Erythema infectiosum
- *Features*: Diffuse erythema and edema of the cheeks

Syphilitic Facies (Fig. 47)[25,66-69]
- *Bulldog facies*:
  - *Conditions*: Late congenital syphilis
  - *Features*:
    - Frontal bossing
    - Saddle nose
    - Small maxilla
    - Bulldog jaw (normal mandible appears large and long)
  - *Cause*: Local effect of syphilitic rhinitis on development of adjacent structure

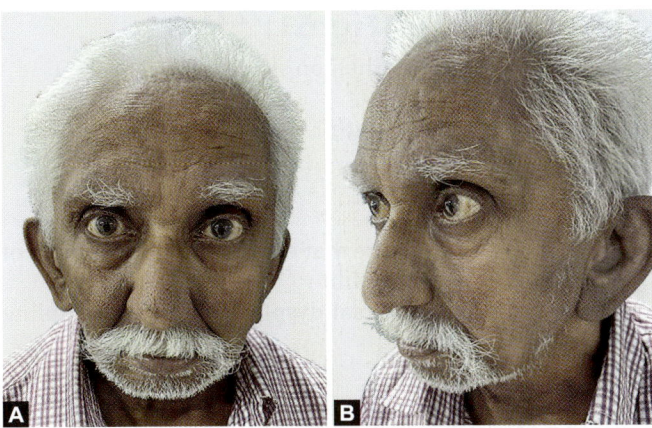

FIGS. 48A AND B: Thyrotoxic facies (Graves' disease).

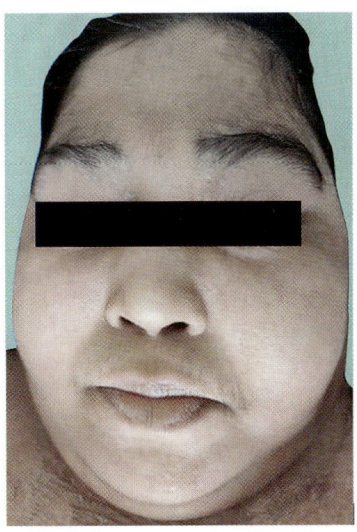

FIG. 49: Torpid or myxedematous (myxedema).

- *Old man facies*:
  ○ Condition: Congenital syphilis with marasmus
  ○ Features:
    – Pot belly
    – Loss of weight produces withered skin
- *Stokes facies*:
  ○ Condition: Many congenital syphilis patients who may lack the gross stigmata
  ○ Features:
    – In-alertness, a sleepy, tired, fagged, clouded, dreaming, or obscured appearance of the upper face
    – Appearance of veiledness as if a smudge had lightly swept across the brows and eyes and the nasal bridge of a crayon portrait
- *Tabetic facies*:
  ○ Condition: Tabes dorsalis
  ○ Characteristics:
    – Bilateral partial ptosis
    – Presence of compensatory wrinkling in the forehead (sad expression)
    – Elevated eyebrow
    – Argyll Robertson pupils

Thyrotoxic Facies (Fig. 48)[16]

- *Condition*: Graves' disease
- *Features*:
  – Alert, startled, flushed, and anxious appearance
  – Protrusion of one or both eyes (exophthalmia) associated with retraction of the upper eyelids (lid lag)
  – Exposure of white conjunctiva above the cornea (Von–Graefe's sign)
  – Eye movements are often diminished in range (Joffroy's sign)
  – Muscle of brow are wasted
  – Wrinkling on raising the eyebrow

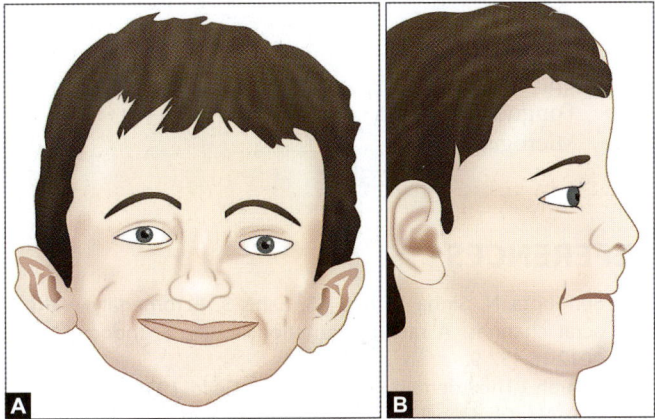

FIGS. 50A AND B: Triangular facies.

Torpid Facies (Fig. 49)[16]

- *Condition*: Myxedema
- *Features*:
  ○ Thickened, coarse, dry, pale, and waxy skin
  ○ Coolness and dryness of skin and hair
  ○ Alopecia
  ○ Periorbital edema
  ○ Xanthelasma
  ○ Swollen lips
  ○ Enlarged tongue
  ○ Broadened nose
  ○ Thickened ears
  ○ Tinted rose-purple flush over each cheek

Triangular Facies (Fig. 50)[21,70,71]

- *Conditions*: Osteogenesis imperfecta, Ehlers–Danlos syndrome, immunodeficiency, centromeric instability, and facial dysmorphism syndrome

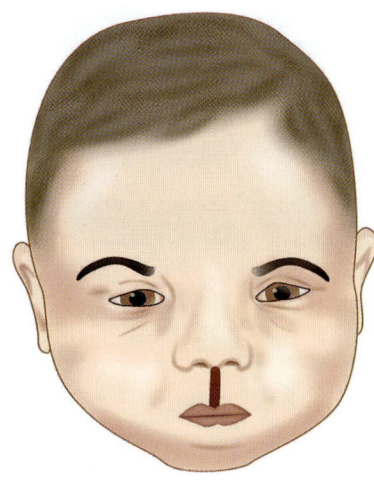

FIG. 51: Whistling facies.

- *Characteristics*:
  - Low-set ears
  - Hypertelorism
  - Flat nasal bridge
  - Epicanthic folds
  - Tongue protrusion
  - Micrognathia

Whistling Facies (Fig. 51)[72,73]

- *Condition*: Freeman–Sheldon syndrome
- *Features*:
  - A small, pursed mouth
  - Long philtrum
  - Small nose
  - Deeply sunken eyes
  - Scar like contracture that extends from the middle of the lower lip to the chin
- *Cause*: Craniocarpotarsal dysplasia and skin dimpling defect

ACKNOWLEDGMENTS

Medicine and Pediatric Departments of LG Hospital, AMC MET Medical College, Ahmedabad, Gujarat, India, for sharing valuable knowledge and clinical photographs.

Special thanks to Dermatology Resident of LG Hospital, AMC MET Medical College—Dr Twinkle C Rangnani for dedicated contribution in illustrative reformatting.

Special thanks to Dermatology Residents of LG Hospital, AMC MET Medical College, Ahmedabad—Dr Tithi B Shah and Dr Tithi R Jain.

REFERENCES

1. Sengupta N, Sinha U, Roy KS, Saha S. Acromegaly without acral changes: A rare presentation. Indian J Endocr Metab. 2012;16:457-9.
2. Ruhrah J. The Adenoid Facies. Am J Dis Child. 1935;49(6):1622-3.
3. Cox AH, Coulson HI. Systemic disease and skin. In: Burns T, Breathnach C, Cox N, Griffiths C (Eds). Rook's Textbook of Dermatology, 8th edition. London: Blackwell Publishing; 2010. pp. 62.162.113.
4. Vorperian VR, Havighurst TC, Miller S, January CT. Adverse effects of low dose amiodarone: A meta-analysis. J Am Coll Cardiol. 1997;30:791-8.
5. Yones SS, O'Donoghue NB, Palmer RA, Menagé Hdu P, Hawk JL. Persistent severe amiodarone-induced photosensitivity. Clin Exp Dermatol. 2005;30(5):500-2.
6. Paller AS, Mancini AJ (Eds). Hurwitz Clinical Dermatology: A Textbook of Skin Disorders of Childhood and Adolescence, 4th edition. Edinburgh: Elsevier Saunders; 2011. pp. 562-79.
7. Gupta V, Ramam M. Monogenic autoinflammatory syndromes in children: Through the dermatologist's lens. Indian J Paediatr Dermatol. 2018;19:194-201.
8. Kanathur S, Sarvajnyamurthy S, Somaiah SA. Characteristic facies: an index of the disease. Indian J Dermatol Venreol Leprol. 2013;79:439-43.
9. Degitz K. Mycobacterial infections. In: Plewig B, Landthaler W (Eds). Braun Falcos Dermatology, 3rd edition. New York: Springer; 2009. p. 190.
10. James WD, Berger TG, Elston DM (Eds). Andrews' Diseases of the Skin: Clinical Dermatology, 10th edition. Canada: Saunders Elsevier; 2006. p. 547-80.
11. Mahadevan B, Karthikeyan K, Bhat BV, Thappa DM. Restrictive Dermopathy. A case report. Indian Pediatrics. 2002;39:1149-52.
12. Bidier M, Salz M, Meyburg J, Elbe-Bürger A, Lasitzschka F, Hausser I, et al. Restrictive Dermopathy: Four Case Reports and Structural Skin Changes. Acta Derm Venereol. 2018;98:807-8.
13. Pape KE, Pickering D. Asymmetric crying facies: an index of other congenital anomalies. The J Paediatrics. 1972;81:21-30.
14. Smith JL, Stowe FR. The Pierre Robin syndrome (glossoptosis, mirognathia, cleft palate): A Review of 39 Cases with Emphasis on Associated Ocular Lesions. Pediatrics. 1961;27:128-33.
15. Chowchuen B, Jenwitheesuk K, Chowchuen P, Surakunprapha P. Challenges in Evaluation, Management and Outcome of the Patients with Treacher Collins Syndrome. J Med Assoc Thai. 2011;94(Suppl. 6):S85-S90.
16. Taj FT, Dash R, Haveri S. Facies in dermatology. Int J Curr Res. 2013;5(08):2270-4.
17. Jacqueline M, Hopkins J, Avram AS, Avram M. Lipodystrophies. In: Bolognia JL, Jorizzo JL, Rapini RP (Eds). Bolognia Dermatology, 2nd edition. USA: British Library Cataloguing in Publication Data; 2008. pp. 1542-8.
18. Nagaraj T, NU U, Devarhubli AR, SN Shankara. B Thalessemia major: A case report. J Int Oral Health. 2011;3(5):68-73.
19. Bangal V, Kwatra A, Raghav S, Modi H. Recurrent pregnancy loss due to Haemoglobinopathy (Thalassemia): Case report. Pravara Med Rev. 2009;1:25-7.
20. Burrows NP, Lovell CR. Disorders of connective tissue. In: Burns T, Breathnach S, Cox N, Griffiths C (Eds) Rook's Textbook of Dermatology, 8th edition. Singapore: Wiley Blackwell; 2010. pp. 45.1-45.70.

21. Paige DG, Gennery AR, Cant AJ. The neonate. In: Burns T, Breathnach S, Cox N, Griffiths C (Eds). Rook's Textbook of Dermatology, 8th edition. Singapore: Willey Blackwell; 2010. p. 17.1-17.85.
22. Judge MR, McLean WH, Munro CS. Disorders of keratinization. In: Burns T, Breathnach S, Cox N, Griffiths C (Eds). Rook's Textbook of Dermatology, 8th edition. Singapore: Wiley Blackwell; 2010. p. 19.42.
23. Sarkany RP, Breathnach SM, Morris AA, Weismann K, Flynn PD. Metabolic and nutritional disorders. In: Burns T, Breathnach S, Cox N, Griffiths C (Eds). Rook's Textbook of Dermatology, 8th edition. Singapore: Wiley Blackwell; 2010. p. 59.1-59.103.
24. Kagalwala TY, Bharucha BA, Khare RD, Kumta NB. Diagnostic approach to coarse facies. Indian J Pediatr. 1988;6:861-70.
25. Master FJ (Ed). Diseases of the Skin, 1st edition. New Delhi: B Jain Publishers; 2003. p. 432.
26. Arenas R. Dengue. In: Arenas R, Estrada R (Eds). Tropical Dermatology, 1st edition. USA: Landes Bioscience; 2001. p. 284.
27. De Berker DA, Messenger AG, Sinclar RD. Disorders of Hair. In: Burns T, Breathnach S, Cox N, Griffiths C (Eds). Rook's Textbook of Dermatology, 8th edition. Singapore: Willey Blackwell: 2010. p. 63.93.
28. Thomas P. Gammopathies. In: Plewig B, Landthaler W (Eds). Braun Falcos Dermatology, 3rd edition. New York: Springer; 2009. pp. 1250-1.
29. Santos G, Lestre S, João A. Do you know this syndrome? POEMS syndrome. An Bras Dermatol. 2013 Nov-Dec;88(6):1009-10.
30. Hacihamdioglu B, Berberoglu M, Şıklar Z, Dogu F, Bilir P, Erdeve SS, et al. Case Report: Two patients with partial DiGeorge syndrome presenting with attention disorder and learning difficulties. J Clin Res Pediatr Endocrinol. 2011;3:95-7.
31. Benneth FC, Laveck B, Sells CJ. The Williams elfin facies syndrome: The psychological profile as an aid in syndrome identification. Pediatrics. 1978;61:303-6.
32. Seemanova E, Rüdiger HW, Dreyer M. Morfan: A new syndrome characterized by mental retardation, pre- and postnatal overgrowth, remarkable face and acanthosis nigricans in 5-year old boy. Am J Med Genet. 1993;45(4):525-8.
33. Zaridoust A, Rabbani A, Sayarifard F, Thiel CT, Rezaei N. Acanthosis nigricans, Abnormal Facial Appearance and Dentition in an Insulin Resistance Syndrome. Iran J Pediatr. 2013;23(3):363-5.
34. Kudur MH, Hulmani M. "Pseudo" conditions in dermatology: Need to know both real and unreal. Indian J Dermatol Venereol Leprol. 2012;78:763-73.
35. Goodfield MJD, Jones SK, Veale DJ. The connective tissue diseases. In: Burns T, Breathnach C, Cox N, Griffiths C (Eds). Rook's Textbook of Dermatology, 8th edition. London: Blackwell Publishing, 2010. p. 51.49-51.
36. Quinn GA, Perkins W. Non Melanoma skin cancer and other Epidermal Skin Tumuors. In: Burns T, Breathnach C, Cox N, Griffiths C (Eds). Rook's Textbook of Dermatology, 8th edition. London: Blackwell Publishing; 2010. p. 52.1-52.48.
37. Kumar R, Kumari S. Evaluation and management of photosensitivity in children. Indian Pediatr. 2008;45:829-37.
38. Hillman RE. Renal Tubular Disorders. Biomed Sci. 2014.
39. Offerman SR, Daubert GP, Clark RF. The treatment of black widow spider envenomation with antivenin latrodectus mactans: a case series. Perm J. 2011;15:76-81.
40. Rufli T. Diseases caused by arthropods. In: Plewig B, Landthaler W (Eds). Braun Falcos Dermatology, 3rd edition. New York: Springer; 2009. p. 341.
41. Jopling WH, Mcdougall AC (Eds). Handbook of Leprosy, 5th edition. New Delhi: CBS publishers; 2005. p. 33.
42. Freitas JA, dos Santos WM, Opromolla DV, Alle N. New criteria for the characterization of facies leprosa. Hansenol Int. 1986;11:7-23.
43. Irvine DA, Mellerio EJ. Genetics and Genodermatoses. In: Burns T, Breathnach S, Cox N, Griffiths C (Eds). Rook's Textbook of Dermatology, 8th edition. Singapore: Willey Blackwell; 2010. p.15.115.97.
44. Burton JL. Disorders of connective tissue. In: Champion RH, Burton JL, Ebling FI (Eds). Textbook of Dermatology, 5th edition. London: Blackwell Scientific Publications; 1992. p. 1814-5.
45. Sowmiya R, Prabhavathy D, Jayakumar S. Progeria in siblings: A rare case report. Indian J Dermatol. 2011;56:581-2.
46. Jagadish R, Mehta DS, Jagadish P. Oral and periodontal manifestations associated with systemic sclerosis: A case series and review. J Indian Soc Periodontol. 2012;16:271-4.
47. Paller AS, Mancini AJ (Eds). Hurwitz Clinical Pediatric Dermatology A Textbook of Skin Disorders of Childhood and Adolescence, 4th edition. Edinburgh: Elsevier Saunders; 2011. p. 497-527.
48. Singh DN. Down's syndrome: A study of clinical features. J Natl Med Assoc. 1976;68:521-4.
49. Chacham OS, Lang TC, Lamaraca ME, Krasnewich D, Sidransky E. Lysosomal storage disorders in the newborn. Paediatrics. 2009;123:1191-207.
50. Manchanda SS. Gargoylism. Report of four cases with a brief review. Indian J Pediatr. 1960;27:281-7.
51. Cohen G, Treherne A. Treatment of facial lipoatrophy via autologous fat transfer. J Drugs Dermatol. 2009;8:486-9.
52. Hunter JA, Savin JA, Dahl MV (Eds). Clinical Dermatology, 3rd edition. Massachusetts: Blackwell Science; 2003. p. 309.
53. Jackson SM, Nesbitt LT (Eds). Differential Diagnosis for the Dermatologist, 1st edition. Berlin: Springer-Verlag; 2008. p. 1323.
54. Marinella MA. On the Hippocratic facies. J Clin Oncol. 2008;26:3638-40.
55. Mukhi SV, Kuruvila M, Pai PK. Generalised cutis laxa. Indian J Dermatol Venereol Leprol. 2002;68:100-1.
56. Inamadar AC, Palit A. Genodermatoses. In: Valia RG, Valia AR (Eds). IADVL Textbook of Dermatology, 3d edition. Mumbai: Bhalani Publishers; 2008. p. 145.
57. Rapini RP. Clinical and pathologic differential diagnosis. In: Bolognia JL, Jorizzo JL, Rapini RP (Eds). Bolognia Dermatology, 2nd edition. USA: British Library Cataloguing in Publication Data; 2008. p. 4.
58. Batra P, Saha A, Kumar A. Infantile onset of Cockayne syndrome in two siblings. Indian J Dermatol Venereol Leprol. 2008;74: 65-7.
59. Senthil Kumar AL, Aruna C, Swapna K, Ramamurthy D. Neonatal onset Cockayne syndrome: A rare photogenodermatosis. Indian J Paediatr Dermatol. 2016;17:297-9.
60. Scheinfeld N. Phenytoin in cutaneous medicine: its uses, mechanisms and side effects. Dermatol Online J. 2003;9(3):6.
61. Patel LM, Lambert P, Gagna CE, Maghari A, Lambert WC. Cutaneous signs of systemic disease. Clin Dermatol. 2011;29: 511-22.
62. Mohanasundaram K, Govidaraj A. Raccoon eyes in cutaneous neonatal lupus syndrome. Eur J Rheumatol. 2020;7(2):92-3.
63. Meshram RM, Dandale AA, Rohadkar LA, Chirag RN. Conradi–Hunermann syndrome: A rare case of chondrodysplasia punctata. Indian J Paediatr Dermatol. 2019;20:255-7.

64. Halpern AV, Heyman WR. Bacterial diseases. In: Bolognia JL, Jorizzo JL, Rapini RP (Eds). Bolognia Dermatology, 2nd edition. USA: British Library Cataloguing in Publication Data; 2008. p. 1079.
65. Wolff K, Johnson RA (Eds). Fitzpatrick's Color Atlas and Synopsis of Clinical Dermatology, 6th edition. New York: McGraw Hill; 2008. p. 807.
66. Sparling PF, Swartz MN, Mushes DM, Healy BP. Clinical Manifestations of Syphilis. In: Holmes KK, Sparling PF, Stammt WE, Piot P, Wasserheit JN, Corey L (Eds). Sexually Transmitted Diseases, 4th edition. New York: McGraw-Hill; 2008. p. 671.
67. Walker GJA. Antibiotics for syphilis diagnosed during pregnancy. Cochrane Database Syst Rev. 2001;3:CD001143.
68. Sanchez M, Luger AF. Syphilis. In: Fitzpatrick TB, Eisen AZ, Wolff K, Freedberg IM, Austen FK (Eds). Dermatology in General Medicine, 4th edition. New York: McGraw-Hill; 1993. p. 2703-43.
69. Saliny M, Joy B, Sridharan R. Laws and signs of congenital syphilis. J Skin Sex Transm Dis. 2020;2(1):62-4.
70. Morais P, Mota A, Eloy C, Lopes JM, Torres F, Palmeiro A, et al. Vascular Ehlers-Danlos syndrome: A case with fatal outcome. Dermatol Online J. 2011;17:1.
71. Constantinou CD, Pack M, Young SB, Prockop DJ. Phenotypic heterogeneity in osteogenesis imperfecta: The mildly affected mother of a proband with a lethal variant has the same mutation substituting cysteine for alpha 1-glycine 904 in a type I procollagen gene (COL1A1). Am J Hum Genet. 1990;47:670-9.
72. Kaissi A, Klaushofer K, Grill F. Severe skew foot deformity in patient with Freeman-Sheldon syndrome. J Clin Med Res. 2011;3:265-7.
73. Paller AS, Mancini AJ (Eds). Hurwitz Clinical Pediatric Dermatology: A Textbook of Skin Disorders of Childhood and Adolescence, 4th edition. Edinburgh: Elsevier Saunders; 2011. p. 10-35.

30
Phenomenon in Dermatology

Pragya Nair, Pratik R Agarwal

INTRODUCTION

Immanuel Kant's work on "Erscheinung" meaning thereby "appearance" implies an immediate object of sensory intuition, the bare data that becomes an object when interpreted through the categories of substance and cause. This is in contrast to "noumena," meaning, a thing in itself to which categories do not apply.

Phenomena[1] are detected through the use of data and are predictable by scientific theories. Bogen and Woodward[2] seem to assume that phenomenon is constructed from data obtained by experimentation, the effects, and processes of which are (1) stable, (2) repeatable, (3) which serve as objects of prediction and systematic explanation by general theories, and (4) which serve as evidence for such theories.

Dermatologic literature is replete with mention of phenomena **(Table 1)**, some that have been extensively studied and some that have faded in oblivion. Further, there has been a tendency to use the term as a synonym for signs in dermatology, some have retained the designation while others have crystallized into "effect," "test," "reaction," "sign," and the likes.

CUTANEOUS PHENOMENON

Table 1: Phenomena that find mention in dermatology.				
Clinical		**Histological**	**Laboratory**	**Therapeutic**
Elicitable	Observable			
Nikolsky phenomenon	Wolff's isotopic phenomenon	Splendore–Hoeppli phenomenon	LE cell phenomenon	Tachyphylaxis phenomenon
Pathergy phenomenon	IPD phenomenon	Borst–Jadassohn phenomenon	Prozone phenomenon	Hoigne phenomenon
Koebner phenomenon*	Halo phenomenon	Pagetoid phenomenon	Reynolds–Braude phenomenon	Jarisch–Herxheimer phenomenon
Brocq phenomenon†	Meyerson's phenomenon		Epitope spreading phenomenon	Castling phenomenon
Delayed blanch phenomenon	Harlequin phenomenon		Meirowsky phenomenon	

Continued

Continued

Clinical		Histological	Laboratory	Therapeutic
Bell phenomenon	Mauserung phenomenon		Mei and Rayleigh scattering phenomenon§	
Raynaud phenomenon	Kasabach–Merritt phenomenon			
Rumpel–Leede phenomenon	Ultraviolet recall phenomenon			
Renbok phenomenon*	Olfleck phenomenon			
Frei–Sulzberger–Chase phenomenon	Lucio phenomenon			
Rebound phenomenon	Phenomene de la Bruno Bloch‡			
Shwartzman–Sanarelli phenomenon	Lyonization phenomenon			
Mandarin phenomenon	Phenomenon of Woronoff ring			
Schultz–Charlton phenomenon of extinction	Nevus aversion phenomenon			
Phenomenon of fluorescence				
Iris phenomenon				

*Although elicitable, it is not usually an office procedure, because of the highly varied latency to show the response.

†Lichen planus, itself being livid or violaceous, it may be difficult to appreciate subepidermal hemorrhage and may require histomorphological observation to appreciate Brocq's phenomenon.

‡Described by Bruno Bloch in zoonotic dermatophytosis, it may be seen as a protective immunity in patches especially caused by geophiles and zoophiles but the claim remains unsubstantiated.

§The understanding of phenomenon is important for understanding the skin and laser optics.

NIKOLSKY PHENOMENON

(Sir Wilhelm Lutz 1957)

Lutz[3] suggested that "on carefully rubbing uninvolved area of skin, the superficial layers of the skin move and a blister is formed after sometime." Although not described by Piotr Vasiliyevich Nikolsky in 1894, Lutz alluded this phenomenon to his name.

The phenomenon is confounded in a cobweb (Table 2) of different definitions and interpretations. Whilst the activity of disease in pemphigus vulgaris is high when direct Nikolsky sign is positive, it is comparably low in Nikolsky phenomenon. The phenomenon is absent during an inactive phase of the disease.

Further, what Braun Falco described as Nikolsky phenomenon I and II are, in fact, Nikolsky sign and Asboe-Hansen sign (also known as Lutz sign as Wilhelm Lutz was the first to describe it), respectively.

NIKOLSKY PHENOMENON

- *Acantholytic (true Nikolsky sign):*
  - Pemphigus vulgaris (mildly active)
  - Ritter von Rittershain disease (SSSS)
- *Nonacantholytic (pseudo-Nikolsky sign):*
  - Acute skin failure [toxic epidermal necrosis (TEN)/Stevens-Johnson (SJ) syndrome]
  - Bullous ichthyosiform erythroderma
  - Bullous lichen planus
  - Burns

Clinically, there is a set of four different signs and one phenomenon summarized in Table 2:

Table 2: Various Nikolsky signs and phenomenon.					
Author	Shear of perilesional skin causes the normal skin to peel	Tangential pressure over normal distant skin causes erosion	Extension of erosion to normal skin on lateral pressure	Extension of intact blister to normal skin on application of pressure	Separation of epidermis from underlying layer on careful rubbing
Nikolsky PV[4] 1896	1	3	2		
Lutz W 1957[3]				Lutz sign	Nikolsky phenomenon
Sheklakov ND[5,6] 1965			Marginal Nikolsky		
Fassmann[7] et al. 2003		Direct Nikolsky		Indirect Nikolsky	
Asboe Hansen G[8] 1960				Asboe-Hansen sign	
O Braun Falco[9] 1991	Nikolsky phenomenon I			Nikolsky phenomenon II	

PATHERGY[10]

(Blobner 1937)

It is a state of altered tissue reactivity, characterized by a nonimmunologic hyperinflammatory response to minor trauma. It appears as a pustular eruption at the site of trauma.

Pathergy can be elicited both in the oral mucosa and on the cutaneous tissue. The former is known as oral pathergy test (OPT), while the latter is known as skin pathergy test (SPT).

Skin pathergy test is regarded as a minor criterion for the diagnosis of Behçet's disease by the International Study Group Diagnostic criteria for Behçet's disease.[13]

DERMATOSES WITH PATHERGY[11,12]

Significant clinical marker:
- Behçet's disease

Consistent clinical marker:
- Pyoderma gangrenosum
- Pyogenic arthritis, pyoderma gangrenosum, and acne (PAPA) syndrome
- Sweet's syndrome
- Erythema elevatum diutinum
- Blind loop syndrome
- Subcorneal pustular dermatosis

Case reports:
- Chronic myeloid leukemia (CML) with interferon α (INF-α) therapy
- Atypical eosinophilic pustular folliculitis
- Neonates with Down syndrome

An intradermal injury is inflicted using a 20–25 gauze needle which is inserted obliquely to a depth of 5 mm. One-tenth of a milliliter, i.e., 0.1 mL, of normal saline is usually injected and the test result is read at 48 hours. An erythematous papule of >2 mm or pustule at the site of injury is considered a positive test.

There is an augmented antigen-independent nonspecific induction phase of inflammatory reaction, the response to epidermal injury showing lack or absence of VCAM-1.

SALIENT FEATURES

- Antigen-independent augmented inflammatory reaction
- *Depth of injury*: Dermal
- *Needle*: Fine needle 20 gauze better than 26 gauze:
  - Blunt needle better than beveled
- *Site*: Forearm better than abdomen
- *Injections*: Normal saline
  - Monosodium urate
  - Streptococcal antigen

While clinical macroscopic changes are restricted to erythema, papule, or pustule formation in a given time period, it is the histological section that shows marked changes and helps in differentiate a positive from negative skin pathergy reaction (SPR) **(Table 3)**.

KOEBNER PHENOMENON

(Heinrich Koebner 1876)

The appearance of new, but similar lesions over normal appearing skin in response to any trauma is termed as *isomorphic* or *Koebner phenomenon*. The injury could be mechanical, chemical, or photo-induced. The phenomenon is "all or none"[14,15] in nature suggesting thereby that patients responding to stimulus will respond to any form of injury and patients who do not react to trauma are likely not to react to another stimuli. In psoriasis, Koebnerization is seen within 10–20 days following a trauma but can manifest over a wide temporal range of 3 days to 20 years.[16]

Because the latency for Koebnerization is varied, there are no attempts to elicit the phenomenon.

Table 3: Histomorphologic changes in cutaneous pathergy.

HP findings	SPR positive	SPR negative
Epidermis	Basal cell and mid-epidermal layers express HLA-DR and ICAM-1 Cell vacuolization ↓ Epidermal thickening ↓ Subcorneal pustulation	
Dermis	Endothelial cells express strong ICAM-1 and moderate e-selectin	Endothelial cells express weak e-selectin
	<5% infiltrate is neutrophil which are present as clusters of elastase positive cells	Increased neutrophils at the site of prick
	Dense mononuclear cells infiltrating around vessels and appendages extending to deep dermis	Few clusters of T cells and macrophages
	T cells express HLA-DR (50%), CD4+, and CD45RO	

There are numerous case reports of *questionable* Koebnerization secondary to herpetiform trauma, viz. eruptive xanthoma, vasculitides, transient acantholytic dermatosis, telangiectatic variant of cutaneous mastocytosis, Still's disease, porokeratosis of Mibelli, pityriasis rubra pilaris, nevocytic nevi, multicentric reticulohistiocytosis, lichen amyloidosis, keratoacanthoma, atopic dermatitis, discoid lupus erythematosus (LE), Duhring disease, pemphigus vulgaris, and anaphylactoid purpura.

DERMATOSES WITH KOEBNERIZATION[17]

Certain Koebnerization:
- Psoriasis
- Vitiligo
- Lichen planus (Fig. 1)
- Psoriatic arthritis

Occasional Koebnerization:
- Erythema multiforme
- Hailey–Hailey disease
- Darier–White disease
- Lichen sclerosus
- Lichen nitidus (Fig. 2)
- Kyrle's disease
- Perforating folliculitis
- Reactive perforating collagenosis
- Kaposi sarcoma

Further, viral exanthems including herpes recidivans, varicella, and variola have been found to have lesions preponderant at sites of sun exposure, phototherapy, and chemexfoliation. Finsen noted that the location of the deepest and most confluent small pox scars was photo exposed. Preventing exposure by using thick red curtains prevented suppuration and scar formation in such patients.[18]

There are cases that may suggest a history trauma followed by eruptions but they are contiguous progression of an infection and can best be termed *pseudo-Koebnerization*. The most common examples are toxicodendron or ivy

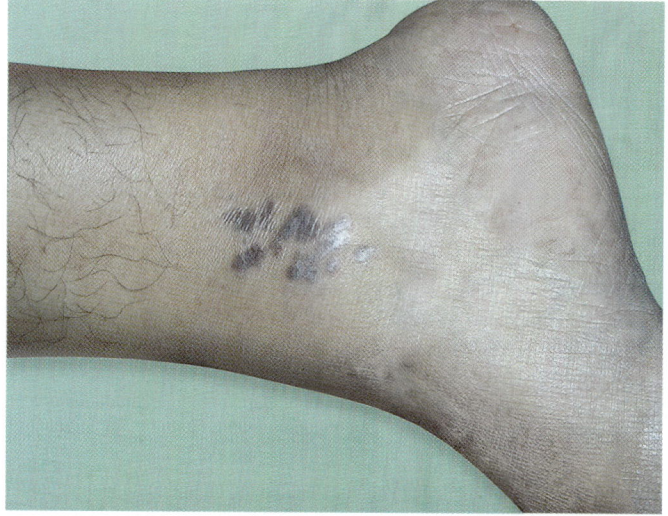

FIG. 1: Lichen planus at the site of continuous irritation caused by anklets.

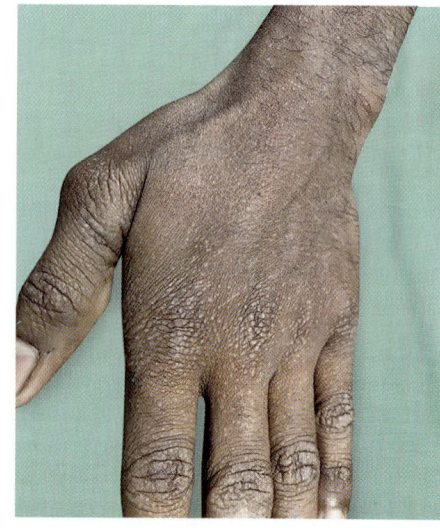

FIG. 2: Koebnerization seen in lichen nitidus.

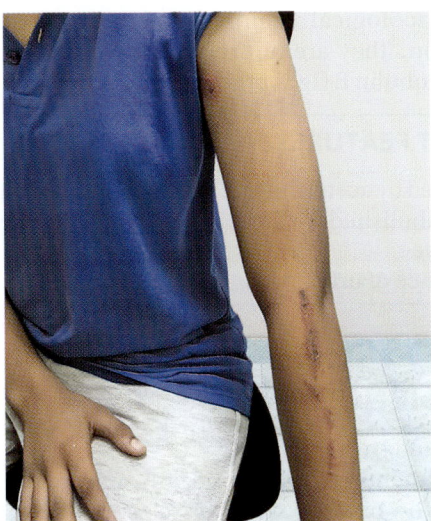

FIG. 3: Pseudo Koebnerization in a case of irritant contact dermatitis.

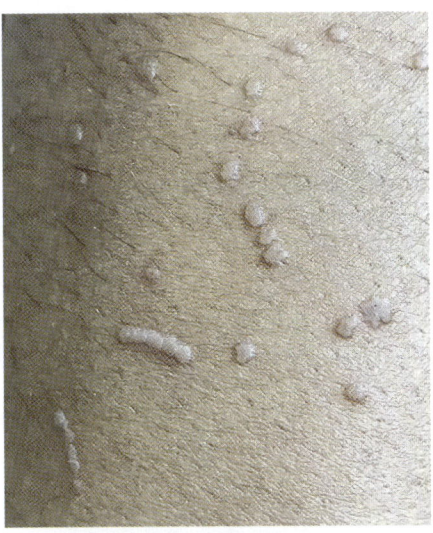

FIG. 4: Discrete verruca plana lesions presenting in a linear fashion due to auto inoculation.

dermatitis **(Fig. 3)**, verruca plana **(Fig. 4)**, verruca vulgaris, and molluscum contagiosum.

Koebner experiment[19] involves either experimental trauma using 2 mm biopsy punch or scarification. Tape stripping is not an effective method, at least for psoriasis, to elicit Koebnerization. However, in vitiligo, Koebnerization can be seen with epidermal injury also.

What causes the eruption has not been fully "understood and elucidated." However, in psoriasis, it is supposed to be either (1) immune-mediated with cytokines and auto-antigens playing a role or (2) T cell-mediated reaction with subsequent keratinocyte proliferation and angiogenesis. Although microvasculature involvement is certain, other neural, genetic, infectious, and hormonal factors could be possible causes.

> **SALIENT FEATURES**
> - Induced by dermal trauma
> - Reproducible
> - Nonspecificity of noxae
> - Histologic concordance with naïve disease

The phenomenon is clinically relevant as it suggests an increased activity of the disease process. In psoriasis, the new lesions tend to erupt at the sites of trauma and also at distant sites. In vitiligo, presence of Koebner phenomenon suggests a higher disease activity as well as a poor prognosticator for the effect of therapy.

Reverse Koebner phenomenon is the disappearance of a dermatosis induced by trauma. The effect could be within the lesion or at distant remote sites when lesions are multiple. The latter is designated as remote reverse Koebnerization. While not much is known about the mechanism by which the lesion disappears, in vitiligo, it has been hypothesized that trauma-induced cytokine release after local secretion may influence melanocytes at distant sites.

> **REVERSE KOEBNER PHENOMENON**
> - Psoriasis
> - Vitiligo (lesional, satellite, and remote)
> - Granuloma annulare[20,21]
> - Alopecia areata
>
> **REMOTE REVERSE KOEBNER PHENOMENON**
> - Vitiligo
> - Generalized granuloma annulare[22]

BROCQ PHENOMENON[23]

(Pautrier 1936)

Pinkus introduced this phenomenon that was common among French dermatologists. Methodical grattage of the surface of a lichen planus lesion leads to turgescence and eventual subepidermal bleeding **(Fig. 5)**. This is known as Brocq phenomenon. Both psoriasis and lichen planus show increased vascularity but there is a suprapapillary thinning in psoriasis with loose parakeratotic scales that can be easily removed exposing the papilla, breaking of the tortuous capillary, and bleeding. In cases of lichen planus, there is a tenuous scale with hypergranulosis and pseudoacanthosis. With basal cell damage, an infiltrate restricted to the papilla and the superficial fine elastic fibers destroyed, mechanical grattage leads to a subepidermal hemorrhage.

DELAYED BLANCH PHENOMENON

(Lobitz WC, Campbell 1953)

A paradoxical vascular reaction showing a blanching response to acetylcholine especially in eczematous and

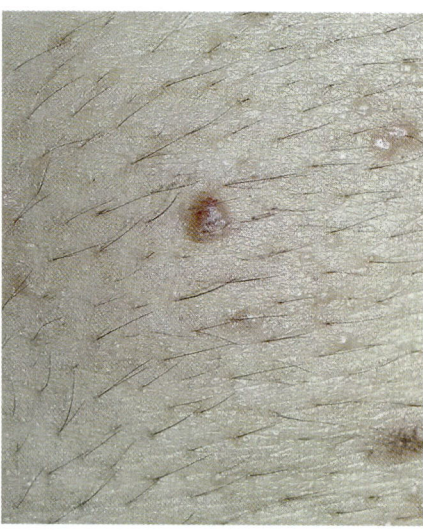

FIG. 5: Gentle grattage causing subepidermal hemorrhage seen over a discreet lesion in a fair skinned individual.

dry skin of atopic dermatitis patients is termed as delayed blanch phenomenon.[24]

This phenomenon can be elicited by injecting 0.1 mL (0.025 mg) of carbachol or pilocarpine into the dermis of the volar aspect of the forearm of a test subject. After a brief 3–5 minutes, up to 30 minutes, there develops a central anemic pallor and persists for more than an hour. The paradox lies in the fact that in a normal individual, the anticipated reaction would be one of erythema rather than pallor.

There are multiple hypotheses for these paradoxical vascular reactions including (1) vasoconstriction due to acetylcholine, (2) vasoconstriction secondary to the vasodilatation-induced wheal, (3) increased liberation of norepinephrine, and (4) arteriolar dilatation.

DERMATOSES WITH DELAYED BLANCH PHENOMENON

Common:
- Atopic dermatitis:
  ○ Lichenified lesions of AD patients
  ○ 50% of atopics with no dermatitis
- Nonatopic individuals (22%)
- Infective lichenified plaques
- Seborrheic eczema

Case reports:[25]
- Disseminated neurodermatitis
- Erythroderma:
  ○ Psoriasis
  ○ Lymphoma
- Second stage of Mycosis fungoides

There is consensus that AD patients do not show redness after a vasodilatory stimulus. The variable response in AD indicates vascular dysregulation in response to the effects of pharmacological agents possibly due to autonomic dysfunction. They are not related to hereditary factors of immunoglobulin E (IgE) production.

SALIENT FEATURES

- Caused by acetylcholine, methacholine, or pilocarpine
- Not abolished by atropine, adrenolytic-like phentolamine
- Absence of urticaria

BELL PHENOMENON[26]

(Charles Bell, 1823)

Bell phenomenon is the upward and outward rolling of eyes attempted on bilateral voluntary closure of eyelids against resistance **(Fig. 6)**.

Although described in relation with a lower motor neuron injury, it is neither a typical upward and outward rolling nor is it universally present in all individuals. Bell phenomenon should not be considered pathognomonic for seventh nerve palsy as it is normally resent in a large set of the population.

BELL'S PHENOMENON ISN'T UNIVERSAL

- Rare in infants up to 8 months
- 90% in <30 years of age
- 74% in 30–50-year-olds
- 34% in >50 years of age

The proposed mechanism involves, in all possibility, (1) pathways of VII cranial nerve in brainstem, (2) pathways of III cranial nerve in rostral midbrain, both of which are integrated by (3) mesencephalic reticular network.

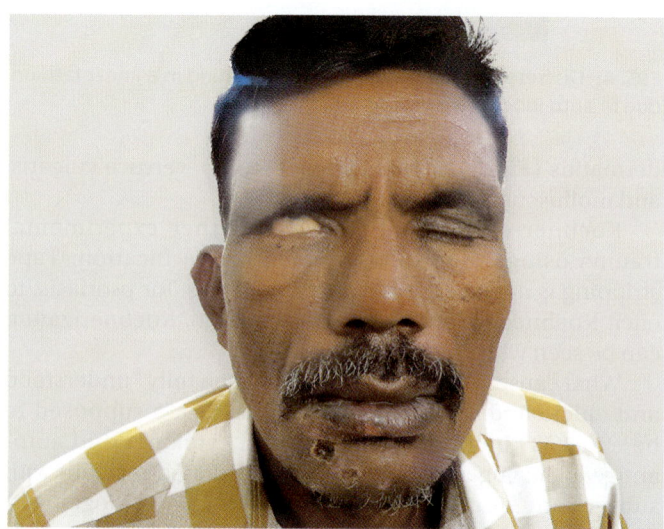

FIG. 6: Upward and outward rolling of eyes displaying Bell phenomenon.

It is elicited as the examiner attempts to elevate the upper eyelids using his finger and thumb of one hand, while the patient tries to close his eyes. The movement of the eyeballs is recorded.

This examination is carried along with assessment for lagophthalmos. Here, the patient is asked to extend the neck and gently close his eyes in an active non-forceful manner. The distance separating the supposedly closed upper eyelid and lower eyelid is measured in millimeters.

BELLS PHENOMENON IN DERMATOSES

- Bell palsy:
  - Herpes simplex infection
  - Lyme's disease
  - Ramsay-Hunt syndrome II
  - Leprosy
  - Infectious mononucleosis
  - Melkersson-Rosenthal syndrome
- Sturge-Weber syndrome
- Tuberous sclerosis

RAYNAUD PHENOMENON[27,28]

(Maurice Raynaud 1862)

A phenomenon characterized by vasospasm-associated episodic changes in the blood flow in the cutaneous vasculature with a triphasic response of pallor, cyanosis, and hyperemia **(Table 4)**.

The phenomenon can be elicited by placing an ice cube wrapped in a mesh cloth on the subject's hand for around 20 minutes and noting the changes in color and sensation.

It is typically present in the hands **(Figs. 7 and 8)** but can also affect the toes, nose, earlobes, or nipples. It may begin in one finger and spread symmetrically to other digits, often sparing the thumb. The phenomenon of intermittent symmetrical painful spasms may be idiopathic wherein it is termed Raynaud disease, while in those with a secondary cause, it is termed Raynaud syndrome.

Apart from the dermatoses, it can be seen in patients with costoclavicular and anterior scalenus syndrome, pneumatic workers and percussionists, syringomyelia, prolapse of nucleus pulposus, fungal, and cyanide poisoning.

Table 4: Clinical and hemodynamic changes in various phases of Raynaud phenomenon.			
Phase	Symptoms and signs	Mechanism	Hemodynamics
First	Color turns pale or dead white	Vasospasm	Decreased blood flow
Second	Blue black with intense pain	Venous engorgement	Stasis of deoxygenated blood
Third	Redness with warmth	Arterial hyperemia	Reperfusion injury

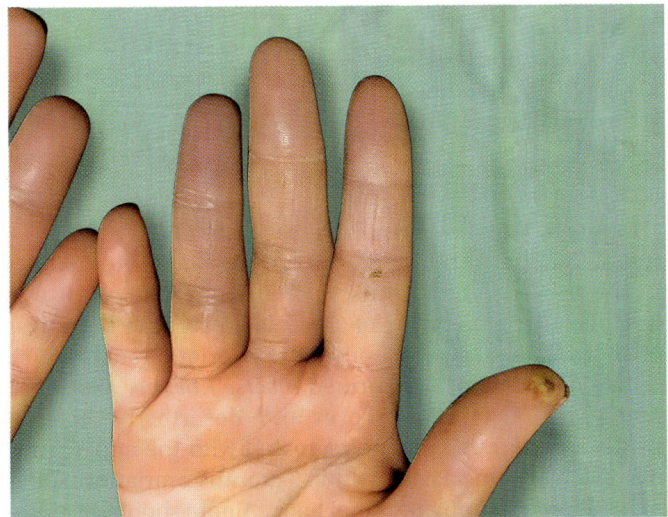

FIG. 7: Lividity seen on the distal phalanges after exposure to cold with digital ulceration on the tip of the thumb.

Courtesy: Dr Jigna Padhiyar.

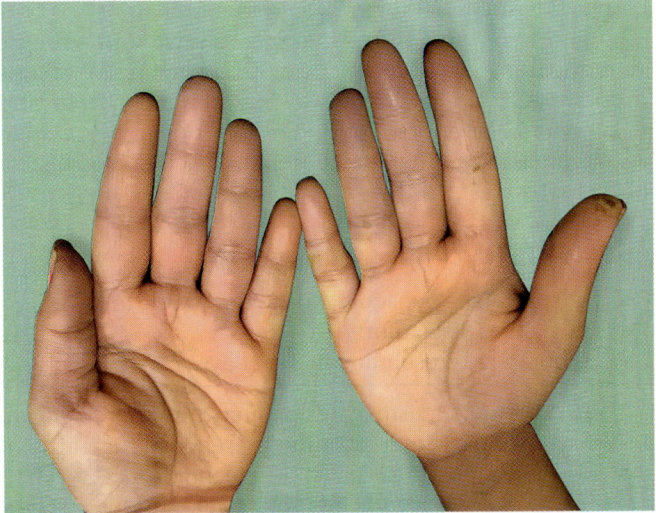

FIG. 8: Dusky bluishness over distal phalanges and livid erythema at the proximal phalanges after exposure to cold. Tell-tale signs of poor circulation include stellate scar over left thumb and digital ulceration on the tip of the right thumb.

Courtesy: Dr Jigna Padhiyar.

COMMON DERMATOSES WITH RAYNAUD PHENOMENON[27,29]

- Progressive systemic sclerosis
- CREST or CRST syndrome
- Acute cutaneous LE
- Dermatomyositis
- Rheumatic arthritis
- Sharp syndrome
- Thromboangiitis obliterans
- Cryoglobulinemia
- Cryofibrinogenemia
- Waldenstrom macroglobulinemia
- Paroxysmal hemoglobinuria
- Polyarteritis nodosa
- Drugs including ergot alkaloids, bromocriptine, clonidine, cyclosporine, methysergide, bleomycin, and vinyl chloride

Raynaud phenomenon should be differentiated from acrocyanosis in young females, the latter characterized by cold and clammy skin, hyperhidrosis, and absence of all three phases of color change. In children, it should be differentiated from Swift syndrome (Feer disease) which is characterized by brick red to blue cyanotic palms and soles which look like raw flesh, itch, and hurt as well. Massive hyperhidrosis, mousy smell lamellar peeling, and muscle flaccidity are usual associations.

RUMPEL-LEEDE PHENOMENON

(Theodor Rumpel 1909, Carl Stockbridge Leede 1911)
An acute efflorescence of petechial lesions distal to the site of compression suggesting acute capillary rupture in the dermis is termed as Rumpel–Leede phenomenon.

The first reports of the phenomenon were in patients suffering from Scarlet fever. It can be elicited by inflating a pressure cuff, to a point midway between the systolic and diastolic pressure. For a period of 5 minutes, the sudden appearance of >20 petechiae per square inch suggests a positive Hess test.

SALIENT FEATURES

- >20 petechiae per square inch distal to the test site
- No pain or discomfort
- Spontaneous resolution in 3–14 days

The exact mechanism of this phenomenon is not known. Increased capillary fragility in the presence of high arterial and/or venous pressure is plausible mechanism.[30]

Increased capillary fragility relates to either a vasculopathy or aberrant quantity or functional quality of platelets.

The most common nondermatological condition that showcases the phenomenon is the coexistence of diabetes mellitus with hypertension as well as uncontrolled hypertension in nondiabetics.

The phenomenon is innocuous excepting hypertension where it may prognosticate uncontrolled malignant hypertension.

CONDITIONS WITH RUMPEL–LEEDE PHENOMENON

- Infants:
  - Infants subjected to tourniquet-like compressive conditions,[31,32]
  - Infantile scurvy[31]
- Children:
  - Scarlet fever
  - Kawasaki disease
  - Liver disease
  - Henoch–Schönlein purpura[33]
  - Kawasaki disease
  - Leukemia
  - Ehlers–Danlos syndrome[34]
- Adults:
  - Adult-onset Still's disease on corticosteroids[35]
  - Dengue fever
  - Drug-induced erythema multiforme[36]

Rumpel–Leede phenomenon needs to be differentiated from all other forms of noninflammatory, nonretiform, nonpalpable purpura, or mixed purpura.

SPARING PHENOMENON[37]

Under the rubric of sparing phenomenon, we have a constellation of phenomena wherein either a dermatosis leads to remission or withdrawal of another or two unrelated dermatoses spare each other.

They include:
- Koebner nonresponse
- Renbock phenomenon
- Isotopic nonresponse

Renbok Phenomenon

(Happle R, Van der Steen P, Perret C 1991)
It is defined as inhibition of or withdrawal of dermatosis in the presence of another unrelated dermatosis. It was first observed in patients of alopecia areata who had a loss of hair in the scalp excepting the psoriatic patch which retained hairs. This was termed *inverse Koebner* or *Renbok phenomenon*. Ovcharenko et al.[38] described a case of psoriasis where the plaque regressed with the appearance of a patch of alopecia and within 3 months psoriatic plaques reappeared retaining terminal hairs. A note should be taken of the fact that alopecia areata usually tends to spare gray or white hairs. The mechanism by which this phenomenon unfolds is the common autoimmune nature of AA and psoriasis. The skew in cytokine milieu from Th1 to Th17 and vice versa leads to interchange between the two disorders.

Table 5: Examples of Koebner nonresponse.		
Sparing nevus	Disorder spared	Reported by
Nevus depigmentosus	Generalized drug reaction	Naik et al.[39]
Melanocytic nevus	Alopecia totalis	Yamamoto et al.[40]
Melanocytic nevus	Alopecia areata	Bon et al.[41]
Melanocytic nevus	Alopecia universalis	Ruiz Maldonado et al.[42]
Becker's nevus	Guttate psoriasis	Weiss and Schultz[43]
Nevus flammeus	Alopecia universalis	Chen[44]
Congenita nevi	Dermatophytosis	Happle et al.[45]

Table 6: Examples of isotopic nonresponse.		
Previous healed disease	New dermatosis	Reported by
Herpes zoster	Contact dermatitis	Katayama et al. 1990[46]
Herpes zoster	Borderline leprosy	Jain et al. 1993[47]
Herpes zoster	CTCL	Twersky et al. 2004[48]
Herpes zoster	Contact dermatitis	Nikkels et al. 2004[49]

Also included are a group of disorders is mosaic phenomenon where both active dermatoses spare the lesions of each other. This is explained by genetic mosaicism suggesting a distinct microenvironment that protects a dermatosis from the other.

Koebner Nonresponse Phenomenon

(Bernhard JD, Haynes HA 1982)
The nonappearance or disappearance of a particular dermatosis at the site of injury is known as Koebner nonresponse. Before Bernhard et al. coined the term, it was reported by Cochrane et al. in a patient who had maculopapular drug reaction sparing the irradiated site for Wilms' tumor. The most common condition to exhibit is alopecia areata **(Table 5)**.

Isotopic Nonresponse Phenomenon

(Wolf R, Brenner S, Ruocco V, Filioli FG 1995)
Absence of an eruption at the site of another, unrelated, and already healed dermatosis is termed isotopic nonresponse **(Table 6)**.

FREI–SULZBERGER–CHASE PHENOMENON

(Frei W 1928, Sulzberger MB 1939, Chase MW 1946)
The abolition of dermal contact hypersensitivity to sensitizing agents, e.g., picryl chloride by prior feeding of the agent is known as Sulzberger–Chase phenomenon.[50]

There are five theorized states of immunological unresponsiveness: Medawar's tolerance, radiation tolerance, Frei–Sulzberger–Chase phenomenon, Felton's immunological paralysis, and Dixon and Maurer's protein overloading. The first three are central failure and essential nonreactivity while the last two represent thwarting if not suppression of immunity.

The subject is slowly exposed to graded doses of allergen that produces a low-grade nonthreatening anaphylaxis-like reaction. At the end of the test period, the mast cell granules are depleted and the patient does not mount an allergic reaction until the cells restore the contents. Not only does resistance develop to contactant-type sensitivity but also to synthesis of immunoglobulins toward hapten-self complexes.[52] Investigations have disfavored the concept of clonal depletion and so do the relative numbers of suppressor and effector cells.

> **SALIENT FEATURES OF CHASE PHENOMENON[51]**
>
> - *Rate of decay of antigen in blood*: Not known
> - *Rate of decay of passive antibody*: Normal
> - *Reactivity restored by normal cells*: ?
> - *Reactivity restored by immune lymphoid cells*: Yes
> - *Behavior of lymphoid cells from unresponsive animals after transplant*: Inert
> - Can an animal already immune or sensitive be made unresponsive? No
> - Is the unresponsive animal making an immune response? No

REBOUND PHENOMENON

The reappearance of symptoms and signs of a disease increasing severity, far more than the original disease, after a drug has been reduced, discontinued, or continued for a longer period.

A plethora of examples of rebound phenomenon abound medical literature, the most common being antihypertensives including β blockers, angiotensin-converting enzyme (ACE) inhibitors, thiazides, hydralazine, clonidine, etc. Similar rebounds are seen with statins, aspirin, and heparin.

Acute exposure to drugs leads to receptor activation and signaling but the opposite effects are observed on chronic exposure of drugs. This possibly explains the mechanism behind rebound phenomenon and also and new interest in paradoxical pharmacology.[54]

REBOUND PHENOMENON*

- Topical or systemic corticosteroids:
  - Atopic dermatitis
  - Seborrheic eczema
  - Psoriasis
  - Perioral dermatitis
  - Rosacea
- JAK inhibitors:[53]
  - Psoriasis (9.6–30.9%)
  - Alopecia areata
- TNF inhibitors:
  - Psoriasis (0.9–16.6%)
- IL17 inhibitor:
  - Psoriasis

*Histomorphological rebound is observed after cutaneous atrophy induced by topical corticosteroids after withdrawal of applications.[55]

SHWARTZMAN–SANARELLI PHENOMENON

(Giuseppe Sanarelli 1924, Gregory Shwartzman 1928)

The phenomenon of necrosis secondary to endotoxin administered on successive occasions in a short interval is termed as Sanarelli-Shwartzman phenomenon. The phenomenon is a coagulopathy secondary to complement activation and further innate reactions. Researchers have ruled out the involvement of adaptive or humoral immune responses.

Histologically, it is similar to arthus reaction or leukocytoclastic angiitis. However, this reaction occurs without antigen-antibody-complexes and complement deposits. Moreover, arthus reaction takes weeks to develop and persists for years.

Three different reactions of this phenomenon are described:[56]
1. Localized Shwartzman phenomenon
2. Univisceral Shwartzman phenomenon
3. Generalized Sanarelli-Shwartzman phenomenon

The clinical presentation and mediators for the three phenomena are given in **Table 7**.

SCHULTZ–CHARLTON PHENOMENON

(Schultz W, Charlton W 1918)

The blanching of erythema developed as a result of bacterial exotoxin on institution of antitoxin from a convalescent patient of Scarlet fever is known as Schultz–Charlton extinction phenomenon.

The test,[57] also known by the same name, is carried out using intracutaneous injections of 0.5–1 cc of serum from normal persons or convalescing patients of Scarlet fever. The test area produces a pallid blanch of 2.5–5 cm around the injection within 5–6 hours, if tested on the erythematous rash within the first 5 days, the diagnostic predictability diminishing with each passing day.

Group A beta-hemolytic streptococci produce three exotoxins SPE A, SPE B and SPE C. They can be mimicked by a few Group C and D streptococci. Once a patient develops antitoxin, he is not likely to develop scarlet fever. The state of immunity decides the response of the patient to exotoxin producing Group A β hemolytic streptococci in three distinct ways **(Table 8)**.[58]

PROBE PHENOMENON OR MANDARIN PHENOMENON

The diagnosis of tuberculosis cutis luposa depends upon the light brown infiltrates in the margins seen on diascopy or vitropression, a positive probe phenomenon, histological findings, and the presence of tubercle bacilli in the culture or in animal experiments.[59]

The primary lupus lesion can scarcely be recognized as lupus vulgaris unless a diascopy is done. The epidermis is not involved early, but a probe easily breaks through it into the corium and leads to mild hemorrhage.

A thin, bunt, or rounded probe[60] or obturator from a fairly wide bored mandril[61] is placed on the center of the lesion and a gentle pressure is applied. With moderate pressure, the probe penetrates the skin easily, and when it is withdrawn, a drop of blood oozes out.

While other lupoid nodules have an intact epidermis, the epidermis in lupus spot is atrophic resulting from the

Table 7: Clinical presentation of various subtypes of Shwartzman–Sanarelli phenomenon.			
Phenomenon subtype	**Target organ**	**Dermatological condition**	**Mediators**
Dermal	Skin	Purpura	Intradermal PS, IL-1, INF-γ, and TNF
Univisceral	• Skin • Adrenal	• Lucio phenomenon • Waterhouse Friderichsen syndrome	IL-1, INF-γ, and TNF
Generalized	Skin	• Moschcowitz syndrome • Purpura fulminans • Sepsis	• ADMTS 13 auto-Ab • Meningococcemia • Staphylococcal superantigens

underlying necrotizing dermal infiltrates that are much more superficial to those of syphilis or sarcoidosis. Although the infiltrate is avascular, it is difficult to judge because the mass of tubercular tissue is meagre and a rich cutaneous vasculature abound the periphery of these nodular infiltrates.[62] Therefore, the probe can be easily negotiated through the epidermis. Further, the positive probe test suggests that the normal dermis is destroyed by the infiltrate.

Positive probe phenomenon helps differentiate lupus spots from syphilides, lichenoid, and granulomatous infiltrates in Boeck's sarcoid, oriental sore, and rosacea.

PHENOMENON OF FLUORESCENCE

Fluorescence is a molecular phenomenon in which a fluorophore radiates light energy instantaneously upon being struck with an incident light. The emission in fluorescence stops when the excitation ceases, whereas it is long lived in phosphorescence. The main emission bands[63] found in skin find mention in **Table 9**.

The clinical applications of fluorescence are varied including fields of diagnosis and therapy. What has been used for years as a dermatologic office procedure is the use of Wood's lamp **(Table 10)**.

The depth of melanin can be estimated by the presence or absence of accentuation of pigmentary contrast in melasma.

Wood's light subjected to skin, teeth, blood, and urine helps in differentiating various forms of porphyria.[70]

Protoporphyrin IX after aminolevulinic acid (ALA) therapy selectively concentrates in epithelial tumors with a high tumor to surrounding ratio.[71] Upon irradiation, the tumor becomes visible.

Red light therapy utilizes protoporphyrin IX at 825 nm to generate ROS/RNS to decrease propionibacterium load in pilosebaceous follicles.

Fluorescence microscopy has also been employed, by Hermann et al., in the detection of atabrine toxicity.[72]

IRIS PHENOMENON

The reestablishment of color from the periphery to the center after pressure-induced blanching is known as iris phenomenon.[73]

Table 8: Interpretation of Schultz–Charlton phenomenon in group A streptococci infection.							
Type-specific antibacterial immunity		**Antitoxin immunity**		**Bacteria**		**Outcome**	
Present	+	Present or absent	+	Group A streptococci	=	No clinical disease	
Absent		Present	+	Group A streptococci	=	Streptococcal pharyngo-tonsillitis	
Absent	+	Absent	+	Group A streptococci	=	Streptococcal pharyngitis Or Scarlet fever	

Table 9: Fluorophores and band characteristics of fluorescence in skin.				
Band characteristics	**Peak emission**	**Excitation wavelength**	**Fluorophores**	**Remarks**
Intense band	340 nm	280 nm	Aromatic amino acids including tyrosine and tryptophan	Found in epidermis
Broad band	360–480 nm	325 nm	• Pepsin digestible collagen cross links (PDCCL) • Collagenase digestible collagen crosslinks (CDCCL) • Elastin and mitochondrial NADPH (weak contribution)	• Base peak around 390 nm and two side peaks around 420 nm and 450 nm • Seen as chalky white or bluish white fluorescence in vitiligo
Weak band or peak	600 nm	400 nm	Unmetalled porphyrins	Diagnostic for tumors after ALA treatment
Variable band	407 nm, 470 nm, 593 nm, 623 nm	365 nm, 635–708 nm	Microbes	Wood's lamp or black light test

Table 10: Clinical applications of wood's lamp in various skin infections.				
Infection	**Agent**	**Fluorophore**	**Dermatoses**	**Fluorescence**
Yeast infection[64-67]	*Malassezia* species	Pityrolactone	Pityriasis versicolor alba	• Yellowish (aqueous) • Blue or green yellow (lipid)
Dermatophyte infection[64,65]	*Microsporum audouinii*	Pteridine	Tinea capitis	Blue green
	Microsporum canis		Tinea capitis	Bright green
	Microsporum distortum		Tinea capitis	Greenish
	Microsporum ferrugineum		Tinea capitis	Bright green
	Trichophyton schoenleinii		Favus	Faint blue
	Microsporum gypseum		Kerion	Dull yellow or apple green
Bacterial infection	*Corynebacterium minutissimum*	Coproporphyrin (623 nm)	Erythrasma	Coral red
	Propionibacterium species[68]	• Zn II protoporphyrin (593 nm) • Coproporphyrin (623 nm) • Protoporphyrin (633 nm)	Acne vulgaris	Red
	Pseudomonas aeruginosa (skin)	Pyoverdine (470)	• Erythrasma • Hot tub folliculitis • Ecthyma • Superinfection in SJS, TEN and pemphigus	Yellow green

Note: Hypopigmentary dermatoses such as pityriasis versicolor alba, idiopathic guttate hypomelanosis, and nevus achromicus show an accentuation on Wood's lamp, vitiligo autofluorescence chalky white in Wood's lamp examination, while psoriatic plaques exhibit red autofluorescence due to protoporphyrin IX.[69]

In a normal subject, on release of pressure from the surface of the skin, blanching gives way to rapid and regular blood flow causing hyperemia from the base upward. However, in cases of acrocyanosis, the flow of the blood is slow and from the periphery to the center. Furthermore, the red hyperemic vermilion spot or cinnabar spot progresses to a cyanosis. This sign is known as the iris shutter sign.

It occurs as a result of functional angiopathy, vasospasm is cutaneous arteries, and arterioles causing the cyanosis while compensatory dilation in the postcapillary venules causing hyperhidrosis.[74] The test and sign differentiate acrocyanosis from Raynaud phenomenon.

OBSERVABLE PHENOMENON

ISOTOPIC PHENOMENON

(Wyburn-Mason 1955, Wolf R, Wolf D 1985, Wolf R, Ruocco V, Brenner FG, Filioli FG 1995)

The appearance of a new unrelated dermatosis at the site of previously healed lesion **(Figs. 9 and 10)** is termed isotopic response or Wolf isotopic phenomenon.[75]

While the exact cause of the phenomenon is elusive, viral, immunological, neural, and vascular have been proposed as possible etiologies. Every disorder would have a different pathomechanism, high C5 in connective tissue sites, interleukin 1 (IL-1), and IL-6 in psoriasis, transforming growth factor β (TGF-β) in neoplasia, and increased traps in *locus minoris resistentiae* of Foretell or what has been conceptually proposed as *immunocompromised cutaneous district*[76] could be putative contributing factors. In most cases, the changed environment after the primary insult sows the seeds for a second disorder **(Flowchart 1)**.[77]

In the proposed isotopic phenomenon described by Ruocco et al., the definition was restricted to exclude diseases appearing in areas of irradiation or exposure of external chemicals. Nonspecific causes such as leg ulcers arising in stasis or squamous cell carcinoma arising in irradiated sites were also excluded.

However, what is included are certain infective conditions arising in scars including molluscum contagiosum, verruca plana, infectious eczematoid dermatitis, furunculosis, tuberculosis cutis, and atypical mycobacterial infections.

Also included is a large group of scars secondary to LE, lupus vulgaris, epidermolysis bullosa, osteomyelitis sinus, and inedible pencil foreign body that may give rise to subsequent cancers.

Isotopic coresponse phenomenon[78] is an unusual phenomenon where the second dermatosis presents over the first one, the latter still showing pathologic activity **(Figs. 11 and 12)**.

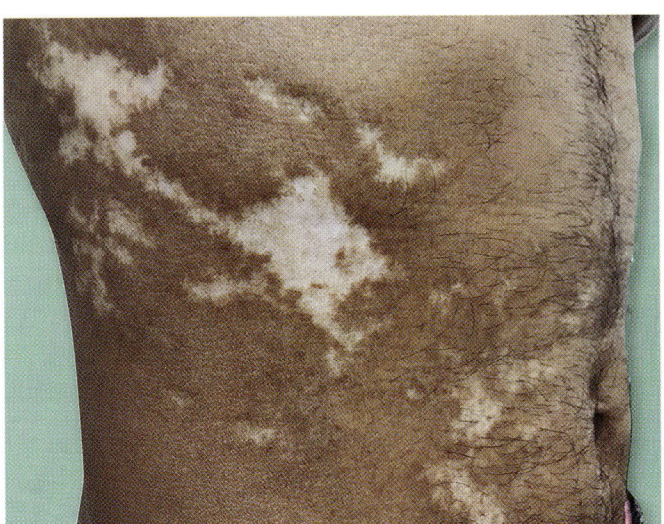

FIG. 9: Vitiligo developing over healed scars of zona cingulata (herpes zoster) after a period of 2 years.

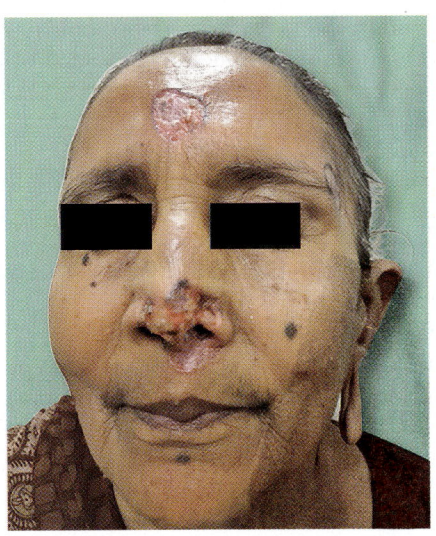

FIG. 10: BCC developing at sites of herpes zoster showing isotopic phenomenon.
Courtesy: Dr Jigna Padhiyar.

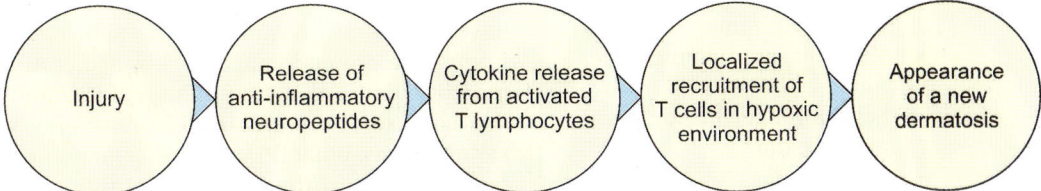

FLOWCHART 1: Schematic representation of pathophysiology in isotopic phenomenon.

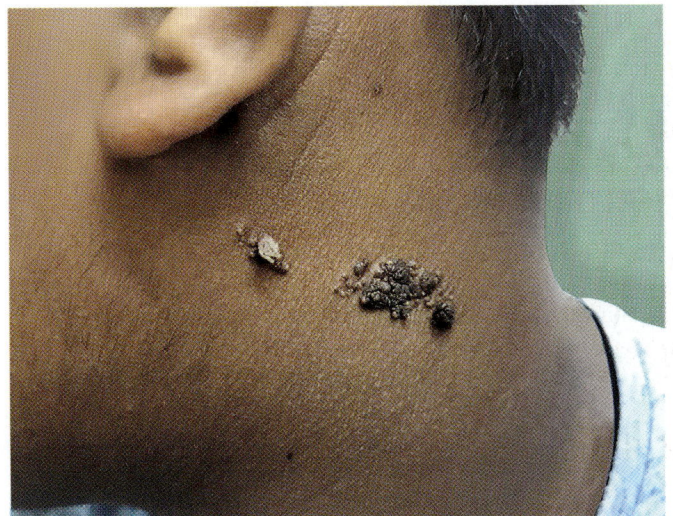

FIG. 11: Keratosis developing over an epidermal nevus.

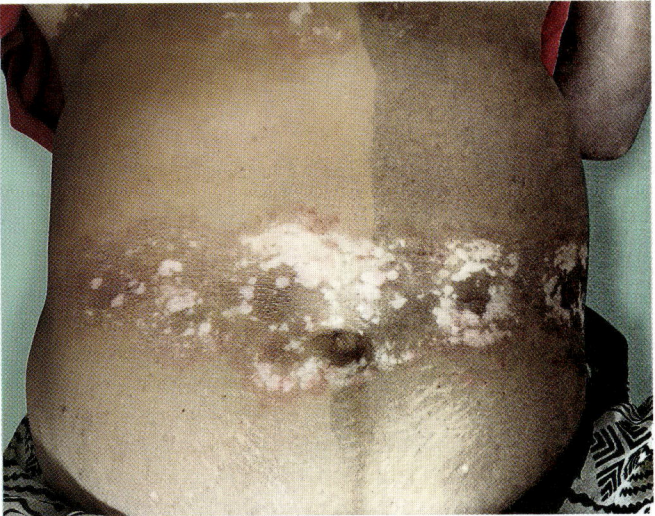

FIG. 12: Vitiligo developing in areas of active tinea corporis suggesting isotopic co-localization.
Courtesy: Dr Jigna Padhiyar.

Isotopic nonresponse[37] or reverse isotopic phenomenon is the sparing of the original site by a second unrelated disease. Stevens–Johnson syndrome (SJS), erythema multiforme (EM), and erythroderma sparing the site of herpes zoster are a few examples.

Anatopic response[37] is the sparing of the first site by another unrelated dermatosis while both of them are active.

EXAMPLES OF ISOTOPIC PHENOMENON

1st dermatosis	2nd dermatosis
Herpes zoster	• Squamous cell carcinoma • Basal cell carcinoma • Basosquamous carcinoma • Breast carcinoma • Larynx SCC • Leukemia cutis • Pseudolymphoma • Granuloma annulare • Sarcoidal granuloma • Angiosarcoma • Dermatophytosis • Kaposi sarcoma • B cell lymphoma • Vasculitic granuloma • Acne • Schwenninger-Buzzi anetoderma
Herpes simplex	Bowen's diseas
Varicella	Verruca Tuberculoid granuloma
Phlebitis	Kaposi sarcoma
Lupus vulgaris scar	Fibrosarcoma
Erythema ab igne	Squamous cell carcinoma

IMMEDIATE PIGMENT DARKENING PHENOMENON

(Hausser 1938)

Sudden appearance of short-lived, ashen, or grayish brown hyperpigmentation on exposure to ultraviolet radiation in the far range between 340 and 450 nm (UVA) is known as immediate pigment darkening (IPD) phenomenon. It is a passive, acellular photochemical reaction resulting from oxidation and/or polymerization of melanin precursors.[79]

Although, photooxidation of "premelanin," changes in the distribution pattern of microfilaments and microtubules, movement of melanosomes to melanocyte dendrites, increased transfer of melanosomes to keratinocytes, and changes in the melanosome distribution pattern in keratinocytes were proposed as possible pathomechanisms, most were discounted, by well-designed experimental studies using ultrastructural morphometry by Honigsmann et al.[79]

Immediate pigment darkening was first studied by Hausser in isolated skin specimens taken from corpses which then were irradiated with a filtered Quartz lamp.

Pigmentation was seen in vitro and in vivo on exposure to UVA light and attempts with 297 nm at high doses failed to elicit darkening.

Immediate darkening also occurred at 0°C, after chemical disruption of tubular structures, repeated freezing and thawing and even after short fixation with formalin.

SALIENT FEATURES OF IPD PHENOMENON

- Observed only with irradiation of UVA rays
- Temperature independent
- Independent of structural integrity of tubular structures
- Reversible only under physiological conditions in undamaged skin
- Does not lead to alterations in cytoskeleton of melanocytes
- Does not result in changes in melanosome distribution pattern in melanocytes and keratinocytes

Although the IPD dose is 10–30 J/cm² at 330–400 nm, fewer joules are required if the skin is already tanned. Immediate protection against ultraviolet A (UVA)-induced radiation damage is the function of IPD and it happens at the expense of the amount of preformed melanin in the keratinocytes. What IPD achieves is an immediate protective response against the UVA spectrum but it fails to prevent ultraviolet B (UVB)-induced erythema.

CONDITIONS DISPLAYING IPD PHENOMENON

- Patients outdoors in natural sunlight in an afternoon
- During PUVA-SOL or PUVA (psoralen and ultraviolet A) therapy
- UVA exposure in tanning saloons

HALO PHENOMENON[80]

(Hebra, Sutton 1916)

Halo phenomena was discovered by Hebra and popularized by Sutton as leukoderma acquisitum centrifugum in 1916. It is defined:
- Clinically with a ring of depigmentation around a pre-existing pigmented lesion (**Figs. 13 and 14**)
- Microscopically with a band-like lymphohisticytic infiltrate and a diminution or absence of melanin pigment at the dermoepidermal junction at the periphery of the nevus.

It can occur either following exposure to actinic radiation, external depigmenting agents, or can be idiopathic.

The halo phenomenon may result from an immune response causing destruction of nevus cell.

CHAPTER 30 Phenomenon in Dermatology

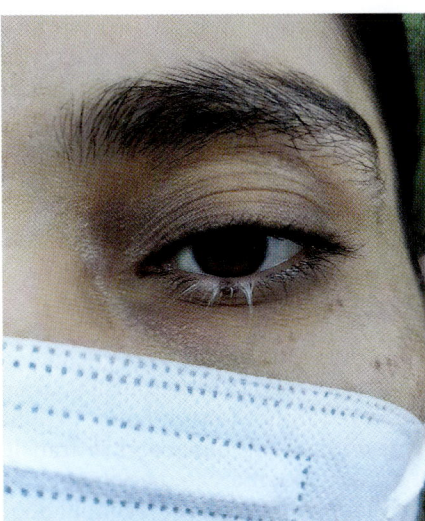

FIG. 13: Hypopigmented halo around a melanocytic nevus on the left lower tarsal plate.

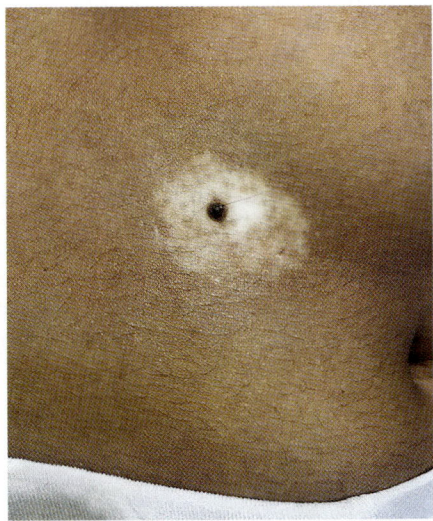

FIG. 14: Perinevoid vitiligo.
Courtesy: Dr Jigna Padhiyar.

Babu et al.,[81] have reported a case of inverse halo phenomenon wherein depigmentation commences within the center of the nevus showing a lighter hue at the center than the periphery.

EXAMPLES OF HALO PHENOMENON

- Halo nevus (Sutton's nevus)
- Perinevoid vitiligo
- Melanocytic:
  - Blue nevus
  - Congenital melanocytic nevus
  - Dysplastic melanocytic nevi
  - Minimal deviation melanoma of the halo nevus-like type
  - Primary cutaneous malignant melanoma or metastases
- Nonmelanocytic:
  - Angioma
  - Basal cell epithelioma
  - Histiocytoma
  - Lichen planus
  - Molluscum contagiosum
  - Neurofibroma
  - Neuroid nevus
  - Psoriasis
  - Sarcoidosis
  - Seborrheic keratosis
  - Spitz nevus
  - Warts

MEYERSON PHENOMENON

(Meyerson 1971)

Meyerson phenomenon is a symmetrical area of erythema and scaling encircling a central lesion which is most commonly a benign melanocytic nevus. Multiple nevi can be involved separately or simultaneously. Nevus presenting with eczematous changes was termed as Meyerson's nevus, halo dermatitis, or halo nevus. It is to be differentiated from halo nevus or Sutton's nevus where melanocytic nevus is surrounded by either hypo- or depigmentation. Progression of Meyerson's nevus into Sutton's nevus has been reported.[82]

The exact mechanism is not known. Proposed mechanisms are:

- The dermatitis is immune-mediated with upregulation of intercellular adhesion molecule-1 (ICAM-1) on keratinocytes and dermal endothelial cell surfaces which initiates an autoimmune reaction against the skin melanocytes. CD4+ lymphocytes are found to be the major cellular infiltrate with a reduced proportion of CD8+ cells.
- Abnormal dermal vasculature and these ectatic vessels possibly cause excessive production of proinflammatory cytokines, promoting the development of eczema.

CONDITIONS WITH MEYERSON PHENOMENON[83,84]

- Melanocytic conditions:
  - Benign melanocytic nevi **(Figs. 15 and 16)**
  - Atypical nevi
  - Dysplastic nevi after interferon alfa-2b therapy
  - Melanoma in situ
  - High-risk melanoma
  - Lentigo

- Nonmelanocytic conditions:
  - Seborrheic keratosis
  - Molluscum contagiosum **(Fig. 17)**
  - Dermatofibromas
  - Stucco keratosis
  - Keloid
  - Insect bites
  - Basal and squamous cell carcinoma
  - Nevus sebaceous
- Vascular malformations such as port wine stain, Klippel–Trénaunay syndrome

Aggravating factors include ultraviolet radiation, chemotherapy, INF-α-2B, laser therapy for vascular malformations. The presence of inflammation in or around a benign lesion can arouse the concern of malignant transformation, though not true in most cases. Halo of eczema cannot be considered a reassuring sign when evaluating melanocytic lesions.

HARLEQUIN PHENOMENON[85]

(Neligan GA, Strange LB 1952)

The harlequin color change is an unusual cutaneous phenomenon observed in newborn infants. The characteristic abnormality is a migratory pink color or transient, benign episodes of a sharply demarcated erythema involving one lateral half of the infant's body, with simultaneous pallor or blanching of the other half.

On axial rotation to the other side, there is a reversal of profound vasodilatation and the pale lateral half turns pink. It spares the head and genitalia and does not involve the mucous membranes.

HARLEQUIN PHENOMENON

- Preterm infants: 15%
- Term infants with low birth weight
- Normal birth weight neonates: 10%
- Neonates with hypoxic injury, intracranial injury

It appears between the second and fifth days of life or may be late as the third week of life. The color changes develop suddenly, without obvious precipitating factors, and persist from 30 seconds to 20 minutes or more.[86]

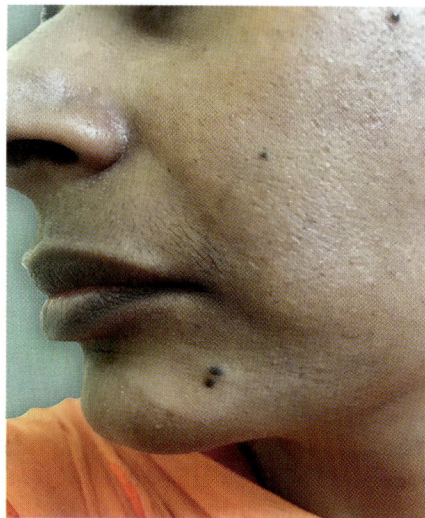

FIG. 15: Eczematization around benign melanocytic nevi suggesting Meyerson's phenomenon.
Courtesy: Dr Jigna Padhiyar.

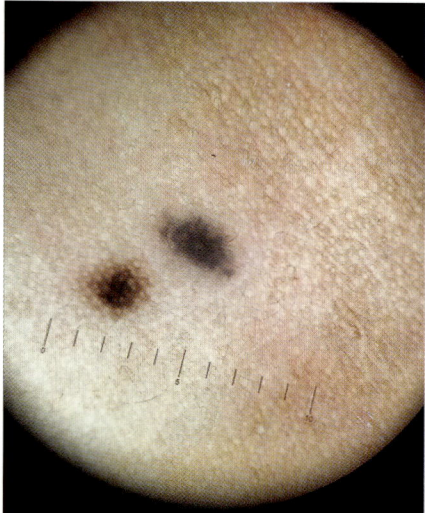

FIG. 16: Dermatoscopic pattern of nevi with erythema in Meyerson's nevi.
Courtesy: Dr Jigna Padhiyar.

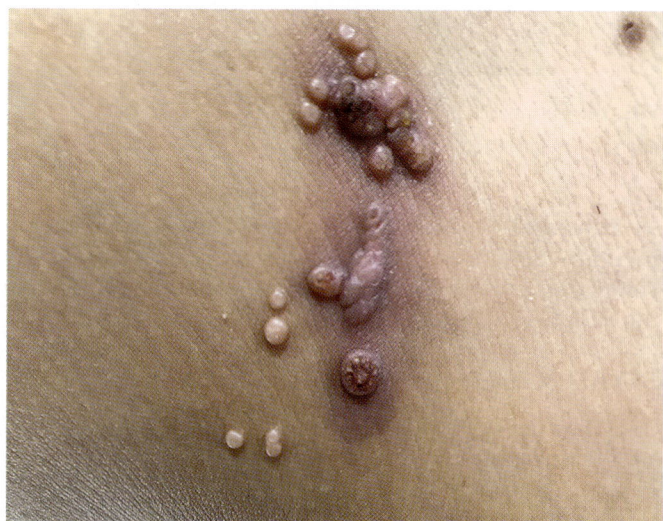

FIG. 17: Intense erythema with slight call around molluscum contagiosum.

Table 11: Differentials of Harlequin phenomenon.		
Harlequin* phenomenon	**Harlequin syndrome**	**Color change in CHD**
• Seen soon after birth • Unilateral • Dynamic color change involving half of the body • Sparing of face, head, and mucosa • Prematurity of hypothalamic centers	• Seen in children • Unilateral warmth and flushing • Dynamic flush involving the face, arms, and chest with warmth and contralateral anhidrosis • Sparing of lower torso and distal limbs • Lesion or tumor affecting autonomic nervous system	• Seen in infants with CHD • Bilateral • Dynamic lower body and acral cyanosis • Spares the upper torso and upper limb

* It needs to be differentiated from harlequin fetus, a severe and uncommon form of ichthyosis manifesting with large, plate-like scales and fissures over the body.
(CHD: congenital heart disease)

Barring isolated reports of an association with tricuspid atresia in a 3½-month-old infant and in an infant with intracranial hemorrhage, there are no usual associations and no specific histologic changes are noted. It may result from immaturity of dysfunction of hypothalamic centers associated with vascular tone in the peripheral vessels.

Harlequin phenomenon[87] should be differentiated from harlequin syndrome and acrocyanosis secondary to ischemic heart disease **(Table 11)**.[85]

MAUSERUNG PHENOMENON[50]

(Siemens in 1937, Traupe 1986)

Mauserung meaning moulting in German is an example of ichthyosis bullosa of Siemens (IBS) that has been reported to be clinically different from bullous congenital ichthyosiform erythroderma of Brocq (BCIE).

The phenomenon is similar to Nikolsky phenomenon, only that is occurs in the superficial epidermis. It is characterized by the absence of erythroderma, localization of dark gray hyperkeratosis to the flexural sites, and areas of peeling of the skin (small patches of bare, apparently normal skin due to regeneration of the epidermis) in the middle of areas of hyperkeratosis.

KASABACH–MERRITT PHENOMENON

(Kasabach HH and Merritt KK 1940)

Kasabach–Merritt phenomenon is a triad comprising of vascular tumors, thrombocytopenia, and bleeding diathesis discovered by Kasabach and Merritt in 1940. It is also known as hemangioma with thrombocytopenia, a rare disease in infants in which a vascular tumor leads to decreased platelets and sometimes other bleeding disorders which can be life-threatening.

It can be seen in different vascular tumors or occurs as a part of syndrome.[80]

The thrombocytopenia associated with vascular lesions is caused by a localized consumption coagulopathy. The vascular lesion triggers an intravascular coagulation with platelet trapping, consequent thrombocytopenia, and fibrinogen consumption and degradation, as well as activation and consumption of coagulation factors, resulting in disseminated intravascular coagulation (DIC). Activation of platelets also promotes further growth of vascular tissue.

Laboratory evidence of the consumptive coagulopathy includes decreased platelets, fibrinogen, and factors II, V, and VIII: Increased prothrombin time, partial thromboplastin time, and fibrin-split products; and microangiopathic hemolytic anemia.[88]

Vascular tumors	Part of syndrome
Common infantile hemangiomas	Klippel–Trénaunay (KT) syndrome
Kaposiform hemangioendothelioma (KHE)	Blue rubber bleb nevus syndrome
Tufted angioma (TA) (syn: angioblastoma)	Gorham-Stout disease
Diffuse infantile or neonatal hemangiomatosis	
Retroperitoneal hemangiomatosis	
Visceral hemangiomatosis	

ULTRAVIOLET RECALL PHENOMENON

(Erythema recall, photo recall, radiation recall)[89,90]
(D'Angio 1959)

Radiation recall dermatitis (RRD) is defined as a "recall" of dermatitis by the skin at the site of previous radiation exposure, in response to administration of certain drugs. It is an acute inflammatory reaction within a previously irradiated or sunburned area after the administration of systemic chemotherapeutic agents such as methotrexate or cytarabine.

First described in 1959 by D'Angio in connection with actinomycin D, radiation recall is commonly seen with

Table 12: Severity of UV recall phenomenon.	
Grade 0	No event
Grade 1	Faint erythema or dry desquamation
Grade 2	Moderate-to-brisk erythema or a patch moist desquamation, mostly confined to the skin folds and creases, moderate edema
Grade 3	Confluent moist desquamation, ≥1.5 cm diameter, not confined to skin folds; pitting edema
Grade 4	Skin necrosis or ulceration of full-thickness dermis; may include bleeding not induced by minor trauma or abrasion
Grade 5	Death (US National Cancer Institute Common Terminology Criteria for Adverse Events – CTCAE V.3)

chemotherapeutic drugs, UV radiation, and megavoltage radiation therapy.

The exact mechanism remains speculative, but it may represent a form of Koebner phenomenon. Vascular damage, epithelial stem cell inadequacy or sensitivity, and idiosyncratic drug hypersensitivity are the probable pathogenic factors. The time interval between radiotherapy and radiation recall dermatitis ranges from 7 days to 15 years. If the interval is short, the reaction is severe **(Table 12)**. It is sometimes difficult to differentiate between radiosensitization (in which the use of a drug makes the tumor cells more sensitive to radiation) from radiation recall dermatitis.

Example: In psoriatics, with the use of methotrexate immediately following PUVA or UVB therapy, thus methotrexate should be introduced after 2 weeks of stopping of any form of phototherapy.

OLFLECK PHENOMENON[91]

"Olfleck" is a German phrase with a literal translation in English as "oil stain." Also known as "*oil spot*" or "*salmon patch*," it is a focal psoriasis of the nail bed characterized by orange area surrounded by a yellow brown margin beneath a paler pink, normal nail plate. Macroscopically, it appears as a brownish discoloration seen over the nail plate as a result of accumulation of parakeratotic columns leading to subungual hyperkeratosis, this is called Olfleck phenomenon.

LUCIO PHENOMENON (ERYTHEMA NECROTICANS)[92,93]

(Lucio and Alvarado 1852)

Lucio phenomenon (LP) first described by Lucio and Alvarado was later confirmed by Latapi and Zamoraas as vasculitis. It is a rare type of reaction with distinct clinical and histopathological features in patients of undiagnosed

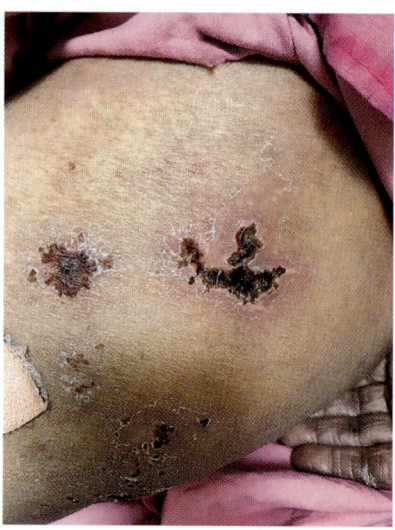

FIG. 18: Irregular necrotic lesion with ragged margins displaying Lucio phenomenon.
Courtesy: Dr Jigna Padhiyar.

and untreated, non-nodular, diffuse, lepromatous, or borderline lepromatous leprosy known as Lucio's leprosy, or pure primitive diffuse lepromatous leprosy.

It is characterized by erythematous, ill-defined, and painful plaques progressing to form ulcers which are extensive, jagged-edged, necrotic, irregular, and geometrically distributed over the legs, thighs, forearms, and buttocks **(Fig. 18)**. Lepromin test gives an intense local response (4–6 hours), the Medina–Ramirez reaction.

Histopathology shows colonization of the endothelial cells by acid–fast bacilli, ischemic epidermal necrosis, changes of vasculitis, and neutrophilic infiltration.

It may clearly imitate or simulate Lucio's reaction and is explained by the Schwartzman type of bacterial hypersensitivity and need to be differentiated from necrotic erythema nodosum.[94]

LYONIZATION PHENOMENON

(Mary Lyon 1961)

X chromosome inactivation occurs early in female mammalian development to achieve dosage compensation with males. The event is random for each cell and is passed on the progeny of the cell in a stable manner.[95]

X inactivation that is unevenly distributed across cell lines with one organism commonly occurs. In X-linked skin disorders, lyonization gives rise to a mosaic pattern along the lines of Blaschko. It is controlled by LINE-1 retrotransposons which are abundant in the region of X-inactivation center (XIC).[96] For male embryos, mutations can be both lethal and nonlethal.

It is unclear whether imprinted (paternal) X-inactivation occurring at 4–8 cell stage occurs in humans. However, random X-inactivation occurs in late blastocyst stage after implantation.

EXAMPLES OF LYONIZATION[97]

- Blaschko lines:
  - Male lethal X-linked traits:
    - Incontinentia pigmenti
    - Conradi–Hünermann–Happle syndrome
    - Gorlin–Goltz syndrome
    - OFD syndrome type I
    - MIDAS syndrome
  - X-linked nonlethal phenotypes:
    - Christ–Siemens–Touraine syndrome
    - IFAP syndrome
    - X-linked Zinsser–Cole–Engman syndrome
    - Hoyeraal–Heidarsson syndrome
- Lateralization:
  - CHILD syndrome
- Checkerboard pattern:
  - X-linked congenital hypertrichosis
- Nonmosaic inactivation:
  - Fabry disease

WORONOFF RING PHENOMENON[98]

(Woronoff DL 1926)

A ring-like achromatic phenomenon characterized by hypopigmented zone around a dermatosis, especially regressing lesions of psoriasis, is called Woronoff ring.

The achromatic rings are pseudoatrophic zones surrounding acanthotic psoriatic plaques. The intermediate zone differs histologically from the surrounding disease and normal skin with marked absence of parakeratosis, a broadened malphigii with hyperkeratotic irregularly shaped papillae without capillary dilation.

It is usually 2–6 mm thick and increases with the size of the lesion.

WORONOFF PHENOMENON

- Regressing psoriasis with treatment:
  - Due to UV therapy
  - Due to dithranol
  - Due to adalimumab[99]
  - Systemic glucocorticoids or fumaric esters
- Corymbiform syphilis
- Varicella infection with Scarlet fever[100]

In addition to what was once thought to be due to an inhibitor of prostaglandin synthesis as well as decreased levels of TGFβ scavenger endoglin, it is now also proposed that human leukocyte antigen (HLA)-class-I restricted autoimmune response of CD8+ T cells produces IL-17, IL-22, and tumor necrosis factor α (TNF-α) which acts synergistically on melanocytes by increasing melanocytes but decreasing melanogenesis. The consequence is that despite healing, the peripheral edge remains hypopigmented.

NEVI AVERSION PHENOMENON[101]

(Norlund JJ)

Certain nevi tend to spare other pigmentary areas of the integument or have an aversion for other nevi is termed as nevi aversion phenomenon.

Whether this phenomenon occurs in all congenital nevi or some of them are still not known. The phenomenon that has been observed so far is a lifelong phenomenon. The biological basis or the phenomenon is still not known and neither have been histologic studies and epidemiological studies been done.

EXAMPLES OF NEVI AVERSION PHENOMENON

- Garment nevi (CMN) sparing the integument:
  - Sparing the areola and nipple
  - Sparing the penis
- CMN sparing a Mongolian spot

HISTOPATHOLOGICAL PHENOMENA

SPLENDORE–HOEPPLI PHENOMENON

Splendore–Hoeppli phenomenon was described by Splendore in sporotrichosis and Hoeppli in schistosomiasis.

It is characterized by intensely eosinophilic material (radiate, star-like, asteroid, or club-shaped configurations) around the microorganisms (fungi, bacteria, and parasites) or biologically inert substances.

The intensely eosinophilic material represents the deposition of antigen–antibody complexes (immunoglobulins and major basic proteins) and debris from the host inflammatory cells.[102]

EXAMPLES OF SPLENDORE HOEPPLI PHENOMENON

Infective causes

- Actinomycosis (Fig. 19)
- Aspergillosis
- Blastomycosis
- Botryomycosis
- Candidiasis
- Eumycetomas
- Majocchi's granuloma
- Nocardiosis
- Pityrosporum folliculitis
- Sporotrichosis
- Strongyloidiasis
- Zygomycosis

Noninfective causes

- Allergic conjunctival granulomas
- Hypereosinophilic syndrome

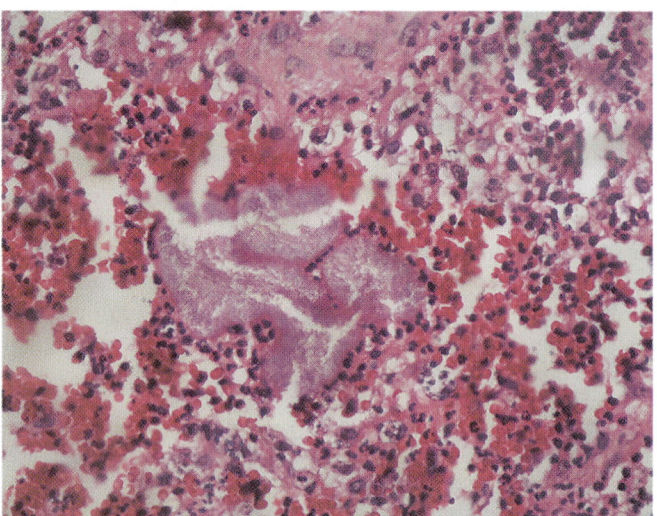

FIG. 19: Splendore–Hoeppli phenomenon in a case of actinomycosis.

THE BORST–JADASSOHN PHENOMENON

(Borst 1904)
In 1904, Borst observed nests of malignant cells at the edges of carcinoma of the lip, sharply defined from the surrounding hyperplastic epidermis, being a secondary intraepidermal growth of the carcinoma. In 1926, Jadassohn described epidermal nests occurring in the absence of dermal invasion as intraepidermal basal cell carcinomas.[103]

Smith and Coburn proposed that the typical Jadassohn lesion is sweat gland origin, and coined the name as hidroacanthoma simplex characterized by well-demarcated nests of uniform, basaloid cells confined within the epidermis, contained large amounts of glycogen, and stained positively with PAS, suggesting differentiation toward eccrine ducts.

EXAMPLES OF BORST–JADASSOHN PHENOMENON

- Actinic keratosis
- Bowen's disease
- Melanoma in situ
- Paget's disease and
- Epidermotropic metastatic carcinomas

Mehregan and Pinkus concluded that Borst and Jadassohn had described quite different biological phenomena, and that the term "Borst-Jadassohn intraepidermal epithelioma" therefore should be discarded. According to them, this phenomenon can be seen in benign lesions such as seborrheic keratosis (especially if irritated by infection or trauma) or entirely intraepidermal sweat gland tumors (hidroacanthoma simplex of Smith and Coburn).

PAGETOID PHENOMENON

Pagetoid refers to "upward spreading" of melanocytes into the epidermis.

A pattern with upward growth of the melanocytes so that they are no longer confined to the basal layer is pagetoid phenomena and is pathognomonic for melanoma.[104]

EXAMPLES OF PAGETOID PHENOMENON

Apocrine gland carcinoma

LABORATORY PHENOMENA

LUPUS ERYTHEMATOSUS CELL PHENOMENON[105]

(Hargraves et al.)
It is due to the action on leukocytic nuclei by autoantibodies (serum factor, LE cell factor) present in patient serum. These altered nuclei are extruded from the affected cells, which are then phagocytosed by viable leukocytes.

LE cells are polymorphonuclear leukocytes (neutrophils, macrophages) that have ingested nuclear material from the degenerated white cells.

Three ingredients are necessary for the LE cell phenomenon to take place, which include:
- Serum factor (autoantibodies, previously called as LE cell factor)
- Nuclei to be altered
- Leukocytes capable of phagocytosis

Method of Elicitation

About 5 cc of heparinized blood is added to a conical flask containing glass beads and then the flask is agitated (to induce trauma to the white blood cells and to make contact between the traumatized cells and the serum factor) manually for about 20–30 minutes. After incubating the flask at 37°C for 30 minutes, the sample is centrifuged for 1 minutes at 8,000 g or 700 g for 5 minutes. The Buffy coat is separated from the centrifuged sample and it is stained with either Wright's stain or Giemsa stain and observed under a microscope.

EXAMPLES OF LE CELL PHENOMENON

- LE
- Rheumatoid arthritis
- Lupoid hepatitis
- Scleroderma
- Dermatomyositis
- Polyarteritis nodosa
- Pernicious anemia

- Hemolytic anemia
- Multiple myeloma
- Miliary tuberculosis
- Drugs such as hydralazine, penicillin, INH and hydantoin, and procainamide

REYNOLD'S BRAUDE PHENOMENON

Incubation of the culture of *Candida* species with human or sheep serum at 37°C produces germ tubes which originate from the pseudohyphae of *Candida albicans* within 2–4 hours called as Reynolds-Braude phenomenon.

It helps to distinguish pathogenic *C. albicans* and *C. dublinensis* from other pathogenic strains such as *C. pseudotropicalis* and *C. parapsilosis*.[106]

EPITOPE SPREADING PHENOMENON

Epitope spreading phenomenon explains the progressive formation of antibodies against more than one antigenic determinant during the course of an autoimmune disease.[107]

As the disease progresses, progressive tissue injury caused by primary antibodies results in the unmasking of neighboring proteins to which secondary antibody responses are generated.

In pemphigus vulgaris, epitope spreading occurs as a result of an immune response against the endogenous target antigens secondary to the release of self-antigen during the chronic autoimmune response. Antigen-specific autoimmune responses can spread to different epitopes on one protein (intramolecular epitope spreading) or to epitopes on other structural proteins (intermolecular epitope spreading). The formation of new antibodies may result in an atypical clinical picture.

EXAMPLES OF EPITOPE SPREADING

- Transformation of pemphigus foliaceous into pemphigus vulgaris
- Change from the mucosal form of pemphigus vulgaris to mucocutaneous form
- Paraneoplastic pemphigus
- Lichen planus pemphigoides

In pemphigus vulgaris, epitope spreading occurs as a result of an immune response against the endogenous target antigens secondary to the release of self-antigen during the chronic autoimmune response. Antigen-specific autoimmune responses can spread to different epitopes on one protein (intramolecular epitope spreading) or to epitopes on other structural proteins (intermolecular epitope spreading). The formation of new antibodies may result in an atypical clinical picture.

PROZONE PHENOMENON[108]

The prozone phenomenon refers to a false-negative serologic test in which very high antibody titers interfere with the antigen–antibody lattice network necessary to visualize a positive flocculation test venereal disease research laboratory/treponema pallidum hemagglutination (VDRL/TPHA). Thus, a higher dilution of the serum sample should be made to elicit a true positive flocculation test.

The prozone phenomenon occurs in 1–2% of cases of secondary syphilis, hence when clinical evidence for secondary syphilis is strong and serum VDRL is reported negative, the VDRL test should be repeated in higher dilutions to rule out the prozone phenomenon.

Example: Human immunodeficiency virus (HIV)-positive patients exhibit B-cell dysregulation, which leads to hypergammaglobulinemia, giving high antibody titers, thereby showing the prozone phenomenon. It is increasingly seen in patients coinfected with syphilis than in syphilitic patients who are negative for HIV, other infections such as brucellosis, typhoid, and hepatitis B.

MEIROWSKY PHENOMENON[109]

(Meirowsky 1909)

The phenomenon of darkening of epidermis on exposure to heat at a given temperature on changing the redox potential is termed as Meirowsky phenomenon.

In vitro experiments have shown that fresh skin epidermis on being subjected to heat leads to irreversible darkening.

The time requires for consistent unequivocal results was 1–3 days, care being taken to avoid desiccation. Apart from being temperature dependent, the darkening varied with the change in redox potential, low redox potentials giving pale color.

The response is dependent on the tissue fixation and oxygenation.

SALIENT FEATURES

- Irreversible
- Temperature specific:
  - Effect at 56°C > 37°C > 100°C
  - No change at 0–20°C
- Fresh specimen required
- Oxygen dependent:
  - Higher redox potential causes greater darkening

THERAPEUTIC PHENOMENA

TACHYPHYLAXIS

Tachyphylaxis is defined as a rapid decrease in response to repeated doses over a short period of time.

Repeated administration of the same dose over a short interval leads to a diminution of the physiological effect. Moreover, stoppage of therapy reverses the short-lived tolerance like effect of the drug.

Re-administration of the drug after a holiday is recommended with potent steroid use as well as with conventional antihistamines **(Table 13)**.

EXAMPLES OF TACHYPHYLAXIS

- Hydroxyzine* especially in atopic
- Class I and II topical corticosteroids[110]
- Anesthetics
- Ephedrine[111]
- Substances–alcohol, opioids,[112] and nicotine[113]

*No tachyphylaxis noted with newer second-generation antihistamines.[114]

HOIGNE PHENOMENON (PROCAINE PSYCHOSIS)[115]

(Hoigne and Schoch, 1959)

Hoigne phenomena is an acute, nonallergic, psychiatrically based reaction occurring with a wide list of medications, mainly antibiotics ("pseudoanaphylactic reaction to procaine penicillin," "acute psychotic syndrome after penicillin," or "antibiomania").

First described by Hoigne and Schoch in 1959 with antimicrobials but very rare in dermatology.

Table 13: Characteristic features differentiating tachyphylaxis from tolerance.

Characteristics	Tachyphylaxis	Tolerance
Dose of drug	Not dose-dependent	Larger dose required to produce same effect
Rate sensitive	Yes	No
Effect	Short-lived	Relatively longer
Pharmacokinetic clearance	No effect	Increases on repeat dosing
Physiological tolerance	No physiological adaptation	Adaptation of unrelated systems as compensatory mechanism
Behavioral tolerance	Not seen	Learned compensation diminishes drug effect

Psychotic symptoms arising as a complication of treatment with procaine penicillin given for primary and secondary syphilis having classic features of anxiety/panic and hallucinations are called as Hoigne phenomenon. Accidental intravascular injection of procaine penicillin results in mental confusion, visual and auditory hallucination, sense of impending doom, headache, and hypotension.

This symptom complex occurs due to the lipid-soluble procaine moiety, which readily crosses the blood–brain barrier. There are two theories about the cause of nonallergic procaine penicillin reactions.

The vascular theory was first proposed by Batchelor et al. Hoigne also proposed that microembolization of the small vessels in the lungs and brain by microcrystals of procaine penicillin dislodged from the site of injection.

The toxic theory proposes that the reaction is caused by the toxic action of procaine on the central nervous system.

JARISCH–HERXHEIMER PHENOMENON[116]

(Adolf Jarisch 1885, Karl Herxheimer 1902)

This is a pathophysiological phenomenon attributed to the endotoxins released from the dying microbe following treatment against it.

Jarisch–Herxheimer phenomenon is a sudden intensification of existing symptoms after institution of therapy associated with systemic signs and symptoms.

The reactions are characterized by:
- Fluctuation of body temperature
- Symptom flare an
- Physiological changes

It is transient, occurs within 12–24 hours of institution of therapy, and may show polymorphonuclear leukocytosis, lymphopenia, and raised erythrocyte sedimentation rate (ESR).

A massive release of bacterial constituents following antibacterial therapy leads to a cytokine storm with elevations of TNF-α, IL-6, and IL-8 leading to systemic flare up.

A similar phenomenon is seen after treatment of dermatophytosis with griseofulvin, ketoconazole, and itraconazole. The authors have seen inflammatory reactions to be not uncommon with terbinafine therapy. Similar phenomenon is seen in onchocerciasis treated with ivermectin leading to Mazzotti reaction.

JARISCH–HERXHEIMER PHENOMENON

- Jarisch-Herxheimer reaction:[117]
  - Syphilis (in decreasing order)
  - Neurosyphilis (64–79%)

- Early syphilis (40%)
- Cardiovascular syphilis
- Vincent's infection
- Relapsing fever
- Leptospirosis
- Lyme's disease
- Brucellosis treated with aureomycin, chloramphenicol, terramycin, or sulfonamide-streptomycin combination
- Herxheimer-like reactions:[117]
  - Glanders treated with streptomycin
  - Tularemia treated with streptomycin
  - Leprosy treated with dapsone
  - Anthrax treated with aureomycin
- Mazzotti reaction:[118]
  - Onchocerciasis and Scabies treated with ivermectin
- Inflammatory reaction:[119]
  - Dermatophytosis treated with griseofulvin, azoles, and terbinafine[120]

CASTLING PHENOMENON[121-123]

(Happle et al.)

Castling is characterized by the appearance of hair growth in areas remote to the treated site following treatment by immunosensitizers such as dinitrochlorobenzene (DPCB), squaric acid dibutylester (SADBE), or diphencyprone (DCP). Also known as *"rochade"* or *"crossing,"* the effect of the topical agent crosses beyond the boundary of application and hair growth is observed in different parts of the scalp or different sites such as the face, eyebrow, eyelashes, torso, axillae, and the pubis.

CONCLUSION

While newer data is being accumulated, newer appearances shall be identified and corroborating theories shall define newer phenomenon. Established phenomenon shall transform into measurable signs, effects, tests, and reactions in the future.

REFERENCES

1. Machamer P. Phenomena, data and theories: A special issue of synthese. Synthese. 2011;182(1):1-5.
2. Bogen J, Woodward J. Saving the phenomena. The philosophical review. 1988;97(3):303-52.
3. Lutz W. (1957) Pemphigus chronicus vulgaris. Lehrbuch Der Haut- Und Geschlehts- Krankheiten, 2nd edition. Basel: Karger; 1957. pp. 198-9.
4. Nikolskiy PV. The Materials on the Study of Pemphigus Foliaceous Cazenavi. Kiev (Ukraine): St. Vladimir Emperor University; 1896.
5. Sheklakov ND. On so-called mechanical symptoms in certain bullous dermatoses. Vestn Dermatol Venereol. 1967;41:28-31.
6. Sheklakov ND. Symptom of Perifocal Subepidermal Separation. Vestn Dermatol Venereol. 1965;39:38-41.
7. Asboe-Hansen G. Blister-spread induced by finger pressure, a diagnostic sign in pemphigus. J Invest Dermatol. 1960;34:5-9.
8. Fassmann A, Dvovrakova N, Izakovivcova Holla L, Vanvek J, Wotke J. Manifestation of pemphigus vulgaris in the orofacial region. Case report. Scripta Medica (Brno). 2003;76:55-62.
9. Braun-Falco O, Plewig G, Wolff HH, Winkelmann RK. Vesicular and bullous diseases. In Dermatology, 3rd edition. Berlin: Springer-Verlag; 1991. pp. 467-501.
10. Rahman S, Daveluy S. Pathergy Test. StatPearls. Treasure Island (FL): StatPearls Publishing; 2020.
11. Baker MR, Smith EV, Seidi OA. Pathergy Test. Practical neurology. 2011;11(5):301-2.
12. Hatemi I, Hatemi G, Celik AF, Melikoglu M, Arzuhal N, Mar C, et al. Frequency of pathergy phenomenon and other features of Behçet's syndrome among patients with inflammatory bowel disease. Clin Exp Rheumat. 2008;26(4): S91.
13. Davatchi F, Assaad-Khalil S, Calamia KT, Crook J, Sadeghi-Abdollahi B, Schirmer M. International Study Group for Behçet's Disease. Criteria for diagnosis of Behçet's disease. Lancet. 1990;335(8695):1078-80.
14. Weiss G, Shemer A, Trau H. The Koebner phenomenon: Review of the literature. J Eur Acad Dermatol Venereol. 2002;16(3):241-8.
15. Dos Santos Camargo CM, Brotas AM, Ramos-E-Silva M, Carneiro S. Isomorphic phenomenon of Koebner: Facts and controversies. Clin Dermatol. 2013;31(6):741-9.
16. Ahad T, Agius E. The Koebner phenomenon. Br J Hosp Med. 2015;76(11):C170-2.
17. Boyd AS, Neldner KH. The isomorphic response of Koebner. Int J Dermatol. 1990;29(6):401-10.
18. Urbach F. The negative effects of solar radiation: A clinical overview. Compr Ser Photosci. 2001;3:39-67.
19. Van Geel N, Speeckaert R, Taieb A, Picardo M, Böhm M, Gawkrodger DJ, et al. Koebner's phenomenon in vitiligo: European position paper. Pigment Cell Melanoma Res. 2011; 24(3):564-73.
20. Levin NA, Patterson JW, Yaoc LL, Wilson BB. Resolution of patch-type granuloma annulare lesions after biopsy. J Am Acad Dermatol. 2002;46(3):426-9.
21. Srinivasan S, Karthikeyan SA, Thomas J. Reverse Koebnerization in a case of granuloma annulare: a case report. Int J Sci Res. 2019;8(12):29-30.
22. Naveen KN, Pai VV, Athanikar SB, Gupta G, Parshwanath HA. Remote reverse Koebner phenomenon in generalized granuloma annulare. Indian Dermatol Online J. 2014;5(2): 219.
23. Pinkus H. Lichenoid tissue reactions. A speculative review of the clinical spectrum of epidermal basal cell damage with special reference to erythema dyschromium perstans. Arch Dermatol. 1973;107(6):840-6.
24. Rajka G. Pathomechanism: The altered skin. In: Essential Aspects of Atopic Dermatitis. Berlin: Springer Science & Business Media; 2012. pp. 172-202.
25. Gandhi G, Vasani R. White dermographism. Indian J Paediatr Dermatol. 2018;19(2):173-5.

26. Francis IC, Loughhead JA. Bell's phenomenon: A study of 508 patients. Aust J Ophthalmol. 1984;12(1):15-21.
27. Braun-Falco O, Plewig G, Wolff HH, Burgdorf WH. Diseases of connective tissue. In: Dermatology. Berlin, Heidelberg: Springer; 2000. pp. 751-832.
28. Klippel JH. Raynaud's phenomenon. In: Freedberg IM, Eisen AZ, Wolff K, Austen KF, Goldsmith LA, Katz SI (Eds). Fitzpatrick's Dermatology in General Medicine. New York: McGraw Hill; 2003.
29. Dowd PM. Reactions to cold. In: Burns T, Breathnach S, Cox N, Griffiths C (Eds). Rook's Textbook of Dermatology. Oxford: Blackwell Publishing; 2004.
30. Khan HQ, Adil M, Amin SS, Mudassir M. Petechiae over face: A case of Rumpel-Leede phenomenon. Indian Dermatol Online J. 2020;11(4):658-9.
31. Vinod CE, Saju SJ, Moudgil K. The phenomenon of external pressure Rumpel Leede sign: A review. J Pharm Sci Res. 2020;12(3):433-5.
32. Nguyen TA, Garcia D, Wang AS, Friedlander SF, Krakowski AC. Rumpel-Leede phenomenon associated with tourniquet-like forces of baby carriers in otherwise healthy infants: Baby carrier purpura. JAMA Dermatol. 2016;152(6):728-30.
33. Lava SA, Milani GP, Fossali EF, Simonetti GD, Agostoni C, Bianchetti MG. Cutaneous manifestations of small-vessel leukocytoclastic vasculitides in childhood. Clin Rev Allergy Immunol. 2017;53(3):439-51.
34. Wiesmann T, Castori M, Malfait F, Wulf H. Recommendations for anesthesia and perioperative management in patients with Ehlers-Danlos syndrome (S). Orphanet J Rare Dis. 2014;9(1):1-9.
35. Lambdin JT, Mackenzie C. Rumpel-Leede phenomenon in a patient with adult-onset Still's disease. BMJ Case Rep. 2017;2017: Bcr2016217290.
36. Gross AS, Holloway RJ, Fine RM. The Rumpel-Leede sign associated with drug-induced erythema multiforme. J Am Acad Dermatol. 1992;27(5):781-2.
37. Pakran J. Sparing phenomena in dermatology. Indian J Dermatol Venereol Leprol. 2013;79(4):545-50.
38. Ovcharenko Y, Serbina I, Zlotogorski A, Ramot Y. Renbök phenomenon in an alopecia areata patient with psoriasis. Int J Trichol. 2013;5(4):194.
39. Naik RP, Srinivas CR. Generalized drug reaction sparing nevus depigmentosus. Arch Dermatol. 1986;122(5):509-10.
40. Yamamoto T, Okabe H, Hoshi M. Alopecia totalis sparing congenital melanocytic nevus: Renbok phenomenon. Dermatologica Sinica. 2019;37(3):176-7.
41. Bon AM, Happle R, Itin PH. Renbök phenomenon in alopecia areata. Dermatology. 2000;201(1):49-50.
42. Ruiz-Maldonado R, Tamayo L, Duran C. Hairy pigmented congenital naevocellular naevus in a patient with alopecia universalis. Clin Exp Dermatol. 1993;18(2):162-3.
43. Weiss RM, Schulz EJ. Guttate psoriasis sparing becker's melanosis: a case report. Dermatology. 1990;180(3):160-2.
44. Chen W. Alopecia areata universalis sparing nevus flammeus. Dermatology. 2005;210(3):227-8.
45. Happle R, Wollina U, Verma SB. Two examples of Renbök phenomenon in dermatophytosis sparing congenital nevi. J Eur Acad Dermatol Venereol. 2021;35(10):e695-7.
46. Katayama H, Karube S, Ueki Y, Yaoita H. Contact dermatitis sparing the eruption of herpes zoster and its periphery. Dermatology. 1990;181(1):65-7.
47. Jain R, Dogra S, Kaur I, Kumar B. Leprosy and herpes zoster; an association or dissociation? Indian J Lepr. 2003;75(3):263-4.
48. Twersky JM, Nordlund JJ. Cutaneous T-cell lymphoma sparing resolving dermatomal herpes zoster lesions: An unusual phenomenon and implications for pathophysiology. J Am Acad Dermatol. 2004;51(1):123-6.
49. Nikkels AF, Sadzot-Delvaux C, Piérard GE. Absence of intercellular adhesion molecule 1 expression in varicella zoster virus–infected keratinocytes during herpes zoster: Another immune evasion strategy? Am J Dermatopathol. 2004;26(1):27-32.
50. Madke B, Doshi B, Pande S, Khopkar U. Phenomena in dermatology. Indian J Dermatol Venereol Leprol. 2011;77(3):264-75.
51. Wolstenholme GE, O'Connor M (Eds). Cellular aspects of immunity. New York: John Wiley & Sons; 2009.
52. Chase MW. The induction of tolerance to allergenic chemicals. Ann N Y Acad Sci. 1982;392:228-47.
53. Garcia-Melendo C, Cubiró X, Puig L. Janus kinase inhibitors in dermatology: Part 1—general considerations and applications in vitiligo and alopecia areata. Actas Dermo-Sifiliográficas. 2021;112(6):503-15.
54. Teixeira MZ. Therapeutic use of the rebound effect of modern drugs: "New homeopathic medicines". Revista Da Associação Médica Brasileira. 2017;63:100-8.
55. Zheng P, Lavker RM, Lehmann P, Kligman AM. Morphologic investigations on the rebound phenomenon after corticosteroid-induced atrophy in human skin. J Invest Dermat. 1984;82(4):345-52.
56. Chahin AB, Opal JM, Opal SM. Whatever happened to the Shwartzman phenomenon? Innate Immun. 2018;24(8):466-79.
57. Birkhaug KE. Studies in scarlet fever: I. Studies concerning the blanching phenomenon in scarlet fever. J Clin Invest. 1925;1(3):273-94.
58. Braun-Falco O, Plewig G, Wolff HH, Winkelmann RK. Diseases of blood vessels. In: Braun-Falco (Ed). Dermatology. Berlin, Heidelberg: Springer; 1991. pp. 13-60.
59. Korting GW, Denk R. Differential Diagnosis in Dermatology. Philadelphia: WB Saunders Company; 1976. p. 527.
60. Braun-Falco O, Burgdorf WH, Plewig G, Wolff HH, Landthaler M. Mycobacterial infections. In: Braun-Falco (Ed). Dermatology. Berlin, Heidelberg: Springer; 2009. pp. 176-201.
61. Braun-Falco O, Plewig G, Wolff HH, Winkelmann RK. Diseases caused by bacteria. In: Braun-Falco (Ed). Dermatology. Berlin, Heidelberg: Springer; 1991. pp. 64-202.
62. Pinkus H, Mehregan AH. Predominant mononuclear granulomas. In: A Guide to Dermatohistopathology. New York: Appleton-Century-Crofts; 1981. pp. 225-46.
63. Morvova Jr M, Jeczko P, Šikurová L. Gender differences in the fluorescence of human skin in young healthy adults. Skin Res Technol. 2018;24(4):599-605.
64. Rativa D, Barbalho JP, Martins Filho JF, Araujo RE, Gomes AS, Souza Filho LG. Perspectives on in vitro fungal diagnosis with UV light. Rev Bras Eng Biomed. 2007;23(1):25-30.
65. Remya VS, Arun B. Diagnostic efficacy of wood's lamp examination compared with KOH wet mount for diagnosis of pityriasis versicolor cases. Int J Health Sci Res. 2019;9(4):27-30.
66. Boekhout T, Guého-Kellermann E, Mayser P, Velegraki A (Eds). Malassezia and the Skin: Science and Clinical Practice. Berlin: Springer Science & Business Media; 2010.

67. Raugi G, Nguyen TU. Superficial Dermatophyte Infections of the Skin. Innetter's Infectious Diseases. Philadelphia: WB Saunders; 2012. pp. 102-9.
68. Putra IB, Jusuf NK, Dewi NK. The role of digital fluorescence in acne vulgaris: Correlation of ultraviolet red fluorescence with the severity of acne vulgaris. Dermatol Res Pract. 2019;2019:4702423.
69. Bissonnette R, Zeng H, Mclean DI, Schreiber WE, Lui H. Psoriatic plaques exhibit red autofluorescence that is due to protoporphyrin IX. J Invest Dermatol. 1998;111(4):586-91.
70. Halprin KM. Diagnosis with Wood's light: II. The porphyrias. JAMA. 1967;200(6):460.
71. Bäumler W, Abels C, Szeimies RM. Fluorescence diagnosis and photodynamic therapy in dermatology. Med Laser App. 2003;18(1):47-56.
72. Mescon H, Grots IA. Fluorescence microscopy in dermatology. J Invest Dermatol. 1963;41(4):181-96.
73. Braun-Falco O, Plewig G, Wolff HH, Winkelmann RK. Diseases of Blood Vessels. In: Braun-Falco (Ed). Dermatology. Berlin, Heidelberg: Springer; 1991. pp. 607-48.
74. Kurklinsky AK, Miller VM, Rooke TW. Acrocyanosis: The flying dutchman. Vasc Med. 2011;16(4):288-301.
75. Wolf R, Brenner S, Ruocco V, Filioli FG. Isotopic response. Int J Dermatol. 1995;34(5):341-8.
76. Piccolo V, Baroni A, Russo T, Schwartz RA. Ruocco's immunocompromised cutaneous district. Int J Dermatol. 2016;55(2):135-41.
77. Sahl Jr WJ, Clever H. Cutaneous scars: Part II. Int J Dermatol. 1994;33(11):763-9.
78. El Jouari O, Senhaji G, Douhi Z, Elloudi S, Baybay H, Mernissi FZ. The isotopic response phenomenon. J Derm Surg Res Ther. 2019;2(1):1-3.
79. Hönigsmann H, Schuler G, Aberer W, Romani N, Wolff K. Immediate pigment darkening phenomenon. A reevaluation of its mechanisms. J Invest Dermatol. 1986;87(5):648-52.
80. Atherton DJ, Moss C. Naevi and other developmental defects. In: Burns T, Breathnach S, Cox N, Griffiths C (Eds). In: Rook's Textbook of Dermatology, 7th edition. Oxford: Blackwell Publishing; 2004. pp. 15.57-15.60.
81. Babu A, Bhat MR, Dandeli S, Ali NM. Throwing light onto the core of a halo nevus: A new finding. Indian J Dermatol. 2016;61(2):238.
82. Ramon R, Silvestre JF, Betloch I, Banuls J, Botella R, Navas J. Progression of Meyerson's naevus to Sutton's naevus. Dermatology. 2000;200(4):337-8.
83. Vasani R. Meyerson phenomenon. Indian J Paediatr Dermatol. 2019;20:78-80.
84. Dawn G, Burden AD. Meyerson's phenomenon around a seborrheic keratosis. Clin Exp Dermatol. 2002;27(1):73.
85. Ichenfield L, Larralde M. Neonatal skin and skin disorders. In: Schachner L, Hnsen RC (Eds). Pediatric Dermatology, 3rd edition. Amsterdam: Elsevier; 2003. pp. 205-62.
86. Tang J, Bergman J, Lam JM. Harlequin colour change: Unilateral erythema in a newborn. CMAJ. 2010;182(17):E801.
87. Elboukhari K, Baybay H, Elloudi S, Senhaji G, Douhi Z, Mernissi FZ. Idiopathic Harlequin syndrome: A case report and literature review. Pan Afr Med J. 2019;33:141-4.
88. Hall GW. Kasabach–Merritt syndrome: Pathogenesis and management. Br J Haematol. 2001;112(4):851-62.
89. Azria D, Magné N, Zouhair A, Castadot P, Culine S, Ychou M, et al. Radiation recall: A well recognized but neglected phenomenon. Cancer Treatment Reviews. 2005;31(7):555-70.
90. Patil S, Nadkarni N, Shende S. Recalling the recall phenomenon. Indian J Dermatol Venereol Leprol. 2015;81(2):214.
91. Sehgal VN (Ed). Psoriasis. In: Textbook of Clinical Dermatology. New Delhi: Jaypee Brothers Medical Publishing; 2006. p. 128.
92. Costa IM, Kawano LB, Pereira CP, Nogueira LS. Lucio's phenomenon: A case report and review of the literature. Int J Dermatol. 2005;44(7):566-71.
93. Saoji V, Salodkar A. Lucio leprosy with lucio phenomenon. Indian J Lepr. 2001;73(3):267-72.
94. Ranugha PS, Chandrashekar L, Kumari R, Thappa DM, Badhe B. Is it Lucio phenomenon or necrotic erythema nodosum leprosum? Indian J Dermatol. 2013;58(2):160.
95. Lyon MF. X-chromosome inactivation and developmental patterns in mammals. Biol Rev Camb Philos Soc. 1972;47(1):1-35.
96. Happle R. Mosaicism and epidermal nevi. In: Braun-Falco O, Burgdorf WH, Plewig G, Wolff HH, Landthaler M (Eds). Dermatology. Berlin, Heidelberg: Springer; 2009. pp. 776-94.
97. Happle R. X-Chromosome inactivation: Role in skin disease expression. Acta Paediatrica. 2006;95:16-23.
98. PRINZ JC. The Woronoff ring in psoriasis and the mechanisms of post-inflammatory hypopigmentation. Acta Dermato-Venereologica. 2020;100(3):adv00031.
99. Park KK, Swan JW, Eilers D, Tung R, Koo J. Woronoff ring associated with adalimumab therapy for psoriasis. Cutis. 2014;93(2):E1-2.
100. Penneys NS. Varicella lesions and Woronoff's Ring. Clin Infect Dis. 1993;17(5):928.
101. Norlund JJ. Nevus aversion phenomenon. Rare benign neoplasms of melanocytes. In: Norund JJ, Boissy RE, Hearing VJ, King RA, Oetting WS, Ortonne JP (Eds). The Pigmentary System: Physiology and Pathophysiology. New York: John Wiley and Sons; 2008. pp. 1148.
102. Hussein MR. Mucocutaneous Splendore-Hoeppli phenomenon. J Cutan Pathol. 2008;35(11):979-88.
103. Larsson A, Hammarström L, Nethander G, Sjögren S. Multiple lesions of the lip exhibiting the 'Jadassohn Phenomenon' review of the literature and report of a case. Br J Dermatol. 1977;96(3):307-12.
104. Usui K, Ochiai T, Abe I, Nishio H, Togo K, Yamagata M. Apocrine gland carcinoma of the mammary skin concomitant with Pagetoid phenomenon. J Dermatol. 2010;37(4):350-4.
105. Holman HR. The LE cell phenomenon. Ann Rev Med. 1960;11(1):231-42.
106. Rimek D, Fehse B, Göpel P. Evaluation of Mueller-Hinton-Agar as a simple medium for the germ tube production of Candida albicans and Candida dubliniensis. Mycoses. 2008;51(3):205-8.
107. Tchernev G, Orfanos CE. Antigen mimicry, epitope spreading and the pathogenesis of pemphigus. Tissue Antigens. 2006;68(4):280-6.
108. Jurado RL, Campbell J, Martin PD. Prozone phenomenon in secondary syphilis: Has its time arrived? Arch Int Med. 1993;153(21):2496-8.
109. Findlay GH, Van Dee Merwe LW. The Meirowsky phenomenon. colour changes in melanin according to temperature and redox potential. Br J Dermatol. 1966;78(11):572-6.

110. Singh S, Gupta A, Pandey SS, Singh G. Tachyphylaxis to histamine-induced wheal suppression by topical 0.05% clobetasol propionate in normal versus croton oil-induced dermatitic skin. Dermatology. 1996;193(2):121-3.
111. Cowan FF, Koppanyi T, Maengwyn-Davies GD. Tachyphylaxis III. Ephedrine. J Pharm Sci. 1963;52(9):878-83.
112. Ehrman R, Ternes J, O'Brien CP, Mclellan AT. Conditioned tolerance in human opiate addicts. Psychopharmacology. 1992;108(1):218-24.
113. Zuo Y, Lu H, Vaupel DB, Zhang Y, Chefer SI, Rea WR, et al. Acute nicotine-induced tachyphylaxis is differentially manifest in the limbic system. Neuropsychopharmacology. 2011;36(12):2498-512.
114. Del Cuvillo A, Mullol J, Bartra J, Davila I, Jáuregui I, Montoro J, et al. Comparative Pharmacology of the H1 antihistamines. J Investig Allergol Clin Immunol. 2006;16(1):3-12.
115. Kryst L, Wanyura H. Hoigné's syndrome—its course and symptomatology. J Maxillofac Surg. 1979;7(4):320-6.
116. Scott V, Maxwell RW, Skinner JS. The Jarisch-Herxheimer phenomenon in late syphilis: Probable fatal reactions to penicillin. J Am Med Assoc. 1949;139(4):217-20.
117. Heyman A, Sheldon WH, Evans LD. Pathogenesis of the Jarisch-Herxheimer reaction: A review of clinical and experimental observations. Br J Vener Dis. 1952;28(2):50.
118. Ito T. Mazzotti reaction with eosinophilia after undergoing oral ivermectin for scabies. J Dermatol. 2013;9(40):776-7.
119. Nikkels AF, Nikkels-Tassoudji N, Piérard GE. Oral antifungal-exacerbated inflammatory flare-up reactions of dermatomycosis. Am J Clin Dermatol. 2006;7(5):327-31.
120. Hryncewicz-Gwóźdź A, Wojciechowska-Zdrojowy M, Maj J, Baran W, Jagielski T. Paradoxical reaction during a course of terbinafine treatment of trichophyton interdigitale infection in a child. JAMA Dermatol. 2016;152(3):342-3.
121. Van Der Steen PM, Happle R. The «Castling» phenomenon in topical immunotherapy of alopecia areata. Eur J Dermatol. 1992;2(3):151-3.
122. Orecchia G. The castling phenomenon: a possible explanation. Eur J Dermatol. 1994;4(2):161.
123. Sharquie KE, Ahmed RK, Sharquie IK. Targetoid polycyclic concentric hair regrowth pattern is a sign of immunological recovery in alopecia areata. J Cosmet Dermatol Sci Appl. 2018;8(3):151.

Distinguished Appearance or Pattern and Named Signs in Dermoscopy

Jigna Padhiyar

INTRODUCTION

Dermoscopy is a noninvasive technique which is helpful in routine practice to diagnose and differentiate various entity in dermatology. It might also help us for deciding the site of biopsy.

Various terminologies have been described pertaining to various sites like trichoscopy, onychoscopy, capillaroscopy, dermatoscopy, etc.m while other terminologies like inflammoscopy, entomodermoscopy, etc., have been described for underlying etiology of various dermatoses. We have tried to enumerate all possible described signs, but as it is an evolving field of dermatology, few might have been missed.

SIGNS IN DERMOSCOPY[1,2]

- *Blink sign*: While using a dermoscope which have both the mode polarized as well as nonpolarized; switching from one mode to other during examination demonstrates this blink sign. Structures such as comedo-like opening and milia-like cysts in seborrheic keratosis which are visible in nonpolarized mode appear to blink when we switch over to polarized mode.
- *Blue pseudo-veil sign*: Whitish blue halo surrounding a macrocomedone is known as blue pseudo-veil sign **(Fig. 1)**.
- *Bonbon toffee sign*: This sign refers to central depression surrounded by whitish-yellow globules in sebaceous hyperplasia.
- *Cumulus sign*: In sebaceous hyperplasia whitish-yellow globules seem to be aggregated which is described as cumulus sign **(Fig. 2)**.
- *Handlebar sign*: This refers to a curved hair attached to both ends in pseudofolliculitis barbae.
- *Iceberg sign*: Arctic blue keratotic plug seen in cases of actinic keratosis neglecta is described as iceberg sign.
- *Jelly sign*: Pigmentary pseudonetwork sparing follicular ostia in melasma which is having various shades of brown have concave borders resembling borders of jelly.
- *Lightening sign*: Parallel ridged pigmentation and cracks of blood on acral part giving appearance of lightening is seen in post-traumatic hemorrhage.
- *Pore sign*: It refers to keratin filled opening in epidermal cyst.
- *Ring scale sign*: Circular ring-shaped scales are seen in polymorphic light eruption.
- *Rosette sign*: Though described in actinic keratosis, it can be seen in many other dermatoses and is not specific for it. It refers to four white points like four leaf clover inside folliclular ostia.

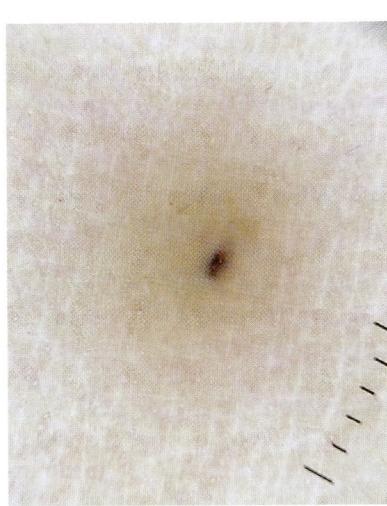

FIG. 1: Whitish blue halo surrounding macrocomedone.

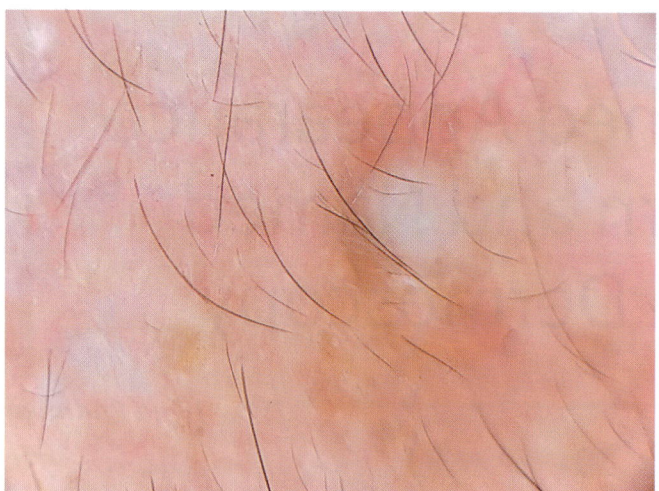

FIG. 2: Cumulus sign of sebaceous hyperplasia where yellowish sebaceous lobules seem aggregated.

- *Setting sun sign*: Orange yellow background with erythematous border and linear vessels resembling, setting sun sign can be seen in juvenile xanthogranuloma, sebaceous hyperplasia, spitz nevus, mycetoma, and histiocytic sarcoma.
- *St. Tropez sign*: Topical tanning products giving appearance of bizarre pigmentation on dermoscopy is known as St. Tropez sign.
- *Translucency sign*: Because of translucent nature of membrane in membranous aplasia cutis on dermoscopy reddish background with vessels and hair bulb are seen which is described as translucency sign.

SIGNS IN INFLAMMOSCOPY[1,3-5]

- *Collarette sign*: Peripheral whitish scaling with irregularly spaced and distributed red dots is characteristically observed in pityriasis rosea.
- *Dermoscopic Auspitz sign*: In cases of marked hyperkeratosis in patients of psoriasis, after removing scales it is easy to see regularly spaced red globules representing capillaries is known as dermoscopic auspitz sign **(Fig. 3)**.
- *Diamond necklace sign/white track or lines of volcanic crater*: This refers to peripheral double-edged white border in case of porokeratosis representing the coronoid lamella.
- *Inverse strawberry pattern*: Follicular red dots with surrounding white hallo are seen in early stages of discoid lupus erythematosus.
- *Peppering pattern*: This is described in lichen planopilaris and ashy dermatosis where larger and brownish pigmented dots in "hem" like pattern are found in former while smaller and gray-bluish dots are found in later.
- *Pseudo-Wickham striae*: This can be seen in lupus erythematosus, prurigo nodularis, and nodular scabies.

- *Rail-like appearance*: Asteatotic eczema occasionally shows double-edged scales which is described as rail-like appearance.
- *Red globular ring pattern*: This vascular arrangement is sometimes observed in psoriasis.
- *Strawberry pattern*: This refers to white follicular keratotic plugs over a background of erythema seen in discoid lupus erythematosus.
- *Sulci and gyri pattern*: Brownish flat globules separated by whitish striae resembling sulci and gyri are seen in Gougerot–Carteaud syndrome.
- *Trizonal concentric pattern*: From center to periphery three color zones are seen: (1) brownish/greenish, (2) whitish, and (3) erythematous—in acquired reactive perforating collagenosis.
- *Wagyu beef appearance*: In ashy dermatosis, papillomatosis along with pigment incontinence gives this appearance on dermoscopy **(Fig. 4)**.

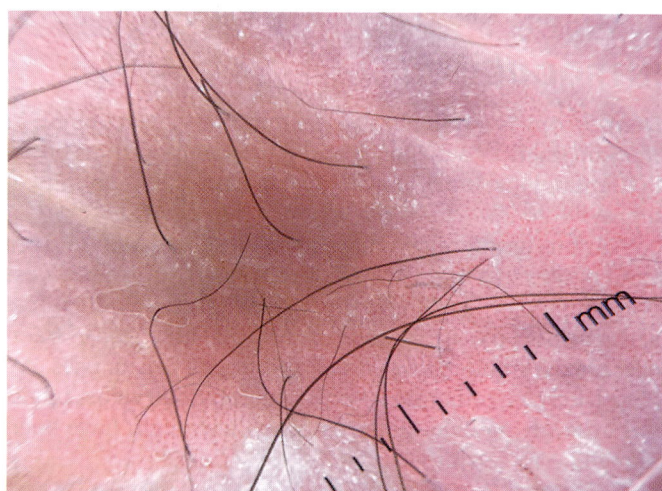

FIG. 3: Regularly spaced red dots representing capillaries seen in a plaque of psoriasis after removing scales.

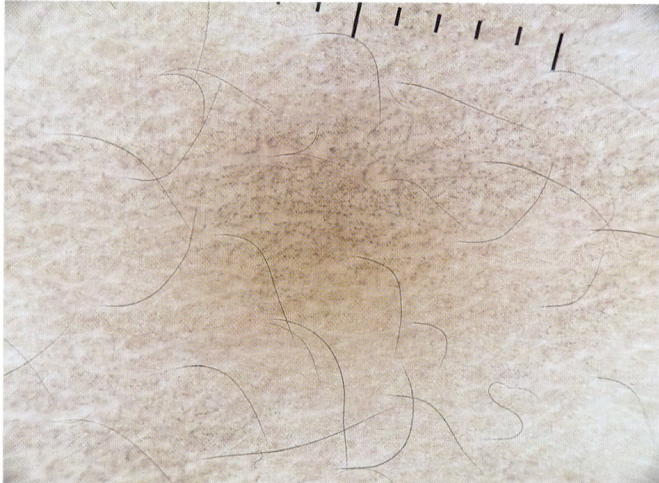

FIG. 4: Wagyu beef appearance in ashy dermatosis.

- *White starburst pattern*: It refers to radially arranged white striae over a reddish or brownish background seen in prurigo nodularis.
- *Yellow clod sign*: In nummular eczema, serum exudates are seen as yellow clods in dermoscopy which are absent in psoriasis and dermatophytosis.

SIGNS IN TRICHOSCOPY[1,6]

- *Broom fiber appearance*: Multiple hair shaft emerging from single follicular opening breaking at same distance described as broom fiber appearance are seen in lichen simplex chronicus of scalp.
- *Burnt matchstick sign*: In trichotillomania, darkening bulbous proximal part of hair shaft is known as burnt matchstick sign.
- *Color transition sign*: This sign is seen in alopecia areata incognito where proximal end of hair shaft is lighter or clear compared to distal part which might help us to differentiate it from telogen effluvium.
- *Eastern pan cake sign*: Dilated follicular opening along with comedo-like openings in alopecic and aseptic nodules of scalp is known as eastern pan cake sign.
- *Flambeau sign*: Multiple white linear tracts in continuation with hair posterior to the fringe in traction alopecia give appearance like flame.
- *Fried egg sign*: This sign refers to multiple yellow dots with whitish halo corresponding to detached epidermis from follicular ostia in cases of pemphigus.
- *Golf club set sign*: Hair bulbs are radially arranged at the periphery of a lesion in a case of bullous aplasia cutis congenita.
- *Mace sign*: Bulbous distal end of broken hair shaft resembling a mace is seen in trichotillomania which is helpful to differentiate it from alopecia areata.
- *Peripilar sign*: Perifollicular lymphocytic infiltrate giving peripilar brownish hallo in dermoscopy of androgenic alopecia is described as peripilar sign.
- *Pigtail hair*: Presence of this helps us to differentiate alopecia areata incognito from diffuse alopecia areata apart from other dermoscopic features related to alopecia areata which is usually seen in both.
- *Pluck out sign*: This sign describes the characteristic hemorrhagic halo surrounding hair shafts in trichotillomania.
- *Regularly bended ribbon sign*: In monilethrix regular constrictions resembles bended ribbon.
- *Starry night sky sign*: Ultraviolet (UV) light enhanced trichoscopy in frontal fibrosing alopecia demonstrates fluorescent follicular ostia due to propionibacterium resembles starry night sky.
- *V sign*: This sign is characteristically seen in trichotillomania where two hairs emerging from same ostia are broken at same length by pulling force.

SIGNS IN ONYCHOSCOPY[7-10]

- *Aurora Borealis pattern*: Parallel bands of varying color are seen in onychomycosis which resembles northern lights.
- *Lamellar microsplitting*: it is a new finding described in onychomycosis.
- *Pseudo-Hutchinson's sign*: Because of translucent cuticle, nail plate pigmentation is visible in dermoscopy of melanonychia or benign nevi.
- *Ruin appearance*: It refers to subungual keratosis with longitudinal spikes in distal subungual onychomycosis.
- *Scaly cuticles*: This has been seen in association with alopecia areata along with longitudinal ridging and pitting.

SIGNS IN SKIN NEVI AND TUMORS[1,7,11]

- *Adherent fabric fiber sign*: Because of microulceration adherent fabric fibers may be seen in case of benign lesions turning malignant.
- *Beauty and beast sign*: This refers to overall symmetry and benign look of melanocytic nevi versus asymmetrical and worrisome look of melanoma on dermoscopy.
- *Bolognia sign*: In acquired melanocytic nevi, small dark dots are eccentrically situated on one side of the nevi.
- *Double-edge sign*: In cases of Bowen's disease, peripherally parallel two lines of pigmentation are described as double-edge sign.
- *Hypopyon sign*: This refers to purple-red color seen at the bottom of yellow and red clods in angiosarcoma. It is also seen in lymphangioma circumscriptum.
- *Isobar sign/circle within circle sign*: Concentric pigmented circles surrounding a follicular opening in lentigo maligna is known as isobar sign.
- *Little red riding hood sign*: When a melanocytic nevus looks benign from a distance but show few changes of malignancy on dermoscopy is referred as little red riding hood sign.
- *Micro-Hutchinson's sign*: This sign refers to micro-extension of pigment in cuticle or submatrix which is not seen on naked eye in case of subungual melanoma.
- *Mistletoe sign*: Pseudopods seen in melanoma in situ and inflammatory melanocytic nevi are known as mistletoe sign.
- *Mushroom cloud sign*: In melanoma, hyperpigmented area extends in one direction beyond the border of lesion is described as mushroom cloud sign.
- *Pink glow sign*: It describes characteristic of pink glow as seen on UV light dermoscopy of glomus tumor.
- *Pink rim sign*: Pink colored rim surrounding a melanocytic lesion is suggestive of malignancy.
- *Poppy field bleeding sign*: It refers to appearance of droplets of blood while pressing of dermoscope on melanoma lesion.

- *Rainbow sign*: This is used to describe whitish structureless area, whitish crystalline area, and multicolored structureless area in dermoscopy of basal cell carcinoma.
- *Red planet sign*: Red to maroon exophytic lesions with delicate vascular network resembling blood moon is seen in angiomyxoma.
- *Sagrada Familia sign, digitations, and mirror sign*: Multiple, regularly spaced and arranged, hyperbolic cavities in the ventral aspect of the nail is termed as "Sagrada Familia sign," while finger like area and symmetry of onychomatricoma is termed as "digitation and mirror sign".
- *Spermatozoon-like structures*: Red dots with linear vessels resembling spermatozoa are observed in mycosis fungoides.
- *String of pearls sign*: In clear cell acanthoma, coiled and dotted vessels are arranged in a serpiginous pattern is known as string of pearls sign. It has also been observed in lichen planus like keratosis and seborrheic keratosis.
- *Triangular sign*: Progressive proximal enlargement of pigmentary band giving triangular appearance has been described in both nail matrix melanocytic nevi and melanoma.
- *White ring around ulceration*: This finding has been described in aneurismal dermatofibroma and it might be a helpful feature to differentiate it from melanoma.
- *Wobble sign*: Papillomatous part of melanocytic nevi moving with tangential movement of dermoscope is known as wobble sign.

SIGNS IN ENTOMODERMOSCOPY[1]

- *Anal groove sign*: In ixodes tick, crescentic depression is noted anterior to anus which helps in differentiating it from other tick where it is located posteriorly.
- *Delta wing jet with contrail sign/delta glider/triangle sign/jet plane/spermatozoid appearance*: It refers to triangular fore part of Sarcoptes scabiei seen on dermoscopy. This triangular appearance along with presence of burrow is known as "jet with contrail' appearance.
- *Radial crown sign*: Zone of columnar hemorrhagic parakeratosis situated between central black pore and peripheral pigmented rim corresponding to anus and posterior abdomen of Tunga penetrans.
- *Yellow tears and white star burst pattern*: These two are most characteristic features of leishmaniasis referring to white/yellow keratotic plug and peripheral white projections.

REFERENCES

1. Bothra A, Das S, Maheswari A, Singh M, Bhargava S. Evolving eponymous signs in diagnostic dermoscopy. IP Indian J Clin Exp Dermatol. 2021;7(2):98-106.
2. Kaliyadan F, Kuruvilla J, Al Ojail HY, Quadri SA. Clinical and dermoscopic study of pseudofolliculitis of the beard area. Int J Trichol. 2016;8:40-2.
3. Bhat YJ, Jha AK. Dermatoscopy of inflammatory diseases in skin of color. Indian Dermatol Online J. 2021;12:45-57.
4. Errichetti E. Dermoscopy of Inflammatory Dermatoses (Inflammoscopy): An Up-to-date Overview. Dermatol Pract Concept. 2019;9(3):169-80.
5. Lallas A, Argenziano G, Apalla Z, Gourhant JY, Zaballos P, Di Lernia V, et al. Dermoscopic patterns of common facial inflammatory skin diseases. J Eur Acad Dermatol Venereol. 2014;28(5):609-14.
6. Alessandrini A, Starace M, Bruni F, Brandi N, Baraldi C, Misciali C, et al. Alopecia Areata Incognita and Diffuse Alopecia Areata: Clinical, Trichoscopic, Histopathological, and Therapeutic Features of a 5-Year Study. Dermatol Pract Concept. 2019;9(4):272-7.
7. Grover C, Jakhar D. Onychoscopy: A practical guide. Indian J Dermatol Venereol Leprol. 2017;83:536-49.
8. Nirmal B, Krishnaram AS, Sudhagar R. Rainbow sign in dermatoscopy of nodular basal cell carcinoma. Indian J Dermatopathol Diagn Dermatol. 2019;6:107-8.
9. Kayarkatte MN, Singal A, Pandhi D, Das S, Sharma S. Nail dermoscopy (onychoscopy) findings in the diagnosis of primary onychomycosis: A cross-sectional study. Indian J Dermatol Venereol Leprol. 2020;86:341-9.
10. Darwish HM, Galal SA, Tawfik YM. Dermoscopic evaluation of nail changes in alopecia areata. Sci J Al-Azhar Med Fac Girls. 2021;5:690-8.
11. Kelati A, Aqil N, Baybay H, Gallouj S, Mernissi FZ. Beyond classic dermoscopic patterns of dermatofibromas: a prospective research study. J Med Case Rep. 2017;11:266.

32
Named Appearance, Cell, or Sign in Dermatopathology

Jigna Padhiyar, Krina Bharat Patel

INTRODUCTION

Dermatopathology is of vital importance in day-to-day practice in diagnosing a patient. First, we will go through the general signs. We have tried to list most of named signs and appearance. But list may be incomplete as new terminologies are continued to describe as well as even after extensive search few might have come to author's attention.

- *Signs of sun-damaged skin on histopathology*: Laminated stratum corneum, proteinous material in stratum corneum, cell heterogenicity in stratum spinosum, fibrorhexis, and fibrolysis in dermis along with elastotic changes.[1] Dermal atrophy can also occur on long term.
- *Signs of degeneration on histopathology*:
  - *Colloid degeneration*: Hyaline-like degeneration of the collagen bundles of the dermis[2] commonly seen as colloid milium.
  - *Hyalinization of collagen*: Degeneration of collagen in papillary dermis which appears smooth pink seen in lichen sclerosus et atrophicus.
  - *Reticular degeneration/ballooning degeneration* **(Fig. 1)**: Swelling and rupture of keratinocytes followed by death of cell which is commonly seen in viral and eczematous disorders.
  - *Filamentous degeneration*: Theory of generation of civatte bodies.[3]
  - *Fibrinoid degeneration*: Degenerated connective tissue or blood vessels which resembles fibrin on staining.
- *Signs of apoptosis*: Civatte bodies, satellite cell necrosis, hyaline bodies, and pyknotic nucleus.
- *Signs of dysplasia or malignancy on histopathology*: Loss of polarity, nuclear polymorphism, increased mitotic figures, and altered nuclear cytoplasmic ratio.

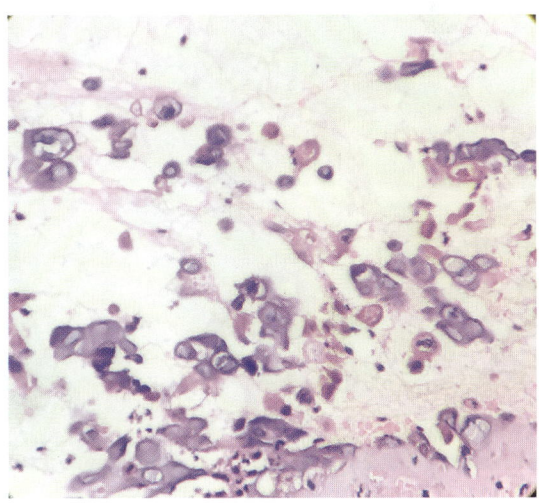

FIG. 1: Ballooning degeneration and giant cell formation in a case of herpes zoster.

- *Signs of vasculitis*: Erythrocyte extravasation, endothelial cell swelling, vessel wall damage, angiocentric infiltrate, leukocytoclasis, and fibrin deposition.[4]

APPEARANCES IN DERMATOPATHOLOGY

- *Antler-like/staghorn appearance*:[5] In Dowling–Degos disease, epidermis shows finger-like irregular elongation of rete ridges with melanin concentration at the tip which resembles deciduous horn (antler) of deer **(Fig. 2)**. Same changes can be seen in Haber's syndrome, Galli-Galli disease, and pigmented actinic keratosis.

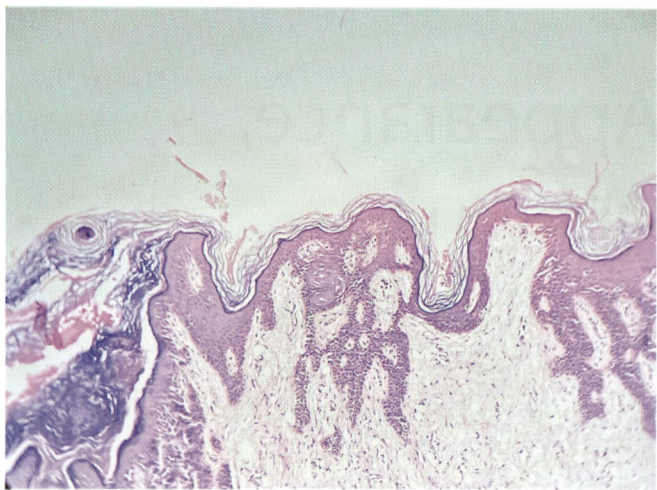

FIG. 2: Antler like proliferation extending from rete ridges with pronounced melanin deposit.

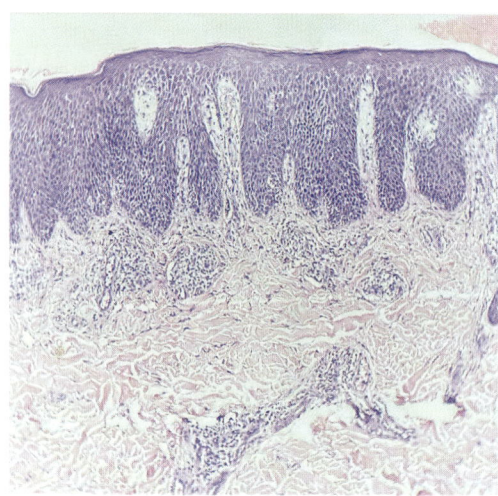

FIG. 4: Camel foot appearance of rete ridges in psoriasis.

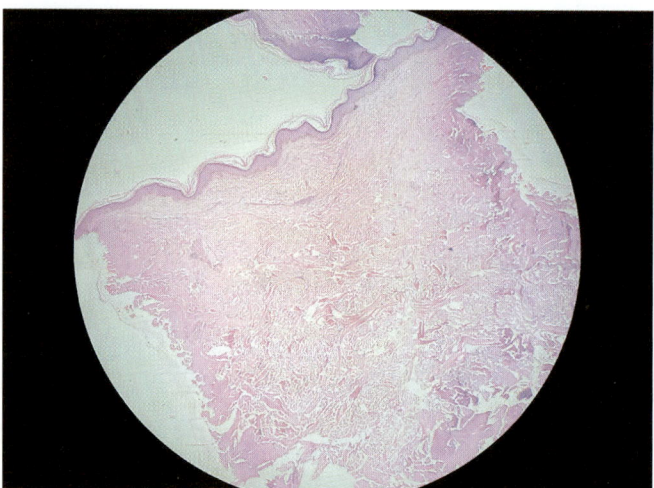

FIG. 3: Scanning view of biopsy specimen in a case of morphea giving square appearance with parallel lateral borders.

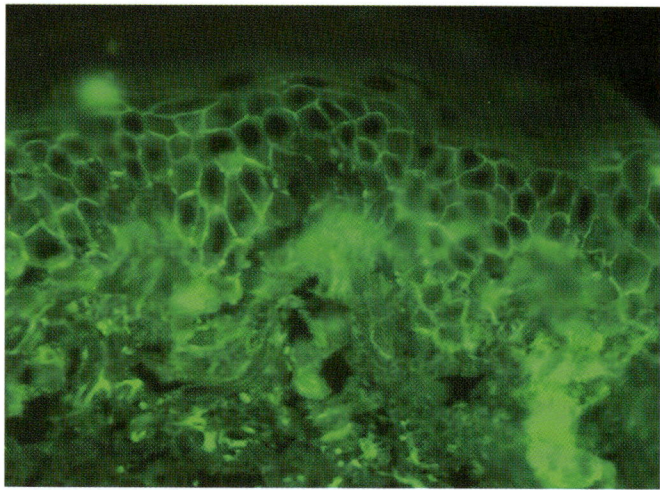

FIG. 5: Fishnet appearance of intercellular deposits consisting of immunoglobulin G (IgG) and C3 in a case of pemphigus.

- *Box-shaped/squared off appearance*: Sclerosis of collagen involving dermis and subcutis gives appearance of square appearance to dermis is classically seen in localized scleroderma **(Fig. 3)** but may be observed in morphea-lichen sclerosus overlap and scleredema as well.
- *Camel foot appearance* **(Fig. 4)**: This has been used to describe bulbous appearance of rete ridges in histopathology of psoriasis along with regular acanthosis.
- *Cannon ball appearance*: Clusters of angiomatous tufts and lobules scattered in the dermis in a "cannon ball" pattern is classically seen in acquired tufted angioma. However, similar tufts of thick-walled capillaries are frequently seen in pseudo-Kaposi's sarcoma (acroangiodermatitis of Mali).
- *Chicken wire/fish net pattern* **(Fig. 5)**: Intercellular deposition of immunoglobulin G (IgG) and C3 between epidermal cells give this type of appearance in immunofluorescence.
- *Church spire appearance* **(Fig. 6)**: Hyperkeratosis, hypergranulosis, and acanthosis together with papillomatosis leading to numerous digitate upward extensions of epidermis-lined papillae, giving the appearance of "church spires." It is classically seen in acrokeratosis of Hopf. Similar changes can also be seen in epidermal nevus, seborrheic keratosis, tar keratosis, and acanthosis nigricans.
- *Claw clutching ball appearance*: Well-circumscribed lymphoid infiltrate that are clutched by surrounding hyperplastic rete ridges, giving the overall "claw clutching ball" appearance is characteristic histopathology finding in lichen nitidus.

- *Coat sleeve appearance*: Inflammatory lymphohistiocytic infiltrate tightly surrounding superficial vessels in coat sleeve appearance is described in erythema annulare centrifugum and syphilis.[6]
- *Dilapidated brick wall appearance* **(Fig. 7)**: Prominent suprabasal clefting and extensive loss of intercellular bridges (acantholysis) with partial coherence of cells between keratinocytes, giving the whole epidermis a "dilapidated brick wall" appearance. It is classically seen in Hailey–Hailey disease.
- *Festooned papillae appearance*: Subepidermal bulla with minimal inflammatory infiltrate and dermal papillae protruding upward into the blister cavity giving "festooned papillae" appearance is seen in porphyria cutanea tarda.
- *Flame-thrower-like appearance*: The presence of bright red trichilemmal keratin bordering the club hair results in a "flame-thrower like" appearance of telogen hair in vertical hematoxylin and eosin sections.
- *Fried egg appearance*: A mast cell on H&E stain appears like fried egg because of centrally located nucleus and partial staining of cytoplasm. This appearance has been noted in few other nondermatological disorders also.[7]
- *Hobnail (matchstick) appearance*: In Retiform hemangioendothelioma elongated, arborizing blood vessels lined by monomorphic bland endothelial cells with prominent apical nuclei and scanty cytoplasm which resemble "matchstick" or hobnail.[8]
- *Hourglass appearance*: Histopathological finding with perifollicular fibrosis and epithelial atrophy at the level isthmus and infundibulum giving hourglass appearance.
- *Jigsaw puzzle appearance*: Cylindroma is composed of irregularly shaped islands of basaloid cells arranged in a mosaic-like mass molding together in a "jigsaw puzzle" pattern.
- *Mariner's Pilot Wheel appearance*: Paracoccidioidomycosis (also known as Brazilian blastomycosis, South American blastomycosis, Lutz-Splendore-de Almeida disease) is caused by the thermally dimorphic fungus *Paracoccidioides brasiliensis*. The tissue phase of the fungus is seen as multiple buds surrounding the whole surface of the mother yeast cell. This configuration is described as a "Mariner's pilot wheel" or "Mickey Mouse" appearance.
- *Owl's eye appearance* **(Fig. 8)**: Histopathology of verruca plana shows hyperkeratosis, acanthosis, diffuse vacuolization of cells in the upper spinous, and granular layer. The nuclei of the vacuolated cells lie at the centers of the cells giving owl's eye appearance.
- *Picket fence appearance*: Direct immunoflourescence (DIF) of noninvolved perilesional skin in dermatitis herpetiformis shows deposit of immunoglobulin A (IgA) alone or in combination with C3, which are arranged in a granular pattern at the dermoepidermal junction over tips of dermal papillae. These granular deposits may be vertically elongated, giving a "picket-fence" appearance.

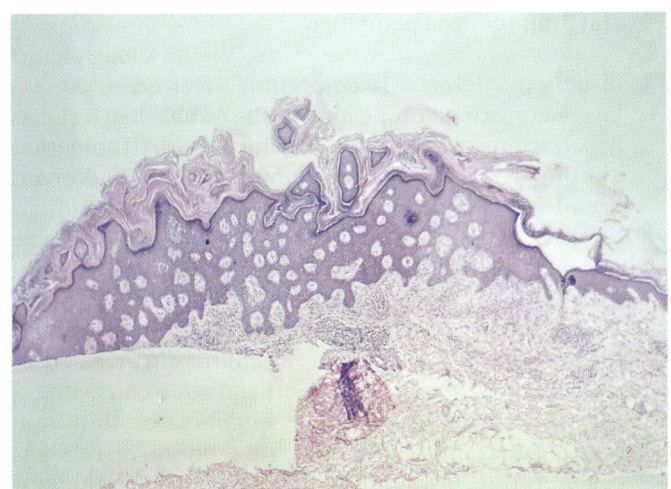

FIG. 6: Church spire appearance in a case of seborrheic keratosis.

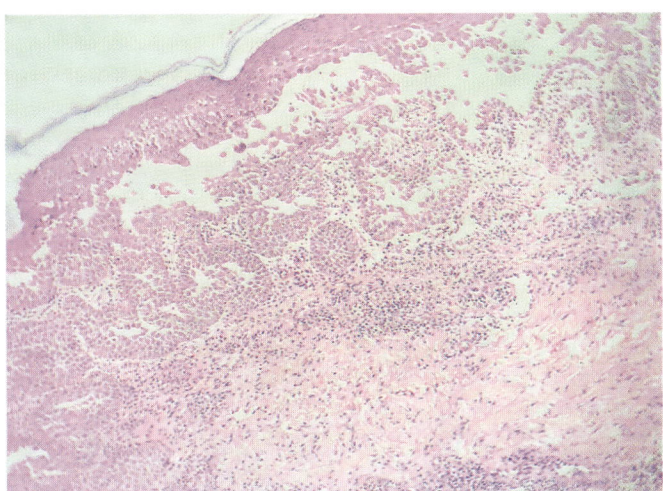

FIG. 7: Dilapidated appearance in a case of Hailey–Hailey disease.

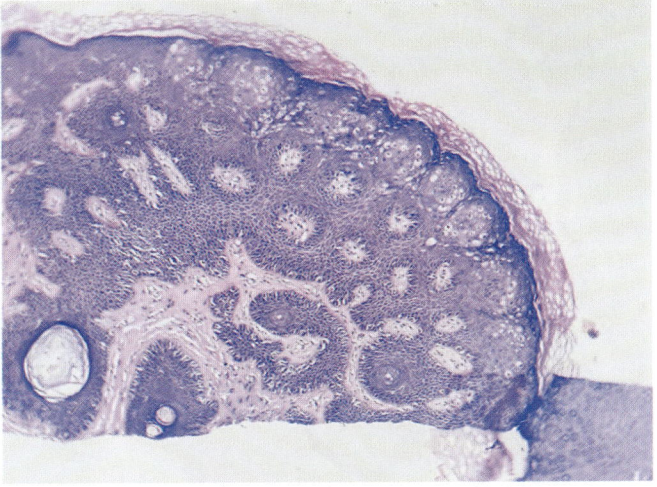

FIG. 8: Owl eye appearance in histopathology of verruca plana.

- *Ravelled wool appearance*: Biopsy from a lesion in pseudoxanthoma elasticum (PXE) will show small, fragmented, wavy and clumped eosinophilic elastic fibers, giving a "ravelled wool/tangled threads" appearance.
- *Septate tomato appearance* **(Fig. 9)**: In molluscum contagiosum, scanner view of hematoxylin and eosin-stained sections shows an epidermal invagination with several closely spaced lobules of epidermal proliferation leading to a septate tomato appearance. The septum of this appearance is formed by normal dermis and not by epidermal proliferation.
- *Sieve-like appearance*: Kaposi sarcoma (KS) is a low-grade malignant tumor of vascular origin associated with human herpes simplex virus 8 (HHV-8) infections. Biopsy from the plaque stage of KS shows spindle cells arranged in fascicles with slit-like dense and irregular vascular spaces, creating a sieve-like appearance.
- *Shotgun appearance*: Pagetoid pattern as well as epithelioid atypical melanocytes with hyperchromic nucleus and pale cytoplasm with dusty melanin, in superficial spreading melanoma, imparts a shotgun appearance.[9]
- *Spaghetti and meatball appearance (banana and grape appearance)*: Hematoxylin and eosin-stained biopsy from the lesions of pityriasis versicolor shows slender septate hyphae and spores resembling the spaghetti and meatball appearance.
- *Storiform appearance*: This is classically described in dermatofibrosarcoma protuberans (DFSP), but is also seen in the frequently seen dermatofibroma. DFSP is a rare, locally aggressive dermal tumor composed of interwoven bundles of spindle cells with plump nuclei arranged in a "storiform" or pinwheel pattern.
- *Swarm of bees' appearance*: Histopathology in active alopecia areata shows peribulbar infiltrates composed of predominantly lymphocytes around anagen hair follicles. This pattern of infiltrate is referred to as "swarm of bees" appearance.
- *Tadpole/comma-shaped appearance*: Classically seen at scanning magnification in histology of syringoma. This benign tumor of eccrine lineage comprises numerous ducts lined by two rows of epithelial cells embedded in a fibrous stroma. The epithelial component is arranged in nests, cords, or tubules of relatively uniform size. Depending upon the plane of section, some nests of syringoma can assume a morphology that closely resembles a comma or tadpole.
- *Telephone handle appearance*: The deep red nucleus of an eosinophil is composed of two lobes connected by a band of nuclear material which resembles the old-fashioned "telephone receiver".
- *Tomb stone appearance* **(Fig. 10)**: Suprabasal blistering with basal keratinocytes still adhered to basement membrane zone gives appearance of tomb-stones. This characteristic finding is described in pemphigus vulgaris and drug-induced pemphigus.
- *Tri-layered or striped appearance*: The histology picture of lichen sclerosus is commonly referred to as "tri-layered or striped" appearance. The established lesion of lichen sclerosus shows three distinct zones: (i) epidermal atrophy with surface hyperkeratosis, (ii) an underlying broad zone of subepidermal edema in the papillary dermis, and (iii) homogenization and ground glass appearance of collagen, which becomes more sclerotic over time.

A similar trilayered appearance can be seen in the histology of soft chancre (chancroid) caused by *Haemophilus ducreyi*: (i) superficial zone consisting of necrotic tissues and an acute inflammatory infiltrate, (ii) the mid-zone containing new blood vessels and regenerating granulation tissue on one hand and

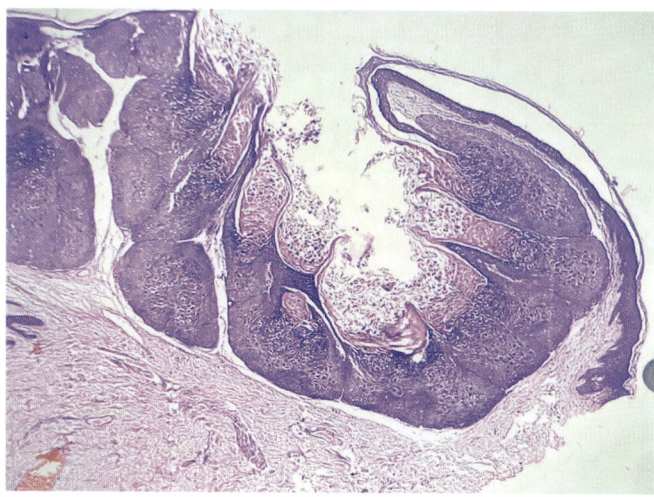

FIG. 9: Septate tomato appearance in scanning view of a biopsy from mollucum.

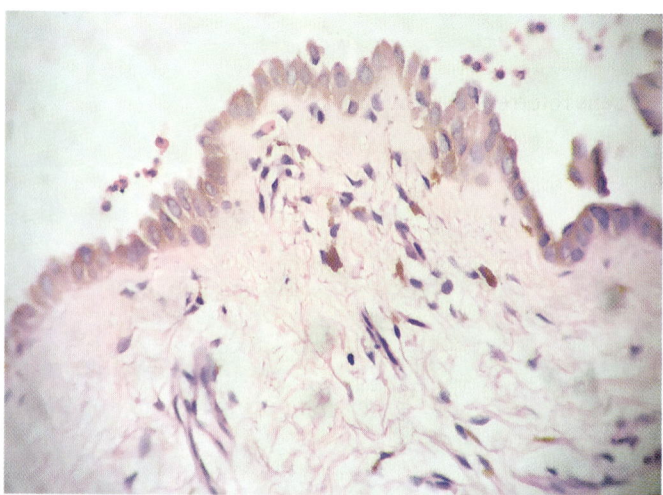

FIG. 10: Classical tombstone appearance of pemphigus vulgaris.

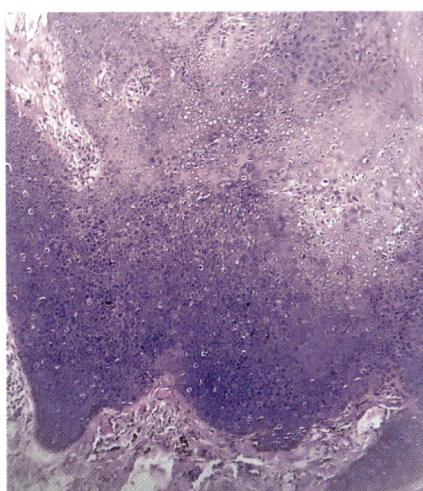

FIG. 11: Windblown appearance in a case of Bowenoid papulosis.

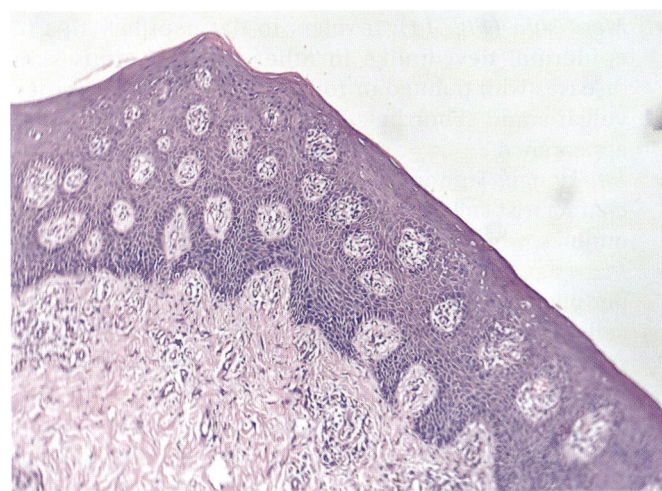

FIG. 12: Handholding sign in a specimen of psoriasis which was tangentially cut.

degenerative changes on the other, and (iii) the deeper zone shows a chronic inflammatory infiltrate of plasma cells and lymphocytes.

- *Windblown appearance* **(Fig. 11)**: A descriptive term for the enlarged, crowded, haphazardly arranged neoplastic cells that show loss of polarity, enlarged and hyperchromatic nuclei and atypical mitoses in the epithelium of Bowen's disease and Bowenoid papulosis of the genitalia. This overall appearance in the epithelium of Bowen's disease is referred to as "windblown appearance".

NAMED SIGNS IN DERMATOPATHOLOGY

- *Bare underbelly sign*: Lymphocytic infiltrates are concentrated more around the superficial vascular plexus in mycosis fungoides while there is very scant infiltrate in underlying dermis. It is an inconsistent sign suggesting epidermotropism.[10]
- *Brass knuckles sign*: Histopathologic examination of lobomycosis shows chains of thickly walled, yeast-like cells referred to as the brass knuckles sign.
- *Checkerboard sign*: Histopathology of pityriasis rubra pilaris (PRP) shows alternations of orthokeratosis and parakeratosis in a vertical and horizontal direction resembling the checkerboard and, therefore, referred to as the checkerboard sign.
- *Cookie-cutter sign* **(Fig. 3)**: Punch biopsy specimens of the fully developed lesions of morphea have distinct straight lateral edges called cookie-cutter signs.[11]
- *Cornflake sign*: A ruptured epidermoid cyst that invokes foreign body reaction with neutrophils, macrophages, and multinucleated giant cells, sometimes with the inclusion of scales, is known as the cornflake sign.
- *Eyeliner sign*: Bowen's disease, also referred to as an in situ squamous cell carcinoma, is characterized by full-thickness epidermal atypia but basal keratinocytes are spared. This normal appearing basal cell layer over the layers of full-thickness atypia resembles eye liner. But it can be relatively absent also in orthokeratotic Bowen's disease.[12]
- *Flag sign (also known as the pink-and-blue sign)*: This type of sign appears in actinic keratosis as alternating orthokeratosis above the spared ostia of acrosyringium and acrotrichium and parakeratosis above the interadnexal epidermis.[13]
- *Floating sign*: Histiocytes wrapping the individual collagen fibers in middle and deep layers of the dermis, giving floating appearance is observed in morphea[14] and interstitial granulomatous scarring alopecia.[15]
- *Goggle sign*: Central centrifugal cicatricial alopecia demonstrates perifollicular fibrosis of compound follicles on histology, resembling the frame of glasses, and fused outer root sheaths, resembling the lenses of goggles.
- *Hairy palm sign*: This sign refers to palmar surface like presence of thick compact stratum corneum in histopathology of prurigo nodularis along with presence of pilosebaceous unit which is generally absent on palmar surface.
- *Hand-holding sign* **(Fig. 12)**: Tangential cut in a biopsy from psoriatic plaque gives appearance of interdigitating epidermis resembling hand-holding.
- *Line sign*: In morphea, the demarcation between the dermis and the subcutaneous layer becomes sharp and horizontally straight due to the loss of the rounded contour of subcutaneous fat lobules because of sclerosis.[11]
- *Lowenbach's sign*: Attenuation of the granular cell layer in pityriasis rosea is known as Lowenbach's sign.
- *Marquee sign* **(Fig. 13)**: In leishmaniasis, amastigotes are seen at the periphery of macrophagic cytoplasm. The marquee sign was named for its resemblance to the light bulbs arranged around a dressing room mirror.

- *Mesa sign* **(Fig. 14)**: It refers to flat papillary tips in epidermal nevi unlike in other papillomatous skin diseases with pointed or rounded tips, such as verruca vulgaris and seborrheic keratosis giving church spire appearance.
- *Murky sign*: Tumor cells in Merkel cell carcinoma have characteristically sparse cytoplasm and blurred cellular outlines, which are referred to as the murky sign.
- *Pizza sign*: A trichoblastoma consists of two zones: (1) the peripheral zone with dark palisading basophilic basaloid cells and (2) the central zone with pale eosinophilic squamous cells. This arrangement is described as pizza sign.
- *Promontory sign*: Proliferation of irregular jagged vascular channels which surrounds the preexisting small vessel gives appearance of that small vessel protruding into an abnormal vascular space which has been termed "promontory sign." It has been described in KS as well as patch and plaque stage of angiosarcoma.[16]
- *Purple fiber sign*: Elastotic fibers in acquired melanocytic nevi, often have a purple tincture. This finding is not present in case of melanoma.
- *Recovery sign (also known as the last week's sign)*: A normal lamellar stratum corneum is seen underlying parakeratosis or orthokeratosis with mild dermal inflammation indicating prior inflammation in a case of recovering from scabies.
- *Sabouraud's sign*: Erythrocyte extravasation in papillary dermis and occasionally in epidermis in histopathology of pityriasis rosea is known as Sabouraud's sign.
- *Salute sign (teapot spout sign/the teapot lid sign/the teapot sign)*: Pityriasis rosea involves an angulated parakeratosis attached at one end and free on the other, which very much resembles a salute. Similar findings can also be sometimes observed in histopathology of psoriasis, subacute eczema, and pityriasis lichenoides chronica (PLC).
- *Sampaio sign*: This is a manifestation of pseudopelade of Brocq where a gelatinous mass observed close to the bulbar portion in histopathology sections.
- *Sandwich sign*: In dermatophytosis, fungi are seen in the stratum corneum, sandwiched between the upper zone of the normal basketweave layer and the lower zone of parakeratosis and orthokeratosis **(Fig. 15)**, sharing features of psoriasis such as psoriasiform epidermal hyperplasia and neutrophilic collections.

  This sign is also seen necrobiosis lipoidica where infiltrate and necrobiosis forms alternate layers like sandwich.[17]
- *Screeching halt sign/vertical line sign*: Incompletely excised acquired melanocytic nevi (pseudo-melanoma) reveal a melanocytic proliferation over the scarring.

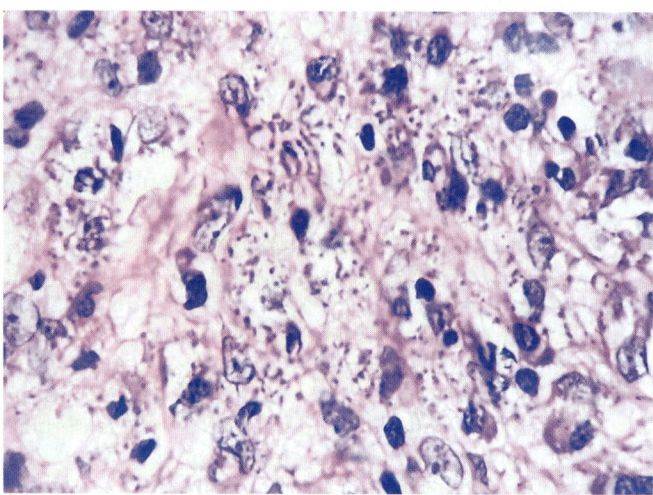

FIG. 13: Amastigotes of leishmaniasis are seen at the periphery of macrophagic cytoplasm.

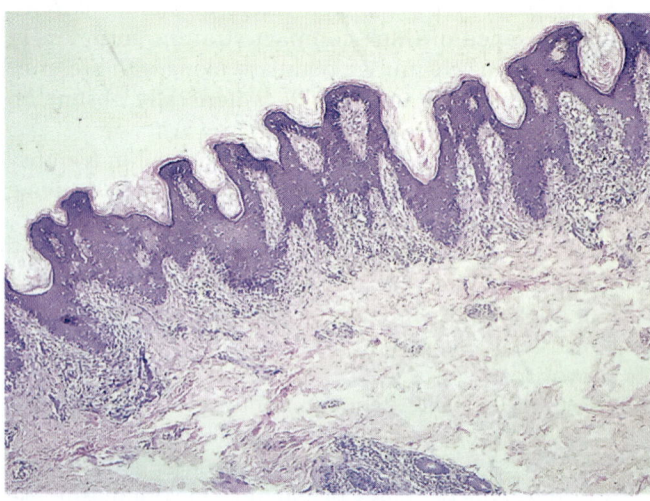

FIG. 14: Mesa sign in epidermal nevus.

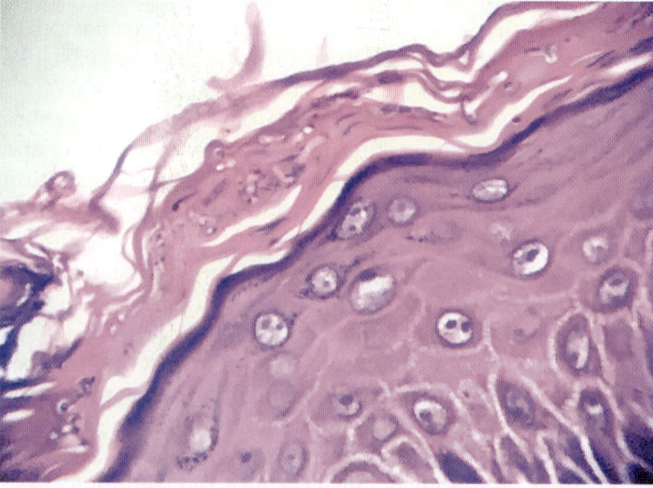

FIG. 15: Dermatophytes sandwiched between lower parakeratotic and upper orthokeratotic layers.

These regrowing melanocytic nests do not spread beyond scarring. It seems like scarring is halting the proliferation beyond a line where melanocytes and the scarring meet.
- *Toy soldier sign*: Malignant T lymphocytes in mycosis fungoides line up like soldiers along the dermoepidermal junction, hence known as toy soldier sign.
- *Tram track sign*: Plump CD34+ spindle or epithelioid cells are arranged parallel to elastic fibers and collagen bundles to produce a parallel pattern like tram track in nephrogenic fibrosing dermopathy/nephrogenic systemic fibrosis.
- *Tricolor sign*: This sign occurs in orf and milkers' nodules and owes its name to the three different colored layers on histology: (1) the red cornified layer, (2) the white necrotic epidermis, and (3) the blue basophilic dermal infiltrate.
- *Umbrella sign*: The pattern of solar elastosis carries some diagnostic importance between benign melanocytic nevi and melanoma. In melanocytic nevi, elastic fibers are present in between melanocytes to receive protection from solar damage and are, for this reason, referred to as the umbrella sign. This pattern is absent in melanoma, wherein elastotic fibers are pushed downward in the dermis by the expansion of malignant melanocytes.
- *Unna's sign*: The eczematoid pattern in pityriasis rosea was first described by Unna in 1894 and is known after his name.

NAMED CELLS IN DERMATOPATHOLOGY

- *Bean-bag cells* **(Fig. 16)**: Cytophagic histiocytic (phagocytic macrophages) packed with white blood cells, red cells, nuclear fragments, and platelets thus giving a characteristic "bean-bag" appearance are seen in cytophagic panniculitis. They can also be seen in hemophagocytic lymphohistiocytosis.[18]
- *Clue cells* **(Fig. 17)**: It seen in bacterial vaginosis where epithelial cell is studded with infective organisms.
- *Sezary cells/mycosis cells/cerebriform cells/monster cells*: It is characteristically seen in mycosis fungoides and Sezary syndrome referring to an atypical lymphocyte with cerebriform nuclei.[19]
- *Touton giant cells*: These are seen in histiocytic disorders.[20]
- *Tzanck cell*: It refers to acantholytic cells which has hypertrophic nucleus with peripherally condensed basophilic cytoplasm (mourning edged cells) seen in pemphigus vulgaris.[21]
- *Virchow's cell* **(Figs. 18 and 19)**: It is a name given to a foamy macrophage with many lepra bacilli after the name of a scientist who discovered it.

There are many other named cells like Langerhans cell, Toker cells, Pakin cells, LE cells, Tart cell, Paget cell, balloon cells, signet-ring cells, spiderweb cells, strap cells, tadpole cells, etc. which are not included in above list.

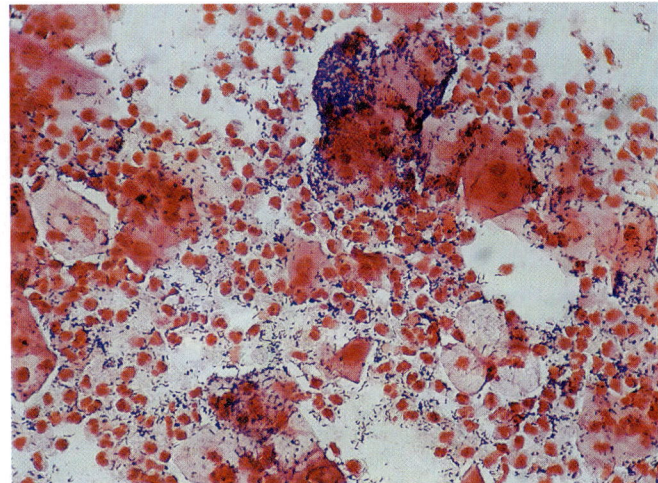

FIG. 17: Clue cells in a case of vaginal discharge.

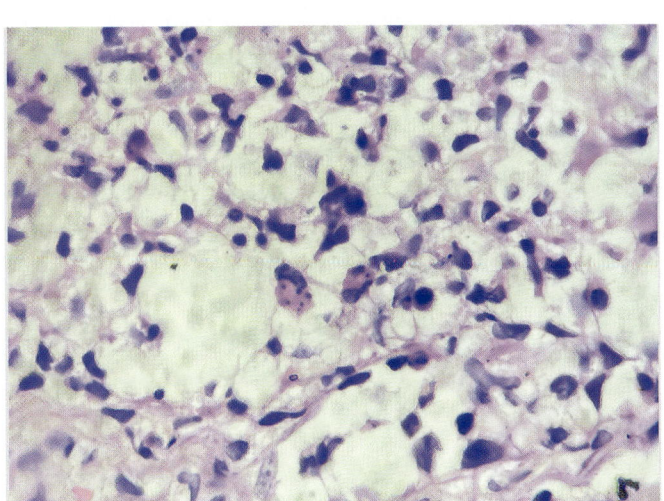

FIG. 16: Bean-bag cells in cytophagic panniculitis.

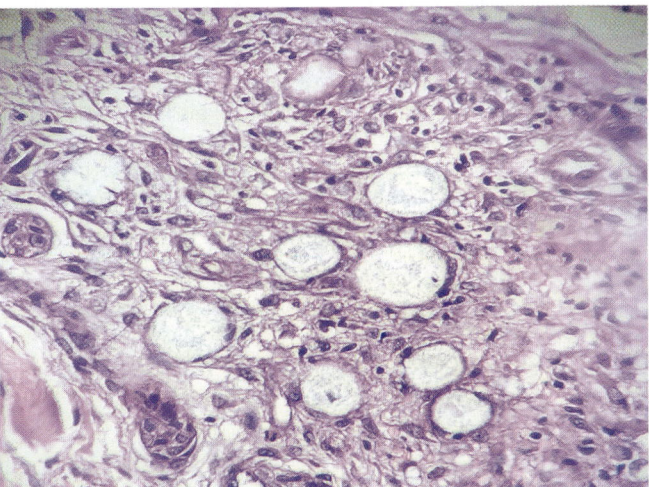

FIG. 18: Virchow's cell in a case of lepromatous leprosy.

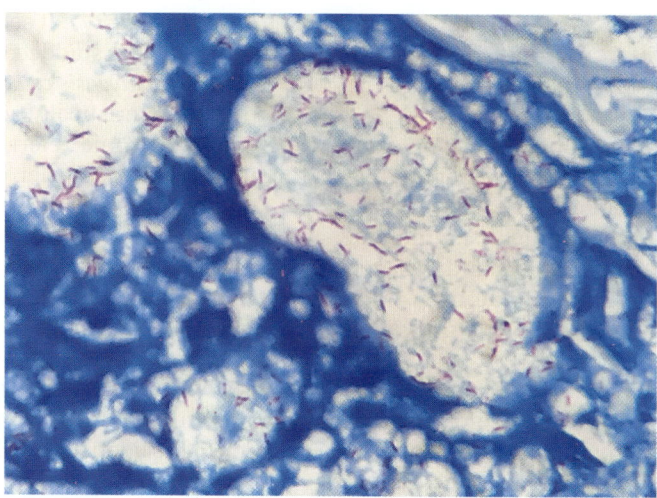

FIG. 19: Acid-fast bacillus (AFB) stain showing Virchow's cells with lepra bacilli.

REFERENCES

1. Montagna W, Kirchner S, Carlisle K. Histology of sun-damaged human skin. J Am Acad Dermatol. 1989;21(5 Pt 1):907-18.
2. Reuter Mj, Becker SW. Colloid Degeneration (Collagen Degeneration) of the Skin. Arch Derm Syphilol. 1942;46(5):695-704.
3. Pranay T, Kumar AS, Chhabra S. Civatte bodies: A diagnostic clue. Indian J Dermatol. 2013;58(4):327.
4. Tirumalae R. Histopathologic approach to cutaneous vasculitis. Indian J Dermatopathol Diagn Dermatol. 2014;1:2-6.
5. Madke B, Doshi B, Khopkar U, Dongre A. Appearances in dermatopathology: The diagnostic and the deceptive. Indian J Dermatol Venereol Leprol. 2013;79:338-48.
6. Engelkens HJ, ten Kate FJ, Vuzevski VD, van der Sluis JJ, Stolz E. Primary and secondary syphilis: a histopathological study. Int J STD AIDS. 1991;2(4):280-4.
7. Vimal M, Nishanthi A. Food eponyms in Pathology. J Clin Diagn Res. 2017;11(8):EE01-EE06.
8. Requena L, Kutzner H. Hemangioendothelioma. Semin Diagn Pathol. 2013;30(1):29-44.
9. Ferrara G, Improta G. The Histopathological Diagnosis and Reporting of Melanoma: A New Look at an Old Challenge. Austin J Dermatolog. 2016;3(1):1044.
10. Long V. Clothing-related Eponyms and Signs. Indian J Dermatol. 2016;61(2):234.
11. Jindal R, Shirazi N, Chauhan P. Histopathology of morphea: Sensitivity of various named signs, a retrospective study. Indian J Pathol Microbiol. 2020;63:600-3.
12. Idriss MH, Misri R, Böer-Auer A. Orthokeratotic Bowen disease: a histopathologic, immunohistochemical and molecular study. J Cutan Pathol. 2016;43(1):24-31.
13. Reinehr CPH, Bakos RM. Actinic keratoses: review of clinical, dermoscopic, and therapeutic aspects. An Bras Dermatol. 2019;94(6):637-57.
14. Perez-Chua TA, Kisel YG, Chang KH, Bhawan J. Morphea and its variants and the "floating sign"—an additional finding in morphea. Am J Dermatopathol. 2014;36(6):500-5.
15. Tiwary AK, Kumar P. Anthology of dermatopathological signs. Our Dermatol Online. 2021;12(2):224-9.
16. Lazova R, McNiff JM, Glusac EJ, Godic A. Promontory sign: present in patch and plaque stage of angiosarcoma! Am J Dermatopathol. 2009;31(2):132-6.
17. Kota SK, Jammula S, Kota SK, Meher LK, Modi KD. Necrobiosis lipoidica diabeticorum: A case-based review of literature. Indian J Endocrinol Metab. 2012;16(4):614-20.
18. Millsop JW, Ho B, Kiuru M, Fung MA, Sharon VR. Cutaneous Hemophagocytic Lymphohistiocytosis: Bean Bags from the Bone. JAMA Dermatol. 2016;152(8):950-2.
19. Cyriac MJ, Kurian A. Sezary cell. Indian J Dermatol Venereol Leprol. 2004;70:321-4.
20. Sequeira FF, Gandhi S, Kini U, Bhat I. Named cells in dermatology. Indian J Dermatol Venereol Leprol. 2012;78:207-16.
21. Gupta LK, Singhi MK. Tzanck smear: A useful diagnostic tool. Indian J Dermatol Venereol Leprol. 2005;71:295-9.

Index

Page numbers followed by *b* refer to box, *f* refer to figure, *fc* refer to flowchart, and *t* refer to table.

A

Acanthosis 354*f*
   nigricans 403, 403*f*
Acetazolamide 56
Acid peptic disease 332
   incidence of 332
   warning signs for 332*b*
Acid-fast bacillus stain 122, 454*f*
Acne 106
Acneiform 48
   eruptions, steroid-induced 49*f*
Acquired immunodeficiency
   disease 211, 215
   syndrome 47, 211, 215
Acquired palmoplantar keratoderma 193*t*
   causes of 198*t*
Acrocyanosis 13
   keratoderma of 199
Acromegalic facies 397, 397*f*
Acrylic acid 131
Actinic freckles 107
Actinic keratosis 211, 218
Actinic lentigines 107
Actinic porokeratosis, disseminated
   superficial 211
Actinic purpura 26
Actinic reticuloid 216*f*
Actinomycosis 436*f*
Activated partial thromboplastin time 31, 32, 284
Acute cutaneous lupus erythematosus 43, 202, 211, 214, 215
Acute fulminant hepatic failure 359
Acute generalized exanthematous pustulosis 51*f*, 55, 359
Addison's disease 109, 168, 403, 403*f*
Adenitis 183
Adenoid
   facies 397, 398*f*
   hypertrophy 397
Adherent fabric fiber sign 445
Adverse drug reactions 328, 329, 333
   cutaneous 46, 47
   management of 55
   plethora of 324
Alanine aminotransferase 359
Albinism 116, 307, 309*f*
   differential diagnosis of 116*t*
Albright's sign 370, 376
Alcohol wipe sign 378
Alkylamines 56
Allergic salute sign 369

Alopecia 48
   areata 127, 128, 128*t*, 147, 166, 394*f*
      diffuse 126*f*, 142, 144
      incognita 142, 144
   extent of 151
   mucinosa 154
Aluminum acetylacetonate 131
Amifostine 191
Amine test 229
Amiodarone facies 398
Amitriptyline 244
Amlodipine 49*f*
Amoxicillin 48*f*
Amyloidosis 27, 28*f*
Anagen effluvium 141, 142*t*, 144
Analgesic sensitivity 57
Anaphylaxis 49, 55
Androgen secreting tumors 134
Androstenedione 137
Anemia, pernicious 118
Anesthetic induction drugs 56
Angel's wing sign 392, 392*f*
Angelic facies 398
Angioedema 16, 48, 48*f*, 320
Angiotensin-converting enzyme inhibitor 48
Angiotensin-receptor blocker 334
Ankyloblepharon-ectodermal defects 283
Annular atrophic lesion 84*f*
Annular erythemas 87
Annular erythematous scaly lesions 83*f*
Annular hyperpigmented patch 83*f*
Annular lesions 74, 75*t*, 76*t*, 81*f*, 82, 84, 87, 89, 89*b*
   frequency of 75 fc
Annular skin lesions 74, 77*fc*, 79*t*, 85*t*
Anogenital lesions 248, 262*f*
Antenna sign 371, 371*f*
Antibiotics, topical 179
Antibody
   antinuclear 8, 22, 37, 39, 94, 95, 95*f*, 146, 154, 183
   antiphospholipid 13, 177
   tests 190
Anticonvulsant drugs 56
Antifungal agents, topical 359*t*
Antifungal drugs 358*f*
   compatibility of 359*t*
   systemic 358*t*
Antihistamines 56
Antineutrophil cytoplasmic antibody 12, 16, 22, 94
Antipruritic agents, symptomatic 54
Antipsychotic drugs 109

Anti-Ro antibodies 41*f*
Antistreptolysin O 8, 95
Antitrypsin 98
Antonine facies 398, 398*f*
Aphthous stomatitis 183
Aplasia cutis 150
Apoptotic panepidermolysis, acute syndrome of 43
Argyria, facies of 403, 404*f*
Arthralgia 14, 41
Arthropod infections 371
Arthrospore 337
   formation 353
Asboe-Hansen sign 377
Ash leaf macules 117
Ashy dermatosis 108, 444*f*
Asiatic porcelain doll facies 398, 399*f*
Aspartate aminotransferase 359
Asthma 13, 319
Asymmetric crying facies 399, 399*f*
Ataxia telangiectasia 309, 320*f*
Atopobium vaginae 232
Atrophic vaginitis 232
Atrophy
   cutaneous 426
   steroid-induced 348*f*
Auricular dermatophytosis 344*f*
Aurora borealis pattern 445
Auspitz's sign 77, 371
   dermoscopic 444
Autoimmune connective tissue disorders 58, 59
Autoinflammatory syndromes 181
Axillary ecchymosis sign 378
Azathioprine 23
Azelaic acid 131

B

Bag sign 146
Ballooning degeneration 447, 447*f*
Ball-site sign 378
Bamboo hair 394
Bandaid sign 378
Barber pole sign 382
Bare underbelly sign 451
Barnett's sign 367
Basal cell carcinoma 150, 202, 211, 216, 218
Basement membrane zone 22, 156, 188
Basophilic hyphae 354*f*
Bateman herpes iris 34
Battle's sign 378
B-cell lymphoproliferative malignancy 13
Beaded hair 394

Bean-bag cells 453, 453f
Beau's line 392, 392f
Beauty and beast sign 445
Bedside tests 145, 145b
Bees' appearance, swarm of 450
Behavior modification 242
Behçet's syndrome 181
Bell phenomenon 422, 423
Benediction sign 384
Benzocaine 56
Benzodiazepines 56
Bergen syndrome 406f
Beta-hemolytic streptococcal infection 238
Betamethasone 326
Biett sign 382, 382f
Billard sign 379
Biochemical tests 137
Biopsy 22, 242, 450f
   small 11
   technique 18, 218
Bird facies 399, 400f
Black dot sign 369
Black urine 166
Blanch sign 379
Bleeding tendencies 91
Blink sign 443
Blood
   glucose monitoring 329b
   hound facies 409
   investigations 52, 128
   meals 371f
   pressure 17
   urea nitrogen 22, 288
Bloom syndrome 309, 311, 312
Blue dot sign 379
Blue pseudo-veil sign 443
Body
   fluids, composition of 286fc
   surface area 71, 278, 287, 348
Bologna sign 445
Bonbon toffee sign 443
Bone
   marrow examination 322
   mineral density 331
Borda sign 375
Borderline tuberculoid 211, 213f
   leprosy, annular plaques of 82f
   plaque of 213
Borrelia burgdorferi 87
Borst–Jadassohn phenomenon 436
Bovine facies 399, 400f
Bowen's disease 240f
Bowenoid papulosis 451f
Brachioradial pruritus 68
Brain tumors 68
Brass knuckles sign 451
Breast cancer 168
Brenner's sign 376
Brittle nails 127
Brocq's phenomenon 418, 421
Brocq's pseudopelade 159f
Bronchopneumonia 317
Broom fiber appearance 445
Brownish macular coalescing lesion 111f

Bruises 27
Bryant sign 379
Bulla spread sign 377
Bulldog jaw sign 382
Bullous fixed drug eruption, generalized 39, 43, 43f
Bullous ichthyosiform erythroderma 282t
Bullous impetigo 80, 82, 83f, 262f
Bullous pemphigoid 41, 42f, 59, 182, 184
Burns, third-degree 152
Burnt matchstick sign 445
Burton line 393
Buschke–Ollendorff sign 382
Butterfly sign 369
Buttonhole sign 370

C

Cachectic facies 399, 400f
Cadaverous hair 394
Café-au-lait tint sign 383
Calcium-channel blockers 334
Camel foot appearance 448, 448f
Cancer treatments 67
Candida albicans 88
   treatment for 231
Candidal intertrigo 257f
Candidal vulvovaginitis 223t, 225, 226, 228, 229, 231
Candidiasis, congenital 279
Cannon ball appearance 448
Carbamazepine 50f, 56
Carbamoyl phosphate synthetase 285
Carbonic anhydrase inhibitor 56
Cardiovascular adverse events, glucocorticoid-related 333
Cardiovascular system 283, 328, 329
Carpet tack sign 367
Casal sign, necklace of 375, 376f
Cat tongue sign 367
Caviar tongue 393
Celecoxib 56
Central centrifugal cicatricial alopecia 157
Central dell sign 376
Central nervous system 211, 265, 283
Cerebriform cells 453
Cerebrovascular accident 69
Certain koebnerization 420
Cervical test 230
Chanarin–Dorfman syndrome 282
Chase phenomenon, salient features of 425
Checkerboard sign 451
Chemical injury 152
Chest pain 14
Chicken wire 448
Chickenpox 5-7, 300f
Chik sign 374f
Chikungunya 297, 299, 302
   fever 5, 6, 10
Chipmunk facies 400, 401f
Chlamydia trachomatis 223
Chloroquine 164
Chlorpheniramine maleate 55
Chromobacterium 316

Chronic inflammatory dermatomes, treatment for 243
Church spire appearance 448
Churg–Strauss syndrome 11
Cicatricial alopecia 150, 151t, 152t, 153t, 157, 157f
   causes of 159
   differential diagnosis of 150t
Cicatricial pemphigoid 154
Cigarette facies 400, 401f
Citalopram 244
Civatte poikiloderma 110, 115
Classical tombstone 450f
Claw clutching ball appearance 448
Cleft
   lip 283
   palate 283
Clindamycin 232
Cloacal defect 274f
Clobazam 56
Clobetasol propionate 232
Clofazimine 168
Clown nose sign 376
Clue cells 453, 453f
Coarse facies 400, 401f
Cockayne syndrome 310, 312
Cold abscess 281
Collagen, hyalinization of 447
Collarette sign 444
Colloid degeneration 447
Colposcopy 237
Complete blood count 22, 39, 69, 167, 170, 183, 360
Compression therapy 179
Concentric lesions 81f
Congenital disorders 116, 166
Conidia, barrage of 337
Conjunctivitis 304
Connective tissue
   disease 22, 175, 177
   disorder 92, 183, 367
Conradi–Hünermann–Happle syndrome 280
Contrast paper method 146
Cookie-Cutter sign 451
Coombs test, direct 128
Coral bead sign 379, 392
Cornflake sign 371, 451
Coronary artery disease 176
Coronavirus disease 2019 (COVID-19) 9f, 141, 297, 347
   cutaneous manifestations of 303t
   infection 6, 10
Coronoid lamella 219f
Corticosteroids 23
   systemic 54
   topical 267, 426
Cortisone 326
Cotrimoxazole 49f
Coudability sign 394, 394f
Cough 14
C-reactive protein 22, 37
Creatine
   phosphokinase 71
   transporter deficiency 98

Crowe' sign 370
Cryoglobulinemic vasculitis 15, 23
Cullen' sign 379
Cumulus sign 443, 444f
Cushing syndrome 134, 334
Cushingoid facies 401, 402f
Cutaneous lupus erythematosus, chronic 37, 151, 152, 157f
Cyclical neutropenia 182
Cyclophosphamide 23
Cyclosporine 23
Cyproheptadine hydrochloride 56
Cyproterone acetate 139
Cyrano sign 379
Cystic fibrosis 293
Cytochrome P450 346
Cytomegalovirus 17, 47, 184, 186
Cytophagic panniculitis 453f
Cytotoxic drugs 109

D

Darier's sign 281, 379, 379f
Deck chair sign 379, 380f
Deep leg ulcer 173f
Dehydroepiandrosterone sulfate 135, 137, 143, 146
Delmege sign 385
Dengue 297, 299
   facies 401, 402f
   fever 5, 6, 7f, 10
Dennie sign 369
Dennie–Morgan sign 369
Deoxyribonucleic acid 166, 306
   double-stranded 39, 95f
Depigmentation, intralesional steroid-induced 347f
Dermal vasculitis 41
Dermatitis 106, 369
   atopic 235, 301f
   herpetiformis 63
   severe 282, 283
Dermatological disorders 125
Dermatology
   phenomena in 417, 417t
   signs in 367
Dermatomyositis 22, 215, 359, 368, 404, 404f
Dermatopathology 451, 453
Dermatophytes 338t, 452f
   chlamydospore of 337
Dermatophytic lesion 346f
Dermatophytosis 344, 346f, 351f, 352f, 358f
   chronic 348
   recalcitrance in 348 fc
   recurrent 338, 354f
   relapsing 338
   severe recalcitrant 350t
   severity grading of 348t
Dermatoscopy 217f
Dermatosis 419, 420, 422
   generalized 250fc
Dermoepidermal junction 22, 59
Dermoscope 78
Dermoscopy 98, 98f, 129t, 216, 217t, 443
   signs in 443

Dexamethasone 326
Diabetes mellitus 63, 69, 176, 236, 328, 329
Diamond necklace sign 444
Diathesis, atopic 166
Diazepam 56
Diffuse hair loss
   differential diagnosis of 141b
   management of 148t
Dihydrotestosterone 132
Dimple sign 379
Diphenhydramine 56
Diplopia 14
Direct immunofluorescence 22, 37, 39, 72, 156, 183
Dirty neck sign 369
Discoid lupus erythematosus 17, 83, 84f, 152, 183, 188, 188f, 211, 214-216, 218, 369f
Dixyrazine 164
Doll's hair 395
Dopa oxidase 165
Dory flop sign 383, 393, 393f
Double-edge sign 445
Doughnut sign 375
Down syndrome 408f
Doxepin 244
Doxycycline 83f
Dracula's sign 375
DRESS syndrome 8f
Dressings, types of 179t
Drip sign 380
Drug
   hypersensitivity syndrome 46, 50, 51f
   reaction 46, 47, 50, 283, 325
      morphological pattern of 48t
Dubois sign 383
Dusky bluishness over distal phalanges 423f
Dysgeusia 359
Dysmorphic facies 402, 402f
Dysplasia, signs of 447
Dyspnea 14

E

Earlobe sign 369
Eastern pan cake sign 445
Eczema 318, 319fc, 369
   coxsackium 301f
Elbow sign 384
Electrolytes 52
Elfin facies 403, 403f
Elicitation, method of 436
Elliot sign 383
Emollients 290
En coup de sabre 212f
   morphea 154f
Enamel paint sign 375
Enanthem 296
Endocrine disorder 59, 69, 375
Entomodermoscopy, signs in 446
Enzyme 52
   linked immunosorbent assay 72, 183
   replacement therapy 293
Eosinophilia 4, 50, 54, 283, 325
Epidermal dermal separation 43f
Epidermal necrolysis 54

Epidermal nevus 429f, 452f
Epidermal niche 338t
Epidermis 74
Epidermodysplasia verruciformis 318
Epidermolytic ichthyosis 94
Epilepsy 54
Epistaxis 14
Epitestosterone 137
Epstein–Barr virus 17, 88, 302
Erlotinib 168
Erythema
   annulare centrifugum 75, 88
   dyschromicum perstans 108
   gyratum repens 87, 88
   induratum 6, 7, 94
   lacy pattern of 300f
   marginatum rheumatica 89
   migrans 87
   multiforme 5f, 34, 35, 37, 40, 41f, 48, 80, 82, 182-184, 301
      recurrent 185f
   necroticans 434
   nodosum 93, 97f, 98
      leprosum 91, 92f, 94, 97f, 213
      nodule of 95f
      stages of 93f
   over face 308f
   toxicum neonatorum 279f
   types of 88t
Erythematous macules coalescing 279
Erythematous nodules 92f
Erythematous papules 88
Erythematous plaque 94f
Erythrocyte sedimentation rate 17, 22, 37, 52, 59, 69, 71, 146, 167, 190
Erythroderma 51f, 278, 281, 282t, 284t, 285fc, 287t, 318
   childhood 278
Erythrose peribuccale pigmentation 109
Escherichia coli abscess 247
Ethanolamines 56
Ethinylestradiol 137
Exanthema 302t
   infective 47t
Exanthematous drug rash 47t
Exclamation hair 394, 395f
Exogenous ochronosis 108, 111f, 113
Extragenital lichen sclerosis et atrophicans 118
Eyebrow hair loss 151
Eyeliner sign 451
Eyes displaying Bell phenomenon 422f

F

Face
   diffuse hyperpigmentation of 301f
   signs in 384t, 385t
Facial
   hypermelanosis 105
   hyperpigmentation 110
   hypopigmented lesions 119
   melanosis 105
   nerve dysfunction 398
   plaque 202, 202t, 216fc

cutaneous examination of 204t
general examination 215t
systemic symptoms in 214t
Facies
asymmetrical 411
lactrodectismica 405, 405f
leprosa 405, 406f
types of 397
Factitial panniculitis 95
Factitious purpura 26f
Familial mediterranean fever 182, 183
Fat embolism syndrome 30
Fat
lobules, lipophagic necrosis of 93f
necrosis 178
subcutaneous 91
Faun tail nevus 395
Female pattern hair loss 141
types of 143t
Festooned papillae appearance 449
Fever 6t, 14, 175, 296, 304t
causes of 4t, 297t
infectious causes of 296t
viral hemorrhagic 29
Fibrinoid degeneration 447
Fibula sign 384
Filamentous degeneration 447
Finasteride 139
Fitzpatrick sign 379
Fixed drug eruption 48, 50, 80, 83, 182-184, 261
Flag sign 394, 451
Flat facies 407, 408f
Floating sign 451
Fluid and electrolyte
balance 286
maintenance of 286
therapy 287fc
Fluid loss 286, 286t
insensible 287t
Fluid resuscitation 288t
Fluorescence, phenomenon of 427
Fluorophores 427t
Fluoxetine 244
Flutamide 139
Fluvoxamine 244
Follicle stimulating hormone 146
Follicular
mucinosis 154
pustulation 342f
Folliculitis
bacterial 151
decalvans 162f
eosinophilic 248
Folliculotropic mycosis fungoides 218
Forchheimer's sign 394
Fournier's sign 371, 383
Fox's sign 380
Frank's sign 380
Free testosterone 137
Frei-Sulzberger-Chase phenomenon 425
Freund sign 369, 385
Friar tuck sign 394
Frictional melanosis 110, 115

Fried egg
appearance 449
sign 445
Froment sign 384
Frontal fibrosing alopecia 158f
Functional itch disorders 68
Fungal infection 118, 247, 317, 373
Furosemide 56
Furunculosis 347f

G

Gabapentin 56, 244
Gangrene 13
Gardnerella vaginalis, virulent strains of 232
Gargoyle facies 408, 408f
Gastrointestinal endoscopy 95
Gaucher's disease 280, 282
Gaunt facies 408, 409f
Generalized pruritus 58, 59, 62, 62t, 66t, 70, 71, 72fc
treatment of 71t
Genital dermatosis, erosive 263
Genital lesions 249fc, 250fc
Genital papular lesion, causes of 248
Genitalia, developmental anomalies of 263
Genodermatoses 306, 312t, 370
Gentle grattage 422f
Geographic tongue 394
Gianotti-Crosti syndrome 299, 303b
Giant melanocytic nevus 108
Gingivitis, desquamative 187f
Gliclazide 56
Glimepiride 56
Glomerulonephritis 41
Glucocorticoid 325, 330, 334
systemic 324
therapy 324t, 326b
Goggle sign 451
Gonadotropin releasing hormone agonists 139
Gonococcal infection, disseminated 270
Goose bumps sign 380
Gorlin's sign 370
Gorlin's syndrome 404, 404f
Gottron sign 367, 368
Graft-versus-host disease 39, 43, 44f, 150, 154, 182, 185, 223, 282
Graham-Little-Piccardi-Lasseur syndrome 158f
Gram stain 229
Gram-negative enteric bacteria 247
Granulation tissue 173f
Granulocyte colony-stimulating factor 39
Granuloma 319
annulare 84
eosinophilic 22
gluteale infantum 257, 262
Granulomatosis 13, 15-17, 19, 22, 23, 213-215
eosinophilic 13, 15, 17, 22, 23
Granulomatous disease
chronic 316
congenital 317f
Granulomatous invasive aspergillosis 211
Graves' disease 413f

Gray hair 164, 165
repigmentation of 168
Graying severity score 167
Greek warrior helmet facies 408, 409f
Grey Turner sign 380
Griscelli syndrome 167f
Groove sign 383
Gubler sign 380
Gulliver's sign 380

H

Haemophilus
ducreyi 247, 450
influenzae 247
Hailey-Hailey disease 449f
Hair 281
bearing sites examination 152
collar sign 380, 395
color 168, 169t
dark 164
density 151
eumelanotic 164
examination 76
fall, progress of 143t
follicles 143
graying, rate of 167
loss 143
count 145
diffuse 141, 146
on scalp, patches of 166
patch of 160t
pigmentation 165
pull test 145, 152
reduction, permanent methods of 138
signs 392, 394
white forelock of 117
Hairy palm sign 451
Half nail 392
Halo phenomenon 430, 431
Halsted's sign 380
Hamburger sign 395
Hand-foot-mouth disease 262f, 300f, 302
severe 301f
Hand-holding sign 451
Handlebar sign 443
Hard palate 188f
Harlequin phenomenon 432, 433t
Hartnup disease 404, 405f
Headache 359
Headlight sign 369
Heart disease, congenital 433
Heliotrope sign 368
Helix sign 381
Helminthic infections 247
Hemangioma, infantile 212f, 274f
Hematological disorders 27, 31t
Hematoma 27, 27f
Hematuria 15
Hemidysplasia, congenital 283
Hemoglobin 22, 32
Hemolytic uremic syndrome 12
Hemophilia 27f
Hemoptysis 14
Hemorrhagic edema, acute 37, 40

Henoch–Schönlein purpura 32
Hepatic pruritus 63, 67
  treatment modalities for 68t
Hepatitis 49
  autoimmune 359
  B
    surface antigen of 227, 360
    virus 23
  C 13
    virus 23
  viral 63, 64
Herpes
  genitalis 262f
  labialis 40f
  progenitalis 238, 240f
  simplex virus 37, 64, 183, 261, 265, 318
    infection 10
    lesions, recurrent 185f
  zoster 429f, 447f
Herpetiform recurrent aphthous ulcers 185f
Hertoghe's sign 380
Herxheimer reactions 439
Heugh-Gottron sign 368
Hidradenitis suppurativa 249
Hidradenoma papilliferum 238
Higoumenakis sign 383
Hiker's feet sign 381
Hildreth's sign 376
Hippocratic facies 409, 409f
Hirsutism 132, 136f
  causes of 133, 133t
  score, abnormal 132
Histamine gels 191
Hobnail appearance 449
Hodgkin's lymphoma 63, 88
Hoigne phenomenon 438
Holster sign 368
Honeycomb pigment 152
Hot cross bun skull 383
Hound dog facies 409, 409f
Howel-Evans syndrome 196f
Human herpesvirus 302
Human immunodeficiency virus 47, 62, 64, 69, 92, 102, 150, 177, 183, 211, 214, 215, 226, 282, 349
  infection 42, 63, 64, 108
Human leukocyte antigen B 39
Human papillomavirus 236
Hutchinson's nail sign 392
Hutchinson's teeth 394
Hydroa vacciniforme 310
Hydrocortisone 55, 232, 326
Hydroxy ethyl starch 70
Hydroxychloroquine 23, 37, 39, 164, 188
Hydroxyethyl starch 62
Hydroxyprogesterone 137
Hymenal tag 275f
Hyperandrogenic insulin-resistant-acanthosis nigricans 133
Hyperglycemia
  developing 329t
  glucocorticoid-induced 327
Hyperimmunoglobulin
  D syndrome 183

E syndrome 282
  syndrome 317f
Hyperkeratosis 354f
Hyperkeratotic lesions 192
Hypermelanosis, classification of 105t
Hypernatremic dehydration 287
Hyperpigmentation 109t
  causes of 106t
  investigations for 112t
  treatment for 113t
Hyperpigmented plaque 376f
Hyperprolactinemia 135
Hypertension 328, 329
Hyperthermia, management of 289b
Hypertrichosis 48
Hypocomplementemic urticarial vasculitis syndrome 15, 17, 22
Hypoesthesia 118
Hypopigmentation
  causes of 106t
  investigations for 120t
  treatment for 122t
Hypopigmented halo 431f
Hypopyon sign 372f, 445
Hypothalamic pituitary adrenal axis 334, 334b
Hypothermia
  management of 288
  prevention of 288

I

I love you sign 381
Iatrogenic hirsutism 134
Iceberg sign 443
Ichthyosiform erythroderma 283
Ichthyosis 290
  congenital 290
  hystrix 280f
Igneous rock sign 371
Imatinib 168
Immune dysregulation 283, 292
Immune thrombocytopenic purpura 32
Immunodeficiency, severe combined 283, 318f
Immunofluorescence 22
Immunoglobulin 283, 292
  A 18, 35, 75, 77, 325
    pemphigus 84
    vasculitis 18f
  E 37, 165f, 167, 170
  G 39, 156
  intravenous 23, 39, 267, 293
  M 147, 188
Immunohistochemistry 244
Impetigo 106
In vitro tests 52
Incontinentia pigmenti 150
Indirect immunofluorescence 72, 188
Infections 59, 66, 118, 219, 371
  bacterial 118, 175f, 316, 372
  dermatophytic 238
  treatment for 243
  viral 47, 247, 317, 374
Infective discharge, symptoms of 225t

Infestations 59, 66, 371
Inflammation, signs of 152
Inflammatory bowel disease 92, 188t
Inflammatory dermatoses, chronic 242t
Inflammatory disorders 154
Ingram's sign 368
Injection, conjunctival 14
Insect bite 297
Insensible water loss 286, 287
Insulin
  like growth factor 135, 137
  sensitizers 139
Intense erythema 432f
Intense pulsed light 115
Interferon 23
Interleukin 39, 325
Intestinal whipworm infestation 108
Intrauterine device 226
Intravascular coagulation, disseminated 12, 29
Invasive aspergillosis
  acute 211
  chronic 211
Inverse strawberry pattern 444
Iris
  lesion 34
  phenomenon 427
Iron
  deficiency 165f
    anemia 66, 66fc
  metabolism, disorders of 59, 66
Irritant contact dermatitis 257, 347, 421f
Irritant diaper dermatitis, chronic 257
Isotopic nonresponse
  examples of 425t
  phenomenon 425
Isotopic phenomenon 428, 430
  pathophysiology in 429fc
Itch
  acute 58
  chronic 58
Itraconazole 352, 359
  monitoring of 360t

J

Jacquet erosive dermatitis 257, 257f, 263
Jarisch-Herxheimer
  phenomenon 438
  reaction 438
Jeanne's sign 375, 384
Jelly sign 443
Jessner's lymphocytic infiltration 78, 86, 87
Jewel sign, cluster of 378, 378f
Jigsaw puzzle appearance 449
Juvenile spring eruption 306

K

Kaposi sarcoma 450
Kaposi-Stemmer sign 381
Kasabach-Merritt phenomenon 433
Kawasaki disease 12, 41, 299, 304b
  diagnosis of 304
Keel like facies 409, 410f
Keining sign 368

Keratinization disorders 371
Keratitis ichthyosis-deafness 283
Keratoacanthoma 216
Keratoderma
  thickened 196f
  transgradient diffuse 194f
Keratolysis, mechanical 290
Keratolytics 290
Keratosis
  developing 429f
  follicularis spinulosa decalvans 152
Kerr's sign 381
Kidney disease, chronic 178
Kindler syndrome 308f
Kirmisson sign 381
Knotty-cypress wood-grained 88
Koebner phenomenon 419, 425, 425t
  remote reverse 421
Koebnerization 420, 420f
Koilonychia 63t
Koplik's spot 394
Krisowski's sign 383

L

Lactate dehydrogenase 69
Lactic acid 131
Lamellar ichthyosis 150, 280f
Lamotrigine 56
Langerhans cell histiocytosis 211, 214, 215, 219
Lantern jaw sign 375
Laser
  therapy 191
  treatment 138
Latanoprost 168
Latrodectus facies 405, 405f
Laugier–Hunziker syndrome 109, 115
Leathery palm sign 381
Leg ulcer 173, 175f
  causes of 173t
  chronic 173
  clinical assessment of 175
  management of 179
  measurement tool 178
  treatment for 180
Leishmaniasis 178, 213f
  amastigotes of 452f
Lekocytoclastic vasculitis 42f
Lentigo maligna 211
Leonine facies 410, 410f
Leopard syndrome 109
Lepra bacilli 454f
Lepromatous leprosy 92f, 211, 453f
Leprosy 118
  borderline 81
  signs in 384
Leser–Trélat sign 376, 377f
Lesions 35, 76, 174f
  duration of 182
  erosive 258t, 263
  hypopigmented 119t, 120t
  morphology of 309
  nature of 307

number of 184, 184t
progression of 35
site of 184
types of 76, 184, 185t
Leukemia 168
Leukocytoclastic vasculitis 22f, 41
Leukoderma 119
  colli 118
  syphiliticum 118
Leukorrhea 222
Leukostasis 30
Levodopa 168
Lichen nitidus 248, 420f
Lichen planopilaris 151, 152, 157f
  trichoscopic features of 157f
Lichen planus 79, 82, 106, 127, 127f, 128, 128t, 129t, 156, 184, 188, 239, 418, 420f
  erosive 186f
  pigmentosus 107, 111f, 115
Lichen sclerosus 154, 239
  et atrophicus 116, 118-120, 122, 236, 239f, 271f
Lichen scrofulosorum 248
Lichen simplex chronicus 236, 239f
Lichenoid 48
  drug reaction 49f
  lesions 343f
Liddle's sign 375
Light treatment 138
Lightening sign 443
Limb defects 283
Limburger sign 381
Line sign 451
Linear immunoglobulin A dermatoses 41, 42f, 87, 182, 184, 186
Lip tip vitiligo 118
Lipodermatosclerosis 95f
Lipschutz ulcers 271f
Livedo reticularis 13, 91
Liver
  cirrhosis of 403, 404f
  function 39
  test 39, 128, 146, 282
Local anesthetic agent reaction 56
Loose anagen hair syndrome 142, 144
Love's sign 376, 393
Lowenbach's sign 451
Lower parakeratotic layers 452f
Lucio phenomenon 434
Ludwig's type 143
Lupus erythematosus 37, 39, 44f, 76, 83, 151, 152, 156, 183, 185, 188, 214, 406, 406f
  cell phenomenon 436
Lupus panniculitis 97f, 212f
Luteinizing hormone 137, 146
Lyell's syndrome 42
Lymph node examination 297
Lymphadenopathy 304
Lymphocyte 354f
  rich perivascular infiltrate 23f
Lymphoid tissue, absence of 321
Lyonization 435
  phenomenon 434

M

Mace sign 445
Maculopapular drug rash 303t
Maculopapular exanthema, management of 10
Maculopapular lesions 299f
Maculopapular rash 4t, 6t, 48, 301f
  ampicillin-induced 9f
  drug-induced 4, 9f
Magnan's sign 381
Malassezia furfur 118
Malassezia infection 353f
Malignancy 67
  Trousseau sign of 377
Mandarin phenomenon 426
Maple syrup urine disease 284
Marfan syndrome 370
Marie-Unna hereditary hypotrichosis 151
Mariner's pilot wheel appearance 449
Marquee sign 451
Marshall's sign 375
Matchbox sign 381
Mauserung phenomenon 433
Mazzotti reaction 439
McCune–Albright syndrome 109
Measles 6, 298, 299f
Median canaliform dystrophy 393
Median raphe cyst 275f
Medium vessel vasculitis 13
Meffert's sign 381, 394
Meirowsky phenomenon 437
Melanin, location of 105, 106t
Melanocytes 165
Melanocytic nevus, congenital 213, 218
Melasma 105, 106, 111f
Mephenesin 164
Mesa sign 452, 452f
Metabolism, inborn error of 282, 283, 284t, 285fc, 293
Methotrexate 23
Methylprednisolone 326
Metronidazole 49f, 231
Meyerson's nevi 432f
Meyerson's phenomenon 431, 432f
Mickey mouse facies 410
Microbial endothelial damage 29
Micro-Hutchinson's sign 445
Microscopic polyangiitis 13, 17, 22, 23
Miescher's granuloma 93f
Mild recalcitrant dermatophytosis 350t
Milian's ear sign 202
Minimal erythemtopapular lesions 343f
Minimum inhibitory concentration 358
Minor aphthous ulcer 181f
Mirtazapine 244
Mistletoe sign 445, 368
Modified wash test 145
Molluscum
  contagiosum 432f
  pendulum necklace sign 370
Mongoloid face 407
Monkey like facies 410
Monomorphic papular lesions 301f

Mononucleosis, infectious 6, 7, 10
Monster cells 453
Moon facies 401
Morbilliform drug eruption 299, 303
Morphea 448*f*
Morphine 56
Moth eaten alopecia 395
Mottled hyperpigmentations 308, 309*f*, 310
Mottled hypopigmentation 308, 309*f*, 310
Moyamoya syndrome 166
Mucocutaneous candidiasis, chronic 318*fc*
Mucosa 185*t*, 281
Mucosal lesions 297
Mucosal signs 392, 393
Mucositis, chemotherapy-induced 191
Mucous membrane
    examination 152
    pemphigoid 182, 184-186
Muehrcke's line 393
Mulberry molars 394
Multi-annular rings 342*f*
Multibacillary-multi-drug treatment 122
Multiple allergies 282, 283
Multiple annular lesions 81*f*
Multiple biopsies 159
Multiple depressed atrophic lesions 212*f*
Multiple discrete symmetrical
    hyperpigmented macules 382*f*
Multiple endocrine neoplasia 406
Multiple freckles 111*f*
Multiple pneumatoceles 317*f*
Multiple sclerosis 68
Mupirocin 243
Murky sign 452
Mushroom cloud sign 445
Myasthenia gravis 412*f*
Myasthenic facies 412, 412*f*
Mycobacteria, atypical 177
Mycobacterial infections 317, 373
Mycophenolate mofetil 23, 39, 122
Mycoplasma pneumoniae 267*t*
Mycosis
    cells 453
    fungoides 119, 122, 215, 218
        hypopigmented 119
Myeloid leukemia, acute 317*f*
Myopathic facies 410, 411*f*
Myxedema 413*f*

N

Nail 129*f*, 281
    destruction 125
    examination 76, 152
    floating 393
    lichen planus 129*f*
    plate 128*f*, 152
    psoriasis 129*t*
    scrapping 128
    signs 392
Naïve dermatophytosis, differential diagnosis
    of 349
Naïve tinea
    corporis 341*f*
    inguinalis 341*f*

Naranjo adverse drug reaction 51*t*
Narrow band ultraviolet B 122
Nasal leprosy 406*f*
Natiform skull sign 383
Nazzaro sign 376
Necrobiosis lipoidica 154, 178
Necrobiotic xanthogranuloma 211, 214-216
Necrotic lesion 434*f*
Necrotizing sialometaplasia 182
Neisseria gonorrhea 223
Neodymium-doped yttrium aluminum
    garnet 115
Neonatal alloimmune thrombocytopenia
    12
Neonatal candidiasis 279
Neonatal lupus 311
    erythematosus 87
Neonatal onset multisystem inflammatory
    disease 183, 398
Neoplasia 224
    treatment for 243
Neoplastic conditions 242, 242*t*
Neuritic pain 14
Neurodermatitis 168
Neurogenic itch 58
Neurogenic pruritus 63, 64
Neuropathic itch 58
Neuropathic pruritus 68
    causes of 69*t*
Neurosyphilis 438
Neutral lipid storage disease 282-284
Neutropenia, severe congenital 316*f*
Neutrophils 97*f*
    exocytosis of 354*f*
Nevi aversion phenomenon 435
Nevirapine 51*f*
Nevoid conditions 263
Nevoid lesions over perineal region 272*t*
Nevus depigmentosus 117
Nevus of Ota 108, 112*f*, 113, 115
    classification of 109*t*
Nicoladoni–Branham sign 378
Nikolsky phenomenon 418
Nikolsky sign 377, 418, 419*t*
Nodular basal cell carcinoma 218
Non-albicans *Candida*, treatment for 231
Nonbullous impetigo 80
Nondermatological disorders 125
Nondermatophyte infection 349
Noninfective discharge, symptoms of 225*t*
Nonpalpable purpura 32*fc*
Nonpruritic urticarial erythema 398
Nonsexually acquired genital ulcers 266*t*
Nonsteroidal anti-inflammatory drug 23, 35,
    37, 46, 48, 50, 106, 182, 188, 329
Noonan syndrome 406, 407*f*
Normal nail matrix function 125
Nose sign 369
Notalgia paresthetica 68
Nucleic acid amplification test 224, 229,
    270
Nummular eczema 80, 83
Nutrition 289
Nutritional disorder 375

O

Oblaten sign 371
Obstructive pulmonary disease, chronic 17,
    22
Occasional koebnerization 420
Oil drop sign 393
Olfleck phenomenon 434
Olympian brow sign 383, 385
Omega nail 393
Omenn's syndrome 321
Omnibus sign 383
Onchocerciasis 63
Onychogryphosis 393, 393*f*
Onychomycosis 127, 129*t*
Onychoscopy, signs in 445
Opaque nails 127
Opera glass nose sign 383
Opioid reaction 56
Optic neuropathy, anterior 359
Oral bisphosphonate therapy 331*b*
Oral contraceptive 138
    pills 91, 102, 226
Oral desensitization protocol 55*t*
Oral erosive lichen planus 190
Oral leukoplakia 196*f*
Oral penicillin desensitization protocol 55*t*
Oral ulcerative lesions 188*f*
Oral ulcers 184*fc*, 186*t*, 190, 191
    case of 182*t*
    chronic 181
    progression of 183*t*
    recurrent 181, 182*t*
Orentreich sign 394
Organic anion transporting polypeptide 346
Ornithine transcarbamylase 285
Orofacial granulomatosis 189*f*
Osler nodes 381
Osler sign 381
Osteonecrosis 331, 331*fc*, 332*b*
    glucocorticoid-induced 330, 331
Ota nevus 108, 112*f*, 113, 115
Owl's eye appearance 449, 449*f*

P

Packed parakeratotic column 219*f*
Paget's disease 242
Paget's eczema sign 369
Pagetoid phenomenon 436
Pain, nature of 175
Paired ear creases 381
Palifermin 191
Palmar psoriasis 199*f*
Palmoplantar keratoderma, hereditary 192*t*,
    194, 195*t*, 198*t*, 200*t*
Palpable purpura 11, 13, 14*t*, 16, 17*t*, 20*f*, 21
    examination of 17*fc*
Panda sign 381
Panniculitides, types of 95
Panniculitis 91, 93*t*, 98, 98*fc*, 175
    classification of 92*b*, 93
    histopathological classification of 96*t*
    infectious 97
    infective 97, 97*f*

plaque of 93f
 types of 99t
Papillae, loss of 186f
Papillon–Lefèvre syndrome 196
Papular acrodermatitis, infantile 299
Papular lesion 248, 251t
Papulonodular lesion 248, 251t
 causes of 248
Papulosquamous dermatoses 250, 254t
Para-aminobenzoic acid 168, 169
Paracetamol 48f
Paradoxical hair 395
Paradoxical reactions 56
Paranasal sinus 211
Paraphenylenediamine 168, 169
Parasitic diseases 373
Parasitic infections 63, 247, 318
Paresthesia 14
Parkinsonian facies 410, 411f
Paroxetine 244
Parvovirus B19 infection 6, 7, 300f
Patchy cicatricial alopecia 154
Pathergy 419
 test 190
 cutaneous 420t
Pathological vaginal discharge 223
Patrick Yesudian sign 370, 370f
Pavithran nose 369
Pearls sign, string of 446
Pediatric genital dermatoses, classification of 248
Pelvic inflammatory disease 225, 282
Pemphigus 448f
 foliaceus 281f
 paraneoplastic 35, 43
 vulgaris 184, 187f, 189f, 450f
 ulcers of 187f
Penicillin allergy 56
Penile dermatophytosis 344f
Perianal erythema, recurrent toxin-mediated 257f
Perianal pseudoverrucous papules 257, 263
Perilesional erythema 300f
Perinevoid vitiligo 431f
Periodic acid-Schiff 39, 312, 353f
Periodic fever 183
Perioral pigmentation 110
Periorbital erythematous rash 308
Periorbital hyperpigmentation 107
Periorbital pigmentation 107t
Periorbital purpura 28f
Peripilar sign 445
Persistent traumatic ulcer 181
Peutz–Jeghers syndrome 109, 115
p-glycosylation, products of 346
Pharyngitis 183
Phenobarbitone 56
Phenothiazines 56
Phenylketonuria 166
Phenytoin 56
 facies 411, 411f
Photoexacerbated skin disorders 306
Photopatch test 311
Photosensitive genodermatoses 309t

Photosensitivity 306, 307
 disorders, classification of 306b
Phototoxic reactions 106
Physiological skin flora 118
Physiological vaginal discharge 222
Phytophotodermatitis 310
Picket fence appearance 449
Piebaldism 117
Pig tail hair 395
Pigment, color of 111
Pigmentary deficiencies 307
Pigmentary demarcation lines 110, 113, 115
Pigmented basal cell carcinoma 212f
Pigtail vellus hair 394f, 445
Pincer nail 393
Pinch sign 379
Pink glow sign 445
Pink sign 382
Pinkus yellow line 393
Pinworm infestation 238
Piperazines 56
Pitaluga sign 395
Pityriasis
 alba 89
 amiantacea 154
 rosea 48, 49f, 79, 81, 81f, 299
 pilaris 199f, 282
 versicolor 118
Pizza sign 452
Plantar ecchymosis sign 382
Plaque, diffuse indurated 95f
Plasmapheresis 23
Platelet 12
 abnormalities of 28
 function
 abnormal 28
 defect 12
Pluck out sign 445
Pneumonia, atypical 40
Pneumonitis 49
Pohl-Pinkus constriction 395
Pointing index sign 384
Polyangiitis 11, 13, 15-17, 19, 22, 23, 213-215
 nodosa 13, 15, 17, 19f, 22, 23, 91, 177
 cutaneous 23f
Polycyclic skin lesions 74
Polycystic ovary syndrome 135
Polymerase chain reaction 31, 261, 265, 304
Poppy field bleeding sign 445
Pore sign 443
Porokeratosis 87, 88f
Porphyria cutanea tarda 168
Port-wine stain 213
Post chikungunya
 fever 301f
 hyperpigmentation over face 7f
Posterior trunk 342f
Postinflammatory hyperpigmentation 37, 39, 106, 113, 115, 116
Post-kala-azar dermal leishmaniasis 106, 116, 119, 122
Postmenopausal pregnancy 331
Postoperative pressure-induced alopecia 152
Potassium hydroxide 224, 228, 229, 231

Prayer sign 375
Prednisolone 326
Prednisone 326
Pregnancy, intrahepatic cholestasis of 71
Premalatha sign 378
Premature aging syndrome 406, 407f
Premature hair graying 164, 166, 169, 170fc
Premlatha sign 394
Pressure ulcer 177t
Prevotella bivia 232
Prick and intradermal testing 53
Primary cicatricial alopecia 155t, 157, 159
 classification of 162t
Primary immunodeficiency 292, 315, 316, 320f, 321, 321t
 syndrome 278, 282, 283
 treatment of 292t
 warning signs for 316
Probenecid 56
Procaine 56
 psychosis 438
Prodromal period 42
Progesterone 137
Progressive macular hypomelanosis 122
Progressive osseous heteroplasia 107, 113, 115
 classification 107t
Prolactin 137
Promethazine 56
Promontory sign 452
Prozone phenomenon 437
Pruritic skin disease 58
Pruritoceptive itch 58
Pruritus 58, 70, 70t, 71, 340t
 causes of generalized 58
 classification of 58
 drug-induced 68, 70t
 generalized 58, 59, 62, 62t, 66t, 70, 71, 72fc
 management of 66fc, 69t, 71t
 vulvae, differential diagnoses of 236t
Pseudo groove sign 384
Pseudo-Hutchinson's sign 393, 445
Pseudomonas 316
Pseudo-Nikolsky sign 418
Pseudo-Wickham striae 444
Psoriasiform 48
Psoriasis 78, 79, 106, 127, 128, 128t, 154, 238, 451f
 plaque of 444f
 rete ridges in 448f
Psychiatric adverse events 333, 333b
Psychogenic itch 58
Psychogenic pruritus 63, 64
 diagnostic criteria for 69t
 management of 69t
Psychogenic purpura 26
Psychological pruritus 68
Pterygium formation splitting 129f
Pubic lice 238
Punctate keratoderma 197t
Punctate porokeratotic keratoderma 196f
Punshi's sign 376
Pup tent sign 393
Purple fiber sign 452

Purpura 11, 19*f*, 31*t*
 differential diagnosis of 12*t*
 nonhematological causes of 26, 28*t*
 pathophysiologic categories of 26*t*
 simplex 27, 27*f*
Pus appearance, lake of 393
Pustular psoriasis 75
Pustulation, steroid-induced 346*f*
Pyoderma 247
 gangrenosum 178, 267*t*

Q

Q tip test 227
Quadrichrome vitiligo 118

R

Raccoon facies 411, 411*f*
Raccoon sign 368
Racquet nail 393
Radiological tests 146
Rail-like appearance 444
Rainbow sign 446
Ram's horn nail 393
Ramirez ashy dermatosis 108
Rash 304*t*
 distribution of 6*t*
 drug-induced 6
 location of 296, 298*t*
 morphology of 297*t*
 progression of 296
 severity of 47
 simple 47
 type of 3*t*
Rasin's sign 375
Ravelled wool appearance 450
Raynaud's phenomenon 13, 15, 76, 175, 423, 423*t*
Raynaud's sign 368
Reactions, contrast media-induced 55
Rebound phenomenon 425, 426
Recalcitrant dermatophytosis 337, 338, 339*fc*, 340*t*, 342*f*, 344*f*, 345*f*, 349*b*, 349*t*, 354*f*, 355*fc*, 355*t*
 management of 348
 pruritus in 340*t*
Recalcitrant disease 341*t*, 351*b*, 358*t*
Red blood cells 11
Red flag signs 47, 303, 304*t*
Red globular ring pattern 444
Red planet sign 446
Red-stained hyphae 353*f*
Rehydration 287*t*
Reinfection 338
Renal disease, severe 19*f*
Renal function test 39, 183
Renbok phenomenon 424
Resistant dermatophytosis 338
Respiratory system 286
Respiratory tract infection 39
Reticular degeneration 447
Retinoids, systemic 290
Reverse Koebner phenomenon 421
Reverse namaskar sign 370
Reynold's braude phenomenon 437

Rheumatoid arthritis 17, 22, 37, 94, 95
Riehl's melanosis 108, 113
Right labium majora 274*f*
Ring scale sign 443
Ringed hair 395
Ringer's lactate 287
Rituximab 23, 187*f*
Roller coaster nail 393
Rope sign 382
Rosette sign 378, 443
Rothmund-Thomson syndrome 309, 310, 312
Round finger pad sign 368
Rounded facies 411
Rowell's syndrome 41
Rubella 6, 298
Ruin appearance 445
Rumpel-Leede phenomenon 424
Rumpled sock appearance 395
Russell sign 382

S

Sabourad's dextrose agar 229
Sabouraud's sign 452
Sad man facies 412, 412*f*
Sagrada Familia sign 446
Saline wet mount 227
Salmon patch 393
Salute sign 452
Samitz sign 368, 393
Sampaio sign 452
Sandpaper nails 125
Sandwich sign 452
Sarcoidosis 74, 84, 154
 hypopigmented 118
Scabetic nodules 240*f*
Scalp 152
 biopsy, examination of 159
 dermatophytosis 345*f*
 local examination of 144*t*, 145
Scaly cuticles 445
Scarlet fever 10, 299
Scarring alopecia, signs of 151
Schamroth's sign 393
School chair sign 370
Schultz-Charlton phenomenon 426, 427*t*
Scleroderma neck sign 367
Sclerosing panniculitis 91
Sclerosis, systemic 17, 22, 63, 406, 407*f*
Scotch plaid pattern 393
Screeching halt sign 452
Screening tests 241
Sebaceous hyperplasia 444*f*
Seborrheic keratosis 211, 218, 449*f*
Seborrheic melanosis 110, 115
Seeping sign 383
Selective estrogen receptor modulator 232
Selective serotonin reuptake inhibitors 69
Senile nails 127
Senile purpura 27*f*
Septate tomato appearance 450
Septicemia 54
Serratia 316
Sertraline 244

Serum folic acid 167
Serum free light chain assay 32
Serum glutamic
 oxaloacetic transaminase 284
 pyruvic transaminase 284
Serum sickness like reaction 37, 40
Setting sun sign 444
Sex hormone-binding globulin 137
Sexually acquired genital ulcerative disease 264*t*
Sexually transmitted
 diseases 383
 infection 226, 250, 261, 271
Sezary cells 453
Sharpei sign 376
Shawl sign 368
Shiny nails dermoscopic 128*f*
Shoulder pad sign 376
Shuster's sign 368, 369*f*
Shwartzman-Sanarelli phenomenon 426, 426*t*
Sickle cell disease 175
Silex's sign 383
Silicon dioxide 131
Silvery hair 167*f*
Simian facies 402, 402*f*
Simple metabolic screening tests 284*t*
Single patch 151
Sjögren-Larsson syndrome 47, 280, 283
Skin
 biopsy 78, 159, 282
 crease sign 377
 derived itch 58
 disorders 75*t*
 examination 281
 failure, acute 286*fc*
 fluorescence in 427*t*
 grafts 179
 infections 316, 428*t*
 internal milieu of 338*t*
 lesions 58, 59*f*, 62*t*, 65*t*, 70*t*, 71*t*
  primary 59
 nevi, signs in 445
 rash 320
Slapped cheek facies 412, 412*f*
Small vessel vasculitis, cutaneous 13, 15-17, 18*f*, 22, 23
Snarling facies 412, 412*f*
Sneddon syndrome 13
Sneddon-Wilkinson disease 87
Sodium valproate 56
Solar urticaria 310
Solenonychia 393
Solitary chronic ulcers 186*t*
Spaghetti and meatball appearance 118
Spangled hair 395
Sparing dorsal spine 117
Spironolactone 138
Splendore-Hoeppli phenomenon 435, 436*f*
Spongiosis 354*f*
Spun glass appearance 395
Squamous cell carcinoma 150, 182, 184, 186, 211, 215, 216, 218, 236
Stafne's sign 368, 394
Staphylococcal scalded skin syndrome 282

Staphylococcus aureus 154, 316
Steinberg sign 370
Steroid 54, 139, 179
    application, topical 257f
    molecules 326t
    systemic 324
Steroidal abuse 343f
Stevens–Johnson syndrome 5, 34, 35, 39, 46, 50, 50f, 110, 279, 293, 303, 359
Storiform appearance 450
Stratified epithelial-specific antinuclear antibody 188
Stratum corneum disjunctum 353f
Strawberry gums 394
Strawberry pattern 444
Strawberry tongue 394
Streptococci infection 427t
Streptococcus viridans 247
Subacute cutaneous lupus erythematosus 37, 80, 83, 211, 214-216
Subcorneal pustular dermatosis 87
Sulfa allergy 56
Sulfamethoxazole 23, 55t
Sulfasalazine 56
Sun-damaged skin, signs of 447
Sunken eyes 308
Superficial basal cell carcinoma 218
Superficial dermatophytosis 339
Surgical therapy 179
Sweets syndrome 41, 213
Syphilide pigmentaire 118
Syphilis 41, 118, 382, 438
    annular lesions of 76
    congenital 262f, 382
    secondary 5, 7, 8f, 10, 42f, 80, 83
Syphilitic facies 412f
Syphilitic vitiligo 118
Systemic disorders 182t
Systemic lupus erythematosus 15, 17, 22, 41, 47, 94, 177, 183, 188, 211, 214, 215, 328
Systemic therapy 130, 200

T

Tachycardia 144
Tachyphylaxis 438, 438t
Tamoxifen 168
Tap sign 384
Targetoid annular lesions 42f
Targetoid lesion 34, 42f
Tay syndrome 395
T-cell lymphoma 78, 87, 154
    cutaneous 87, 150
Teeter-Totter sign 377
Telangiectasia 110, 309f
    conjunctival 320f
Telephone handle appearance 450
Tell-tale signs 423f
Telogen effluvium 141
    acute 142t, 144
    chronic 141, 142t, 144
Temporary hair removal, cosmetic methods of 138
Tent sign 377

Terbinafine 352
    monitoring of 360t
Terry nail 393
Tertiary syphilis 154
Testicular pain 15
Testosterone, topical 137
Tetracyclines 109
Thimble nail 393
Thinker's sign 382
Thrombocytopenia 12
    heparin-induced 30, 32
Thrombocytopenic purpura 28
Thrombosis 30
Thrombotic thrombocytopenic purpura 30, 32
Thumb sign 370
Thyroid
    disorders 63, 69, 135
        interpretation of 71t
    stimulating hormone 59, 71, 135, 137, 146, 167, 170
Thyrotoxic facies 413, 413f
Tiger tail appearance 395
Tin tack sign 367
Tinea
    capitis 150, 154
    corporis 347f, 429f
        extensive 346f
    cruris 257f
        et corporis 348f
    faciei, eczematous 342f
    incognita 343f
    infection 74, 76, 78, 81f
    inguinalis 347f
    pseudoimbricata 344f
Tinidazole 231, 232
Tolbutamide 56
Torpid 413f
    facies 413
Total iron binding capacity 66, 146
Touton giant cells 453
Toxic epidermal necrolysis 35, 39, 42, 43, 44f, 47, 50, 279, 283, 284, 287, 289b, 293, 359
Toxic shock syndrome 10, 41, 279, 282, 283
Toy soldier sign 453
Trachyonychia 125, 126t, 128, 128t, 129, 130fc
    changes of 127f
    etiology of 125t
Tram track sign 453
Transepidermal water loss 287
Transient neonatal dermatoses 279
Translucency sign 444
Trauma, mechanical 152
Treponema pallidum 247
Triamcinolone 326
Triangular facies 413, 413f
Triangular sign 446
Trichogram 145, 152
Trichomonas rapid test 229
Trichomonas vaginalis 223, 225, 226, 228, 229
Trichomoniasis 238

Trichoscopy 152
    signs in 445
Trichotillomania 153, 153f
Trichrome vitiligo 118
Tricolor sign 453
Trimethoprim 23, 55t
Trizonal concentric pattern 444
Trophic ulcer 174f, 176
Trousseau syndrome 377
Trumpet nails 393
Trumpeter's wart 394
Tuberculoid leprosy 81, 211
Tuberculosis 94, 184, 214, 215, 250, 328
    cutaneous 154, 177
    reactivation 324
Tuberous sclerosus 117
Tufted hair appearance 395
Tulip sign 395, 395f
Tumors 376
    necrosis factor 267, 325
        alpha 37
        inhibitors 315
    signs in 445
    solid 67
    specific signs and symptoms 68t
Turner's syndrome 407, 408f
Twycross classification 58
Tyrosine kinase 165
Tzanck cell 453
Tzanck smear 190

U

Ugly duckling sign 377
Ulcers 18f, 182, 188t, 189f
    aphthous 181, 189
    arterial 179
    borders of 176
    causes of chronic 176
    drug-induced 190
    eosinophilic 182
    neuropathic 177t, 179
    progression of 175
    shape of 176
    size of 176
    traumatic 182
    venous 179
Ultrathin adhesive bandage 131
Ultraviolet recall phenomenon 433
Umbilical sign 370
Umbrella sign 453
Unit area trichogram 145
Unna's sign 453
Upper orthokeratotic layers 452f
Upper respiratory symptoms 14
Uppsala monitoring center 51
Uremia 59
Uremic pruritus 63, 66
    treatments for 67t
Urethral discharge 263, 268t
Urinary tract infection 225, 236
Urine
    analysis 241
    testosterone 137

Urschel sign 382
Urticaria 48, 48f, 79, 82, 82f, 89
  bullous pemphigoid 87
  lesions 21
  multiforme 37, 40, 40f
  simple 49
  vasculitis 13, 15, 23, 37, 41, 84

V

V sign 369
Vaginal discharge 222, 240f, 224fc, 263, 268t, 453f
  causes of 224b
  chronic 222, 229
  infective 228t, 229t
    causes of 227f
  nonsexually transmitted causes of 271t
  recurrent 222, 223, 229, 230fc
Vaginal maturation index 231
Vaginal swabs 229fc
Vaginal warts 224
Vaginitis
  desquamated inflammatory 223, 232
Vaginosis, bacterial 223, 225, 226, 228, 229, 231, 238
Valdecoxib 56
Varicella 154
Vascular disorders 378
Vascular lesions 263
Vasculitis 13, 15, 20f, 48, 49
  cutaneous 13
  drug-induced 15, 15t
  lesion of 174f
  management of 19, 23t
  signs of 447
  types of 19
Vector-borne diseases 297
Venereology, signs in 382
Venous leg ulcer 174f
Venus sign, crown of 383
Verruca plana, histopathology of 449f
Verruciform xanthomas 249
Vertical line sign 452
Vesiculation 18f
Vesiculobullous disease 186t

Vesiculobullous disorder 181, 190, 377
Vesiculobullous lesions 258t, 263
Vesiculobullous skin diseases 44
Videodermoscopy 145
Vincent's infection 439
Vinyl acetate, copolymer of 131
Violaceous macular diffuse pigmentation 111f
Viral exanthems 303t
Viral infections, recurrent 319
Virchow's cell 453, 453f, 454f
Virchow's sign 383
Vision, blurring of 14
Vitamin
  B12 165f
  D 165f
    supplementation 292
  E 191
Vitiligo 117, 420f, 429f
  blue 118
  chemical 119
  inflammatory 118
  macular lesions of 117f
Voigt's line 110
Volcanic crater, lines of 444
Vulvar dermatoses, symptoms of 236t
Vulvar intraepithelial neoplasia 236, 239, 242
Vulvar pruritus 235, 244fc
Vulvar psoriasis 240f
Vulvar Q-tip examination 241
Vulvoscopy 237
  evaluation of 241t
Vulvovaginal candidiasis 229, 231, 240f, 271
Vulvovaginitis, erosive 224

W

Waardenburg syndrome 166
Wagyu beef appearance 444, 444f
Walker–Murdoch sign 370
Walzel sign 382
Warfarin skin necrosis 29, 30f
Warning signs 47, 332b
Wartenberg's sign 384
Wegner's granulomatosis 11, 394

Weight loss 14
Whisker hair 395
Whistling facies 414, 414f
White blood cell 8, 37, 167
White starburst pattern 445
White strawberry tongue 394
Whitish blue halo surrounding macrocomedone 443f
Whitish fluorescence 196f
Whitish membrane 189f
Whitish reticular pattern over buccal mucosa 186f
Wickham's striae 78
Widespread fixed drug eruption 49f
Willan's itch 70
Williams facies 403f
Wimberger's sign 383
Windblown appearance 451
Wiskott–Aldrich syndrome 319, 319f
Wood's lamp 428t
  examination 167f, 194, 196f, 312
Woronoff phenomenon 435
Wound dressing 179
Wrist sign 370

X

Xanthogranuloma, juvenile 202, 211, 214, 215, 218
Xanthoma disseminatum 249
Xeroderma pigmentosum 306b, 308, 309f, 310, 312
X-linked recessive ichthyosis 280

Y

Yellow clod sign 445
Yersinia enterocolitica 247
Yoga sign 382

Z

Zigzag hair 395
Zinc 191
Zona cingulata 429f
Zonal parakeratosis 354f
Zoophiles 338